Child Health Care Nursing

Concepts, Theory and Practice

Child Health Care Nursing

Concepts, Theory and Practice

Edited by

Bernadette Carter

and

Annette K. Dearmun

Blackwell Science

© 1995 by
Blackwell Science Ltd
Editorial Offices:
Osney Mead, Oxford OX2 0EL
25 John Street, London WC1N 2BL
23 Ainslie Place, Edinburgh EH3 6AJ
238 Main Street, Cambridge,
   Massachusetts 02142, USA
54 University Street, Carlton,
   Victoria 3053, Australia

Other Editorial Offices:
Arnette Blackwell SA
   1, rue de Lille, 75007 Paris
   France

Blackwell Wissenschafts-Verlag GmbH
   Kurfürstendamm 57
   10707 Berlin, Germany

   Feldgasse 13, A-1238 Wien
   Austria

First published 1995

Set in 10 on 12pt Garamond
by DP Photosetting, Aylesbury, Bucks
Printed and bound in Great Britain by
The Alden Press, Oxford

DISTRIBUTORS

Marston Book Services Ltd
PO Box 87
Oxford OX2 0DT
(*Orders:* Tel: 01865 791155
          Fax: 01865 791927
          Telex: 837515)

North America
Blackwell Science, Inc.
238 Main Street
Cambridge, MA 02142
(*Orders:* Tel: 800 215-1000
          617 876-7000
          Fax: 617 492-5263)

Australia
Blackwell Science Pty Ltd
54 University Street
Carlton, Victoria 3053
(*Orders:* Tel: 03 347-0300
          Fax: 03 349-3016)

A catalogue record for this book is
available from the British Library

ISBN 0–632–03689–3

Library of Congress
Cataloging in Publication Data

Child health care nursing: concepts, theory, and practice/edited by
   Bernadette Carter and Annette K. Dearmun.
      p. cm.
   Includes bibliographical references and index.
   ISBN 0–632–03689–3
   1. Pediatric nursing. I. Carter, Bernadette. II. Dearmun,
Annette K.
   [DNLM: 1. Pediatric Nursing. WY 159 C5362 1995]
RJ245.C4737 1995
610.73′62—dc20
DNLM/DLC
for Library of Congress   95-22040
                                                      CIP

Contents

Foreword

Sue Burr

The United Nations Convention on the Rights of the Child (1989), The World Summit for Children (1990) and advances in scientific knowledge have helped society to recognize that children are individuals with rights, whose physical, psychosocial and physiological needs are unique. Adults have a responsibility to ensure that children's rights and needs are met. Within health care services it is children's nurses who have a particular responsibility.

The development and health of children are easily affected by adverse changes in the family, community or society in which they live. The health care needs of children, the setting and the system which provides health care is undergoing rapid and radical change worldwide. This presents a real challenge, particularly to those nurses who have specifically chosen to provide child health care nursing.

Nurses are meeting the challenge by changing the focus of nursing children to one of empowering parents and children to become real partners in family centred care as well as expanding their own professional role. Whatever the changes it is paramount that children, are first and foremost, considered as children.

Child Health Care Nursing: Concepts, Theory and Practice reflects these changes, the wide range of issues which need to be addressed and the knowledge which must be acquired in order for nurses to enhance the quality of child health care nursing.

Sue Burr, FRCN
Royal College of Nursing's
Adviser in Paediatric Nursing (1995)

Acknowledgements

The illustrations on pages 1, 77 and 191 are of sculptures produced by Barbara Holgate and photographed by Jon Sparks. They are reproduced here by their kind permission. The photographs are © Jon Sparks. The titles of the sculptures are as follows: page 1: *Piggy Back:* page 77: *Family:* page 191: *Three Legged Race*. Barbara Holgate has been a professional sculptor since 1970 and specializes in modelling images of childhood. She lives in Lancaster.

The following photographs are reproduced by kind permission of Jon Sparks: Figures 3.1, 7.2, 9.2, 9.3, 9.4, 10.1, 12.1, 16.4, and 21.3.

Chapter 1 includes extracts from DHSS (1972) *Report of the Committee on Nursing (Briggs Report)*; DHSS (1976) *Fit for the Future: Report of the Committee on Child Health Services (Court Report)*; and DoH (1991) *Welfare of Children and Young People in Hospital*. These are Crown Copyright and are reproduced with the permission of the Controller of Her Majesty's Stationery Office.

Figure 4.9 is reproduced with the kind permission of the Brighton Health Care NHS Trust.

Chapter 6 includes tables compiled from data published and © to the Central Statistical Office which are reproduced with permission.

Figure 9.1 is reproduced from *Basic Developmental Screening* by R. S. Illingworth, published by Blackwell Science Ltd in 1973, with kind permission.

Figure 12.2 is reproduced with the kind permission of The Yorkhill NHS Trust, Glasgow.

Figure 12.5 is reproduced with the kind permission of J. Norden, Nursing Research Associate, Children's Research Institute, Children's National Medical Center, Washington DC.

Figure 12.6 is reproduced with the kind permission of Dr Annie Gauvain-Piquard, Unité de Psychiatre et d'Oncopsychologie, Institut Gustave-Roussy, Cedex, France.

Figures 12.7 and 12.8 are reproduced with the kind permission of Dr Joann Eland, Associate Professor, University of Iowa, USA.

Figure 12.10 is reproduced with the kind permission of Reckitt & Colman (Disprol) Products, Dansom Lane, Hull.

Figure 12.11 is reproduced with the kind permission of Dr G. D. Champion, Division of Paediatrics, The Prince of Wales Children's Hospital, Randwick, Australia.

Figure 16.8 is reproduced with the kind permission of J. P. Lippincott Co., USA. The illustration is taken from *The Lippincott Manual of Paediatric Nursing* 3rd edn, (Eds) L. S. Brunner & D. S. Suddarth (1991), Harper Collins Nursing, London.

Chapter 18 includes an illustration from Doris Smith Suddarth (1991) *The Lippincott Manual of Nursing Practice* 5th edn. This is reproduced by permission J. B. Lippincott Co., USA. Also included is tabular material from A. V. Hoffbrand & J. E. Pettit (1992) *Essential Haematology* 3rd edn, published by Blackwell Science Ltd, Oxford. This is reproduced with permission. Table 18.9 is reproduced with permission from AIDS Education and Research Trust, original published in D Gibb & S. Walters (1993) *Guidelines for Management of Children with HIV Infection*, 2nd edn.

Figures 21.1, 21.2, 22.4, 24.1 and 24.2 are reproduced with permission.

Appendices:
The material in Appendix 1, *Vital Signs*, is reproduced with the permission of The National Heart, Lung and Blood Institute (1977) Report of the task force on blood pressure control in children, *Pediatrics*, **59** (Supplement 5, part 2), pp 797–820; and the permission of the American Academy of Pediatrics for material from de Sweit *et al.* (1980) Systolic blood pressure in a population of infants in the first year of life, *Pediatrics*, **65**, pp 1028–35.

The nomograms are reproduced by permission of Ciba Geigy Ltd. These originally appeared in *Scientific Tables (Documenta Geigy) Ciba-Geigy Ltd* (1982) edited by C. Lentner, published by Ciba-Geigy Ltd, Basel, Switzerland.

Appendix 2 *The NAWCH Charter for Children in Hospital* is reproduced by kind permission of Action for Sick Children (National Association for the Welfare of Children in Hospital Ltd), Argyle House, 29–31 Euston Road, London NW1 2SD. Tel: 0171 833 2041; Fax: 0171 837 2110.

Appendix 3 *The United Nations Convention on the Rights of the Child* is reproduced by kind permission of the Children's Rights Department.

Editorial Advisers and Manuscript Reviewers

Imelda Charles-Edwards, *RSCN, RGN, MA, DipN, DipEd*, Director, School of Paediatric Nursing & Child Health, South Bank University, London.

Janice M. Colson, *MA, RSCN, RGN, Dip NEd*, Senior Education Manager, Childcare, Buckinghamshire College of Nursing and Midwifery, and Chair of the ABPN Nurse Teacher Group.

Sue Hooton, *BSc (Hons), Cert Ed, RGN, RSCN*, Course Manager (Children's Nursing) School of Nursing and Midwifery, Chester College of Higher Education.

Leslie C. Robertson, *MSc, SRN, RSCN, RNT*, President ABPN, Education Officer, Adult & Children's Nursing, English National Board for Nursing, Midwifery and Health Visiting, London.

Janet M. Turner, *MEd, BEd (Hons), RGN, RSCN, DipN (London), RNT*, Nurse Educationalist.

List of Contributors

Tony Andrews, *CQSW, BA(Hons)*, formerly Services Manager, Muscular Dystrophy Group, London.

Jan Barlow, *RGN, RSCN*, Clinical Nurse Specialist – Child Health, Scarborough General Hospital.

Pamela A. Barnes, Member of NAHPS, Chairman, Hospital Play Staff Examination Board (Hospital Play Staff Education Trust), London.

Kathy Bird, *RGN, RSCN*, Clinical Manager, Paediatrics, Kettering General Hospital.

Steve Campbell, *BNurs, RGN, RSCN, RHV, NDN Cert, Cert Ed, FRSH*, Clinical Editor of *Child Health*, formerly Lecturer in Child Health Nursing, University of Southampton.

Bernadette Carter, *RGN, RSCN, BSc (Hons), PGCE, RNT, PhD*, Senior Lecturer, Department of Health Care Studies, The Manchester Metropolitan University.

Imelda Charles-Edwards, *RSCN, RGN, MA, DipN, DipEd*, Director, School of Paediatric Nursing & Child Health, South Bank University, London.

Janice M. Colson, *MA, RSCN, RGN, Dip NEd*, Senior Education Manager, Childcare, Buckinghamshire College of Nursing and Midwifery, and Chair of the ABPN Nurse Teacher Group.

Sandra Day, *MCSP, MIFA, MISPA*, Principal, Sandra Day School of Health Related Studies, Rochdale.

Annette K. Dearmun, *RSCN, RGN, BSc (Hons), DipN (London), DNE, RNT*, Lecturer Practitioner, School of Health Care Studies, Oxford Brookes University and Senior Nurse/SDU Manager, Oxford Radcliffe Hospital.

Marcella De Sousa, *RSCN, RGN*, Peritoneal Dialysis Sister, Paediatric Renal Unit, Guy's Hospital.

Elizabeth Dyer, *RGN, RSCN, Dip Community Nursing*, Paediatric Oncology Community Nurse, Oxford Radcliffe Hospital.

Carolyn Evans, *RGN, ONC*, Family Care Officer, Muscular Dystrophy Group, Oswestry.

Marjorie L. Gillies, *RGN, RSCN, DipN (London)*, Research Nurse, University of Glasgow, Department of Child and Adolescent Psychiatry, Yorkhill NHS Trust.

James E. Hewitt, *BN (Hons), RGN, RSCN*, Senior Nurse, Practice Development, Paediatric Surgical Unit (PSU), Harefield Hospital NHS Trust.

Maggie Hicklin, *RGN, RSCN*, Specialist Clinical Nurse, Paediatric Renal Unit, Guys Hospital.

Angela Hobsbaum, *BA*, Lecturer in Child Development, Institute of Education, London University.

Beryl Holmes, *RGN, HV*, Clinical Nurse Specialist (Paediatric Metabolic Disorders), Birmingham Children's Hospital NHS Trust.

Sue Hooton, *BSc (Hons), Cert Ed, RGN, RSCN*, Course Manager (Children's Nursing) School of Nursing and Midwifery, Chester College of Higher Education.

Gerison Lansdown, Director, Children's Rights Office, London.

Nicki Mackett, *BSc, RGN, RSCN*, Nurse Specialist, Haematology and HIV, Royal Liverpool Children's Trust.

Geraldine Mason, *BA (Hons), RSCN, RGN, RN (Illinois USA), RCNT, CNS, RNT*, Lecturer in Nursing, University of Manchester and Manchester College of Midwifery & Nursing.

Lindy May, RGN, RSCN, Diploma Counselling, MSc Neuroscience, Senior Sister, Neurosurgery, The Great Ormond Street Hospital for Children NHS Trust.

Adele McEvilly, *RGN, RSCN*, Clinical Nurse Specialist, Diabetic Home Care Unit, Birmingham Children's Hospital.

Ruth Mitchell, *MSc, RSCN, RGN, SCM, RCNT Dip CNE, RNT, Cert Ed*, Nurse Teacher, Lothian College of Health Studies, Edinburgh.

Leslie C. Robertson, *MSc, SRN, RSCN, RNT*, President ABPN, Education Officer, Adult & Children's Nursing, English National Board for Nursing, Midwifery and Health Visiting, London.

Anna Sidey, *RSCN, RGN, DNCert, RCN*, Paediatric Community Nurse Specialist, Rockingham Forest NHS Trust, Kettering.

Lynne Styles, *RGN, RSCN*, Clinical Nurse Specialist (Paediatric Endocrinology), Birmingham Children's Hospital NHS Trust.

Anne Taylor, *BSc (Hons), RSCN, RGN*, Lecturer Practitioner, Children's Orthopaedic Nursing, Nuffield Orthopaedic Centre, Oxford.

Ethel E. Trigg, *RGN, RSCN, DMS, MBA*, Patient Services Manager, Royal Alexandra Hospital for Sick Children, Brighton.

Della Wait, *RMN, SRN, RSCN, DipN (Lond), BSc (Hon) Nursing, Cert Ed*, Nurse Teacher, Northern College, Bolton.

Sigrid Watt, *RSCN, SRN, RCNT Dip CNE, RNT, Cert Ed*, Nurse Teacher, Lothian College of Health Studies, Edinburgh.

Rhoda Welsh, *BPharm, MRPharmS*, Deputy Chief Pharmacist with Paediatric Speciality, John Radcliffe Hospital, Oxford.

Carolyn J. White, *RGN, RSCN*, Nurse Manager, Women's and Children's Services, Royal Hull Hospitals NHS Trust.

Maggie Wilson, *BA, PGCE, MA*, Senior Lecturer in Education, Oxford Brookes University, Oxford.

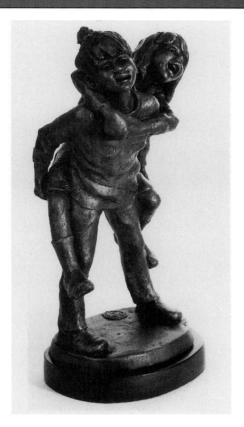

This section introduces the reader to many of the diverse issues which impact on practice. Children's nurses have a responsibility to be aware of these issues and the ways that they challenge and change the nature of nursing itself and the delivery of care. Nursing is, by its very nature, an integral part of society and therefore reflects, responds to, challenges and drives the consideration of health care issues.

Within the following chapters the reader should be able to develop a deeper level of understanding of where changes have arisen from and more importantly of future directions. The range and roles and responsibilities that the children's nurse has to consider and be skilled in are diverse. A sense of commitment to personal and professional development is paramount if the children's nurse is to keep informed and thus continue to make a significant contribution to the dynamic health care scene into the next century.

Chapter 1

Professional Perspectives

Leslie Robertson

INTRODUCTION

Children's nurses are part of the wider profession of nursing. There is therefore a need to have specialist knowledge, attitudes and skills to care for children and their families, and also knowledge of professional issues. Knowledge from both spheres is needed to work in a speciality and is often shared with that of others, as evidenced by Project 2000 programmes with their four branches in adult nursing, children's nursing, caring for those with a mental handicap (learning disability), and in mental health, each of which follows a common foundation programme.

Working in a speciality, maybe in a small unit in a children's ward in a district general hospital, is not without its problems as evidenced historically and more recently by the Allitt Inquiry (DoH 1994). All children's nurses need to keep abreast of changes and to communicate appropriately with their colleagues, be it in a regional or more isolated setting.

This chapter places children's nursing within the wider context of the current National Health Service (NHS) culture, professional practice and education. A knowledge of history can give helpful information as to why certain changes have occurred and where future directions lie for planners and individuals. Being professionally aware and politically astute means that nurses can raise priorities for child care in the right place and at the right time. The author therefore makes no apology for firstly concentrating on wider and historical issues which are then applied to children's nursing later in the chapter and elsewhere in the book.

PROFESSIONAL STATUS AND NURSING KNOWLEDGE

Professional status

Nursing has recently been through some of the most significant changes in the development of its professional status. However nursing has not yet reached full maturity (Deane & Campbell 1985) as this chapter will attempt to elucidate and debate.

Bringing in change is not always a comfortable experience but nursing could not and still cannot 'afford to languish in the *status quo* it has drifted in for so long' (Hendry 1992). It has recognized that there is a need for a different type of practitioner for the future (UKCC 1985a). There will be new health care needs to provide for, resulting from changing disease patterns and social contexts, against a background of political agendas and the introduction of reforming modes of delivery of care.

Children's nursing is but one part of the profession. It too has been through many changes, with the likelihood of more to follow. This chapter will explore these against the wider context of historical and more current events affecting the whole nursing profession and the NHS.

In order to achieve the status of being classified as a profession, an occupation must have acquired 14 characteristics (Houle, cited in Jarvis 1986), including the seeking of a definition of its occupational function and its members having mastery of theoretical knowledge, being capable of using practical knowledge and the ability to problem-solve.

According to Wilinsky (Jarvis 1986; Jolley & Allan 1991) a profession firstly establishes a training school which later integrates with a university – as is currently occurring in nursing. It then seeks legal support for protection of its job territory, with control of licensing and certification for professional registration – the function of the United Kingdom Central Council (UKCC). Practitioners are prepared through controlled education and examinations – the role of the statutory bodies, with a belief in lifelong education thereafter – now being structured (UKCC 1992a). The profession also publishes a Code of Ethics through the UKCC (1992a).

Some of these characteristics can be applied to nursing. If it has not yet reached its full maturity, what stage is nursing at now? Throughout its history, it has not proved easy to provide an occupational definition for a complex profession such as nursing, although more recently there have been attempts to do so (Kim 1983; Griffith & Kenney 1986). Peplau was one of the first, in 1952, in describing nursing 'as an interpersonal process with patients having felt needs' (Griffith & Kenney 1986; Meleis 1991). The most frequently cited definition used though, is probably that by Henderson in 1964, which appears to be internationally acknowledged, and which states that nursing is 'assisting patients in 14 essential functions towards independence' (Griffith & Kenney 1986; Meleis 1991).

In relation to members of the nursing profession having mastery of theoretical knowledge and the abilities to use practical knowledge and problem-solve, the basis of nursing knowledge was previously intuitive (Griffith & Kenney 1986) before becoming dependent on medical models (Clarke 1986). As Meleis (1991) so aptly suggested, there was therefore a need for nursing to progress and ask itself some major questions, so developing a true and particular knowledge base for its nursing theory. It needed to become a scientific discipline in its own right (Adams 1991), more recently taking the form of the creation of a separate body of knowledge, that is nursing theory in its own right. More recently nursing has evolved towards greater professional status (Melat Zieglar *et al.* 1986; Hayne 1992) aided by the introduction of the nursing process, and the increasingly pluralistic theories/frameworks/models of nursing care which have been devised to explain and predict this practice discipline, 'as it develops its knowledge, science and research base' (Hollingsworth 1985).

Nursing process as a theoretical basis for practice?

The theoretical approaches of the nursing process serve as a frame of reference through each of its components, in assisting nurses to understand, analyse and interpret clients' complex health situations, to apply knowledge, and to demonstrate accountability and responsibility to clients in providing a rational basis for their actions (Griffith & Kenney 1986). The nursing process has not always been successfully implemented – having been introduced from America in the 1970s – many seeing it as yet another nursing bandwagon (Robinson 1990). Nevertheless it has changed the emphasis of nursing care from a disease orientated, medical approach, to a patient centred problem-solving model (Hollingsworth 1985; Hurst 1985). Its aim is to give holistic care, as the nursing process is concerned with individualized total patient care and the unique person (Clarke 1990). Nursing care should be based on the individual needs of patients through patient allocation/centredness and the nursing process/problem-solving process which can develop several types of theories and ideas (Kim 1983; Robinson 1990; Hale 1991; Meleis 1991). Benner &

Schön (Champion 1988) advocate the need for professional practice based on holistic knowledge, and acquisition of skills which is role context dependent and which then can be creative in knowledge and action.

The nursing process involves intellectual and decision making skills, observation, and the forming of interpersonal relationships so that the carrying out of systematic nursing actions becomes a deliberate, logical and rational activity (Griffith & Kenney 1986; Bradshaw 1989) (Table 1.1). Using the nursing process is stated to produce confident professional autonomous decision-makers (Hollingsworth 1985) who are no longer doctors' handmaidens but are capable of identifying patient needs in making a nursing diagnosis, and planning, implementing and evaluating the care given.

Models and frameworks as a means of developing knowledge base

The knowledge base of nursing further developed through the introduction of models/frameworks which were devised to further explain and predict the practice discipline of nursing. They included those models of Roper, Logan & Tierney; Orem; Roy; and Johnson for example (Argyris & Schon 1989; Schön 1990). Today, staff often devise their own eclectic model, taking appropriate pieces from various models in order to provide the most individualistic and appropriate care for patients. Whatever the choice, the model and rational basis for care should be an 'articulated and communicated conceptualization of discovered reality . . . in or pertaining to nursing for the purpose of describing, explaining, predicting or prescribing nursing care' (Meleis 1991).

The introduction of formal models, whilst seen to be contributing to holistic individualized patient care, was seen also to be part of an overwhelming desire of nursing to become a profession, and a belief that using such theories was the only way to professionalism (Hardy 1990). There were those however who questioned their application to the real world of practice.

Formalizing the rational base of nursing activities in relation to the human behaviours/science has been another step in explaining/defining nursing practice. The nurse must be both a knowledgeable worker and one who cares. Knowledge is dangerous if it is divorced from caring as 'human existence requires care and caring practices' (Benner & Wrubel 1989).

Table 1.1   The four components of the nursing process (Griffith & Kenney 1986).

Assessment	Involves the collection of data which must be analysed, interpreted and synthesized. It requires a high level of intellectual and communication skills, critical thinking, decision-making and judgement in identifying clients' normal behaviours and health state, and then diagnosing concerns/problems on which to base the next phase of the process. Optional hypotheses for planning and giving care have to be chosen from a number of alternatives.
Care planning	This requires judging priorities of concerns, and then establishing goals and strategies from the nursing diagnosis, based on knowledge and problem-solving, so that the theoretical framework provides scientific rationale for care implementation. The care plan is the tool for documenting and communicating the client's diagnoses, expected outcomes, strategies, nursing orders and evaluation. It also ensures accountability.
Implementation	This is the execution and documenting of the care plan through performing activities/actions. It requires intelligence, reasoning, understanding, knowledge and interpersonal skills as well as technical skills. It should be undertaken competently and efficiently.
Evaluation	This determines progress and the effectiveness of nursing intervention in assessing the stated goals and objectives in meeting patient needs. It requires judgement and should lead to more thoughtful care. It is frequently the most neglected part of the process, nurses seemingly concentrating on the doing aspects of nursing at the expense of the analytical processes of problem-solving (Hurst 1985; Robinson 1990).

Benner's work (Benner & Wrubel 1989), based on Heideggar and a phenomenological approach to caring, concluded that caring is having things matter which involve coping mechanisms, and the setting up of what is described as stressful concerns. Emotions should not be reviewed as a block to rationality, or disruptions that always have to be coped with, but as meaningful integral aspects of practical knowledge embodying intelligence. Without care, Benner suggests (Benner & Wrubel 1989) 'a person is without projects and concerns', meaning that they lack the means for interpreting and understanding. Care 'sets up a world' creating meaningful distinctions and self, so reducing the stress placed on nurses as they become experts in caring, which is not achieved solely by acquiring privileged information. There is therefore a need for nurses not only to know, but to understand and interpret feelings, ideals, choices and purposes, as to how meaning is experienced and expressed through words and responses in caring practices (Meleis 1991). These then become 'organized specific practices related to caring for and about others ... an ethic, a way of knowing and practical knowledge' (Benner & Wrubel 1989).

Caring fuses thought, feeling and action, knowing and being. It enables problem-solving and the relevance

of situations to become clear, as with caring for children and their parents, where mere technique and scientific knowledge are not enough for effective action. Caring is central to a theory of nursing practice (Benner & Wrubel 1989).

Nursing theory should become an intellectual tool to explain the world in which we live and practice. If theory is not applied appropriately through the right choice of models, government and society will perhaps not unsurprisingly intervene (Fish *et al.* 1989; Fish & Purr 1991). Instead of the profession changing itself through judgements and refinements of its own practices, the Government will reform the profession from the outside by imposing models of efficiency and enterprise.

There is now a shift to implementing informal models of care which are personal theories derived from practice: special theories of action that determine human behaviours (Argyris & Schon 1989), vehicles for exploration, prediction or control. These include value strategies and underlying assumptions that express individual patterns of interpersonal behaviours. Human beings in their interactions with each other, as with nurses and their clients, have a responsibility not just to do, but to design their behaviours and to hold theories for doing so (Schon 1990). A practice becomes a sequence of actions undertaken by a person to serve others who are considered clients, where theory becomes related to practice more effectively and meaningfully.

Historically therefore, nurses have evolved from being seen as 'angels of mercy smoothing fevered brows' giving task orientated, medically orientated care within a hierarchical 'profession'. The professional body of nursing knowledge has become increasingly more unique, distinct and clinically research based (Clarke 1986; Akinsanya 1990) in its practice disciplines so that there is now a more rational basis for holistic care. It still needs, however, to become more confident in making its practices explicit in a world of general management, and having an increasingly academic focus as nursing integrates into higher education. This is especially important with the introduction of information technology. The importance of intellectual abilities in caring must be emphasized, so that 'knowing and doing' become reality and each individual's responsibility for formulating their own theories of action – which can be fully espoused – can continue to develop.

PROFESSIONAL KNOWLEDGE – THEORY AND PRACTICE FURTHER EXAMINED

Professional behaviours are characterized by decisions based on a body of professional knowledge and training which involve autonomy and responsibility to society (Deane & Campbell 1985). There has to be some congruence between theory and practice in order for expertise to be acquired.

Historically in nursing there has long been a gap between theory and practice, and between the knowledge taught in schools of nursing (ideal) and learned in clinical areas (real) (Bendal 1975; UKCC 1985a; Elkan & Robinson 1991). Practice in the past has also been seen by some as less prestigious than theory.

New nurse preparation courses have introduced radical changes in the development of the body of professional knowledge for nursing. In particular theory has now been increased, so correcting past deficits, as will be discussed later in this chapter.

'Needs are never static but vary according to individual patients, medical and technical advances and developments... The range of human and technical skills required in nursing is very wide. Outstanding abilities and skills are necessary.' (Briggs 1979)

Types of knowledge

Types of knowledge, how they are taught, and the development of higher cognitive skills are all important to the practice of nursing. Effective practice means making the best judgements in specific contexts; there is no room for error where patients are involved. Practice must not just be based on intuition or by the applying of professional knowledge to concrete situations, but also on problem-solving and the making of rational choices in everyday life, which presents itself in indeterminate situations. Practical knowledge is therefore preparation for action (Orem 1991) and consists of four types of knowledge: knowledge that; knowledge how; knowledge why; and knowing in action (Table 1.2).

The planning of nurse training courses allows for acquiring these types of knowledge. Foundation modules usually consist of introducing basic facts and procedures. Further modules introduce principles of nursing care which are then applied to wider settings. Problem solving and critical incident analysis facilitate the learning and application of rules in the complex world of patient care. Giving the rationale for knowledge acquisition and the taking of a nursing action will provide for knowledge why, meaningful learning and links between theory and practice.

Judgements cannot afford to be based on pure guesswork or on loose suggestions. Knowledge must be true, corresponding to facts, including rules and norms. Critical theories should stand up to scientific discourse and be true statements which together with authentic insights will enable prudent decisions (Viertal 1974) for care to be made.

Research

Research is the process of systematic enquiry (Bradshaw 1989), which facilitates the acquisition, estimation and application of new knowledge. It provides a rationale and scientific research base for practice, creativity, change and professional status. Research is gathering apace in nursing practice and education, now that it has begun to define its own discipline. Priorities have been and are being established for research to underpin nursing activities in university departments and nursing and research development units, as well as in clinical and community areas. Methodologies may be quantitative

Table 1.2 Preparing for action: types of practical knowledge.

Knowledge that	Facts, procedures and repetitive elements. Knowledge can be learned by rote, e.g. learning all the names of the bones in the body, performing procedures such as the taking of blood pressures, but such information is insufficient as nurses cannot just be robots. In addition, therefore, other forms of knowledge are required.
Knowledge how	Intelligent action – thinking through what is being done, interpreting new evidence and making new connections (Ryle 1990); that is, understanding, learning rules, applying them and then even learning when to break them. This type of knowledge is learned through experience. Nurses need to be able to think through many different situations. No patient is the same in their medical, nursing, psychological or family context. Nursing care must be learned and then individualized, that is principles applied in many different settings. Rules of care are learned but they may need to be broken in an emergency or management situation. Knowing when and how to act with authority and accountability comes partly through experience.
Knowledge why	The rationale for action and application of the knowledge base, the when and where to use knowledge, the why of the world and why people make the choices they do. This leads to meaningful learning and action, allows for appropriate judgements, makes sense of what we do and enables practice to be made explicit. Doing things is far easier when there is an understanding of why they are being done.
Knowing in action	The characteristic mode of practical knowledge (Cervero 1988), which requires dynamic knowledge and tacit intelligence, not just the storage of static facts and figures. There is a need to learn through and not from practice, and to 'find out' when in practice placements. Practitioners should incorporate and synthesize new knowledge and skills into practice creatively, so that theories of practice are never static and are ever responsive to new knowledge.

and/or qualitative, and require ethical considerations to be taken into account, especially where children and young people are involved.

Research of particular note related to children's nursing, includes that by Hawthorn (1974), Bendal (1975), and Hutt (1983) who looked into the need for and retention of registered sick children's nurses. There are of course other projects. More still needs to be done in the speciality of children's nursing. There is a need to co-ordinate and develop the research for children's nursing so that it may be truly recognized as originating from a basis of certainty.

Reflection on practice

Practitioners should be able to *reflect* on their practice which is informed by theory, so finding out about themselves, their values and what happens during their actions (Fish *et al.* 1989; Fish & Purr 1991) so behaving differently and managing variables whilst maintaining constancy and eventually teaching others (Argyris &

Schon 1989). Reflection is the process of being conscious of and being aware of making sense of experiences (Mezirow 1991). It is a central dynamic of learning and problem solving, i.e. thoughtful action, and makes for reinterpretation.

It involves critically assessing content, procedures and strategies in solving problems, improving performance and making decisions on predicted insights. We can therefore learn, i.e. interpret our experiences and change our meaning schemes. Reflective action leads to greater accuracy in perception of the unfamiliar, better self concept, greater job productivity, flexibility, innovation and leadership ability.

Professional practice therefore is based on competence, knowledge, skills, attitudes, ideology, creativity and freedom to think. Nursing knowledge if used appropriately in practice can, as research (Perry & Jolley 1991) demonstrates, positively affect patient outcomes and enhance care. Knowledge must underpin practice and practice must underpin education.

PREPARATION OF PRACTITIONERS FOR THE PROFESSION

Nursing, it must be stated, seems not to be the only profession to have contentious issues with regard to the theoretical and practical preparation of its practitioners; developing professional status; implementing problem-solving approaches; and learning from practice. Social work (CNAA 1990; CCETSW 1991), medical, architecture and law schools (Schon 1990) too, have all had to contend with such developments.

Nurse education in this country is currently going through a period of unparalleled change, with the implementation of new nurse education preparatory programmes. The nursing profession has at last been able to create a major opportunity afforded infrequently to few disciplines, in implementing radical change in the way it prepares its practitioners, develops educational processes, and reviews its body of professional knowledge.

The historical context

'Nursing historically has evolved from a simple pupillage to a long apprenticeship, service needs taking precedence over the education needs of students. Nursing has not been able to use the accepted educational methods such as reasoning from first principles and working from the known to the unknown.' (Baly 1980)

Nurses have until recent times traditionally been seen as compliant, unquestioning handmaidens to medical staff (Hayne 1992), who undertook a training which:

'was less important than the element of apprenticeship with its emphasis on obedience, discipline and copying precept which militated against an enquiring mind.' (Baly 1980)

Nurse training syllabuses (GNC 1952) and text books were subject centred, with medically dominated knowledge (Allan & Jolley 1989). Learning theories were behaviourist. Teaching methodologies were seen to be based on knowledge transmission from teacher to learner (Gooch 1984) through didactic teaching (UKCC 1985a), so socializing students into traditional roles in

preparation for working on the wards (RCN 1985). Such pedagogical methods led to compliance in learners (Greaves 1989), with teachers, including doctors, in control of giving information, using a protective shield of authority within a prescriptive system (Townsend 1990).

Until quite recent times, that is the 1970s and 1980s, learners had only nine weeks theory per year during a three year pre-registration programme (Bradshaw 1989). Classrooms were based in small isolated schools of nursing, linked geographically to health authorities. Student introductory period intakes were frequent, often at eight weekly intervals, one starting as another finished like a conveyor belt, in order to meet manpower needs. The implications for the teaching workload are obvious. At the same time as gaining practical experience in hospital wards and supposedly linking theory to practice, learners were required to provide a service for patient care, and were therefore seen as 'pairs of hands' within such a system. Learner wastage rates were often as high as 15–20% (RCN 1985).

Somewhat naturally perhaps, there was disquiet about the academic level of nursing and its image as portrayed to the outside world, with resulting effects on recruitment (Beacock 1989; Bradshaw 1989). The theory/practice gap was wide with learners being told to 'forget all that stuff they told you in the school' (RCN 1985), learning mainly being achieved through trial and error (Bradshaw 1989; Webster 1990).

Various attempts were made to bring about curriculum developments within these constraints (Allan & Jolley 1989) to try and correct educational mismatches between theory and practice and the gap between desired educational ideology and the reality of NHS requirements in meeting patient needs. To try and integrate theory and practice the former study block systems, whereby learning about the heart was often followed by being allocated to a ward to care for patients with 'kidney problems', was replaced by experimental modular schemes in the 1970s. These worked towards having a greater nursing basis and took cognisance of Briggs (1979) who identified the need for 'determining the balance of theoretical and practical work in the learning process itself'.

Many other educational advances continued to be made pre Project 2000, but concerns continued and not only in this country, to the extent that the European Community issued guidelines for reducing the gap between theory and practice (Commission of the European Communities 1986).

Developments in practice came as previously indicated with the introduction from America of the nursing process and problem-solving in the 1970s. There was a wish to increase the knowledge base of learning (Van Hoozer *et al.* 1987) through implementing a systematic approach to individualized patient care. But it had not advanced enough, nor was sufficiently systematized to apply knowledge into the reality of nursing practice (Davis 1989; Greaves 1989). Together with the education problems, according to Bradshaw (1989):

> 'Such developments placed inexperienced student nurses at a considerable disadvantage as they frequently have to respond to the needs of individual patients by instinctive judgement. The present system lacks systematic attempts to show that the skilled practitioner is not programmed to respond to a pre-defined problem in a ritualistic and stereotyped way, but uses creative intellect to seek solutions to each problem.'

So nursing has not always responded well to change, its resistance being well documented (Allan & Jolley 1989). Project 2000 was preceded by other attempts to bring about reform in nurse education through major reports: the Wood Report in 1947, the Platt Report (MoH 1959) and the Briggs Report (DHSS 1972). Their failure to do so was identified by Clay (1987) (cited in Jolley & Allen, 1991) as being due to the impotent influence of nurse leaders on political agendas through 'over cautious and sectional attitudes', together with limited Government financial resources.

Change is brought about

Many factors, including the frustration of members of the profession, resulted in the publication of three major reports in the mid-1980s from the professional (RCN 1985) and statutory (ENB 1985; UKCC 1985a) bodies, who all made fairly similar recommendations. Sufficient at last were the pressures, that the UKCC, after consultation with the profession, formally acknowledged deficiencies within previous training programmes. The UKCC recommended to the Government that radical reform must indeed be introduced, for as the Royal College of Nursing (1985) had pointed out:

> 'Students had the right to an education that will equip them to question as well as to obey, to discover as well as to be taught.'

In 1988 the Government accepted the 1986 UKCC report (which also incorporated some recommendations from the Royal College of Nursing and English National Board reports) proposals, mainly because of the nursing shortage and the absence of compensatory mechanisms in the NHS for recruitment problems (Jolley & Allan 1991) and the NHS not being in a period of growth. Colleges of nursing have now implemented Project 2000, with the aid of some £320m from the government since 1989.

Project 2000

The Project 2000 report is a vigorous attempt to bring about major reform to nurse education. Funding for Project 2000 was confirmed in the spring of 1988 and the first of the new courses was implemented that autumn. Its aim is to produce a different practitioner via a very different pattern of preparation with wider conditions of teaching and learning which will be a long way from those at present (UKCC 1985a) (Table 1.3).

Project 2000 acknowledged the many weaknesses in the previous preparation of nurses, including the gap

Table 1.3 Main Proposals of *Project 2000: A New Preparation for Practice* (UKCC 1985a).

- Links between colleges of nursing and institutions in higher education.
- The award not only of a professional qualification with entry to new parts of the professional register (12–15) but in addition an academic diploma.
- Supernumary status for learners, made possible in part by creating an alternative workforce of health care assistants.
- A new three year educational framework with a broader eighteen month educationally based common foundation programme, together with a more specialist eighteen month branch in care of the adult or child, or in learning disability or mental health (UKCC 1985b).
- New professional competencies to be achieved.

between theory and practice, in stating that there was now a:

> 'need for a fresh look at ... educational preparation for practice ... new thinking about how placements and practical experience could be developed in relation to a whole range of care settings.' (UKCC 1985a)

Placements are seen to be essential and should be systematic so that in future theory can be applied critically by the students in different clinical settings, which is 'where the art and science is best learned'. The report also highlighted a number of fundamental changes in the approach to educating practitioners (Table 1.4).

Table 1.4 Fundamental changes in the approach to educating practitioners in theory and practice.

- A move from being theoretically centred to an applied content approach (UKCC 1985b)
- Modules of concurrent theory and practice, designed to closely link the two.
- Nursing theory so developed that students can apply it in a practice setting under supervision.
- A common foundation programme not solely concerned with theory, but with both theory and practice.
- Branch programmes with a strong element of practice so that practitioners are confident and ready at registration to be accountable for care.
- New approaches to teaching and learning including self-directed learning and the development of the role of nurse teachers.

Content and kind of Project 2000 courses

The aim of Project 2000 is to produce a knowledgeable doer, one who is capable of coping with change, able to think analytically and flexibly and is capable of problem-solving in the real world of health and nursing. Knowledge and action, theory and practice are thus integrated in such aims, as indeed they are within the very title of Project 2000 – A New Preparation for Practice.

Table 1.5 shows points included in the English National Board (ENB) guidelines to curriculum planners in colleges of nursing (ENB 1989).

Teaching and learning strategies are now based more on adult humanistic educational methodologies/processes. Curricula are planned and 'owned' by a team of

Table 1.5 Guidelines to curriculum planners.

Educational processes, outcomes and knowledge content
A wide range of learning strategies should be utilized to encourage the development of critical enquiry and an analytical approach to the practice of nursing.
Learners should demonstrate the application of principles of a problem solving approach to the practice of nursing.
The dynamic nature of nursing should be introduced so enabling students to begin to develop the skills to master their expanding body of knowledge and the challenge of change.
Learners should be enabled to reflect with insight and participate in the delivery of care with knowledge and skill.

Practice
Common foundation programme:
The topic of nursing must be explored conceptually and experienced in practice. There must be opportunities to observe and participate in the assessment of needs and the planning, implementation and evaluation of nursing care.

Branch programmes:
The exploration of the interrelationship of theory and practice throughout is essential, to ensure that understanding of practice is based on theory underpinned by available relevant research. There should be the identification of the nature of knowledge which informs practice.

Project 2000 programmes must also consist of at least 50% practice, to include six months rostered service which must be educationally led.

---

service and teaching staff who have learner input. Courses are developed for conjoint validation by the statutory bodies and higher educational institutions, using broad content and outcome based guidelines issued by the statutory bodies. These have recently been updated to incorporate the principles of lifelong learning (ENB 1994). Fine detailed knowledge is taught in balance with broader principles so that skills and knowledge learned may then be applied in a variety of settings. Responsibility for learning and taking advantage of offered learning opportunities, are placed firmly with the learner, the teaching staff acting as facilitators.

Clinical/community staff have the responsibility for acting as mentors who can aid reflection and learning. They also create conducive learning environments and teach, assess and supervise students on a variety of courses. Developing professionals includes preparing them for these roles, so passing on knowledge and examples of good practice to future generations of practitioners.

Educational courses are evaluated and constantly adjusted to ensure that they are based in the realities of practice and express the dynamics of curriculum planning. Flexibility and adaptability in course planning will hopefully ensure that appropriate 'end products' (Mangan 1993) result, practitioners having the abilities to provide for required patient needs. Project 2000 is currently being evaluated on a national level. There will inevitably be teething problems as a result of such evolutionary changes.

The child branch – the preparation of children's nurse practitioners

Children's nurses were first registered in 1919. The special needs of sick children have been acknowledged by a variety of agencies, together with the recognition that children require specialist provision to meet their needs. Historically children's nurses gained their qualification through either pre- or post-registration courses. The implementation of Project 2000 nursing educational programmes with a child branch recognized these different needs of children too, in preparing nurses to care for sick children (UKCC 1985a) in both community and institutional settings. It also increased the emphasis on preventative medicine and health education. Though Project 2000 confirmed the need for preparing children's nurse practitioners, little specific co-ordinated research has been undertaken as to the need for, value of and preparation of sick children's nurses. In an era of value for money and the need for an appropriate skill mix in the workplace, such research is now beginning to emerge and is vital.

PROFESSIONAL COMPETENCE

The preparation of nurses to enter their profession has been discussed, but what is a professional and how is this status maintained? Much literature has been written on the subject (Baly 1980; Deane & Campbell 1985;

Kershaw 1990; Jolley & Allan 1991; Robinson & Vaughn 1992), but in essence, to be a professional is to enter a vocation and to serve others (Jarvis 1986). Being a professional requires training (and some would argue education!) for the acquisition of knowledge and practical skills which will lead to having expertise, and the ability to make professional decisions working within a team of colleagues, for the provision of client care (Deane & Campbell 1985).

Expertise leads to competence – being effective on the basis of knowledge and the ability to influence others and make changes within the profession and society (Deane & Campbell 1985). Knowledge therefore leads to power (Bendal 1975) and authority. It has to be remembered by the professional that knowledge is an individual property and each person has a responsibility to use it wisely (Robinson & Vaughn 1992) through personal theories of action. These apply in the indeterminate situations of caring for each individual patient, from a variety of backgrounds, where nurses may have to 'think on their feet', i.e. know and do quickly, as an autonomous and accountable practitioner.

Qualified professionals therefore have a responsibility to participate in continuing education (ENB 1985), to keep pace with changing technologies and to keep up to date regarding work practices.

Post-registration education and practice

More recent and major changes in nurse education have concentrated on proposals for post-registration education and practice (UKCC 1991a) including those for staff working in the community (UKCC 1991b) and with children. The changes are a major opportunity to streamline existing provision and encourage integration of parts of relevant and responsive programmes in a flexible and cost-effective framework for innovation. The accent is on core courses to ensure non-repetition of content, on modularization and on the gaining of academic credit. The reports build on the reform of pre-registration education, offering new opportunities beyond the point of registration and throughout professional life. These developments also respond to the changing health needs of the population and the concurrent changes in general education, demography and employment, providing for the context of future professional practice (UKCC 1991a).

The English National Board (ENB) introduced its structured framework for continuing professional education for nurses, midwives and health visitors in 1992 (ENB 1991a). It meets the UKCC requirements, and emphasizes the need for dynamic work based learning and critical thinking practitioners. The framework is research and outcome based, identifying 10 key characteristics which practitioners require and must integrate for knowledge, skill and expertise. Modular courses provide pathways, facilitated by managers, educationalists and practitioners for professional development, including those for children's nurses. Previous learning is recognized and opportunities provided for shared learning (ENB 1991b), for the widening of professional horizons and for the promotion of the understanding of roles. Professionals can gain both recordable professional qualifications and academic credit/degrees/diplomas as the profession works towards graduate status.

Quality assurance mechanisms are integral to course planning. The emphasis is again with the individual post-registration learner practitioner, in having responsibility for planning their learning needs which should be recorded in a reflective professional portfolio. Through such concepts, it is hoped that confidence will emerge in practitioners for teaching others both formally and informally, by sharing their knowledge and providing leadership and a vision for the future.

PROFESSIONAL DEVELOPMENT

Professional development is guided by a Code of Professional Conduct (UKCC 1992a). The practitioner can always be (Kershaw 1990) called into account (UKCC 1989) for what they decide to do, so there is a need for practitioners to recognize abilities and limitations and the expectations of the UKCC, and they should be trained where necessary for any aspect of their practice (UKCC 1992b). Competence must be maintained through structured continuing education, which should start under the auspices of a preceptor providing guidance on completion of pre-registration courses where you 'are on your own', as it were, and no longer 'under the umbrella' of pre-registration learner status.

Continuing education is mandatory for midwives. The UKCC Report on Proposals for the Future of Post-registration Education and Practice (UKCC 1991a) wishes to introduce five days in three years also for nurses; it is a start in the right direction! The economics of introducing such a proposal for such a large workforce are at the time of writing under review by the UKCC and the government. The debate as to who pays for continuing education – the government, managers or employee – continues apace.

Updating/education should provide for adaptability and should cover a wide area of topics for practice embracing management, the clinical spheres, and the legal, ethical, political and professional dimensions of roles. Nurses do need perhaps to concentrate more on politics than ever before, both with a small and large P, in order to keep abreast of changes, keep themselves and others fully informed of the resources and needs of nurses and clients, and so be able to manage and lead the profession.

LEADERSHIP ROLES FOR THE PROFESSION

The Department of Health stated that there will need to be a range of models for leadership in nursing (DoH 1991a). Leaders are vital to ensure effective care and for the future of the profession – clinically, educationally, managerially and in research.

The Oxford Encyclopedia/English Dictionary provides a definition of leading: a person followed by others; guiding; to cause to go with one. Leaders should be able to influence the future and innovate and are vital to any profession, hence the inclusion of a generalist definition. It is in fact a difficult concept to define. Handy (1985) asserts that leaders must organize or co-ordinate the work of others effectively. Through being self-assured, showing initiative and a supportive style, leaders can facilitate commitment and involvement of the workforce. It requires intelligence, initiative, self-assurance, enthusiasm, integrity, imagination and energy, to name but a few traits.

Through confidence in their subordinates and acting as an appropriate role model, leaders are able to 'develop their staff' depending on the demands of their tasks, the organization norms and relationships within the group. Good public relations, coaching, and the building of trust and respect, will influence the roles of their staff.

Roles (Handy 1985) occur in relation to others and are influenced by situations and expectations, legal and cultural. They are affected by conflict, perceptions of and interactions with others, communications, stress, morale and boundaries. Explanations of others' roles should lead to tolerance and understanding, and to prediction of situations. An understanding of role theory will enable you to find your niche in the health care team.

Management, organization styles and structures all involve leadership of others, definition of roles, and effective use of roles, talents and resources. The topic of management will form the focus of a separate chapter in this book.

THE CURRENT CONTEXT AND THE POLITICAL AGENDAS FOR THE NURSING PROFESSION

There are many issues (historical and otherwise) and circumstances affecting both the nursing profession and the future care of children. They have to be contended with and managed successfully in order to go forward in an age of an informed client group with high consumer expectations.

The provision of health care to a large population in an era of sophisticated technology is expensive. A large team of professionals, all with different roles, works in the NHS (Connah & Pearson 1991), accounting for 75% of the NHS budget; nursing and midwifery form the largest group of employees. The funding of the NHS, within what is recognized as an economic recession, is probably the major issue affecting the government, nursing and other professions at the time of writing.

The NHS commenced in 1948 under the principle of being 'free for all at the time of need'. It is, however, paid for by national insurance contributions, the NHS budget being part of the strategic national expenditure of the government. The NHS is thus politically controlled through a statutory basis and acts of parliament. The secretary of state, through wide powers and committees accountable to parliament, has to provide services. There is therefore a political agenda as to the management and control of the NHS according to the government of the day, each political party having its own views on the style of administration, structures and policies. At the time of writing, the Conservative Party is implementing its vision for the future of the NHS.

The NHS was previously medically controlled, with many staff and consumers seeing it as having a 'bottomless pit' for expenditure. Changing disease patterns, increasing technology and escalating costs of manpower, caused the government to reform the management, administration and structures of the NHS, together with its manpower modelling and modes of education, by implementing the recommendations of the DoH report *Working for Patients* (DoH 1989a) and placing an emphasis on executive decision making. Regional and district health authorities were replaced by smaller regional health authorities (still under review), family health service authorities and trusts. The administrators/chief executives hold the powers of authority and are not necessarily nurses. Many, but not all, are doctors and there is a need therefore to make patient and professional priorities clear to them, and to make practices explicit, if the necessary recognition and funding is to be made available for developments.

The provision of care is now through a market scenario, income generation and services through purchasing. Purchasing (Health Publications Unit 1993) anticipates and adapts to change in contracting for services, in an era of competition from the providers, the general practitioner fund holders and health authorities. It is about developing and managing relationships, requiring effective leadership and commitment. It involves doctors and nurses who should influence the content of contracts and know the outcomes. The underlying aims are public accountability, value for money and appropriate resource management.

Any government of the day faces pressures. Currently this government is contending with a demographic increase in the elderly requiring care; higher workloads through higher turnover of patients; and increased requirements for technological skills. This is against a shortage of qualified nurses and a decrease in availability of female eighteen year old school leavers. Policies being devised to deal with such issues and retain staff, include staff grading exercises and a shift in emphasis from hospital to less expensive and psychologically more acceptable community care (DoH 1989b). In the future there will be more patients cared for at home, those in hospital being sicker. A different thinking as to the provision and preparation and type of nurses will be further required. This raises other issues for children who are dependent, and the mentally ill.

Particular issues, such as the distribution of resources around the country in relation to London, as in the *Making London Better* report (DoH 1993a) receive special attention by the Government. Reports are being issued by each government as to how such topics and current concerns are to be managed, for example in the Health of the Nation report (DoH 1991b). Government policies now emphasize more the use of health education models and the promotion of preventative measures rather than always the more expensive aspects of curative care.

Quality assurance measures are all important. One example is the Patient Charter which is being implemented now, whereby a named nurse should be responsible for each patient, who should be able to benefit from a personal relationship with a qualified nurse who gives direct care. Quality issues are the province of the Audit Commission on a national basis but should also be implemented by managers and individuals.

The provision of care is not only through the NHS. There is also the independent and private sector whereby patients may pay, some through private insurance schemes, for care in private hospitals. Increasingly these are becoming more involved in nurse training and education.

Wider political and cultural contexts

In 1977 an Advisory Committee on Training in Nursing was set up by Ministers of the EEC with the terms of reference 'to help ensure a comparably high standard of training'. Nurses can move across national boundaries only through the context of a directive. They do so of right, within the European Community, relating only to recognition of their qualification and eligibility to practice, and have no guarantee of employment or right to a job. It is hoped that rights already available to other professionals will be extended to paediatric nurses at no expense to their professional integrity and to the care given within the totality of the health care system in their own country. There is a need for freedom of movement for authorized paediatric nurses but not every country offers specialist paediatric nurse training, there being no automatic recognition by another country for a paediatric nurse. Such issues are still under discussion in

Brussels; to speed up the systems and bureaucracy they have now been brought under the aegis of general directives. Discussions will continue to ensure generality of standards for the care of children across Europe.

Some colleges of nursing are providing units of learning in clinical placements in Europe. The UKCC has issued guidance facilitating such initiatives. Obviously language barriers have to be overcome when working and learning in Europe.

Manpower planning

The numbers of the workforce have not always been planned for successfully. Manpower models and strategies are now being further implemented at a time when some nurses are completing training with no jobs to look forward to. Some would say that costs of staff seem more important than the numbers, with a decreasing workforce leading to a decrease in the quality of patient care and supervision of learners (Dyson 1992). Waiting times for patients in accident and emergency and outpatients departments, and on lists to come into hospitals for treatment, are now published in the form of 'league' tables to publicize such issues and with a view to encouraging improvement in services through competition.

As to the roles of staff, Caines (Naish 1992) formerly of the Department of Health, warned that professionals would need to be more flexible in their approaches to 'doing work' and in working together. He advocated no place for defensive professionalism. The shape, size and nature of jobs is going to change; in overall form there will be fewer nurses. There may be a growing number of people applying a wider range of skills.

So the key to future care may be in patient-focused hospitals and multidisciplinary approaches, thus eliminating repetition between roles. There will be the need to re-examine boundaries in caring for patients, working together, the different levels of work involved and the integration of training through shared learning.

There are those who believe that the specialist nurse should be replaced by a generic one (Swanwick & Barlow 1993). Is the government being anti-academic and anti the profession in introducing less qualified and expensive staff, those with vocational qualifications or those trained as health care assistants to work alongside the educated Project 2000 nurse? Will there be a return to task allocated care? The secret is in the balance of the skill mix (Elkan & Robinson 1991). Expensive nurses should not be doing nonexpensive tasks – there is a need to go on reviewing job descriptions. Life never presents itself in distinct packages and as these points are being debated, the government is trying to reduce the number of hours that doctors work. Replenishment of this work can in some instances be taken on by nurses who are trained to do so, but not all. Opportunities have to be grasped now by nurses to shape our own professional destiny.

The influences of the professional and statutory bodies: self regulation

Professional bodies such as the Royal College of Nursing influence the nursing profession, report on topical issues and, together with other unions, provide for industrial relations. The Society of Paediatric Nursing (Royal College of Nursing) and the Association of British Paediatric Nurses provide particularly for children's nurses, by publicizing the needs of children and their carers. They provide a vision of the future for children's nursing and for professional development by sharing knowledge and experience through conferences and study days.

The statutory bodies in the UK consist of the UKCC and the four national boards for England, Wales, Scotland and Northern Ireland. A recent review of their function and structure was undertaken by Peat Marwick McLintock (1989), resulting in some changes in 1993. The UKCC is now the appointed and elected body, having the responsibility amongst others for professional conduct functions and maintenance of the professional register.

The national boards (who now have an executive structure) have statutory responsibilities as laid down in the Nurses, Midwives and Health Visitors Act 1979 (Approval Order 1983 amended 1992) (Table 1.6).

Nursing and midwifery were previously overseen by a number of statutory bodies, e.g. General Nursing Council (with its inspectors), Central Midwives Board, Health Visitors Board and so on. In 1983 these were amalgamated into the UKCC and the four national boards. The boards give approval for institutions to conduct courses, with education officers having a role in advising, and monitoring and approving these courses facilitating less prescriptive approaches.

Table 1.6 Statutory responsibilities of the national boards (Nurses, Midwives and Health Visitor Act 1979).

■ Approve institutions in relation to the provision of
  (a) courses of training with a view to enabling persons to qualify for registration as nurses, midwives or health visitors, or for the recording of additional qualifications in the register; and
  (b) courses of further training for those already registered.
■ Ensure that such courses meet the requirements of the Central Council as to the content and standard.
■ Hold or arrange for others to hold such examinations as are necessary to enable persons to satisfy requirements for registration or to obtain additional qualifications.
■ Collaborate with Council in the promotion of improved training methods and perform such other functions relating to nurses, midwives or health visitors as the secretary of state may by order prescribe.

More recent (1992) changes to the legislation enable the further devolution of the centrally managed grant towards the provision of pre-registration nurse education, except in Northern Ireland. Each regional health authority is now strategically responsible for planning for its nurse education requirements and in providing therefore for future manpower needs and the professional development of staff, its funding and siting. As the numbers of required students decrease, smaller colleges of nursing and midwifery are now amalgamating to form larger institutions which link with higher education institutions/universities. The statutory bodies work closely with the Department of Health, and voluntary, professional and other statutory bodies in implementing educational policies.

Nurse education courses now have to comply with fewer rules and regulations. Course lengths are currently set for pre-registration courses by the EC (UKCC 1987) and those rules in evidence are there to protect the public in ensuring that no one enters the professional register who is not fit to do so, or is not adequately trained.

The statutory bodies, together with the academic registrar's department of higher education institutions, are responsible for conjointly validating nursing, mid-wifery and health visiting pre- and post-registration courses for approval periods, and for maintaining acceptable standards of quality education. Members of the profession join board staff in these functions, so incorporating peer review. The profession thereby currently regulates itself. The future may be further affected by higher education influences, general education developments and the Department of Education and Science. It will be important to balance academic with clinical requirements of the practice discipline of nursing in terms of validation criteria, course content, and practice components.

CHILDREN'S HEALTH SERVICES

The United Nations Declaration of Rights (United Nations General Assembly 1959), since superceded by a convention states that mankind owes to the child the best it has to give. Principle 2:

> 'The child shall enjoy special protection and shall be given opportunities and facilities by law and by other means to enable him to develop physically, mentally, morally and socially in a healthy and normal manner and in conditions of freedom and dignity. In the enactment of laws for this purpose – the best interest of the child shall be the paramount consideration.'

Principle 4:

> 'The child shall have the right to adequate nutrition, housing, recreation and medical services.'

Services for providing for child health are influenced by a number of reports and people. Children are different and are not mini adults. They are dependent on adults.

> 'The special needs of children which arise from the fact that they are growing, developing persons should be reflected in the facilities that are provided for them and perhaps more importantly, in the training of those who care for them. Sick children should be cared for by nurses trained to do so.' (DHSS 1976)

Platt (1959) led the way in stating that:

> 'changes of environment and separation from particular people are upsetting and frequently lead to emotional disturbances which vary in degree and sometimes last into adult life.' (Ministry of Health 1959)

The nature of childhood illness has altered. Antibiotics, genetic engineering, transplants, technological improvements and advances in surgical and medical care mean that children can now survive where there was once no hope. However, ethical issues require more contemplation. Indeed issues relating to children may be easily exploited and especially in the media. Stay in hospital is often shorter with more rapid bed turnovers, but the children may be more acutely ill requiring more intensive nursing skills. Less ill children or those with chronic illnesses can be nursed at home with support, as will be discussed later in this book.

The care of children does not centre on them alone but includes their families. Parents want to be involved in their child's care. The media ensure that they can have information relating to medical knowledge and current issues. Competent family-centred care is a must at home, school and in the hospital. Health education and prevention of illness through the work of health visitors, screening, and immunization measures have greater prominence now than expensive curative treatment.

Social science studies ensure understanding of cultures and human behaviours. The Children Act (1989) has helped to ensure that the child has a right to a say in his/ her life and legal procedures. Child protection, the care of children with learning disability and special needs, and the care of the dying child will all form part of the nurse's curriculum. It is important that nurses work closely with other professionals, as evidenced by the Cleveland Report into Child Abuse (DoH 1987) and the Allitt Inquiry (DoH 1994).

Historically, as seen elsewhere, the specific need for children's nurses has not always been understood, Rosemary Hutt's work (Hutt 1983), as previously stated, providing a needed boost for them in the 1980s. The ENB has since created a range of opportunities and courses to increase training of nurses. A recent survey by the ENB (1993) shows that whilst the number of training places for children's nurses has recently doubled, it is possible that 50% of all children in hospital are still not nursed by nurses with the appropriate qualification. This applies especially to accident and emergency departments, out-patients departments, ear, nose and throat and ophthalmic wards. Some children may even be nursed on adult wards where the environment and facilities are not appropriate to their recovery and psychological welfare. These findings are endorsed by the Department of Health (1991c) who provide recommendations in their Guide to the Welfare of Children in Hospital. For those in Scotland, reference should be made to *At Home in Hospital: A Guide to Care of Children and Young People* (1993) Scottish Office Home and Health Department, Edinburgh.

The Audit Commission in 1993 (DoH 1993b) publishes the most up to date findings as to the standard of hospital services for children. Its recommendations are a valuable tool in helping to ensure that these continue to be raised. Caring for Children in the Health Services reports (NAWCH 1987, 1988a, b, 1991) have highlighted the needs of children in relation to day surgery, parents staying overnight in hospital with their children, ward attender provision and admission of children to children's units. They make salutary reading!

The care of both well and sick children requires an integrated service from community and hospital staff in the home, district general hospital and more regional and supra-regional specialist units. In the hospital, clinical specialists and practitioners are responsible for more high technology care in strange environments. Staff require psychological, nursing, high tech, management and leadership skills in tandem with educational skills, working in multidisciplinary teams. Close collaboration with community staff will ensure continuity of care throughout a child's illness. In order to minimize gaps between theory and practice and knowing and doing, lecturer practitioner roles have emerged.

The principles of the science of nursing practice have been discussed earlier in this chapter regarding problem solving, care planning, and knowledge-based research. How these are specifically applied to children's nursing is discussed in the following chapters of this book.

CONCLUSION

This chapter has attempted to set the scene as to the professional nature of the children's nurse in relation to practice and education, working with an organization,

be it in the hospital or community. Children's nurses have to have knowledge relating to both the well and sick child, and be able to manage and lead, as well as knowing about and participating in nursing research. The current political context within which all this takes place has been acknowledged.

Change must not be for change's sake, academia must not take precedence over practice, professional children's nurses must not be superseded by care assistants, or quality care by economics. Idealism and realism, service and education have to be in mutual balance. There is a need to monitor role boundaries and roles; to be political and use various reports and research as tools to increase standards and funding; to communicate with others, evaluate and publish developments; and to plan, innovate and create.

The future will affect all children's nurses, who will see further care of children at home, and the introduction of community children's nursing courses (UKCC 1994), continuing changes in education and effects from closer integration into Europe. It must include regulation of the profession by nurses and new practice initiatives so that practice can be made explicit, including to those who hold powers of authority and who must prioritize, and who hold the purse strings. The individual, more politically astute nurse must develop confidence in autonomous practice and be responsible for personal theories of practice based on sound knowledge and learning in the workplace. In this situation the profession will develop in the right direction by valuing and caring, and having the courage to accept change and to control and direct the challenges. This will result in a pro-active vision rather than a reactive stance for the future, a scientific explanatory rationale for all actions and the right manpower product being produced to meet the needs of children.

REFERENCES AND FURTHER READING

Adams, T. (1991) The Idea of Revolution in the Development of Nursing Theory. *Journal of Advanced Nursing*, 16, 1487–91.

Akinsanya, J. (1990) A Climate of Change. *Nursing Standard*, 4 (33), 32–34.

Allan, P. & Jolley, M. (1989) *The Curriculum in Nursing Edu-*

cation, pp. 6, 149, 210–11, 215–16. Chapman and Hall, London.

Argyris, C. & Schon, D. (1989) *Theory in Practice: Increasing Professional Effectiveness*, pp. 4–6, 148. Jossey-Bass, London.

Baly, M. (1980) *Nursing and Social Change*, pp. 312, 318. W. Heinemann, London.

Beacock, C. (1989) Supporting Nurse Teachers. *Nursing Standard*, 22 April, 29–32.

Bendal, E. (1975) *So You Passed Nurse*, pp. 60, 63, 66–7. Royal College of Nursing, London.

Benner, P. & Wrubel, J. (1989) *The Primacy of Caring*. Addison Wesley, London.

Bradshaw, P.L. (ed.) (1989) *Teaching and Assessing in Clinical Nursing Practice*, pp. 1, 5, 9, 22. Prentice Hall, London.

CCETSW (1991) *Right or Privilege? Post-Qualifying Training with Special Reference to Child Care*, pp. 33–7. Central Council for Education and Training in Social Work, London.

Cervero, R.M. (1988) *Effective Continuing Education for Professionals*, pp. 43, 47, 158. Jossey-Bass, London.

Champion, R. (1988) *Competent Nurse? Reflective Practitioner?* Unpublished paper, Cardiff International Conference on Nursing Education.

Clarke, M. ;(1986) Action and Reflection: Practice & Theory in Nursing. *Journal of Advanced Nursing*, 11, 3–11.

Clarke, S. (1990) Nursing: A Problem Solving or Needs Activity. *Senior Nurse*, 10(2), 13–15.

Clay, T. (1987) *Nurses, Power and Politics*. Heinemann, London.

CNAA (1990) *The Inter-relationships of Theory and Practice in Social and Public Policy Courses*. A discussion paper, pp. 2, 7. Council for National Academic Awards, London.

Commission of the European Communities (1986) *Advisory Committee on Training in Nursing*. Report on Training in the European Community, 111/D/1027/16/84-EN. Brussels.

Connah, B. & Pearson, R. (1991) *NHS Handbook*, p. 55. NAHAT Macmillan Press, London.

Davis, J. (1989) Making the Model Fit: Theory and Practice. *Senior Nurse*, 9(2) 17–19.

Deane & Campbell (1985) *Developing Professional Effectiveness in Nursing*, pp. 4, 6, 7, 9, 10, 12, 62, 207. Reston Publishing Co, Virginia.

DHSS (1976) *Fit for the Future*. Report of the Committee on Child Health Services (Court Report). HMSO, London.

DHSS (1972) *Report of the Committee on Nursing* (Briggs Report). HMSO, London.

DoH (1987) *Report of the Inquiry into Child Abuse in Cleveland* (Chairman E. Butler-Sloss). HMSO, London.

DoH (1989a) *Working for Patients*. Working Paper 10. HMSO, London.

DoH (1989b) *Caring for People; Community Care in the Next Decade and Beyond*. HMSO, London.

DoH (1991b) *The Health of the Nation*. HMSO, London.

DoH (1991c) *Welfare of Children and Young People in Hospital*. HMSO, London.

DoH (1993a) *Making London Better*. Health Publications Unit, Lancs.

DoH (1993b) Audit Commission. *Children First – A Study of Hospital Services*. HMSO, London.

DoH (1993c) *A Vision for the Future*. HMSO, London.

DoH (1994) *The Allitt Inquiry* (Chairman Sir Cecil Clothier). HMSO, London.

Dyson, J. (1992) The Importance of Practice. *Nursing Times*, 88(40), 44–6.

Elkan, R. & Robinson, J. (1991) *The Implementation of Project 2000 in a District Health Authority: The Effect on Nursing Service*. An interim report, pp.74–76, 42–45, 23–25. Department of Nursing Studies, University of Nottingham.

ENB (1985) *Professional Education/Training Courses*. English National Board for Nursing, Midwifery and Health Visiting, London.

ENB (1989) *Project 2000: A New Preparation for Practice*. Guidelines and criteria for course development and the formation of collaborative links between approved training institutions within the NHS and centres of higher education. English National Board for Nursing, Midwifery and Health Visiting, London.

ENB (1991a) *Framework for Continuing Professional Education for Nurses, Midwives and Health Visitors*. Guide to Implementation. English National Board for Nursing Midwifery and Health Visiting, London.

ENB (1991b) *Interim Measures to Link the Process of Validation Programmes Based on Shared Professional Validation and Training at Post-Qualifying Level*. Circular 1991/15/GMB. English National Board for Nursing, Midwifery and Health Visiting, London.

ENB (1993) A Survey to Identify Progress made Towards Meeting the Requirements of ENB Circular 1988/53/ RMLV – Supervision of Students Gaining Nursing Experience in Children's Wards, pp. 6, 7, 15. English National Board for Nursing, Midwifery and Health Visiting, London.

ENB (1994) Creating Lifelong Learners. Guidelines for Midwifery and Nursing Programmes of Education Leading to Registration. English National Board for Nursing, Midwifery and Health Visiting, London.

Fish, D. & Purr, B. (1991) *An Evaluation of Practice Based Learning in Continuing Professional Education in Nursing, Midwifery and Health Visiting*, pp. 6, 7, 15. Report for the English National Board for Nursing, Midwifery and Health Visiting, London.

Fish, D., Twinn, S. & Purr, B. (1989) *How to Enable Learning Through Professional Practice – A Pilot Study*, pp. 8, 11, 15. West London Institute for Higher Education.

GNC (1952) (1962) Guide and Syllabuses of Subjects Examination for the Certificate of General Nursing. General Nursing Council/English National Board for Nursing, Midwifery and Health Visiting, London.

Gooch, S. (1984) No Apples for Teacher. *Senior Nurse*, 1(11), 8.

Greaves, F. (1989) *The Nursing Curriculum: Theory and Practice*, p. 300. Chapman and Hall, London.

Griffith, R. & Kenney, J. (1986) *Nursing Process. Application of Theories. Frameworks and Models*. Mosby Co, St Louis.

Hale, C. (1991) Developing the New Practitioner. *Nursing Standard*, 5(28), 23.

Handy, C.B. (1985) *Understanding Organisations*, pp. 57–92. Penguin Books, Harmondsworth.

Hardy, L. (1990) The Path to Nursing Knowledge – Personal Reflections. *Nurse Education Today*, 10, 325–82.

Hawthorn, P. (1974) *Nurse, I Want my Mummy*. Royal College of Nursing, London.

Hayne, Y. (1992) The Current Status and Future Significance of Nursing as a Discipline. *Journal of Advanced Nursing*, 17, 104–10.

Health Publications Unit (1993) *Purchasing for Health – A Framework for Action*, p. 10. National Health Service Management Executive, Lancs.

Hendry, C. (1992) Critical and Constructive. *Nursing Times*, **88** (39), 36–7.

Hollingsworth, S. (1985) *Preparation for Change*, pp. 21, 29, 39. Royal College of Nursing, London.

Hurst, K. (1985) Traditional Versus Progressive Nurse Education: A Review of the Literature. *Nurse Education Today*, 5, 30–36.

Hutt, R. (1983) *Sick Children's Nurses*. A Study for the Department of Health and Social Security of the Career Patterns of RSCNs. Institute of Manpower Studies, University of Sussex.

Jarvis, P. (1986) *Professional Education*, pp. 20–30. Croom Helm, London.

Jolley, M. & Allan, P. (ed.) (1991) *Current Issues in Nursing*, pp. 1–21, 123. Wesley Chapman & Hall, London.

Kershaw, K. (1990) *Nursing Competence – A Guide to Professional Development*, pp. ix– xvi. Edward Arnold, London.

Kim, H.S. (1983) *The Nature of Theoretical Thinking in Nursing*, pp. 1, 3, 11. Prentice Hall, London.

Manga, P. (1993) The New Game in Town. *Nursing Times*, **89**(15), 52–4.

Melat Zieglar, S., Vaughn, B.C. & Wrubel, J. (1986) *Nursing Process, Nursing Diagnosis, Nursing Knowledge – Avenues to Autonomy*, p. 1. Prentice Hall, London.

Meleis, A. (1991) *Theoretical Nursing – Development and Progress*, pp. 17, 92, 109, 129–31, 160. Lippincott Co, London.

Mezirow, J. (1991) *Transformative Dimensions of Adult Learning*, p. 99. Jossey Bass, Oxford.

MoH (1959) *Report of the Committee on the Welfare of Children in Hospital* (Platt Report). HMSO, London.

Naish, J. (1992) A Vision of the Future in Nursing. *Nursing Standard*, 6(48), 22–3.

NAWCH (1987) Caring for Children in the Health Services: *Where are the Children?* National Association for the Welfare of Children in Hospital (now ASC), London.

NAWCH (1988a) Caring for Children in the Health Services: *Hidden Children*. National Association for the Welfare of Children in Hospital (new ASC), London.

NAWCH (1988b) Caring for Children in the Health Services: *Parents Staying Overnight with their Children*. National Association for the Welfare of Children in Hospital (now ASC), London.

NAWCH (1991) Caring for Children in the Health Services: *Just for the Day*. National Association for the Welfare of Children in Hospital (now ASC), London.

Orem, D. (1991) *Nursing Concepts of Practice*, pp. 86, 88. Mosby Year Book, London.

Peat Marwick McLintock (1989) *Review of the UKCC and the Four National Boards for Nursing, Midwifery and Health Visiting*. Peat Marwick McLintock, London.

Perry, A. & Jolley, M. (eds) (1991) *Nursing – A Knowledge Base for Practice*, p. 32. Edward Arnold, London.

RCN (1985) *The Education of Nurses: A New Dispensation*. Commission on Nursing Education (Chairman H. Judge), pp. 8, 9, 12. Royal College of Nursing, London.

Robinson, D. (1990) Two Decades of 'The Process'. *Senior Nurse*, 10(2), 4–6.

Robinson, K. & Vaughn, B. (1992) *Knowledge for Nursing Practice*, pp. 9, 75, 124, 221. Butterworth Heinemann, Oxford.

Ryle, G. (1990) *The Concept of the Mind*, pp. 30, 46–48, 53, 57–8. Penguin Books, Harmondsworth.

Schon, D. (1990) *Educating the Reflective Practitioner*, pp. 4–21, 255. Jossey Bass, Oxford.

Swanwick, M. & Barlow, S. (1993) A Generic or Specialist Role in Paediatric Nursing. *Paediatric Nursing*, Sept., 10–11.

Townsend, C. (1990) Teaching/Learning Strategies. *Nursing Times*, 86(23), 66–8.

UKCC (1985) *Project 2000: A New Preparation for Practice*. United Kingdom Central Council for Nursing, Midwifery and Health Visiting, London.

UKCC (1985) *The Learner: Student Status Revisited*. Project Paper 2, pp. 5. 6. United Kingdom Central Council for Nursing, Midwifery and Health Visiting, London.

UKCC (1987) *The European Training Programme for Nurses Responsible for General Care*. Professional Standards and Development Division, United Kingdom Central Council for Nursing, Midwifery and Health Visiting, London.

UKCC (1989) *Exercising Accountability*. United Kingdom Central Council for Nursing, Midwifery and Health Visiting, London.

UKCC (1991a) *Report on Proposals for the Future of Post-Regis-*

tration Education and Practice. United Kingdom Central Council for Nursing, Midwifery and Health Visiting, London.

UKCC (1991b) *Report on Proposals for the Future of Community Education and Practice.* United Kingdom Central Council for Nursing, Midwifery and Health Visiting, London.

UKCC (1992) *Code of Professional Conduct.* United Kingdom Central Council for Nursing, Midwifery and Health Visiting, London.

UKCC (1992b) *The Scope of Professional Practice.* United Kingdom Central Council for Nursing, Midwifery and Health Visiting, London.

UKCC (1994) *The Council's Standards for Education and Practice*

following Registration. Programmes of Education leading to the Qualification of Specialist Practitioners. United Kingdom Central Council for Nursing, Midwifery & Health Visiting, London.

United Nations General Assembly (1959) *Declaration of the Rights of the Child.* UNICEF, Geneva.

Van Hoozer, Bratton Ostmoe, Weinholtz Graft & Albanese Giende (1987) *The Teaching Process – Theory and Practice in Nursing,* p. 197. Prentice Hall, London.

Viertal (1974) (Translated) *Theory and Practice,* pp. 254, 281. J. Habermas, Polity Press, Cambridge.

Webster, R. (1990) The Role of the Nurse Teacher. *Senior Nurse,* 10(8), 16–18.

Chapter 2
Historical Perspectives

Sigrid Watt and Ruth Mitchell

INTRODUCTION

Children's nursing has undergone a number of fundamental changes since its professional inception in the mid-nineteenth century. It has reflected not only changes and developments within the context of professional nursing but also in response to the changing attitudes towards children themselves and society's response to the needs of the child. It is in this spirit that this chapter intends to explore and examine a number of important and interlocking themes: the changing concepts of childhood; the developing recognition of children's welfare needs; the training of nurses (1854–1992) to specifically meet the needs of sick children; the increasing awareness of the psychological welfare needs of children and their families; the development of philosophical perspectives and paradigms related to the care of children and their families and the emerging trends in relation to the education of nurses caring for children.

During the past hundred years, society's attitudes towards children have undergone profound change: the difference between the Victorian attitude that 'children should be seen and not heard' and 'spare the rod and spoil the child' to the current climate in which children very definitely have the political and social right to be seen and heard. This is particularly evident when children can and do take legal action against the parent and in some cases have been reported by the media to 'divorce' their parents. This highlights not only changes to the role and rights of children in today's society, but fundamentally reflects the measure of change within the family in society. The introduction of the Children Act 1989 demonstrates the government's and thus society's commitment to the rights of the child. Similarly the needs and rights of children have been recognized within paediatric/children's nursing as the profession has shown an equally deep commitment to a partnership with parents' approach and a philosophy of family centred care. However, despite the changing context in which nursing care is delivered, it is perhaps interesting to reflect that the essential qualities needed to care for and nurse a child have remained unchanged since they were first described in 1854 by Dr Charles West. He identified the essential qualities of a paediatric nurse to be (West 1854):

'Indeed, if any of you have entered on your office without a feeling of very earnest love to little children, – a feeling which makes you long to be with them, to take care of them, to help them, – you have made a great mistake in undertaking such duties as you are now engaged in: and the sooner you seek some other mode of gaining an honest livelihood, the better. I do not mean this unkindly, for you may be very good, very respectable women, and yet be very bad nurses. You may be feeble in health, and then you will be unable to bear the confinement and fatigue upon attending upon the sick; or you may be fretful in temper, and may find your greatest trial to consist in the difficulty of subduing it, and in being as thankful to God for all his daily mercies, and as friendly with those who you live amongst as you ought to be; or you may naturally have low spirits, and a child's prattle, instead of refreshing, may weary you. Now if any of these things are really the case with you, I would advise you not to be a children's nurse, and especially not to be a nurse in a Hospital for Sick Children.'

Similar qualities were identified over 100 years later by Hanton (1981), cited by Fradd (1992), who stated that the qualities required by paediatric nurses at the end of the twentieth century are:

'a genuine love of children, a deep sense of compassion, moral courage, a sense of humour and confidence to provide support for the children and also their parents.'

Perceptions about children and childhood are coloured by the perspective from which they are viewed and writers about childhood rarely reach a consensus. Aries (1962), de Mause (1974) and Arnold (1980) among others have all contributed to the study of childhood and from their work the difficulties and complexities associated with unravelling the concept of childhood. The work of the French historian Aries (1962) has been seminal in understanding the development of our understanding of the ideology of childhood. He recognized that childhood as a concept was invented in the thirteenth century and has traced its progression through art in the fifteenth and sixteenth centuries. He argues that childhood, as it is recognized today, did not exist in medieval time. His purpose in writing was to examine the development of the concepts of childhood through each historical period.

Stone 1977 (cited by Thomas (1989) in Avery & Briggs 1989) shares many of Aries' views and explores similar aspects of childhood, but draws his examples from English families. However, de Mause (1974) presents opposing views to Aries and graphically states:

'The history of childhood is a nightmare from which we have only just begun to awaken. The further back in history one goes, the lower the levels of child care, and the more likely children are to be killed, abandoned, beaten, terrorized and sexually abused.'

He further emphasizes:

'... it is our task here to see how much of this childhood history can be recaptured from the evidence that remains to us.'

It is interesting to note that Thomas (1989) (cited in Avery & Briggs 1989) succinctly summarizes the difficulties encountered by historians and modern writers in their accounts of childhood when stating:

'... they persist in seeking to write *not* the history of children, but the history of adult attitudes *to* children.'

It is important to understand the implications of what Thomas is saying as it demonstrates the skewed perspective that even the key writers may be presenting.

The concept of the family and the extended family is shown to emerge during the fifteenth and sixteenth centuries although there is relatively little literature available that specifically examines the status of children at that time. The modern family, from the pedagogical and moralistic points of view, emerged in the seventeenth century and education was seen as a central focus. Van den Berg (1960, cited in Arnold 1980) highlights the importance of the emerging beliefs of the philosopher Rousseau who proposed that a transition period existed between the 'young person' and the 'grown up'. Laslett (1971) (cited in Arnold 1980) identified that whilst neither the adult nor the child themselves had changed, social circumstances arising from the Industrial Revolution had affected both groups in different ways. Childhood as a concept is constantly evolving and despite the many differences that can be identified, childhood may be universally defined as 'a period of developing body size, structure, function, maturation and learning that are necessary to become a functioning adult' (Cherry & Carty 1986).

CONCEPTS OF CHILDHOOD

The perception of childhood can be traced through the mediums of play, art and literature and each of these themes/media is explored here.

Children's play

Children throughout history and in all cultures play; it is part of the socialization process and through imitation and experimentation they learn and experience social roles and values.

In the fourth century BC Aristotle believed that children up to the age of five should not work as this could be detrimental to their growth. He believed play was essential for healthy development. Greek and Roman artwork portrayed playthings on painted vases, wall paintings and mosaics. However this tolerant attitude towards play was lost in subsequent centuries and although there is little written evidence of children's play, it is inconceivable to imagine that children themselves ceased playing. By the seventeenth century children were depicted in artwork as attempting to understand the adult world through their play. Two children are portrayed by Bourden, for example, playing dice and surrounded by a group of beggars. This imitatory type of play must have continued through history and Singer (1973) highlights that it is more likely that play was not seen as important enough to comment on rather than that children did not play, when he states:

'It seems unlikely that sociodramatic play started only in the nineteenth century ... rather one might surmise that this type of play was more generally common, but simply went unnoticed and unrecorded by an adult world that had not yet begun to show a genuine interest in childhood experience'.

Children in art

Prior to the twelfth century there were no attempts to portray childhood in art (Aries 1962), this being a reflection of the predisposing view of society in which children had no place. The early artwork depicting children portrayed them simply as adults on a miniature scale, as can be seen in the early portrayals of Mary holding the infant Jesus. By the thirteenth century some attempt to portray children as children had been made and by the fifteenth century it had become popular to portray the child in their social context (Arnold 1980). Individual portraits of children become increasingly popular throughout the seventeenth century and reached the height of their acclaim with the work of the Dutch school of art and great masters such as Rembrandt.

Children's literature

There is little evidence of children's literature before the turn of the eighteenth century, although a limited range of school books was available, the most notable being *Orbis Sensualisum Pictus* (Comenius 1658, cited by Dieterich 1991), the first picture book designed for children. In the early eighteenth century books ostensibly written for children were in reality written to appeal to the adult who would be reading them to the children. *The Governess* or the *Little Female Academy*, written by Sarah Fielding in 1749, are good examples (Avery & Briggs 1989). These books not only appealed to adults but also had strong moral overtones (cited by Briggs 1989 Avery & Briggs 1989). *Der Struwelpeter* was written in 1845 and illustrated by Hoffmann-Donner to amuse his sick child because no other suitable material was available. Strong moral messages are also prevalent with all the stories in *Der Struwelpeter*.

In Scotland, Robert Louis Stevenson (1850–94) made a significant contribution to children's literature based on his own childhood experiences, and through his imaginative, creative ability to write, his books immediately appealed to his young readers. An illustration of his ability to appeal to children and identify with their own experiences can be seen in the verse 'The Lamplighter' and in his *A Child's Garden of Verses* published in 1885.

Beatrix Potter (1866–1943) was encouraged to publish letters sent to her godson and thus the highly acclaimed *The Tale of Peter Rabbit* was made available to the young reading public. Both Stevenson and Potter's stories were and continue to be enormously successful and they still retain a universal appeal to children. During this century the writing and sale of children's

literature have become a growth industry. The attempt to socialize children through literature still continues in today's pluralistic society and books today are published which reflect the various moral, religious and cultural differences.

The recognition of child health

During the eighteenth century poverty stricken parents frequently abandoned their children in the hope they would be found by adults who would love and care for them (Schwartzman 1978). Boswell (1988) cited by Davies (1992) notes that the mortality rate among abandoned children was significantly lower than among the children who remained with their natural families.

In Europe the first country to recognize the need for and establish a hospital for children was France. La Maison de l'enfant Jesus opened in 1679 and converted into L'Hôpital des Enfants Malades in 1802. The trend in developing services specifically for sick children continued throughout the nineteenth century as the number of children's hospitals in Europe steadily increased with St Petersburg 1834, Vienna 1837 and Budapest 1839 following in one decade.

As British society became increasingly aware of child health problems the initial response was to open dispensaries. Dr George Armstrong (1719–89) established the first charitable dispensary for the treatment of sick children in 1769. Dispensaries were considered to be appropriate means of treating sick children who were refused admission to many hospitals. Hospitals were viewed as sources of infection and children were acknowledged to be susceptible to infection; also they were often malnourished. Ruesen (1987) states:

'There existed a hesitancy to open children's wards or establish children's hospitals, because of high mortality rate of foundling hospitals. The public viewed children's hospitals as places of death and as a result the medical staff lost credibility.'

The trend to keep children out of hospital was prevalent throughout Europe at the time. Despite seeing the need for special services for sick children, Armstrong (1769) cited in Miles (1985) was strongly opposed to the principle of admitting children to hospital stating that:

'If you take a sick child away from the parents or nurse you break its heart immediately'.

Armstrong's sentiments were to be echoed 200 years later by Bowlby (1951, 1953) and Robertson (1958). However, Armstrong had established the trend for children's dispensaries, and other cities in the UK were soon providing similar services, with Manchester setting up a dispensary in 1829 and Liverpool providing a service by 1851. The need to establish hospital services for children in the UK was apparent to Dr Charles West who founded the Hospital for Sick Children in Great Ormond Street, London, in 1852.

Again the establishment of one service led the way for further hospitals devoted specifically to the care of sick children. Dr Charles Wilson and Dr John Smith founded the Edinburgh Sick Children's Hospital in 1860. The establishment of a second hospital for sick children in Edinburgh was delayed as a result of the ongoing debate about the actual need for services devoted entirely to the care of sick children, as the diversion of funds to meet the needs of children was viewed as an unwise diversion especially since the child was 'after all, an adult in miniature' (Guthrie 1960).

The aims of the Hospital for Sick Children, Great Ormond Street included teaching women 'the special skills of Children's Nursing' (Piller 1966, cited by Arton 1982), and providing advice for mothers. From the time of opening the hospital provided informal training for sick children's nurses. Initially the training took one year and the compulsory textbook for the pupil nurses was West's *How to Nurse Sick Children* (West 1854). West emphasized the need for the 'right motives' for entry and identified many qualities he considered essential for the pupil nurse. A superintendent was appointed in 1865 to oversee the training of pupil nurses and by 1880 the first systematic training for sick children's nurses had been established by Miss Catherine Wood. In *The Training of Nurses for Sick Children*, published in 1888, she recognized that 'Sick children require special nursing and sick children's nurses require special training.'

In 1888 the training was extended to two years, this being almost ten years in advance of the start of training for adult nurses. As interest increased in training sick children's nurses, further centres were established using West's (1854) three aims as their blueprint; these centres were in Liverpool, Norwich and Manchester in 1853, and Edinburgh, Glasgow and Aberdeen in the

1860s. Miles (1986) reports the aims outlined by West in 1854 as being:

'(1) To provide for the reception and maintenance and medical treatment of the children of the poor during sickness and to furnish them with advice, that is, the mothers of those who cannot be admitted into the hospital.

(2) To promote the advancement of medical science generally with reference to the diseases of children and, in particular, to provide for the more efficient instruction of students in this department of medical knowledge.

(3) To disseminate among all classes of the community, but chiefly among the poor, a better acquaintance with the management of infants and children during illness by employing it as a school for the education and training of women in the special duties of children's nursing.'

Children's health care was established as a unique entity requiring specialist services and specialist nurses. In December 1919 the General Nursing Council was formed and the Nurse Registration Act established a sick children's part of the register that was to be of 'equal status to all the other parts of the register' (Burr 1987). Women were attracted to sick children's nursing because the age of entry into training was 21 years as opposed to 23–24 years for general hospitals. This applied to lady pupils and ordinary practitioners. Nursing was held in good social standing and therefore was able to attract sufficient individuals from working class backgrounds. Pay and conditions for nurses varied greatly from centre to centre. Nurse training, recruitment and pay and conditions have been influenced by government reports and one of the early key reports was the Horder Report (RCN 1946) which was published in four sections between 1942 and 1949 (Section 1 – Assistant Nurse 1942; Section II – Education and Training 1943; Section III – Recruitment; and Section IV – Social & Economic Conditions of the Nurse 1949). Despite the far reaching recommendations proposed in the Horder Report, many of them were not implemented because of the post war economic situation. The role of the nurse was again reviewed in the Briggs Report (DHSS 1972) whose terms of reference included a review of the role of the nurse and the midwife in hospital and the community. However, despite changing attitudes to children being cared for in hospital based on the work of Bowlby (1951) and Robertson (1958), no specific child care recommendations emerged from the Briggs Report.

Psychological welfare of children and families

The seminal work on the psychological impact of hospital admission and care on the child is accepted to be Robertson's film *A Two-year-old Goes to Hospital*. Although this work was initially poorly accepted, professional concern and awareness were stimulated.

As concern mounted, the Ministry of Health commissioned a committee in 1956 to investigate care of children in hospital; the subsequent report The Welfare of Children in Hospital – the Platt Report – was published in 1959 (MoH 1959). Shortly after the publication of the Platt Report and the screening of Robertson's film on BBC television, a group of parents formed the group 'Better Care for Children in Hospital' – the group that was to become The National Association for the Welfare of Children in Hospital in 1961. The organization had a multidisciplinary membership with parents and professionals working together to achieve and support the welfare of children in hospital. The organization was also important in disseminating information to parents and additionally in exerting pressure on professionals to improve their standards of care.

NAWCH recognized the importance of the Platt Report and was determined that it should be implemented. NAWCH advocated less restricted visiting and generally improved access for parents to their children in hospital as fundamental to reducing the recognized adverse effects of both separating a young child from their parents and nursing them in hospital. Residential facilities for parents became an increasingly important part of NAWCH's crusade to improve the care of children in hospital. Today many paediatric centres have residential accommodation as a result of the pressure applied by NAWCH.

In 1974 Hawthorn highlighted the fact that in some units paediatric nurses had little knowledge and insights into children's needs. Relevant research findings were not implemented and general theories of child care were not taken into account. The Court Report (DHSS 1976) again established the importance of appropriately educated and skilled nurses in meeting the needs of sick

children and their parents. Emphasis was placed on qualities of communication and involving parents:

> 'Nurses have more continuous and intimate contact with children and parents than doctors do. They must be equipped and ready to meet not only the needs of illness, but also the needs of children and parents for explanations and comfort and they must be skilled at involving parents as fully as possible in the care of children.'

It is perhaps from these tentative beginnings that the commitment to a partnership approach between professionals and parents can be traced. Other key initiatives that NAWCH has been involved in include the role of parents in the anaesthetic room. They have sought to minimize the restrictions imposed on parents and have identified research which stresses the value of parental presence during induction of anaesthesia (NAWCH 1985). Recently the financial implications for parents making long journeys to hospital has been focused on, with NAWCH urging the government to provide special funds to individual hospitals to cover such expenses. Of equal concern to the organization is the way in which the needs of ethnic minority children are met, and research undertaken in 1990 was published as *Health for All our Children* (in 1993). This sought to promote appropriate care for black and minority ethnic children and their families (Slater 1993).

NAWCH has always reflected and been proactive in respect to changes occurring within the context of caring for children, and in response to the increasing emphasis of care in the community the organization changed its name in 1990 to Action for Sick Children (ASC). The name change also reflected the transition from pressure to advisory group. The mission statement highlights the fundamental concerns of the group: 'joining parents and professionals in promoting high quality health care for sick children' (Shelly 1993). The emphasis on the crucial issue of partnership is evident in the ASC 'Ten Targets for the 1990s' (Table 2.1).

The areas investigated by NAWCH and now ASC have reflected the changing directions and nature of caring for children; despite pressure some changes are still required. The needs of adolescents in hospital continue to promote debate and concern and the report *Welfare of Children and Young People in Hospital* (DoH 1991) fuelled the debate when it stated 'adolescents

Table 2.1   Ten targets for the 1990s (ASC).

(1) All children shall have equal access to the best clinical care.
(2) Parents have responsibility for their children and shall receive positive and appropriate support to care for their sick child both in home and in hospital.
(3) Children and their parents shall be given full information about treatments and participate in all decisions.
(4) Whenever possible sick children shall be cared for at home, unless the care they require can only be provided in hospital.
(5) Staff caring for children, whether in hospital or in the community, shall be specifically trained and fully aware of children's emotional and developmental needs.
(6) Children shall be cared for in an environment furnished and equipped to meet their requirements, whether in hospital or in the community.
(7) No child shall be cared for in an adult ward.
(8) Every hospital admitting children shall provide overnight accommodation for parents free of charge.
(9) Parents shall be positively encouraged to be with their child in hospital at all times and participate in their care.
(10) Every child in hospital shall have full opportunity for play, recreation and education.

Table 2.2   Facilities necessary for adolescents in hospital.

Space for privacy in washing and toilet areas with equipment for disposal of sanitary towels, hair washing, shaving, etc.

Space for the use, display and storage of personal belongings.

Space for education, study and socializing, which must be accessible and usable by all categories of patients; youth clubs have been successful at some hospitals.

Kitchen facilities which, by allowing some patients to make snacks and drinks, give them some flexibility in the organization of their day.

Use of a telephone.

Accommodation for members of the patients' families to stay overnight.

have distinctive and different needs from both child and adult patients'. The facilities specifically required by adolescents in hospital were also highlighted in this document (Table 2.2). However it must be recognized that the particular needs of the adolescent have been under review for a number of years. The Platt Report, for example, in 1959 highlighted the need for separate accommodation for adolescent patients and in the situation where this was not possible that they should be cared for with children as opposed to adults. This area highlights that professional, governmental and parental concerns do not necessarily result in change. ASC continues to highlight the issue and in 1990 published guidelines in the form of a checklist for purchasers, providers and users of health care (ASC 1990). The Audit Commission (1993) indicated that the welfare of adolescents in hospital was still a cause for concern.

Changes in the pattern of care delivery are occurring with increasing emphasis on moving away from hospital care to community care. Although children still require admission to hospital the trend is increasingly moving towards short hospital stay. The average length of stay today is just under 3.3 days whereas it was an average of 6.6 days ten years ago (Forfar 1988). Today fewer children are admitted prior to elective surgery and more are managed on a day-care basis (Audit Commission 1990). Although the benefits to the child and family from day-case surgery are well documented (Thornes 1991) the extra pressure placed on the community staff must not be forgotten. This type of change in care management adds to the already considerable workload of paediatric community nurses currently working with and caring for the families of children with ongoing nursing needs (Burr 1992).

Community care for children and families

The concept of home care has received much attention in recent years and is seen as part of forward thinking and innovative care. Increasingly paediatric home care services are replacing traditional hospital provision (Tatman 1994). However, as Lessing & Tatman (1991) suggest, home care was practised in British society prior to the Industrial Revolution. The minutes of a meeting of the Nottingham Children's Hospital in the mid 1800s furnish some of the earliest accounts of paediatric home visiting. The minutes record payment made to a lady matron to visit patients in their own homes after discharge (RCN 1984/5). Similar accounts are to be found in records in Liverpool from 1910; in Rotherham in 1948 the first home care scheme for children emerged. Birmingham followed in 1954 and at the same time St Mary's, London established a home care service involving RSCNs for the first time (Lessing & Tatman 1991; Bergman *et al.* 1965). From the mid 1950s home care schemes have gradually been established and reported upon across the UK (Table 2.3).

Table 2.3 Home care schemes (While 1991).

Rotherham	Gillet 1954
Paddington	Lightwood *et al.* 1957; Bergman *et al.* 1965; Oppe 1971; Jenkins 1974; Martin 1975; Hunter 1977; Jackson 1978; Belson 1981
Birmingham	Smellie 1956
Edinburgh	Hunter 1974; Campbell 1987
Southampton	Atwell & Gow 1985
Brighton	Armitage *et al.* 1975
Gateshead	Jackson 1974; Hally *et al.* 1977; Jackson 1978
Brent	Smith 1977
Basingstoke	Smith 1986
Manchester	Bennett 1988; Couriel & Davies 1988
Nottingham	Dryden 1983; Fradd 1990
East London	Kitson *et al.* 1987
Bloomsbury	Jennings 1986

The most recent edition of the *Directory of Paediatric Community Nursing Services* (RCN 1993) provides evidence of the growth of paediatric community services in the UK over the past ten years. The value of community care is summarized by Dryden (1989) who acknowledges that the paediatric community service gives back to parents control of the care of their children and improves the quality of that care so that children and their families have a lifestyle that is as normal as possible.

DEVELOPMENTS IN PAEDIATRIC NURSING CARE

The changing nature of community care reflects the changing ideology of health care provision. From the time of admission parents are actively encouraged to participate in the care of their child. In all areas of the hospital parents are seen as partners-in-care rather than simply as visitors. Family centred care has gradually evolved from the time when free visiting was first allowed and encouraged. Darbyshire's (1992a) research gives insight into the experiences of parents who live-in with their child in hospital and their relationship with paediatric nurses. Nethercott (1993) emphasizes the importance of the family when she states: 'The child needs consistency of care and the family needs to remain as a functioning whole with prime care-givers remaining as such.'

Parent support groups are helpful as a means of empowering parents and making them feel more confident to approach the role of partner. The transition to a family centred philosophy of care has presented many challenges (and opportunities) to parents and professionals, raising the profile of issues such as children's rights, parental rights and advocacy (Chambers 1992) as well as legal/ethical issues (Brykczynska 1993). Fradd (1991) highlights the nurse's key role in developing and supporting new care strategies when stating:

'As nurses we need to develop the concept of negotiated care, in order that the family can feel free to opt in and out and that nurses can suggest how much they should or should not be involved according to their professional assessment.'

Further support for the centrality of a family based philosophy of care is added by Evans (1992) who states:

'Most paediatric units recommend the continuous presence of a parent while a child is in hospital and in paediatric practice any philosophy which negates this is unacceptable.'

However, the extent to which parents are true partners in care is not entirely clear. Dearmun (1992) concludes from her research that 'there is not sufficient evidence to suggest that parents see themselves as equal partners in the child's care.'

Paediatric models of care have developed to reflect the concept of negotiated, family-centred care (Nethercott 1993). By encouraging parents to develop their knowledge and skills they become empowered and more independent of health professionals.

DEVELOPMENTS IN NURSE EDUCATION

The changes in care delivery and the developing role of the nurse are reflected in the philosophy which underpins Project 2000 education programmes. The child branch (preparation for entry to part 15 of the register) of the current Project 2000 course places increased emphasis on the psychological and sociological aspects of child and family health care, and stress is placed on the facilitation role of the nurse. The programme aims to enhance both the status and potential mobility of the paediatric nurse. Taking into account existing European Union directives the education programmes aim to allow British children's nurses to be able to practise in Europe. However some difficulties do exist as many EU member states do not have a reciprocal training. As stated previously the biggest and most radical change is the shift towards community based care. *The Welfare of Children and Young People in Hospital* (DoH 1991) clearly states that 'children are admitted to hospital only if the care they require cannot be as well provided at home, in a day clinic, or on a day basis in hospital'. Organizations such as the Association of British Paediatric Nurses (established 1936) and the RCN's Paediatric Society (established 1983) enhance the opportunities for paediatric nurses to share their experiences of providing care in a wide range of settings. These associations provide essential forums for nurses to collectively discuss the potential impact and implications of changing government ideologies. They additionally encourage active networking in respect of current developments and recent research.

In conclusion therefore it can be seen that children's nurses have a rich and diverse history, they have responded to an immense number of changes and challenges and their future requires them to demon-strate an increasing level of flexibility. The need for high quality nursing research addressing all aspects of nursing children is fundamental to the development of the profession, and Swanwick & Barlow (1993/4) suggest that this is the way that the delivery of quality care can be ensured. Long (1991) identifies six factors which RSCNs considered to be significant aspects of their role as children's nurses: advocacy; care by family; the child's psychological welfare; parental concerns and cultural differences; stress; and ethical issues. Long (1991) concludes that 'due to the complexity of children's nursing, decisions regarding children's services cannot be adequately informed without representation from RSCNs.'

As members of a profession it is the responsibility of all children's nurses to ensure that optimum nursing care is delivered at home or in hospital and that role development is seen to be crucial so that innovative and creative approaches are developed to meet the health care needs of children and their families. The need for specially educated, highly knowledgeable and skilled children's practitioners is recognized by the government and professional bodies (The Allitt Inquiry 1994; RCN 1994). It is up to individual nurses to take up the challenge and embrace the opportunities.

REFERENCES AND FURTHER READING

The Allitt Inquiry (1994) *Independent inquiry relating to deaths and injuries on the children's ward at Grantham* (Clothier Report). HMSO, London.

Aries, P. (1962) *Centuries of Childhood*. Jonathan Cape, London.

Armitage, E.N., Howat, J.M. & Long, F.W. (1975) A day-surgery programme for children incorporating anaesthetic outpatient clinic. *Lancet*, ii, 21–23.

Arnold, K. (1980) *Kind and Gesellschaft in Mittelalter und Renaissance*. Ferdinand Schoeningh, Paderborn, Germany.

Arton, M. (1982) Children first and always. *Nursing Times*, 78(40), 1687–8.

ASC (1990) *Setting Standards for Adolescents in Hospital*. Action for Sick Children, London.

ASC (1991) *Caring for Children in the Health Services: Just for the Day*. Action for Sick Children, London.

Atwell, J.D. & Gow, M.A. (1985) Paediatric trained district nurse in the community: expensive luxury or economic necessity? *British Medical Journal*, 291, 227–9.

Audit Commission (1990) *A Short-cut to Better Services; Day*

Surgery in England and Wales. HMSO, London.

Audit Commission (1993) *Children First: a Study of Hospital Services.* HMSO, London.

Avery, G. & Briggs, J. (eds) (1989) *Children and Their Books.* Clarendon Press, Oxford.

Baker, S. & Lane, M. (1994) The good father. How is the role of fathers in child care changing. *Child Health,* 2(91), 28–30.

Barlow, S. & Swanwick, M. (1994) Supplementary Benefits. *Paediatric Nursing,* 6(3), 16–17.

Belson, P. (1981) Alternatives to hospital care. *Nursing,* 23, 1015–16.

Bennett, M. (1988) The fibre squad. *Nursing Times,* 84(4), 49.

Berg, J.H. van den (1960) Metabletica. Uber die Wandlung des Menschen. Grundlinien einer historischen Psychologie. Göttingen, Germany.

Bergman, A.B., Strand, H. & Oppe, T.E. (1965) A paediatric home care program in London: ten years' experience. *Paediatrics,* 36(3) part 1, 314–321.

Bird, J. & Podmore, V. (1990) Children's Understanding of Health and Illness. *Psychology and Health,* 4, 175–85.

Boswell, J. (1988) *The kindness of strangers.* In unpublished conference address (R.A. Davis 1992), 26–29 July, Dundee, paper 18, pp. 1–17.

Bowlby, J. (1951) *Maternal Care and Mental Health.* World Health Organisation, Geneva.

Bowlby, J. (1953) *Child Care and the Growth of Love.* Penguin Books, Harmondsworth.

Brykczynska, G. (1993) Ethical issues in paediatric nursing. In *Advances in Child Health Nursing* (eds E.A. Glasper & A. Tucker). Scutari Press, London.

Buchanan, M. (1977) Paediatric hospital and home care, 2. Easing parents' problems. *Nursing Times,* 73(11), 39–40.

Burr, S. (1987) Paediatric Nursing: Past, Present and Future.*Journal of the Royal Society of Health,* 107(4), 155–6, 158.

Burr, S. (1992) Paediatric Nursing in the United Kingdom. *Journal of Paediatric Nursing,* 7(4), 299–302.

Campbell, M. (1987) Children with on-going health needs. *Nursing,* third series 23, 871–5.

Chambers, M.A. (1992) Who speaks for the children? *Journal of Clinical Nursing,* 1, 73–6.

Cherry, B.S. & Carty, R.M. (1986) Changing concepts of childhood in society. *Paediatric Nursing,* 12(6), 421–4.

Couriel, J.M. & Davies, P. (1988) Costs and benefits of a community special care baby service. *British Medical Journal,* 296, 1043–6.

Darbyshire, P. (1992a) *Parenting in public: a study of the experiences of parents who live-in with their hospitalised child and of their relationships with paediatric nurses.* Unpublished PhD thesis, University of Edinburgh, Edinburgh.

Darbyshire, P. (1992b) Parents, nurses and paediatric nursing

– a critical review. *Journal of Advanced Nursing,* 18, 1670–80.

Dearmun, A. (1992) Perceptions of parental participation. *Paediatric Nursing,* 4(7), 7–9.

DHSS (1972) *Report of the Committee on Nursing* (Briggs Report). HMSO, London.

DHSS (1976) *Fit for the Future.* Report of the Committee on Child Health Services (Court Report). HMSO, London.

Dieterich, V-J. (1991) *Biographie: Johann Amos Comenius.* Rowohlt Verlag, Hamburg.

DoH (1991) *Welfare of Children and Young People in Hospital.* HMSO, London.

Dryden, S. (1983) Home healing. *Nursing Times, Community Outlook,* October, 25–26.

Dryden, S. (1989) Paediatric medicine in the community. *Paediatric Nursing,* 1(8), 17–18.

Evans, M. (1992) Extending the parental role. *Professional Nurse,* 7(12), 774–6.

Forfar, J.O. (1988) (ed) *Child Health in a Changing Society.* Oxford University Press, Oxford.

Fradd, E. (1990) Setting up a paediatric community nursing service. *Senior Nurse,* 10 (7), 4–6.

Fradd, E. (1991) An invitation to influence change. *Paediatric Nursing,* 3(6), 6–8.

Fradd, E. (1992) The evolution of the RSCN. *Journal of Clinical Nursing,* 1, 309–14.

Gillet, J.A. (1954) Domiciliary treatment of sick children. *The Practitioner,* 172, 281.

Glasper, A. (1988) Parents in the anaesthetic room. A blessing or a curse? *Professional Nurse,* 3(4), 112–15.

Glasper, A. (1990) Accompanying children. *Nursing Standard,* 4(24), 6–7.

Guthrie, D. (1960) *The Royal Edinburgh Hospital for Sick Children.* Livingstone Ltd, Edinburgh and London.

Hally, M.R., Holohon, A., Jackson, R.H., Reedy, B.L.E.C. & Walker, J.H. (1977) Paediatric home nursing scheme in Gateshead. *British Medical Journal,* 1, 762–4.

Hanton, P. (1981) They are never small adults. *Nursing Mirror,* 152(16), 30–31.

Hawthorn, P. (1974) *Nurse, I Want my Mummy.* Royal College of Nursing, London.

Health Policy Directorate (1993) *At Home in Hospital.* HMSO, Edinburgh.

Hergenrather, J.B. & Rabnowitz, M. (1991) Age related differences in the organisation of children's knowledge of illness. *Developmental Psychology,* 27(96), 952–9.

Hoffman-Donner (1845) *Der Struwelpeter.* Kindlers Literaturlexikon (1974). Deutscher Taschenbuch Verlag, Munchen.

Hunter, M.H.S. (1974) *A Programme of Integrated Hospital and Home Nursing Care for Children.* Unpublished paper presented at NAWCH conference, 16 October.

Hunter, M.H.S. (1977) Paediatric hospital and home care 1. Integrated programmes. Occasional paper. *Nursing Times*, 73, 33–36.

Hutt, R. (1983) *Sick Children's Nurses.* A study for the Department of Health and Social Security of career patterns of RSCNs. Institute of Manpower Services, University of Sussex, Brighton.

Jackson, R.H. (1974) *Gateshead Home Nursing Scheme: an Operation in Co-operation.* Unpublished paper presented at NAWCH conference, 16 October.

Jackson, R.H. (1978) Home care for children. *Journal of Maternal and Child Health*, 3, 96–100.

Jenkins, S. (1974) *The Home Care Scheme in Paddington.* Unpublished paper presented at NAWCH conference, 16 October.

Jennings, P. (1986) The perfect recipe. *Senior Nurse*, 4, 19–20.

Kitson, A., Atkinson, B. & Ferguson, B. (1987) Specialist delivery of care. *Nursing Times*, 83, 36–40.

Lessing, D. & Tatman, M.A. (1991) Paediatric home care in the 1990s. *Archives of Diseases of Childhood*, 66, 994–6.

Lightwood, R., Birmblecombe, F.S.W., Reinhold, J.D.L., Burnard, E.D. & Davia, J.A. (1957) A London trial of home care for sick children. *Lancet* i, 313–316.

Long, A. (1991) *An Investigation of the Factors Contributing to the Unique Role of Children's Nurses.* Unpublished BSc dissertation, Huddersfield Polytechnic.

Martin, F.R. (1975) The nurse's role in the home care unit. *Nursery Mirror*, 141, 70–72.

de Mause, L. (ed) (1974) *History of Childhood.* Souvenir Press (A&E) Ltd, London.

Miles, I. (1986) The emergence of sick children's nursing: Part 1, Sick Children's Nursing before the turn of the century. *Nurse Education Today*, 6, 82–87.

Miles, I. (1986) The emergence of sick children's nursing: Part 2. *Nurse Education Today*, 6, 133–138.

Miles, I. (1986) A suitable case for treatment. *Nursing Times*, 81(18), 48–50.

MoH (1959) *Report of the Committee on the Welfare of Children in Hospital* (Platt Report). HMSO, London.

NAWCH (1985) *The Emotional Needs of Children Undergoing Surgery.* Policy Paper 2. National Association for the Welfare of Children in Hospital, London.

Nethercott, S. (1993) A concept for all the family. *Professional Nurse*, 8(12), 794–7.

Oppe, T.E. (1971) Home care for sick children. *British Journal of Hospital Medicine*, 22, 39–46.

Piller, G. (1966) *The Story of the Hospital for Sick Children.* Great Ormond Street, London.

Price, S. (1994) The Special Needs of Children. *Journal of Advanced Nursing*, 20, 227–32.

RCN (1946) *Report of the Nursing Reconstruction Committee* (Horder Report). Royal College of Nursing, London.

RCN (1984/85) Changing provision for sick children and diseases in childhood in Liverpool since 1850. *RCN Bulletin*, 6. Royal College of Nursing, London.

RCN (1993) *Directory of Paediatric Community Services* (10th edn). Royal College of Nursing, London.

RCN (1994) *Nursing Children.* Royal College of Nursing, London.

Reading, R. (1993) Equity and community child health. *Archives of Disease in Childhood*, 68, 686–90.

Robbins, M. (1987) The Role of the Nurse. *Nursing*, 24, 905–7.

Robertson, J. (1958) *Young Children in Hospital.* Tavistock, London.

Ruesen, M. (1987) *Die Kinderpflege-Ausbildung in der Bundesrepublick Deutschland im Vergleich zu Grossbritainnien.* Unpublished dissertation. Fachhochschule, Marburg, Germany.

Rushforth, H.E. (1994) *A study to investigate some nurses' knowledge, beliefs and reported practice with respect to children's understanding of concepts of health and illness.* Unpublished BA Nursing Education Dissertation, University of Portsmouth.

Schwartzman, H.B. (1978) *Transformations.* Plenum Press, New York and London.

Scottish Home and Health Department (1993) *At Home in Hospital: A Guide to Care of Children and Young People.* HMSO, Edinburgh.

Shelley, P. (1993) Giving Children a Voice. *Child Health*, 1(1), 21–4.

Singer, J.L. (1973) *The Child's World of Make-Believe.* Academic Press, New York and London.

Slater, M. (1993) *Health for all our children: achieving appropriate health care for black and minority ethnic children and their families.* Action for Sick Children, London.

Smellie, J.M. (1956) Domiciliary nursing service for infants and children. *British Medical Journal*, 1, 236.

Smith, J. (1986) The ward moves out. *Nursing Times*, 82, 44.

Smith, J.P. (1977) Brent's paediatric nursing unit. *Nursing Mirror*, 145, 22–24.

Swanwick, M. & Barlow, S. (1993/4) A caring definition. *Child Health*, 1(4), 137–41.

Tatman, M. (1994) Provision of paediatric home care services. *Nursing Times*, 90(12), 12.

ASC (1991) *Just for the Day.* Action for Sick Children, London.

West, C. (1854) *How to Nurse Sick Children.* Longman, Brown, Green and Longmans, London.

While, A.E. (1991) An evaluation of a paediatric home care scheme. *Journal of Advanced Nursing*, 16, 1413–21.

Young, J. (1992) Changing attitudes towards families of hospitalised children from 1935–1975: a case study. *Journal of Advanced Nursing*, 17, 1422–9.

Chapter 3
Community Nursing Perspectives

Anna Sidey

INTRODUCTION

Children need to be nursed by skilled practitioners who understand and can fulfil their emotional care needs as well as their physical care needs (Swanwick & Barlow 1993). It is equally important that the child is able to benefit from such practitioners within both the hospital and community settings. However, many children are unable to gain access to qualified paediatric practitioners in the community and thus their needs are not met (Burr 1990). The importance of Paediatric Community Nurses (PCNs) lies primarily in terms of caring for the sick child and their family within, and as part of, their own 'home' community.

The PCN acts with, and on behalf of, not only the child but the entire family. Acting in a variety of roles ranging from specialist liaison nurse to a member of a team of PCNs caring for the child's more general health care needs, the PCN must be responsive to the individual child's needs. The PCN acts as an advocate for the child when this role is required and as a facilitator of family centred home care. Other aspects of the PCN role include delivering care, teaching, supporting, advising, liaising and counselling. The family is involved as appropriate in all the roles of the PCN, as flexible, dynamic care that is responsive and proactive in terms of paediatric nursing care, is delivered. Burr (1991) states that '... Paediatric Community Nursing represents a very positive response by paediatric nurses to children's and parent's needs ...'.

PCNs have skills not only in delivering care but also in respect to available resources in the community, how to use community networks and how to act as a resource for associated care professionals. However, despite the seemingly obvious need for PCN services there are still gaps in provision and of those services in existence the funding, budgeting and the characteristics are diverse.

HISTORY OF PAEDIATRIC COMMUNITY NURSING

The desirability of children being nursed at home whenever possible has been on governmental and professional agendas since the Platt Report (MoH 1959) stated that 'children should only be admitted to hospital when the care they require cannot be given at home without real disadvantage.'

However, despite the identified need to move care into the community, The Audit Commission's report, *Children First: a Study of Hospital Services* (1993), identified that three quarters of health authorities had no paediatric community services, and many of the schemes in existence had only one or two nurses. Although this report may suggest that little has happened in the years since the Platt report, much progress and innovation in terms of delivering care for children at home has occurred.

In the early part of the century most sick children were cared for by their family in their own home. Hospital care for sick children became more commonplace as the century progressed, partly in an attempt to reduce the appalling child mortality rate. Child mortality had more to do with ignorance about the spread of infectious diseases than with the specific place of care. For most of this century families have taken their sick children to be cared for by strange people in a strange place, and have left them there alone, relinquishing care and control in the expectation that they would recover. The fact that children did recover owes much to their tenacity, despite the emotional harm they undoubtedly suffered as a result of separation from the carers they loved and trusted. From the 1930s studies by psychologists demonstrated that sick children (especially the young who experienced weeks or even months of this loss and separation whilst in hospital) suffered emotional trauma to a greater or lesser extent and it was invariably long lasting. Since the 1950s a number of reports have continued to acknowledge the need that sick children have both the right and the need to be nursed by suitably qualified paediatric nurses in their own home environments whenever possible (MoH 1959; Bowlby 1965; Hawthorn 1974; DHSS 1976; Rutter 1981; Robertson 1989).

The first PCN services were established in the 1950s in Rotherham (Gillet 1954), Paddington (Lightwood 1956) and Birmingham (Smellie 1956). The advantages of home care schemes were identified in 1957 in the paper published as a result of a two year paediatric home care trial at St Mary's Hospital, London. It identified that home care was less expensive than hospital care; and that both hospital personnel and GPs benefited through a higher degree of co-operation in care. The results of this scheme were published in the Lancet in 1957 as 'A

London Trial of Home Care of Sick Children', and the audit found that over a quarter of children were unnecessarily admitted to hospital as they could have been managed at home if the resources and skills had been available. Additionally it was found that children's length of stay in hospital could have been shorter (At Home 1994). It is interesting to note that despite the success of these early schemes no further paediatric homecare services were established in the UK between 1954 and 1969 (At Home 1994).

However, in recent years the range of services offered

would otherwise have to be admitted to hospital. Some areas achieve this ratio and thus they fulfil recommendations. District nurses provide a comprehensive home nursing service for adults, and children require the same. The RCN acknowledges that the paediatric community nurse is best placed to provide this care due to the range of skills and knowledge they possess (RCN 1993) and the diversity of service offered (see Table 3.1). Family centred home care is most appropriately delivered through a national network of paediatric community nursing services.

Table 3.1 Potential contributions of PCNs (RCN 1993).

Assess the particular needs of a family which has a sick child within it.
Enable children to be nursed in all community settings, for example, playgroup, nurseries, residential homes, respite care facilities and their own homes.
Enable children with a debilitating disease to fulfil their potential, enhancing their quality of life.
Provide opportunistic health promotion for the whole family.
Plan, in co-operation with the family, the special needs of the ill child.
At the end of life, enable the child to die with dignity in the place of their choice.
Provide crisis intervention, thus offering continual support to families who live with a high level of stress associated with caring for a child with chronic illness.
Enable parents to feel confident and competent when caring for their child.
Teach families to carry out specific nursing care, including high-tech procedures.
Act as an interface between community, hospital and all other agencies, for example cubs, school camps or sports camps, providing continuity of care and facilitating the normal activities of childhood and adolescence.
Help families network with others, reducing feelings of isolation and despair.
Offer appropriate support and help following bereavement.
Prevent hospital admission and attendance. Paediatric community nurses can also facilitate early discharge while the option of day care is made more available.
Teach student nurses, community nurses, medical students, GP trainees and others.
Act as a specialist resource for all health care workers.
In common with district nurses and health visitors, paediatric community nurses will be able to prescribe certain medicines once the regulations are in place.

to sick children and their families in the community has increased and there is a strong professional impetus for the range, extent and diversity of services to increase (RCN 1993). Whiting (1994) highlights the development of services when he indicates that there were only eight generalist PCN schemes in the UK in 1981 but that this number had increased to 61 by April 1993. Despite the increase in services many health authorities still do not have a PCN. Work indicates that 4.4 PCNs and 0.5 clerical assistants for every 50 000 children can facilitate home care for up to 20% of children who

FAMILY CENTRED CARE AND PARTNERS IN CARE

Family centred care occurs when carers, and where possible the sick child, are involved as active partners with the health care professionals in management, decision making, treatment and care. Carers should be acknowledged by the nurse and other health care professionals as not only the expert in relation to their well child but also in respect of their child when sick. Parents may not readily accept the role of expert but with support can acknowledge the special and unique contribution they can make. The impact that a child's illness, whether acute or chronic, can have on the family should not be underestimated. Family dynamics are changed and challenged and parents will often feel inappropriately guilty about their child's illness. Anxiety and stress are commonly experienced by all members of the child's family/support network. The child at the centre of this family crisis senses this and this adds to the strangeness of their experience of being ill.

For a child admitted to hospital where health care professionals can so easily take over and disempower the parents, the sense of shock can be profound; care and support in their own home can be infinitely preferable. Without a commitment to a partnership approach the health care professional will never achieve an understanding of what makes individual families 'tick'. In most families, one or more carers protect, clothe, house, wash, feed, care in countless ways, and become the expert on their child. How this role is achieved and maintained varies according to the style of parenting and circumstances. Each family is unique. These carers then are the experts on the normal physical, psychological, social, spiritual and maybe sexual needs of their child, most of which remain unchanged during illness (Jolly 1981). This must be respected by the nurse so that the family can maintain this input. Family centred care can lead to parents as partners, who are consulted, share in the decisions and are able to help in the care.

By working with, teaching and supporting families the nurse can assist acceptance of the nursing care aspects as an extension to their usual caring role. A relaxed, comfortable family can greatly assist in managing a child's care and even potentially unpleasant situations such as injections or tracheostomy tube change can be less stressful for the child if performed by someone they love and trust. Parents as partners in care can be helped through the emotions of shock, grief and guilt, by the fulfilment of the role. Parents may grieve for the loss of a healthy child even in what may be considered to be a commonplace disorder (Sidey 1989, 1990, 1991). No family should be made to feel that partnerships and nursing care are roles they have to take on. 'Bridges' can be built, no matter how wide the gaps, to facilitate a unique and appropriate package of care for each family.

Family centred care at home is a natural extension to family centred care in hospital and is often the first choice of the PCN in planning care. Home care is now available for children who, even a few years ago, could not have been nursed at home. Children who previously would have died are surviving in the 1990s and many have complex care needs requiring support with sophisticated knowledge, technology and medications. These children require skilled support to ensure they have a good quality lifestyle within their peer group rather than languishing in an acute ward. Life for these children is what home care services offer them and the system needs to be able to facilitate this. All but the most intensive care may be delivered at home providing the appropriate package of care and commitment is present.

PATTERNS OF CARE

Paediatric care in the 1990s will be characterized by relatively short hospital admissions and increasing numbers of acute and chronically sick children requiring home care. The paediatric community nurse leading a mixed skill team of PCNs will plan and implement the community care. Teams attached to acute units and working in the community will be funded, organized and managed in a variety of ways dependent on local needs, skills, and financial resources and on the experiences of past, present and future collaboration, communication and commitment.

Schemes have evolved over the past thirty years; in the past few years the majority have developed in response to local needs and resources. Some provide sophisticated home care, others provide less acute care, such as post operative follow up after elective surgery and support for children with asthma and diabetes. Specialist children's nurses attached to regional and supra-regional centres provide outreach services for a variety of specialities including renal and oncology. Nationally there is a mix of generic and specialist PCNs who may practise within teams or in relative isolation.

The majority of sick children based at home who require the support of a PCN are attached to district general hospitals where the least numbers of PCNs are as yet employed. Nationally a comprehensive network of paediatric community nursing services is required which would provide teams of generic nurses managed by a specialist PCN holding a child focused community nursing qualification. Within these teams individual nurses tend to develop different areas of interest, expertise and knowledge, for example diabetes, neonates, respiratory disorders and oncology. Currently home care is not always available to all children requiring it, due to either a complete lack of available service or due to inadequately funded need services. Home care should only be denied in specific or exceptional family or home circumstances; PCNs can assess, negotiate and facilitate home care in the majority of types of health crisis at home providing they are not coerced into taking over their child's nursing needs. Packages of care can be provided to support the family through crises, such as providing care for the terminally ill child, the child with a chronic disorder or an acute change in health status. Many children are motivated and encouraged by their ability to be cared for either totally at home or mostly at home and with short hospital admissions. The paediatric community nurse can act as professional friend, carer, advocate and educator as well as knowledgeable expert and partner in care.

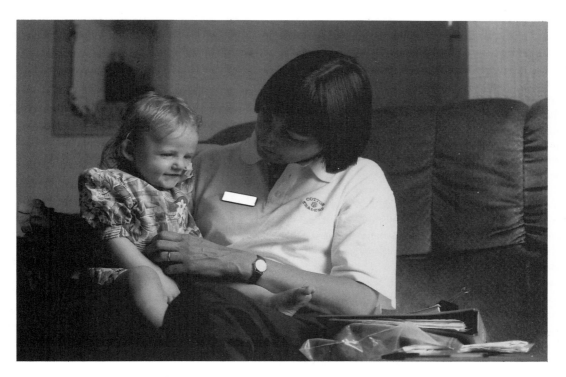

Fig. 3.1 A professional friend, advocate and partner in care. Support at home by a community paediatric nurse. *(Reproduced by permission of Jon Sparks.)*

situations and settings. Caseloads are controlled depending on number of staff, skill mix, density of care required, geography and funding with staff working geographically where possible (Sidey 1990; ASC 1993; Audit Commission 1993).

The rewards of caring for children and their families in the community are immense and the quality of the children's lives can be greatly improved. Families with appropriate help and support can and do manage many

FUNDING AND MANAGEMENT

Currently PCN schemes are funded mainly from acute paediatric budgets although in some areas by community budgets. Community care reduces the need for acute care and where the scheme is funded by the community the money should follow the patient from acute budgets. Few plans exist as yet for purchasers to purchase paediatric community nursing services as a separate entity. Indeed very little work has been undertaken on separate costing of services and the generation of income which in turn would finance the expansion of services. Nursing sick children at home is not necessarily a cheap option although it can be demonstrated to be cheaper than the cost of the child occupying an acute bed.

Both purchasers and providers of health care will be able to demonstrate their commitment to the needs and rights of sick children by negotiating the most appropriate packages of home care. The extra cost of setting up community services is transitional expenditure. A significant part of the comprehensive scheme developed in Nottingham in the past decade has been financed by the closure of paediatric beds (Atwell & Gow 1985; Lessing & Tatman 1991; Fradd 1992; Audit Commission 1993).

Paediatric community nursing services are currently managed by the unit that funds them. Managerially this may be appropriate if management respects the information received from staff about staff needs and can identify and appropriately manage such services. In reality acute management units are unlikely to have community knowledge or experience and community management units are unlikely to possess skills in paediatric nursing. PCNs can be inappropriately managed and their needs and those of their patients inadequately understood.

Appropriately staffed and funded schemes could be managed by a budget holding senior PCN accountable to a director of service similar to other managers within trusts and directorates. PCNs with a community qualification have experience of acute and community paediatric nursing and can practise in and between both settings. Acute based nurses often have little, if any, experience of paediatric community care and even if they do this is unlikely to have been with sick children with the type of sophisticated care needs that are now nursed at home. The nursing of a sick child in the community presents unique challenges and problems. It is unrealistic and unsafe to expect unsupervised acute setting nurses to move out to this type of community nursing. It is equally impractical to expect district nurses, health visitors and practice nurses who do not hold a child nursing qualification to care for sick children in the community.

COMMUNICATION

Good communication is based on many factors including good liaison, administration, documentation and networking. Clerical support is vital for the smooth running of the service and helps to ensure that PCNs spend their time with the children and their families rather than with the paperwork. Multifaceted liaison and communication between professionals and non-professionals involved with a family is vital and this can be achieved by both direct and indirect contact.

Direct contact can be achieved through regular service meetings involving acute carers and community workers as appropriate. The need for an effective contact system should not be underestimated and mobile telephones, answerphones and message pagers can greatly assist interprofessional and family communication; these systems are ultimately cost effective. Telephone triage has been an accepted practice for PCNs for many years. Daily visits to and/or surgeries held within the hospital setting by one of the team produce quality liaison; regular input on the community aspect is vital. Non-direct communication may be through a variety of methods: regularly updated summary cards which fit in GPs' notes; individual patient summary sheets held in a paediatric community nursing service information folder on the paediatric wards; and joint care plans or access to the PCN care plans held in their office based adjacent to the paediatric unit.

Patient care plans and records are evolving in a variety of forms: shared with wards or families; based on wards or in homes; or in service offices. They may be maintained by the family or the child, PCN maintained or a combination of both. The structure depends on individual nurse preference and knowledge, the aim of the record or plan and who maintains it. It may be a one-off sheet for a one-off visit or a detailed document which enhances family centred care. A family held record of care and treatment which accompanies the patient through the 'minefield' of scattered health service options may be the best option (UKCC 1993a).

ORGANIZATION OF SERVICE

The organization of PCN services is complex and reflects the nature of individual schemes. However, a number of issues including referrals, caseload numbers and content, shared care, medical and nursing cover, interprofessional conflict, provision of equipment and supplies and statistical information apply to most if not all services. In a fully staffed service referrals can be accepted from a number of sources and assessed for their appropriateness and the required level of intervention. The referral can then be either redirected, or accepted and allocated to the nurse with the relevant skills within the team. In less or inappropriately staffed services the team leader will need to identify if the team can manage the referral within their resources. In this situation a need to limit the sources of referral may well result.

Only fully staffed services can provide 24 hour, seven day a week cover. Caseload numbers should be realistic to allow safe practice, good quality care with an appropriate amount of time spent with the families, and the ability to accept emergency referrals. Additionally, the need for staff development through in-service education and consolidation of experience is an important time consideration. The limited pool of suitably qualified and experienced PCNs means that holiday, sickness and out of hours cover can be difficult to provide and places additional strains on existing members of the team or service if these issues are not appropriately considered. Crises can be avoided by developing a shared care approach and this has already been established within some services. An important aspect of organization lies in explaining the role of the PCN to other health care professionals such as hospital based staff, health visitors and generic district nurses who may misunderstand the role and this can give rise to a degree of interprofessional conflict.

Medical responsibility for sick children in the community is a partnership between paediatricians and GPs; the ultimate legal responsibility lies with the GP. These partnerships vary in balance and quality and can be confusing to families. A pattern of responsibility should be made explicit to families so that parents know who is managing their child's clinical care at every stage and know where to go for clinical help (ASC 1993).

Provision of equipment and supplies for the treatment and care for sick children in the community greatly varies. A minority of PCNs have access to unlimited resources and either purchase or are provided with both stock and nonstock items as required, with major equipment purchased as either one-off items or available via medical loan departments. These major items are often donated from locally raised monies or voluntary organizations. Managers of services should ensure that supplies and equipment are provided to facilitate home care as managers of inpatient services are obliged to do. Sick children should not be in hospital simply because resources are unavailable in the community. Health authority contracts established with companies such as Caremark, facilitate home provision and delivery of everything necessary for parenteral and enteral nutrition, intravenous antibiotic therapy, chemotherapy, treatment with gammaglobulins and patient controlled analgesics. This reduces the work of the PCN and provides an efficient service for the families and the GPs who supply some of the prescriptions.

Computer-harvested and held statistics of services provide valuable information including caseload content, time allocation according to disorder, numbers of acute bed days saved, patterns of referral and discharge and nurse activities, which illustrate cost effectiveness. Such statistics can assist in the evaluation, justification, forward planning and costing of paediatric community nursing.

Stress management is an important issue for the PCN and the service environment should be supportive so that stress can be identified and managed. Some PCNs have experienced excessive stress and burnout. Sharing and discussing problems and their possible solutions should be seen as a strength and not a weakness (Miller 1992). The nature of the caseload, the numbers and the geographical distribution can all have an effect on the individual's stress levels.

Children's nursing, unlike adult, mental health or learning disabilities nursing, has no nationally implemented community service. However the existing schemes (Whyte 1990, 1991, 1992; RCN 1994a) together with the reports *Bridging the Gaps* (ASC 1993) and *Children First* (Audit Commission 1993) and recent research (Lessing & Tatman 1991; RCN 1994b) clearly demonstrate the value of, and need for, a comprehensive network of PCNs similar to the provision available for adults.

EDUCATION OF PAEDIATRIC COMMUNITY NURSES

Paediatric community nursing modules/options/pathways are now offered at degree and diploma level in Southampton, Oxford, Birmingham, Ulster and Manchester. The child branch of the Project 2000 courses aims to educate students in the care of sick children in both hospital and community settings although difficulties are experienced in providing suitable community experience of caring for the sick child at home. The English National Board's criteria for district nursing diploma provides for a nurse who is registered as an RGN and RSCN to be educated to nurse adults and children in the community, but few nurses are aware of this and few colleges or universities provide the required educational facilities.

Most PCNs who hold a community qualification have either attended an adult oriented district nursing course or health visiting course. A small number of paediatric community Lecturer-Practitioner roles have been established. Paediatric nurses who do not hold an adult qualification have limited means to a community education. Paediatric nurses who wish to become PCN require appropriate education linked with practice experience obtained under the individual supervision and monitoring of experienced PCNs.

The rigour associated with the practice must be reflected in the education. This will be time consuming but essential and achieved by intensive self-questioning, placement and experience. The recommendations and provision of the UKCC for the Education and Practice of the Childrens Community Nursing have been established (UKCC 1994), following their earlier acknowledgement of paediatric community nursing as a separate entity (UKCC 1986; ENB 1990; Lindsay 1993; Muir 1993; Rogers 1993; UKCC 1993b; Whiting 1994).

Children's nurses together with paediatricians appreciate that carers are already the experts on their well child and their everyday needs do not change when they are sick. Carers, children and health professionals in partnership can provide the most appropriate packages of care and treatment for a sick child, each benefiting from the others expertise. This level of co-operation/family centred care can work in many situations, varying from a short term self limiting illness to a longer term chronic or terminal illness. Today sick children can spend more of their time at home with the support of a paediatric community nurse who can teach the families to carry out the necessary treatment and care, provide the equipment needed and can be the link worker between the GP and the community and hospital staff, thus ensuring the child's lifestyle is not dictated or dominated by their illness (Miller 1992; Whyte 1992).

Home care for many sick children should not be an alternative; it can and should be the first choice for many children. When an emotionally and socially beneficial environment is provided the benefits to the mental and physical health for the sick child and family are obvious. Good morale and positive self esteem cannot be prescribed. Home care helps in the development of these essential ingredients, which when present make such a difference to the outcome of childhood illnesses. High dependency, sophisticated, quality care can be safely undertaken at home and ultimately this means that sick children need only be admitted to hospital when the care they need cannot equally well be provided at home (Whyte 1990, 1992).

CONCLUSION

Paediatric community nursing is in itself an autonomous role demanding a high degree of individual accountability. It is the nurse's responsibility to transmit skills and confidence to the families. The child's safety depends largely on the nurse's ability to assess and facilitate unique and appropriate packages of care. PCNs invariably find themselves being the child's advocate, convincing the sceptical in the acute setting that a child could be nursed in the community, particularly when the carers and child are requesting it. This community includes school, shopping or playing and all the usual activities associated with childhood.

REFERENCES AND FURTHER READING

ASC (1993) Caring for Children in the Health Services: *Bridging the Gaps*. Action for Sick Children, London.

At Home (1994) Pioneering Paediatric Homecare. *At Home*, 7, 2–4.

Atwell, J. & Gow, M. (1985) Paediatric trained district nurses in the community, expensive luxury or economic necessity? *British Medical Journal*, 291, 222–9.

Audit Commission (1993) Children First: a Study of Hospital Services. *NHS Report No. 7*. HMSO, London.

Bowlby, J. (1965) *Child Care and the Growth of Love*. Penguin, Harmondsworth.

Burr, S. (1990) Change in the 1990s. *Nursing Standard*, 4(22), 9, 50–51.

DHSS (1976) *Fit for the Future*. Report of the Committee on Child Health Services (Court Report). HMSO, London.

DoH (1989) *The Children Act*. HMSO, London.

DoH (1991) *Welfare of Children and Young People in Hospital*. HMSO, London.

Douglas, J. (1993) *Psychology and Nursing Children*. Macmillan BPS Books, London.

ENB (1990) *Regulations and Guidelines for the Approval of Institutions and Courses*. English National Board, London.

Fradd, E. (1990) Setting up a community paediatric nursing service. *Senior Nurse*, 10(7), 4–8.

Fradd, E. (1992) Working with Specialists. *Community Outlook*, 2(6), 29–30.

Gillet, J.A. (1954) Domiciliary Treatment of Sick Children. *Practitioner*, 177, March, 281–3.

Gray, R. (1993) Defining roles for today: community development and health visitors. *Child Health*, 1(2), 79–82.

Hawthorn, P.J. (1974) *Nurse, I want my Mummy*. Royal College of Nursing, London.

Hennessy, D. (1993) Purchasing community nursing care. *Paediatric Nursing*, 5(2), 10–12.

Jolly, J. (1981) *The Other Side of Paediatrics*. Macmillan, London.

Lessing, D. & Tatman, M.A. (1991) Paediatric Home Care in the Nineties. *Archives of Diseases in Childhood*, 66, 994–6.

Lightwood, R. (1956) The home care of sick children. *Practitioner*, 177, July, 10–143.

Lindsay, B. (1993) Fit for the Community? *Paediatric Nursing*, 5(2), 13–15.

Marland, J. (1994) Back where they belong – caring for sick children at home. *Child Health*, 2(91), 40–42.

Miller, S. (1992) The Cost of Caring. *Paediatric Nursing*, 4(9), 15–16.

MoH (1959) *Report of the Committee on the Welfare of Children in Hospital* (Platt Report). HMSO, London.

Muir, J. (1993) Community based practise and education. *Paediatric Nursing*, 51(7), 25–7.

RCN (1993) *Buying Paediatric Community Nursing*. An RCN guide for purchasers and commissioners of health care. Royal College of Nursing, London.

RCN (1994a) *Directory of Paediatric Community Nursing Services*. Royal College of Nursing, London.

RCN (1994b) Paediatrics Community Nurses' Forum. *Wise Decisions: Developing Paediatric Home Care Teams*. Royal College of Nursing, London.

Robertson, J. & Robertson, J. (1989) *Separation and the Very Young*. Free Association Books, London.

Rogers, R. (1993) Making the Grade. *Paediatric Nursing*, 5(2), 8.

Rutter, M. (1981) *Maternal Deprivation Reassessed*. Penguin, Harmondsworth.

Sidey, A. (1989) Intravenous Home Care. *Paediatric Nursing*, 1(3), 14–15.

Sidey, A. (1990) Co-operation in Care. *Paediatric Nursing*, 2(3), 10–12.

Sidey, A. (1991) The Management of Gastrostomies. *Paediatric Nursing*, 3(7), 24–6.

Smellie, J.M. (1956) Domiciliary nursing service for infants and children. *British Medical Journal*, 5 May, p. 256.

Swanwick, M. & Barlow, S. (1993) A caring definition. Defining quality care in paediatric nursing. *Child Health*, 1(4), 137–41.

UKCC (1986) *Project 2000: a new preparation for practice*. United Kingdom Central Council, London.

UKCC (1993a) *Standards for Record and Record Keeping*. United Kingdom Central Council, London.

UKCC (1993b) *Consultation on the Council's Proposed Standards for Post Registration and Education*. United Kingdom Central Council, London.

UKCC (1994) *The Councils Standards for Education and Practice following Registration. Programmes of Education leading to the Qualification of Special Practitioners*. United Kingdom Central Council, London.

Whiting, M. (1994) Meeting needs: RSCNs in the community. *Paediatric Nursing*, 6(1), 9–11.

Whyte, A.E. (1991) An evaluation of a paediatric home care scheme. *Journal of Advanced Nursing*, 16, 1413–21.

Whyte, A. (1992) A family nursing approach to the care of a child with a chronic illness. *Journal of Advanced Nursing*, 17, 317–27.

Whyte, D. (1990) The family with a chronically ill child. *Paediatric Nursing*, 2(8), 20–23, 2(9), 21–23.

Chapter 4
Management and Quality Perspectives

Ethel Trigg

INTRODUCTION

Nurses at all levels of the organization are increasingly exposed to the effects of management decisions and in many cases actively contribute to them (Fig. 4.1). This chapter introduces some of the relevant principles and terminology, but further reading will be required to develop a more in-depth understanding of the concepts.

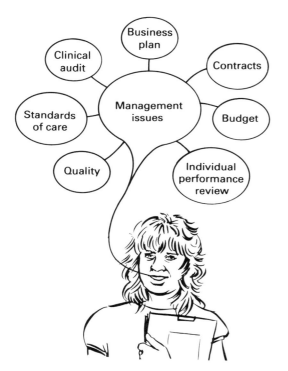

Fig. 4.1 Management issues for nurses.

The first part of the chapter gives a brief overview of health service reforms, thereby putting into context some of the initiatives which are prevalent in the National Health Service of the 1990s. Quality assurance issues, for example standard setting, total quality management and clinical audit, are then discussed and the third section looks at aspects related to business planning, including contracting and the formulation and management of budgets. The final section is focused upon issues related to appraisal and individual performance review.

Although many of these subjects are often treated as 'stand alone topics', it will be seen that they overlap, and optimum delivery of health care may be attained by integrating aspects of all of them.

A BRIEF OVERVIEW OF THE HEALTH SERVICE REFORMS

In April 1991 the government introduced 'Working for Patients' which brought changes, new concepts and challenges to those working within the health service. Many of these were related to the future funding of the service.

The reforms had several underlying principles (Fig. 4.2). First, that competition would be created between hospitals, community and private sector; this competition would be regulated by drawing up contracts of levels of service agreements. Second, there would be a redistribution of money nationally; this would be more equitable to suit population requirements. Third, health authorities would have greater autonomy; this would enable them to plan their own activities. Finally, there would be an increased emphasis on the formal multi-disciplinary auditing of the quality of services delivered to the patient.

By introducing these principles it was anticipated that individuals would be able to respond more actively to health care initiatives, and there would be improvements in the quality of care and greater emphasis on gaining value for money.

By opting for 'trust status' and independence from the district health authority, the hospital and community units could have a greater control over their own affairs. It was predicted that this would promote competition and lead to increased motivation to improve the efficiency and effectiveness of services. The overall focus was upon forward planning to meet health needs, although difficult to define, rather than historic service patterns, and on primary care and health promotion rather than tertiary care and sickness.

Another component of the reforms was the concept of devolved management responsibility and decision making to those providing care to the patients. Subsequently many health authorities and trusts undertook reviews of current arrangements and removed the traditional hierarchical structures that fragmented decision

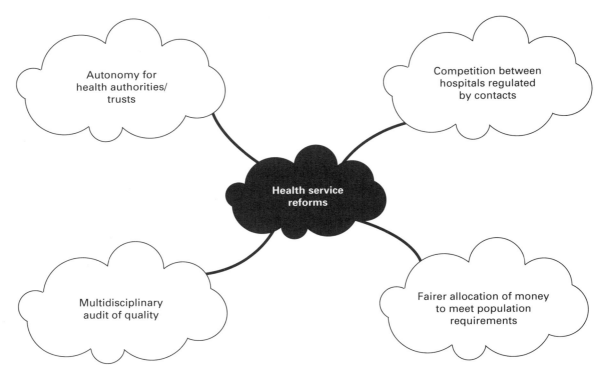

Fig. 4.2 Principles of the 1991 Health Service Reforms.

making. In order to enhance communication a flatter organizational approach was selected.

This restructuring, emphasizing the concept of devolved responsibility, creates a management culture where it is necessary for nurses at all levels to appreciate the implications of the reforms and to have an understanding of quality assurance initiatives, business planning, contracting processes and budgeting. In this way they are better able to consider ways in which they can contribute to the managerial aspects of the service.

THE QUALITY PERSPECTIVE

It could be argued that providing a high standard of care is the remit of every children's nurse; however, there appears to be ambiguity surrounding definitions, terminology and ways of measuring quality. This section addresses the notions of standard setting, total quality management, quality circles and clinical audit.

A significant aim within 'Working for Patients' was 'to bring all parts of the service to the highest level'. In order to achieve this it is necessary to review the quality of the service offered to patients/clients. Whilst quality is seen as a major element of patient care and an implicit and essential component of nurse education, in the last few years it has been formally recognized as an organizational managed process.

A general dictionary definition of quality refers to 'a degree of excellence' and Lang (1976) suggests that 'quality is the process for the attainment of the highest degree of excellence in the delivery of patient care'. Quality has several dimensions. Commonly, people judge the service they receive on their previous experience but customer satisfaction is only one element. Other aspects include:

- Identifying the characteristics of the service.
- Developing quality control systems.
- Implementing strategies to assess deviations from the agreed standards.
- Quality improvement.

- Enhancing positive aspects of the service.
- Quality assurance.

Øvretveit (1992) suggests that 'poor quality results from a badly designed and operated process, not from incompetent health care workers'. So it could be argued that quality is not just about improving customer service and auditing the process of agreed standards, but should also include initiatives for promoting staff development and utilizing new ideas and methods, which build upon good practices and introduce new ones. This will raise customer satisfaction and may at the same time reduce costs and improve efficiency. Quality does not only relate to the needs from the consumer perspective but also requires professional judgement, particularly when there are ethical, legal and contractual implications.

Øvretveit (1992) describes three dimensions of health service quality (Fig. 4.3). The first relates to client quality by giving the customer what they want or expect. The second refers to professional quality achieved through the carrying out of correct technical practice and procedures. The third involves the management of quality to ensure cost effectiveness and efficiency. He suggests that by categorizing quality into these three elements all perspectives are integrated, in this case the child, the parents, and the professional nurses and managers.

This focus on quality of care seems to have come at a difficult and challenging time. The limitations of resources are increasingly recognized and the demand for services may be greater than supply. There may be a reduction in experienced qualified children's nurses to care for more dependent children with complex health needs. All this requires the need to do more with less. Nevertheless it is important to prioritize quality because poor quality may be expensive, especially if it is measured by the cost of 'doing things wrong'. This is especially pertinent in the 1990s when the consumer of the service can be said to be more empowered and thus less reticent to voice their criticisms and concerns, and in some cases proceeding to litigation.

It is incumbent upon the nurses to contribute to organizational strategies which promote a concept of quality. These are sometimes driven or supported by government initiatives, such as the Patients Charter (DoH 1991) and the Health of the Nation (DoH 1992), and incorporate initiatives based upon an analysis of local needs and research.

Shaw (1986) summarized the six key elements to quality as:

- Effectiveness.
- Acceptability.
- Efficiency.
- Access or accessibility.
- Equity.
- Relevance or appropriateness.

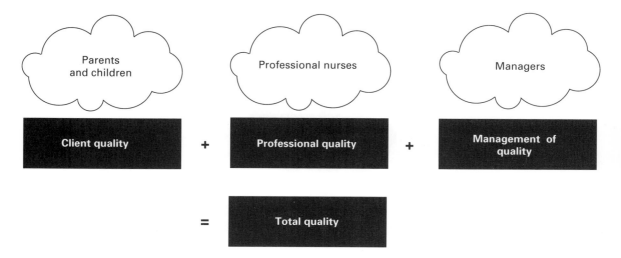

Fig. 4.3 Three dimensions of health service quality (adapted from Øvretveit 1992).

Overall there is a need to encourage a proactive and reflective approach by:

- Promoting discussion.
- Enhancing commitment to the quality concept.
- Translating good ideas into practice.
- Placing emphasis on teamwork.
- Evaluating rituals and barriers to change.
- Applying the six dimensions outlined by Shaw (1986).
- Developing formal systems to measure quality and encouraging a wider perspective on quality.

The impetus for developing quality measurements may come from two directions:

(1) As a response to a perceived deficit or shortcoming with the service, recognized via a complaint or in some cases a serious error; in such cases the response could be said to be reactive.
(2) By applying the principles of total quality management and thus adopting a more proactive stance to quality.

Both these approaches may utilize quality circles.

Quality circles

This concept was first developed in Japan in 1962. A

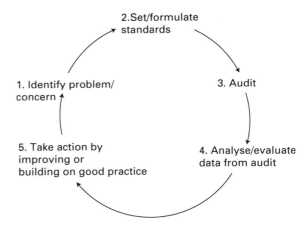

Fig. 4.4 Quality cycle.

quality circle (Fig. 4.4) is a group of staff who meet periodically to solve any problems that relate to the service they deliver. This method can be used to formulate a philosophy, standards or audit tools. Quality circles are based on the premise that staff 'at the grass roots' are best placed to identify and devise solutions to their own work problems and that each staff member has a valid point of view (Ford & Walsh 1994). There are several advantages of this approach (Fig. 4.5), but overall it promotes and values staff participation by providing a forum in which nurses at all levels can

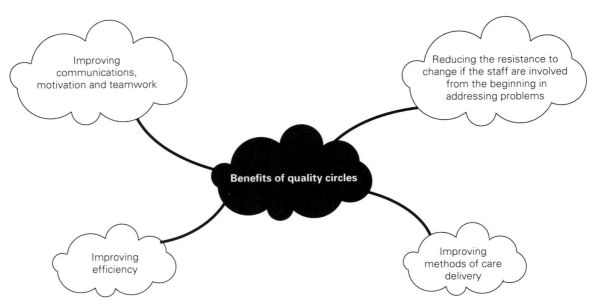

Fig. 4.5 Benefits of quality circles.

analyse, communicate and solve problems in the interest of the child and family.

Devising a philosophy or mission statement

Perhaps a precursor to the success of the quality circle approach is for the team to agree upon the philosophy of care for the service they want to deliver. In essence a philosophy, or mission statement, is a written expression of the beliefs and values held by the team. This sets the strategic direction and should influence and drive subsequent practice developments; 'it translates practice into writing' (Mawdsley 1992). For example, a philosophy which encompasses ideas about partnership may provide the foundation for a scheme to introduce collaborative care planning with parents.

There are several benefits to having a philosophy (Fig. 4.6).

Writing a philosophy can be a challenge (Mawdsley 1992). It will be necessary to gather together the multidisciplinary team, brainstorm ideas, and share their common beliefs and values about care. This vital information will become the building blocks for the philosophy. The statements should reflect the perspective of all the individuals within the team. A succinct statement of three or four sentences will achieve a wider commitment (Table 4.1).

Sometimes a philosophy statement can be incorporated into a 'user friendly' charter for parents and children (Table 4.2). The philosophy should be reviewed in the light of any changes to ensure that it continues to reflect the values and beliefs of the team. Another step in the quality circle is setting standards.

Setting standards

The World Health Organisation (cited RCN 1990) defined a standard in health care as 'an agreed level of care required for a particular purpose'. It is suggested that standards should be a yard stick for comparison (Manley 1992) (Fig. 4.7).

There are persuasive reasons for nurses' involvement in setting standards. The recent health service reforms devolved the responsibility for quality to nurses working

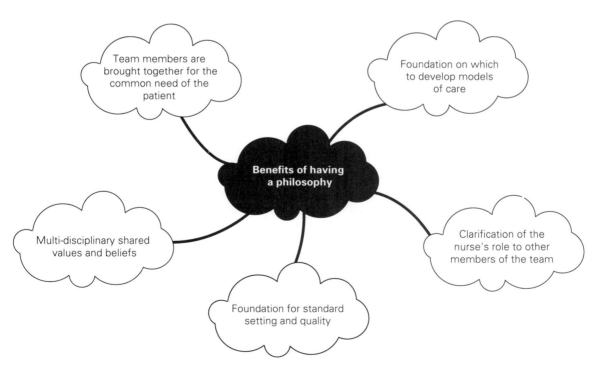

Fig. 4.6 Benefits of a philosophy of care.

Table 4.1   Example of a philosophy of care.

■ Fundamental to our process of caring for children should be the basic assumption that children have essential needs and rights.

■ As professionals we aim to provide an accountable service for children and their families within our care.

■ One of our aims of care is to enable the child and their family to be informed participators in all decisions involving their care.

■ As professionals we aim to provide the continuing care and support to the family and child whether in hospital or at home.

■ Children should be cared for in an environment which is equipped to meet their unique individual needs.

Table 4.2   Example of a parents' charter.

■ We will provide a ward in which you and your child can feel comfortable, relaxed and safe.

■ All members of the ward team will work together to ensure that the best possible care is given to your child.

■ Whenever possible we will provide you with a named nurse and the same group of nurses to look after you throughout your hospital experience. If you would like to discuss any particular aspects of the care please speak to your nurse.

■ We will encourage you to visit as often as possible and if you wish to stay all day and/or night we will provide facilities for you.

■ As we believe that you are the central person in giving care to your child we will support and encourage you in doing this.

■ We will encourage your child, whenever possible, to be involved in decisions about their care.

■ We will provide play and education to encourage your child's development and help them to cope whilst in hospital.

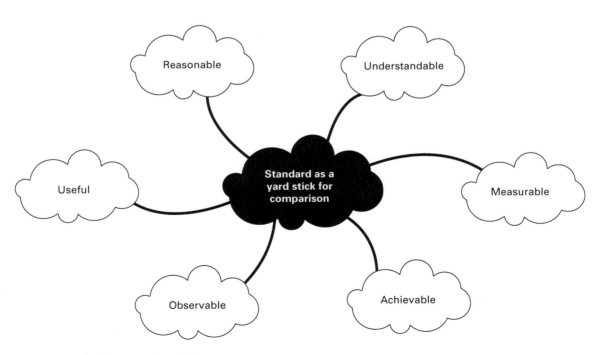

Fig. 4.7   Standards as a yard stick for comparison.

in direct contact with patients. Along with other health care workers they are not only required to agree and document measurable standards of care, but also to account for their actions. Patient's rights are outlined and supported by the Patient's Charter, so the consumer is more conversant about the level of care they can reasonably expect and is more prepared to demand that to which they are entitled.

Standard setting is not new and it has been part of the nursing world since Nightingale, although it seems to have had more obvious significance since the 1980s. The RCN (1990) introduced the Dynamic Standard Setting System (DySSy) and summarized at least three reasons to support the need to set standards (Fig. 4.8).

from management – may be more successful. Standards should reflect both the trust's or unit's mission statement and the previously agreed philosophy of care. The core team can co-opt other personnel who may be instrumental in supporting the effective outcome of a particular standard. For example, if setting standards about nutrition, the dietitian should be included, or when considering standards pertaining to parents in the anaesthetic room, the anaesthetist would be involved.

Setting standards can be a lengthy process and, in fact, as a cyclical exercise it may also be a continuous process as the standard will need to be reviewed, altered, and re-audited (Table 4.3). It has been suggested that standards are more effective if they are integrated within a quality cycle.

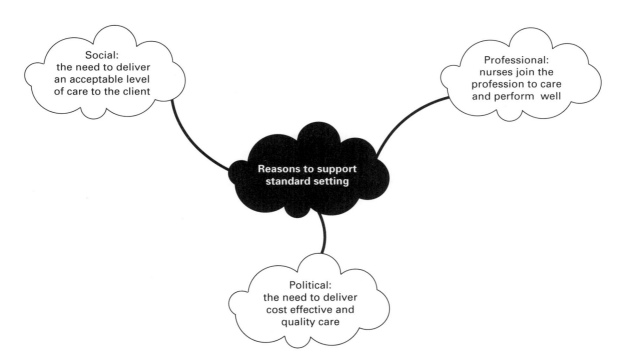

Fig. 4.8 Reasons to support standard setting.

Standard setting requires enthusiasm, stamina, co-operation and teamwork (Glasper & Tucker 1993). A bottom up approach – in other words where the standards should be determined by those delivering the service and complemented by support and commitment

Table 4.4 provides an example of a written standard using the Donabedian (1966) approach of structure, process, outcome. This standard statement is simple, understandable and measurable. It outlines the structure, the process and the expected outcome.

Table 4.3 Setting a standard.

- Organise a meeting of the ward team co-opting appropriate personnel.
- Identify a topic.
- Devise a method to write a standard statement that the team will own.
- Identify aims and desired outcomes.

Ask the following questions:
- How will I achieve the aims?
- What do I require to happen?
- What is needed to make it happen? (Process)
- What is causing the deficit – is it staff, environment, information?

Structure:
- Develop an audit tool.
- Agree an implementation and audit date.

The theme of communication can be used to provide an illustration of integrating standards within a quality circle. In one hospital the overall aim was to improve the quality of verbal and written information given to the patient and parent. A patient's advocate or patient's representative, independent of the health care setting, was asked to interview parents and children to elicit any concerns and relay these back to the nursing teams. Parents and children were approached at random two weeks after discharge. In general, they welcomed the opportunity to talk about their experience of the hospital stay and referred to it as 'fabulous' and a 'second home' but were concerned by the lack of written information available about the ward and their child's condition. The communication standards were reviewed, in line with the quality cycle, in order to improve upon this aspect of care.

Initially it may be important to keep the standards simple in order to maintain enthusiasm and commitment, as standards that are perceived to be achievable will be more successful in their implementation. Complex standards may be seen to be more manageable if they are subdivided into simple objectives.

Assessment/audit tools

Audit tools need to be devised to evaluate that the standard has been achieved. The assessment audit tool to support the communication standard is described in Fig. 4.9. There are ten overall questions. Each have a 10% mark used to score the achievement of the standard. The acceptable score is determined as 90% or above and any score below 70% may require either a review of the standard or of the care delivered or both. Each of the ten questions is subdivided to allow the standard to be evaluated in greater detail. In this example, number eight in the audit was addressed. This involved evaluating the child's and parents' understanding of the information provided by using a further five questions (a–e) on this specific aspect.

Auditing of the standard can be performed by a member of the ward team, but may be more objective if undertaken by a colleague from another area. The audit results will be confidential to the area but the results may provoke discussion and continuous improvement via the quality cycle.

Several authors have addressed standard setting in paediatric nursing, for example, MacDonald (1990), Tucker (1990), Hotton (1991), Swanwick & Barlow (1993). There are also many documents which contain standards for the care of children which can be used to generate local standards; examples of these include:

- The NAWCH Children's Charter (NAWCH 1985) supported by the NAWCH review 1989.
- The Department of Health (DoH 1991b) *Welfare of Children and Young People in Hospital.*
- *Setting Standards for Adolescents* (NAWCH 1990).
- *Children First* (Audit Commission 1993).
- *Just for the Day* (ASC 1991).
- *Setting Standards for Children Undergoing Surgery* (Hogg 1994).
- *Standards for Children in the Accident and Emergency Department* (Harris & Cummings 1992).

Total quality management

Total quality management (TQM) takes quality strategies in health care delivery one step further. It is a systematic method which enhances continuous quality improvement. It involves a change of culture from a tendency towards crisis management aimed at standard setting in response to previous mistakes, towards a proactive preventative approach. Reed (1992) suggests that:

Table 4.4 Example of written standard.

The child on traction will achieve optimum healing with minimal discomfort		
Structure	Process	Outcome
Standard statement 2 for admission of child.	Staff are aware and practised in the implementation of standard.	The child is assessed by an RSCN prior to the traction being established.
Skill mix. Training.	Duty rota reflects supervisory responsibility. Educational/practical teaching available to staff. Opportunity for study days/training.	Transfer of the child to traction is supervised by an RSCN with orthopaedic nursing knowledge and experience.
Ward philosophy. Standard statement 5 for child's participation in decisions.	Staff will identify fears/anxieties related to the traction. Recognize the individual needs of the child.	The child demonstrates a positive adaptation to the traction.
Correct traction equipment. X-ray facilities. Local model of care. Ward round/communication.	Staff practised and safe in the use of equipment. Care plan reflects nursing practise. Regular communication with orthopaedic team.	Correct alignment of the affected limb is maintained. The affected limb exhibits optimum peripheral perfusion. General skin integrity is maintained.
Pain assessment indicators. Research material available Analgesia in a form acceptable to the child.	Assessment of discomfort by staff. Observation of nonverbal indicators. Analgesia offered as prescribed.	The optimum level of comfort is maintained. The child verbalizes/ exhibits behaviour to indicate a relief of pain.
Physiotherapy facilities. Exercise leaflet.	Instruction of family/child on frequency and type of exercises to be undertaken.	Muscular strength/joint mobility is maintained by performing exercises to maintain muscle tone.
Environment suitable. Equipment.	Teaching child/family about new skills/changes required to undertake their normal daily activities.	Activities of daily living are performed independently/safely within the limitations imposed by the traction.
Catering facilities. Choice of food available.	Monitoring of nutritional and fluid intake. Consideration of child's likes and dislikes when planning meals.	Optimum fluid and nutritional intake is maintained to promote health and growth.
Privacy. Equipment – bottles/bedpans etc.	Child and family practised in the use of equipment.	A normal elimination pattern is achieved.
Standard statement 6. School teachers. Play.	Staff recognize the importance of continued development and the effects of restricted mobility.	Developmental/age appropriate activities are undertaken to promote growth and development.
Standard statement 12. Discharge standard.	Preparation of child and family physically and psychologically for discharge. Staff aware of facilities.	The family demonstrates a knowledge/understanding of the rehabilitation required/plan of care.

Standard statements – each statement has a 10% mark.

(1) Does the care plan reflect care to be undertaken?   Yes   No   N/A
        Observe

(2) Did the child receive effective analgesia prior to application?   Yes   No   N/A
        Observe

(3) Is the traction weight hanging clear of the floor?   Yes   No   N/A
        Observe

(4) Does the child appear comfortable?   Yes   No   N/A
        Ask child, observe

(5) Has the affected limb maintained good peripheral circulation?   Yes   No   N/A
        Shown by colour, movement and sensation to the limb.
        Observe

(6) Have the child and parents been taught the appropriate   Yes   No   N/A
        exercises?
        Ask child and parents

(7) Does the allocated nurse know the exercises which the child   Yes   No   N/A
        should undertake?
        Ask nurse

(8) Does the child/family understand the reason why traction has   Yes   No   N/A
        been applied?
        Ask child/family

(9) Is the child maintaining a normal elimination pattern?   Yes   No   N/A
        Observe chart, ask nurse, ask child/family

(10) Is the child able to undertake activities suitable for age/   Yes   No   N/A
        development?
        Observe

Standard statements
(a) Does the child/family know where the fracture/injury site is?
(b) Does the child/family know the approximate time to be spent on traction?
(c) Can the child/family describe how the traction works?
(d) Does the child/family understand the need to keep the weight hanging freely?
(e) Does the child/family feel they have been adequately informed about care of traction?

Fig. 4.9 Audit tool for communication standard *(Reproduced by permission of Brighton Health Care NHS Trust.).*

'TQM goes far beyond simplistic measurements. It is about continually striving to find swifter, more cost effective ways of meeting the required standards with the ultimate aim not just of satisfying the customer but of delighting the customer.'

This concept also arose in Japanese industry in the 1950s (Holloway & Hobbs 1992). Planned quality initiatives are beginning to feature highly in the agreed contracts with purchasers and GP fund holders.

TQM is usually built on the principles shown in Fig. 4.10.

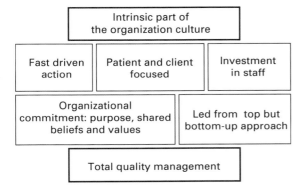

Fig. 4.10 Total quality management is built on several principles.

TQM needs four components to be effective:

- A timed framework.
- Supportive information technology.
- Teamwork.
- Careful management.

The Department of Health is supporting some national pilot schemes but there are suggestions (Freemantle 1992) that the implementation of TQM is costly and this has been perceived as a disadvantage. However, it may be important to consider the cost when quality is poor and results in litigation.

Clinical audit

Clinical audit within the health care setting is relatively new and, to many health workers, still unfamiliar.

Medical staff often informally audit the medical care that patients receive but an audit is rarely performed within a structured framework. The NHS reforms have given particular impetus to audit and have promoted it as a valuable tool to improve the quality of professional care delivered to the patient.

According to the Department of Health (DoH 1989) medical audit is:

'usually defined as the systematic, critical analysis of the quality of medical care, including the procedures used for diagnosis and treatment, the uses of resources and the resulting outcome for the patient. It encompasses all aspects of care planning, care delivery, staffing and organizational and support services, as they affect medical care.'

The Department of Health (DoH 1991a) has defined nursing audit as:

'part of a cycle of quality assurance. It incorporates the systematic and critical analysis by nurse, midwives and health visitors, in conjunction with other staff, of the planning, delivery and evaluation of nursing and midwifery care, in terms of their use of resources and the outcomes for patients/clients, and introduces appropriate change in response to the analysis'.

The Department of Health supports multi-disciplinary audit involving all health care professionals working together in peer review. In essence audit, being another method of quality control (Tucker 1991), is a systematic and critical analysis and peer review of the quality of the total care given to patients, the services provided and the resources used, measured against the actual and expected outcome.

Audit and research are similar in some respects but there are important differences. Retrospective information is collected using medical or nursing notes, questionnaires, surveys or observation. The audit will usually be carried out within a specified time, in one location, and the results will apply specifically to the population examined. It requires voluntary participation and the process is ongoing with results being fed back to the department for discussion in order to determine appropriate action or expose the need for further research.

If audit is used effectively it may offer real, lasting and significant improvements in health care by encouraging peer review, challenging traditional methods of working and enhancing flexible research based care.

Table 4.5 The stages of clinical audit.

- Select the project.
- Assess the subject, topic, proposal for suitability and priority.
- Create an audit methodology measurement tool, e.g. questionnaire.
- Agree objectives.
- Decide how the data will be collected, and the type of analysis required.
- Estimate costings for the project.
- Agree a time frame.
- Implement the audit.
- Discuss the results.
- Change practice as necessary.
- Evaluate the audit against stated objectives and costs in order to establish success and the improvement in care delivery.
- Reflect on the process and outcomes in order to learn lessons for the future (Tomalin 1992).
- Assess need.

Summary

Overall the aim of quality management is for continuous improvement to the care given to patients/clients. Quality is the responsibility of all nurses and should be an intrinsic component of their daily work. A clear strategy, management structure and commitment are required to promote a robust quality culture which is an integral part of the business planning and contracting processes. An effective quality approach will reduce the costs of poor quality.

It may be seen that there are several dimensions to the attainment of a quality service. This section has offered an overview of some of the approaches and identified the features of each. Through an understanding of these, children's nurses at all levels can reflect on their contribution to these initiatives.

BUSINESS PLANNING

This section considers business planning, contracting and some aspects of budget management. Nurses at all levels should have a basic understanding of these processes in order to appreciate the ways in which they influence the service that is offered to patients. They should seek opportunities to be actively involved in decision making.

Prior to 1991 there were few if any formal annual plans. One of the requisites of the reforms was to encourage a more businesslike approach to the management of the service. Business planning creates a common system for documenting proposed objectives and monitoring progress and achievements.

The business plan is a management tool which, used in a systematic way, enables strategic or forward long term planning. The plan identifies what is provided now, what can be planned for, and how it will be achieved (Fig. 4.11). The plan may be used to secure resources, monitor government initiatives or review the effectiveness of any capital development plans. Overall it may help staff to share in the economic and business aspects of care delivery. There is an annual review to monitor the achievements and to generate forward planning for the next year. In order to encourage a sense of ownership the plan should integrate the views of both consumers of the service and the professionals.

CONTRACTING

Generally a trust may derive income from contracts and/or rental of land space or particular clinical or other services.

Since 1992, NHS trusts (providers) have been required to contract for their services in order to secure payment for the care they deliver. The purchasers – usually the health authority or a GP fund holder – and providers – generally the hospital or community unit – meet annually to agree the ways in which the service will be provided, the subsequent cost of that provision for one financial year and plans regarding subsequent development.

Contracts provide information on the total number of cases to be treated, or consultant episodes, against an agreed cost within which the trust has promised to deliver. Many contracts also include evidence of quality assurance strategies and standards, for example application of the Patient Charter principles of named nurse and minimum waiting times in the outpatients department. Thus contracts reflect both government initiatives and cost efficiency strategies.

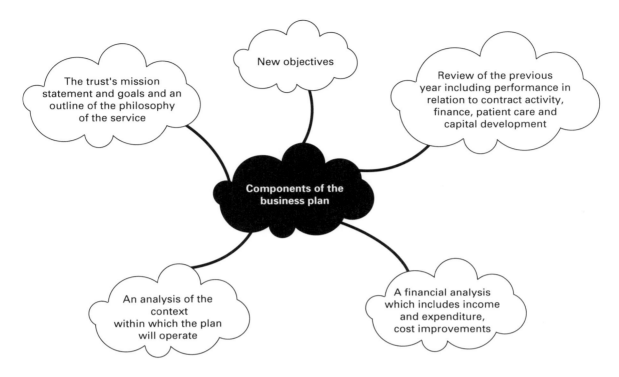

Fig. 4.11   The process and information required to set and develop a business plan.

At present there are three main types of health care contract. It is likely that the contracting process will become more refined as information technology in the health service increases in sophistication.

The block contract

Currently block contracts are the most common form of agreements; the purchaser and provider agree upon blocks of service. These are based on an agreed cost, for example during financial year 1995–6 the purchaser may contract to pay for 300 circumcisions at £300 per case. The number of cases is usually based on past records or referral patterns, seasonal fluctuations and activity. During the contracting process the number of cases may be increased or reduced; this will depend upon the purchaser's requirements and the provider's ability to deliver the level of work required. The purchaser pays for the work in twelve monthly instalments.

Block contracts have several advantages, not least that they guarantee cash flow providing the agreed

targets are achieved by the trust. They can be implemented with ease and monitoring them requires minimal effort. However, there are limitations in that they offer few incentives to either the purchaser or the provider to change their levels of agreement or to increase their efficiency by exceeding the number of cases treated.

Cost and volume contracts

These contracts motivate the provider to increase their activity by rewarding them financially. There is a guaranteed block element to be achieved, as described previously, but there is still incentive to maximize efficiency, exceed the contract levels and receive additional funding for extra activity. This type of contract relies upon sophisticated information technology to record activity accurately.

Cost per case contracts

These contracts recover the cost of each completed

consultant episode. They are useful in specialized services, for example renal and bone marrow transplants or cardiac surgery. However, complex costing and billing systems are required to ensure the provider is not being financially compromised.

Extra contractual referrals

The provider unit may also receive income from extra contractual referrals (ECRs). These come from several main sources: the admission of patients from areas that do not hold a contract with the provider unit; GP fund holders; or emergency referrals such as neonatal or intensive specialized care. Income may also be derived from private patients.

Contracting is a fast growing area in the NHS and if nurses are to be involved, they need knowledge of marketing and to enhance their negotiating skills. It is an area that relies on accurate information and refined information technology.

INCOME AND EXPENDITURE

Financial resources within the reformed NHS provider units are controlled or limited to a great extent by the amount of income that is achieved from contracts. Expenditure budgets fall into two categories: capital and revenue. Capital budgets cover major site developments or the purchase of expensive machinery. Revenue budgets are related to the day to day running expenses of the department, ward or service, for example staff wages, electricity or food.

Budgets

A budget is a costed plan expressed in financial terms. These plans are used as tools to assist budget holders in exercising control over the resources they manage. Many nurses perceive budgeting to be a complex activity and believe that they lack the skills required, but really it is very similar to managing a household or a bank account (Shafer 1991). Budget management is an essential part of the business planning process and the business plan

will include details of the budget available, and information regarding activity and agreed contract levels. In line with the changes brought about by the NHS Act 1991, budgets are now being increasingly linked to contracting activity and this means that money should follow patients and will in some cases actually influence the number of patients that can be cared for.

In many trusts/hospitals the responsibility for effective management of the budgets has been devolved to nursing ward managers (Hicklin & Chantler 1989; Palmer 1991; Rye 1991; Bateup 1992). In the community, budgets may be devolved down to local or sector managers. The budget is set for a twelve-month period commencing on 1 April.

Budgets are traditionally divided into two categories: pay and non-pay. Pay budgets are based on staff establishments expressed as whole time equivalents (WTEs) and take into account grade mix, pay increments, and where appropriate enhancements for working unsociable hours, evenings and weekends, and they include employer contributions of national insurance and pensions.

Pay budgets are more difficult to profile especially in smaller departments because of the lack of flexibility within a small workforce. However, this model allows flexible use of manpower resources to match activity as it occurs, because money can be put in reserve for contingency and used to employ temporary staff during busier periods.

Nonpay budgets are all the other running costs unrelated to pay and include consumables, for example medical and surgical equipment or travelling costs in the community.

Different approaches to budgeting

Result based or incremental budgets

Overall, the most common method of budgeting in the NHS is result based or incremental budgets using historical information to prepare future budgets. This method makes two main assumptions

(1) That each year there will be similar levels of activity, thus they are based on historical information from the previous year.
(2) That recurring activity levels require similar financial resources.

Non-recurring expenditure, for example money for short-term projects or a special piece of equipment, will need to be budgeted for as a separate item.

Many health authorities and trusts use this method of 'roll over', which means that the budget for the previous year is used with changes for inflation, pay awards and planned alterations in establishments of staff.

Zero-based budgeting

This type of budget is established independently from the service being provided and starts at zero, hence the name, and is then constructed by, for example, determining optimum staffing levels, using nursing dependency data, consumables required, and all other revenue and capital costs. This method may be an excellent way to set up the costs of a new project, but is time consuming and is dependent upon accurate data (Wilson 1992).

Activity-based budgets

These are concerned with matching resources to activity levels. Budget calculations are undertaken to identify each unit of workload and activity. Again, dependency data may be used to estimate nursing activity. Other activities can be measured in a number of ways, for example by calculating the number of pathology tests, X-rays or square metres cleaned. Each budget holder is expected to achieve a target of income and expenditure and thus will be concerned with value for money and the efficient use of resources.

Contracts are set according to 'finished consultant episodes' (FCEs), in other words when a patient is referred to hospital for treatment and the treatment is completed. Within this system it is recognized that at various points in the financial year, the FCEs may fluctuate and the activity budgets are profiled to match these changes, for example by introducing a phased budget which takes account of particular trends in paediatric activity, such as an increase in medical admissions during the winter.

Summary

A trust, directly managed unit or community unit will have both an income and expenditure budget. Income is the financial resource generated from contracts to pay for the costs of running the unit. It is generally con-

sidered that the budget control is achieved effectively at ward or department level and the budget holder is often a nurse. However, overall responsibility may rest with the clinical director who in many cases will be a member of the medical staff. Budget proposals are ultimately agreed by the chief executive who is responsible for ensuring that all activity and budgets within the hospital are co-ordinated.

Analysing variances

The budget holder usually has an in depth knowledge of expenditure, activity, sickness and absence and therefore the monitoring process is usually carried out monthly. Financial reports are sent to the budget holder from the finance department and information will include the total annual budget, the cumulative budget and the actual expenditure incurred. The report will also indicate variances between expected (planned) expenditure and actual expenditure. For example:

Annual budget	Budget for period	Actual expenditure	Variance (difference)
£12 000	£4000	£3900	−£100 2.5%

The above example considers the fourth period of the financial year (July). The annual budget is £12 000. The budget is profiled in twelfths, so the budget for the period is £4000 (four-twelfths). The actual money expended is £3900. The difference between the budget and actual expenditure is £100 under budget.

At a glance, this report would indicate a budget that is being well controlled with a small favourable variance. However, with the following activity patterns, the picture changes:

Activity budget	Budget for period	Actual hernias	Variance (difference) hernias
£10 000	£33 333	£30 900	−£2422 7.29%

Now the picture is completely different – it can be seen that the department is 7% under planned activity levels, and yet it is only 2% less in expenditure – indicating that the resources are not being used efficiently.

If a budget is constantly overspent this usually means one of two things: either the ward is under-resourced or the budget is ineffectively managed. Before asking for increased resources nurses should critically appraise the service they offer, explore creative strategies to use the resources they already have, and collect data to support the case for additional resources. If nurses are prepared to become involved in these aspects they will be in a prime position to influence and develop services. When nurses are aware of the expenditure in relation to the agreed budget they will be better able to make a significant contribution to these processes.

INDIVIDUAL PERFORMANCE REVIEW

In tandem with the monitoring of quality and caring for patients/clients, the needs of the staff should be met (de la Cour 1992; Coates 1993). One way of achieving this is through an appraisal system (Herbert & Evans 1991; Northcott 1993). A form of appraisal commonly used in the NHS is individual performance review (IPR) (Bateup & Herbert 1991). This was introduced in the 1980s to encourage a more participative approach to management. Nurses are already required to keep up to date in order to expand their knowledge and skills (UKCC 1994). IPR systems can complement this because they are a means of identifying training needs and future career development. However, staff development does not just benefit individual nurses but also the organization as a whole because job satisfaction and staff motivation will increase if they feel they are valued and are helped with their professional and personal development.

In IPR the post holder's current role is reviewed against their job description and the current and future key objectives of the post. Targets or objectives are defined and agreed and set within a time frame. The objectives should be realistic and measurable, for example within the next six months they agree to carry out an audit of the named nurse initiative within their unit.

Review meetings between the manager and staff member are held at regular intervals to discuss the objectives and the progress in achieving them, and a major review of all objectives is held at the end of each year. During these reviews, the individual will be assisted in their individual development and progress by identifying what is required to achieve the objectives; this may include training staff or resources.

The success of IPR can be enhanced by ensuring that both manager and staff member understand the process and receive appropriate preparation. It is not intended as a disciplinary tool, but rather as a valuable opportunity for open discussion regarding both personal development and development of the clinical area. It is not a panacea, however, but by encouraging staff to work together it may encourage positive change and growth.

Performance-related pay

Links have been made between IPR and performance related pay (PRP). PRP is a system of relating pay rewards to quantifiable achievement, rather than subjective judgements of personal qualities. In one system of PRP each objective is numerically rated on a scale of one to five, one being excellent, five being poor. A pay scale is agreed, based on the numerical weighting, and this is reviewed annually through the IPR process. Few trusts are in favour of PRP and they are looking at alternative ways of rewarding staff for effective performance.

Summary

IPR is regarded as a key to improvement of staff performance and the development of the service. It may be a systematic way of ensuring that employees understand the key objectives of the organization. It enables the individual to appreciate the level of performance that is expected and receive feedback on their performance. It is a vehicle through which career development and profiling might take place.

CONCLUSION

As a result of the reforms and the ensuing changes, the NHS is required to adopt a proactive stance to ensure that all the underlying principles are implemented. In a service that is publicly funded, it is likely that demand will always be greater than supply. With increasing awareness and a raised expectation there is a greater requirement for formalized written standards, quality measurements, budget valuing and development of staff. If managed well, these issues will contribute to a cost effective and efficient service. They will match the contractual, budget, and quality specifications, and allow for innovation in practice. Purchasers of paediatric services require information on the care they are buying and its delivery and will increasingly require proof of purchase or a guarantee.

The areas described in this chapter have a significant impact on the NHS service provisions and on nursing as a whole. They are very topical and require understanding to ensure both the effectiveness and efficiency of the service.

Traditionally it has been acceptable for the nurse to know how to manage a ward, team or caseload. Now this must be complemented with skills of resource management and knowledge of strategies to enhance cost effectiveness or value for money and balance this with the demands of providing quality care.

These issues appear to be well established on the agenda and therefore need to be afforded due attention. Nurses may seek opportunities to offer a major contribution and promote the image of professional nursing.

REFERENCES AND FURTHER READING

ASC (1991) *Caring for Children in the Health Services: Just for the Day.* Action for Sick London, London.

Audit Commission Review (1991) *The Virtue of Patients.* HMSO, London.

Audit Commission (1993) *Children First.* HMSO, London.

Bateup, L. (1992) Managing the nursing service in clinical directorates. *Senior Nurse*, 12(2), 10–12.

Bateup, L. & Herbert, R. (1991) Staff appraisal and individual performance review. *Senior Nurse*, 11(5), 8–10.

Coates, M. (1993) Give the team something back. Developing and implementing staff development programmes. *Professional Nurse*, 8(10), 651–4.

de la Cour, J. (1992) Assessment of staff appraisal systems. *British Journal of Nursing*, 1(2), 99–102.

DoH (1989) *Working For Patients.* HMSO, London.

DoH (1991a) *The Patients Charter.* HMSO, London.

DoH (1991b) *Welfare of Children and Young People in Hospital.* HMSO, London.

DoH (1992) *Health of the Nation: A Strategy for Health in England.* HMSO, London.

DoH (1993) *Clinical Audit.* Redhouse Lane Communications, Heywood, Lancs.

DoH (1993) *A Vision for the Future:* The Nursing, Midwifery and Health Visiting Contribution to Health and Health Care. HMSO, London.

DoH (1994) *Patient's Charter to be expanded and improved.* Press release 94/175. Department of Health, London.

Donabedian, A. (1966) Institutional and professional responsibilities in quality assurance. *Quality Assurance in Health Care*, 1(1), 3–11.

DTI (1990) *Total Quality Management.* HMSO, London.

Ellis, R. (1992) *Handbook of Quality Assurance for Health Care.* Edward Arnold, London.

Ford, P. & Walsh, M. (1994) *New Rituals for Old: Nursing Through the Looking Glass.* Butterworth Heinemann, London.

Fradd, E. (1994) A broader scope to practice. *Child Health*, 1(6), 233–8.

Freemantle, N. (1992) Spot the flaw. *Health Service Journal*, 9 July, p.24.

Girvin, J. & Baker, C. (1990) Standard Setting. *Paediatric Nursing*, 4(13), 26–8.

Glasper, A. & Tucker, A. (1993) Quality in Action. In *Advances in Child Health Nursing.* Scutari, London.

Hancock, C. (1990) Can it work for patients? (Clinical Audit) *Senior Nurse*, 10(7), 8–10.

Harris, A. & Cummings, J. (1992) An environment fit for child care – setting standards in A & E. *Professional Nurse*, 7(7), 461–4.

Herbert, R. & Evans, A. (1991) Staff appraisal and development. *Senior Nurse*, 11(6), 9–11.

Hicklin, M. & Chantler, C. (1989) Resource management at ward level. *Paediatric Nursing*, 1(6), 6–7.

Hogg, C. (1989) *Setting Standards for Children in Health Care.* Quality Review Series. National Association for Welfare of Children in Hospital (now ASC), London.

Hogg, C. (1994) *Setting Standards for Children Undergoing Surgery.* Quality Review Series, Action for Sick Children, London.

Holloway, B. & Hobbs, D. (1992) A challenge we can all achieve; total quality management in health care. *Professional Nurse*, 8(2), 79–83.

Horne, E. & Cowan, T. (eds) (1992) *Ward Sister's Survival Guide, Professional Nurse.* Wolfe Publishing, London.

Hotton, P. (1991) Working for Children. *Paediatric Nursing*, 3(7), 6–7.

Johns, C. & Kingston, S. (1990) Implementing a philosophy of care on a children's ward using action research. *Nursing Practice*, 4(1), 2–9.

Jolly, M. & Brykcznska, G. (eds) (1992) *Nursing Care: The Challenge to Change.* Edward Arnold, London.

Lang, N.M. (1976) *Issues in quality assurance in nursing.* Issues in Evaluation Research, American Nurses Association, Kansas.

MacDonald, A. (1990) Setting Standards. *Paediatric Nursing*, 2(6), 6–7.

Manley, K. (1992) Quality Assurance, the Pathway to Excellence. In *Nursing Care: The Challenge to Change* (eds M. Jolly & G. Brykcznska). Edward Arnold, London.

Mawdsley, D. (1992) Who needs nursing philosophies. *Professional Nurse*, 7(2), 78–82.

Morris-Thompson, P. (1993) Focusing on the future health service reforms and the roles of paediatric nurses in management. *Child Health*, 1(4), 148–50.

NAWCH (1985) *Children's Charter*. National Association for Welfare of Children in Hospital (now ASC), London.

NAWCH (1990) *Setting Standards for Adolescents*. National Association for Welfare of Children in Hospital (now ASC), London.

NHS (1988) *IPR Document* (Revised edn.) HMSO, London.

NHS Management Executive (1991) *Framework for Audit of Nursing Services*. HMSO, London.

Northcott, N. (1993) Appraisal: development tool or bureaucratic nightmare? *Senior Nurse*, 13(1), 14–16.

Øvretveit, J. (1992) *Health Service Quality – Introduction to Quality Methods for NHS*. Blackwell Science, Oxford.

Palmer, B. (1991) Ward Managers and Technology. *Senior Nurse*, 11(1), 18–19.

Parsley, K. & Corrigan, P. (1994) *Quality Improvements in Nursing and Health Care – A Practical Approach*. Chapman and Hall, London.

RCN (1990) *Quality Patient Care: the Dynamic Standard Setting System* (DySSy). Royal College of Nursing, London.

Reed, S. (1992). Bear Necessities. *Health Service Journal*, 20 August, p. 26.

Robertson, L. (1992) *Quality Assurance for Nurses: A Guide to Understanding and Implementing*. Longman, Harlow.

Rowden, R. (1990) Quality of Care. *Nursing Times*, 86(8), 28–30.

Rowe, H. (1992) How am I doing, where am I going: individual performance review in staff appraisal. *Professional Nurse*, 7(5), 288–91.

Rye, D. (1991) Managing clinical services. *Senior Nurse*, 11(1), 3.

Schofield, J. (1990). Practical Standards. *Nursing Times*, 86(8), 31–2.

Shafer, W. (1991) Management in practice; managing a budget at ward level. *Professional Nurse*, 6(11), 677–80.

Shaw, C.D. (1986) *Introducing Quality Assurance*. Kings Fund Project Paper no 64. King's Fund Centre, London.

Swanwick, M. & Barlow, S. (1993) A caring definition: defining quality in paediatric nursing. *Child Health*, 1(4), 137–41.

Teasdale, K. (1992) *Managing the Changes in Health Care*. Wolfe Publishing, London.

Tomalin, D. (1992) *Operational Plan*, Appendix 4, p. 2. Department of Clinical Audit, Brighton Health care.

Tucker, A. (1990) Standards of care. *Paediatric Nursing*, 2(2), 8.

Tucker, P. (1991) *Guidelines to Clinical Audit*. Mersey Regional Health Authority.

UKCC (1994) *The Future of Professional Practice – the Council's Standards for Education and Practice following Registration*. United Kingdom Central Council for Nursing, Midwifery and Health Visiting, London.

Wallace, M. (1990) Prepared for practice. *Paediatric Nursing*, 2(10), 6.

Walshe, K. & Tomalin, D. (1993) Rain check. *Health Service Journal*, 29 April, pp. 28–29.

Wilson, J. (1992) Data systems can boost nursing care; nurse management information systems in resource management. *Professional Nurse*, 7(5), 325–8.

Chapter 5
Moral, Ethical and Legal Perspectives

Imelda Charles-Edwards

INTRODUCTION

This chapter introduces some of the ethical and legal dimensions of children's nursing. The first part gives an overview of the moral basis for decisions, ways of resolving ethical problems and the challenges for nursing practice. Section two outlines legal principles. The focus is on English law and as Scottish law may differ readers should refer to Scottish sources for clarification. Discussion on professional standards, consent to treatment and the Children Act are included. Section three considers ethical principles and their application. Section four integrates the ethical and legal principles and discusses informed consent in further detail. Section five debates the morality of using children as research subjects. Section six addresses issues related to telling the truth to children and the final section explores some of the ethical dilemmas related to allocation of resources for children's health care.

THE MORAL BASIS FOR DECISIONS

Everyday life is governed by moral decisions. Whether conscious or not, decisions are based on a personal moral code arising from beliefs about what is right or wrong. A personal moral code is developed following guidance within the family and at school and as part of progress towards maturity. Although personal, an individual's morality is usually compatible with other members of a society. Any great divergence in belief about what is right or wrong amongst its members threatens a society's cohesion.

Influential moral philosophers, for example Kant or Mill, may influence a whole society's subsequent views. Moral philosophers seek a coherent, logical understanding of right and wrong and thus provide a framework within which others can be helped to reach similarly coherent decisions. However, this is a framework, not a blueprint for every moral dilemma, and does not provide a ready made answer to what is right. The resolution of the ethical dilemmas demands that each individual conscientiously thinks a problem through.

In health care ethics an attempt is made to apply the principles of moral philosophy to practice. It is the major ethical problems in health care, about life and death

issues, which catch general attention. However, there are many, apparently less important, decisions which confront nurses every day that may also have a profound affect upon those cared for and upon carers themselves.

The study of ethics is essential for all nurses because of a responsibility for patients/clients who may be vulnerable. They may be feeling unwell and may feel ill-equipped to understand their condition. Such factors help to contribute to potential inequality of power between the professional and patient/families, thereby disempowering the patient. The study of ethics may help nurses to understand their own perceptions, values and prejudices in relation to such issues, as well as to develop the ability to use reasoned arguments to help resolve moral dilemmas.

The UKCC's Code of Professional Conduct (1992) was developed in the recognition that nurses need guidance in order to help them behave to the standard expected by the profession and to encourage society to have confidence in nurses. The code is an important statement by the nursing profession to the public about the standards of behaviour that the public should expect from nurses. As the title indicates, this is a code of conduct not of ethics and it does not have the status of law. The code is based on accepted views of right and wrong held by the profession.

The resolution of ethical dilemmas

When nurses discuss the ethical problems they face in practice, the multidisciplinary nature of many ethical dilemmas becomes clear. Decisions made by professionals have consequential effects on colleagues, and the resolution of problems is best resolved by the multidisciplinary team working together. This is illustrated by the following example:

The problem concerns a nine year old boy with a poor prognosis. The debate centres over whether he should be given more information about his illness and be included in decisions about further treatment. This could be a difficult problem to resolve without information which may be available, for example, from the boy's teacher and play leader about his intellectual development; his parents may be able to describe the extent to which they have fostered his independence and decision making ability and be able to share their unique understanding of their child; the nurses may know whether he is asking penetrating questions. The wisest decision in a situation such as this is likely to be reached by the parents, doctors, nurses, play leader and teacher discussing together what might be best for the child.

Current challenges to practice

Nurses need to continually review their practice, both as individuals and as a profession, to ensure that, despite ever changing challenges, they continue to comply with moral and legal principles. Three contemporary examples of such changes are:

(1) An increasing awareness of the limitation of resources available to the health service.
(2) Innovations in treatments and care.
(3) A redefinition of professional accountability within the UKCC's code (UKCC 1992).

Uncritical, complacent continuation of work practices from one year to the next is not acceptable. Moral, legal and professional demands require nurses to keep up to date and to be able to justify their actions.

The implementation of the philosophy of family centred care and working in partnership with parents requires professionals working with children and families to face any consequent moral, legal or professional issues which may arise. Two examples of these are:

(1) A potential to covertly coerce parents to participate in care and treatment (Charles-Edwards & Casey, 1992).
(2) The potential danger of forgetting that it is to the child that nurses owe a duty of care, and not to the parents or family unit.

The reform of the health service initiated by the white paper *Working for Patients* in 1989 has instituted a business, market approach within the service. There are times when the dictates of business success are in conflict with professional standards and accountability. Although the duty of professionals to uphold standards is recognized, individuals may have considerable anxiety that, in expressing the view that standards of care are low, they risk their own future and employment. This contemporary challenge can be prepared for by understanding the nature of professional duty, the demands of the code of professional conduct and the support systems available within the profession.

LEGAL PRINCIPLES

Two general principles underpin the law in relation to children and health care:

(1) The requirement to preserve life, where possible, and at least until a child attains sufficient maturity to make their own decision.
(2) To promote a child's best interests.

In some rare cases this leads the law to take action against those normally invested with the duty to care for children: the family.

Another important area of health care law is malpractice.

'The law relating to medical errors ... operates on two basic principles:

(1) The patient must agree to treatment.
(2) Treatment must be carried out with proper skill and care...' (Brazier 1987)

The application of the first of these principles to paediatrics raises a number of particular problems, while the second, concerning standards of practice, is the same for patients of all ages.

Standards of care

Confidence in *professional* standards of care is essential where individuals entrust themselves or their children into a nurse's care. The nurse has a legal duty of care to the patient by virtue of the nurse/patient relationship (Dimond 1990). Such a duty is necessary in recognition of the potential vulnerability of the patient:

'... a duty of care can be said to exist if one can see that one's actions are reasonably likely to cause harm to another person.' (Dimond 1990)

When a nurse harms a patient, with care falling below the expected standard, the patient or parents may sue for negligence. English law sets standards of acceptable performance according to the Bolam test. In the case of *Bolam* v. *Friern Hospital Management Committee* (1957) 2 All ER 118, (1957) 1 WLR 582, Mr Bolam accused a doctor of negligence after he sustained a fracture during electroconvulsive therapy. In rejecting the case, the expected standard of care was defined by the judges as '... practice accepted as proper by a responsible body of medical men skilled in that particular art'. The exact meaning of the judgment is widely debated, but, simply put, a nurse is unlikely to be found negligent if a number of experienced, respected nurses give evidence that they would have acted in the same way in the same situation.

One is not expected to be a world expert, but on the other hand, as in the case of *Wilshire* v. *Essex Area Health Authority* (1987) QB 730, (1986) 3 All ER 801 shows, to plead inexperience is no protection against an accusation of negligence. Clause four of the Code of Professional Conduct (UKCC 1992) states that, in the exercise of professional accountability, a nurse must 'acknowledge any limitation in your knowledge and competence and decline any duties or responsibilities unless able to perform them in a safe and skilled manner'.

Consent to treatment

It is important to recognize that consent is required before any 'bodily touching'. Touching another person, whether patient or not, without consent could be held to be an assault. In many situations consent is implied rather than explicitly requested. However, the giving or refusing of consent is not confined to situations where a signed consent form, giving evidence of consent, is required, but to all forms of care and treatment.

Three ingredients must be present for consent to be legally valid:

(1) Sufficient information.
(2) The capacity to understand the information.
(3) That consent be given voluntarily, without coercion.

Any question about the legal validity of consent given for care or treatment, as a result of which a patient is harmed, can lead to an action for negligence.

How much information qualifies as sufficient information is a vexed issue which has frequently been tested in the courts, notably in the case of *Sidaway* v. *The Bethlem Royal Hospital Governors* (1984) 1 All ER 1018, CA; (1985) 1 All ER 643 HL. As with the *Bolam* case, the exact meaning of this judgment is much debated. Mrs Sidaway took an action for negligence on the basis that, had she been given 'sufficient' information, she would not have given consent to a procedure which, in her case, led to harmful complications. The *Sidaway*

judgment defines sufficient information as that which a responsible body of medical opinion would feel was appropriate. This definition of 'sufficient' includes the amount of information given about the nature and risks of a procedure.

Although it is a doctor's duty to inform a patient about medical procedures, nurses are expected to reinforce this information and act as the patient's advocate, helping them (child and parent) to ask questions and voice concerns. Nurses must also explain nursing procedures. As with doctors, nurses must ensure that they correctly represent the facts.

In paediatric practice parents usually demand, and professionals are glad to give, detailed information about a child's condition, treatment and care. Where a child's illness is complex and decisions are difficult, parents may spend many hours, over weeks and months, discussing available information and options with professionals in order to decide what would be in their child's best interests. Alderson (1990) describes the experience of a 'lawyer father who compared giving consent to his own recent back surgery with the greater responsibility of consenting to his son's heart surgery'. This example illustrates the extra anguish which may be experienced by parents who have to decide what is in their child's interests.

The second ingredient required for a valid consent is the capacity to understand. This relates to the concept of legal competence. The Family Law Reform Act 1969 stated that, in relation to consent to medical treatment, young adults at 16 should be regarded as if they were 18 and had reached the age of majority. The age of 16 is usually, but not invariably, taken as a cut-off point after which an individual's ability to give or refuse consent is not questioned. The issue of whether minors are able to give or refuse consent will be discussed in detail below.

The voluntary nature of consent mainly presents a problem in relation to consent to medical research. Parents may also feel under pressure to comply with the views of professionals over the best treatment option for their child and therefore the approach taken towards parents in any discussion about either treatment or participating in research is extremely important.

The best interests test

Decisions made on behalf of children must be seen to be

in their best interests. This is an imperfect measurement but is the best available. Making decisions on behalf of another person is always more difficult than making up one's own mind. It is even more difficult where the other person is a child. Young children do not have known values and opinions to guide those making decisions on their behalf.

Legal decisions taken in court about what is in a child's best interests attempt to be objective, i.e. what would a reasonable person (parent) in the situation decide (Kennedy & Grubb 1989). However, actual decisions are rarely made by objective third parties in a court, but by emotionally involved parents. The paradox is that it is because parents are usually lovingly involved with their child, that society invests them with the duty to make decisions for their child. While the best interests test makes claim to objectivity, actual decisions made by parents are inevitably and rightly complicated by the love they have for their child and other family concerns.

The Children Act 1989

Although the state invests parents with the duty to care for their children, there are times when, for the child's sake, the state must intervene. The recent history of child abuse cases well illustrates the inherent tension between the parent's duties/rights and family privacy on one hand, and on the other the state's duty to protect vulnerable children. Such tension between the state and the individual are replicated in many other spheres of life. (See also Freeman 1983; Sutherland & McCall Smith 1990).

The Children Act 1989 attempted to address this problem and, through its provisions, reconcile the first three principles embodied in the act:

(1) The welfare of the child is the paramount consideration in court proceedings.
(2) Wherever possible, children should be brought up and cared for within their own families.
(3) Children should be safe and protected by effective intervention if they are in danger.

The Act establishes the child's right to be personally represented in order to allow their view to be expressed in court proceedings. It also increases both the child and parent's right to be involved in local authority decisions about a child's care. Hence the power of the local authority is counterbalanced by the family's right to be heard.

There is an interesting debate over whether the Children Act 1989 is committed to children's rights as the rights of potentially autonomous individuals (autonomy rights) or to the children's right to have their welfare recognized as the prime objective (welfare rights). The Children Act therefore should not be seen as a straight triumph for the children's rights lobby, but at least in part it exemplifies the law's strong motivation to protect children (Montgomery 1994).

ETHICAL PRINCIPLES

Introduction

Viewing the rightness or wrongness of an action by either its consequences or by reference to moral rules represents two main approaches to moral philosophy and ethical decision making. Within both these approaches, or schools of philosophy, philosophers hold that there are some principles which are central to health care ethics: autonomy, justice, nonmaleficence, beneficence and veracity. These principles can be applied within the context of consequential (utilitarian) or non-consequential (deontological) philosophies to provide a framework for the exploration of ethical dilemmas in health care.

Consequentialist (or utilitarian) philosophy seeks to judge the morality of an act by its consequences. In simple terms the right act is that which gives the greatest happiness to the greatest number. Rather than merely being cheerful, happiness here means total wellbeing and fulfilment. One of the most obvious difficulties in applying a consequentialist argument lies in knowing what action will produce the 'best' outcome.

The deontological school of philosophy holds that there are rules which govern actions and which tell us whether acts are inherently right or wrong, irrespective of the consequences. Examples of such rules are: murder is wrong, telling the truth is right. Although such rules may intuitively appear right, an obvious problem with deontological arguments lies in knowing which rules to value and follow.

This is not the place to discuss the relative values of these two schools of moral philosophy; the interested reader will find such exploration elsewhere (Gillon, 1985). However, a tendency to see consequences as of central importance, or to hold to a set of moral rules, will affect the way we apply moral principles, such as autonomy or justice, to ethical problems.

The ethical principle of autonomy

The word autonomy means self rule or self-determination. The notion of respect for autonomy expresses the view that individuals have a right to freedom of thought, will and action and equally are responsible for their thoughts, intentions and actions. The concept of autonomy arises from the concept of personal liberty. Liberty is a central value of the moral, legal and social life of the UK and of many other countries.

Personal liberty is not absolute. It is limited by the fact that people live in social groups with other autonomous individuals, where each person needs to respect the liberty of others. In other words, my freedom is limited by my need to respect the freedom of thought, will and action of my family, friends, colleagues and fellow passengers on the bus to work. Their freedom is equally limited by their respect for my liberty.

When applied to health care, respect for autonomy requires gaining a patient's, or parent's, consent to any proposed treatment or care. A professional's autonomy is limited by the requirement that the autonomous decisions of patients/parents should be respected. As a consequence, there is always potential for tension between a nurse's own autonomy of thought and will or action, and that of the patient, where their views differ. However, it is important to remember that a health care professional is not required to give treatment or care that they consider to be wrong because a patient demands it. The autonomy of patients' or parents' decisions will also be limited by the context of their lives and their relationships.

A similar sort of tension can develop between nurses and other professionals where views and self-interest conflict. The ability to think rationally and express a considered opinion is essential for nurses who wish to challenge their colleagues.

Those who care for children confront the problem of the development of autonomy during childhood.

Children thrive in an environment where their developing autonomy is nurtured, but a young child cannot be said to be autonomous. Children depend on their parents (or other care givers) to make wise decisions on their behalf. In order to fulfil their duties to their child, parents have the right to be the main decision makers for their child. When children are young such paternalistic behaviour is needed but, as children develop towards maturity, the right of parents to make decisions declines and the right of the children to make their own decisions correspondingly increases. It is this changing balance between the developing autonomy of the child and the right of parents to act paternalistically, that makes the application of a respect of autonomy to children so difficult. The dilemma is well illustrated by the issue of consent and the mature minor. This notion of autonomy is explored further by Dworkin (1988).

Non-maleficence

Non-maleficence is derived from Latin and means 'do no harm'. As has already been suggested, one of the responsibilities that nurses and other health care professionals carry is the requirement to avoid harming vulnerable patients. All medical interventions carry the risk of harm and avoidance of harm is not always easy to achieve; for example, when there is a difficult balance to be struck between doing good or doing harm in a decision about health care. The moral duty to avoid harming others (a negative duty) applies not only to health care professionals but to everyone in society. Both the law and moral rules demand that harming others is avoided and such a demand is an example of a way in which autonomy or freedom of action may be curtailed.

Beneficence

Beneficence, which also derives from Latin, means 'do good'. The moral duty to do good does not apply to everyone and to every situation in society; such a demand would be beyond anyone's ability. However, the duty to do good to another (a positive duty) may be required where one enters into a special relationship with the other person: for example, in the duty of parents towards their children and nurses towards patients. Nurses entering the profession knowingly take on the duty to do for patients whatever good lies within their power. A parental and a professional's duty of care arises from this ethical principle. However, it should be remembered that the indiscriminate application of beneficence can lead to unjustified paternalism and the disregard of another's autonomy. In other words: 'I know what is best for you (best treatment) and you will accept my judgement'. Berlin (1969) discusses beneficence and liberty in more detail.

Justice

The principle of justice applied to health care most usually relates to the fair and equitable use of resources. There is an inherent tension between the desire and duty to do one's best for each patient and conflicting claims for resources between patients. (This issue is raised by Gillon 1985.)

Veracity

Veracity means truth. Philosophical writers (for example Gillon 1985) subsume the ethical principle of veracity within the other ethical principles explained above. The reason for this is that either telling or not telling the truth can harm, do good, uphold justice and show respect for autonomy. However, it is in attempting to respect the principle of veracity that many ethical dilemmas arise for nurses in their day to day practice. Nurses therefore need to recognize the importance and relevance of veracity.

The application of ethical principles

As the definitions of ethical principles above suggest, part of an ethical decision making process is not only to apply the relevant principles to the problem case, but also to decide which relevant principle is, in each case, most important. The application of different principles may suggest contrary solutions.

A review of medical ethics over the last 50 years reveals a shift from a tendency for the doctor to 'know what is best' for a patient, what will be 'good', in other words a paternalistic application of beneficence, towards much greater value being accorded to the view of the patient, or parent, in other words a respect for autonomy.

There are a number of ethical decision making models (for example, Seedhouse 1988). These models teach the need to analyse problems in a coherent manner, assembling the facts, identifying those who will be affected by any decision, and applying ethical principles within the context of a utilitarian or deontological philosophy.

CONSENT

Introduction

The issue of consent is central to health care. The patient's consent is required before care and treatment can be given and consent is required before an individual can become a research subject. Seeking consent respects a patient's autonomy. Horror over the uses to which medical science was put during World War II helped to initiate a greater awareness of the need to harness professional power to the aims of care and treatment agreed between the individual patient and professional.

The main issue in relation to children and consent revolves around the fact that autonomy and legal competence are developed during childhood and adolescence. The problems associated with consent that arise with the nonautonomous, noncompetent baby and young child are different from those which occur as autonomy and competence develop in later childhood and adolescence, and children become, to use the legal term, mature minors.

Ethical and legal principles

As identified earlier, three ingredients must be present for consent to be legally valid:

(1) Sufficient understanding.
(2) Sufficient information.
(3) Given voluntarily.

Debate about children and consent therefore concerns their capacity to understand enough information, and, associated with this, whether they are legally competent and morally autonomous.

Society invests parents, through the law, with the responsibility to care for their child. If parents are asked to consent to needed treatment and care, it is their duty to make the best decision for their child, avoiding harm (non-maleficence) and promoting good (beneficence). However, as a child matures, developing understanding and autonomy, the parents' right to decide on behalf of the child correspondingly decreases (Fig. 5.1).

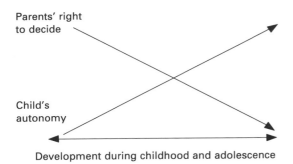

Fig. 5.1   Parents' and child's right of consent.

The basis for all consent decisions is an analysis of risks and benefits. Autonomous children, parents and adult patients all judge the information given to them about risk and benefit in the light of their own values and circumstances. A respect for autonomy must recognize that such decisions are personal. For example, a grandmother might decide to postpone urgent life saving treatment to allow her to attend her grand-daughter's wedding. For parents, balancing risk versus benefit is critical to deciding what is in their child's best interests (Fig. 5.2).

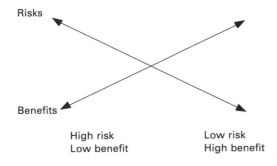

Fig. 5.2   Balance of risks and benefits.

The balance of risk to benefit can also become important in measuring an older child's autonomy or competence. If a mature minor wishes to refuse treatment that is known to be of high risk and low benefit, for example a second heart and lung transplant where the first had failed, competence to decide may be accepted without question. If the same 14 year old refused treatment which was of low risk and high benefit, for example an appendicectomy, competence to decide might be rejected. This illustrates an ambivalence which can arise over recognizing young adults' rights to make decisions which are potentially seriously harmful.

The problem of consent for pre-autonomous children lies in the parent's difficulty in deciding, on behalf of another, albeit their child, what is in the child's interests. This difficulty is made even more acute where the risks are high.

Once children reach two or three years they have a right to information given in a way that is appropriate for their age and about the things that trouble them (Alderson 1991), such as what the child will see, hear and feel and about separation from their parents. Given skilled communication, young children can discuss complex issues. Take the example of six year old Gwen. A psychologist sought to discover Gwen's under-standing of her prognosis. He used Gwen's experience of tests at school and marks out of 10. He then asked Gwen to give marks out of 10 that it would be Wed-nesday tomorrow (today was Tuesday); and then to give marks out of 10 that it would be raining tomorrow; and thence to marks out of 10 that she would be alive in a year's time. Gwen's answer to this last question was five out of 10. The doctors gave her a 50/50 chance of being alive in a year.

During childhood some children start to ask ques-tions and wish to participate with their parents in decisions (Alderson 1991). Individual children react differently and should be allowed to take an active or passive role in decision making as they wish; the child's developing autonomy is thereby respected and nurtured.

As a child grows to adolescence and becomes a mature minor, complex and controversial legal situa-tions arise. From an ethical viewpoint one might wish to respect the autonomous decision of a young adult. Weithorn & Campbell (1982) showed that most four-teen year olds are as able to make health care decisions as most adults. The trouble is that there is no neat test for autonomy or legal competence. Kennedy (1988) suggests that competence lies in an individual's ability to understand the nature and consequence of a procedure.

The case of *Gillick* v. *West Norfolk and Wisbech AHA* (1984) 1 All ER 365; revsd (1985) 1 All ER 4533, CA; revsd (1985) 3 All ER 402, HL, ruled that, if a minor had sufficient understanding of the nature and consequences of treatment, they should be considered competent to consent without reference to their parents. Although the Gillick case was concerned with contraceptive advice and treatment, the ruling has since been applied to all forms of treatment.

The spirit of the Gillick case was replicated in the Children Act 1989, in its recognition that children should participate in decisions about their futures. In the clauses of the act concerning care and supervision orders, there are clear statements that medical treatment may not be included in these orders unless the court is satisfied that a child with sufficient understanding agrees to their inclusion (schedule 3, clauses 4 and 5).

At this point in the history of consent, in 1989, one might have thought, with justification, that it was clear that the consent (or refusal of consent) given by an autonomous, competent under sixteen year old was valid. To ignore such valid consent could risk a claim of assault or negligence against the professionals. However, since 1989 the courts have retreated from this position, leaving ambiguous the minor's right to dispute with parents and/or doctors and refuse treatment. This retreat is illustrated by two recent cases: Re R (1991) 7 BMLR 147, (1992) Fam 11; and Re W (1992) 4 All ER 627 (Kennedy & Grubb 1994). This situation is an example of the potential fluidity of the law where legal opinion is required to adapt to encompass the latest legal case, as discussed by Kennedy & Grubb (1994) and Montgomery (1994).

As has already been suggested, the law in the UK seeks to safeguard the long term interests and the life of children. It is this pressure which may have influenced the courts to withdraw from recognizing a minor's right to refuse treatment recommended by doctors.

Consent in practice

A few cases concerning minors and consent are tested in the courts, but in practice most children, parents and health professionals agree about the best course of action. Discussion and sharing of views may be necessary to achieve such agreement and it is the nurse's role to assist in the harmonious resolution of any disagreements. This is easy to state but may be difficult to achieve where a strong minded young adult and parents disagree over a potentially serious decision.

Alderson (1991, 1993) describes how children of all ages can be helped to participate in decisions about their treatment. The importance of using play preparation, informed by a knowledge of child development, is critical. Alderson (1991) also discusses important differences in attitudes amongst professionals towards children's ability to understand and decide:

'Some of the most child centred professionals were among the most respectful of children's independence. Several nurses said that after years of caring for children, they now trusted the decisions of much younger children.'

Another interesting point is that children with chronic, long term illness may be in a better position to understand and make decisions based on their unique personal experience of illness. Although the nurse may not have experienced cytotoxic therapy, a child receiving treatment for leukaemia will have an indepth knowledge of the side effects.

The tension at the heart of involving children in such difficult decisions is between the desire to protect children and the desire to respect their views and burgeoning autonomy.

RESEARCH AND CHILDREN

Ethical and legal discussion

The morality of using children as research subjects is a complex issue. It is generally accepted, for example by the British Paediatric Association (BPA 1992) that children should only be used for research if all other suitable forms of testing, including using animals and adult humans, have been completed. The research proposal must be scientifically valid and approved by a research ethics committee. Given these provisions, there are some research enquiries which require the inclusion of children.

Using any subject for research gives rise to concerns

over consent and risk, but in the case of young children, who are unable to make an informed assessment of the risk and then give consent for themselves, these concerns are magnified. The problem of balancing risk against benefit has already been referred to within the discussion on consent for treatment. Where treatment is proposed, there is an inherent expectation that the treatment will benefit the child. Whether or not an individual child will benefit from being a research subject is much more problematic.

Most discussions classify research as therapeutic (clinical trials) or nontherapeutic. The aims of therapeutic research are to acquire new knowledge and to provide treatment for the child. For example, the inclusion of a child already receiving treatment for asthma in a study of drugs to treat asthma, may be classified as therapeutic research, even though any benefit for the individual child may be uncertain. The inclusion of children without asthma in a study of drugs to treat asthma is an example of nontherapeutic research. The aim of nontherapeutic research is solely to acquire new knowledge. The child research subject cannot benefit.

Nontherapeutic research

Nontherapeutic research using children who are pre-autonomous and not legally competent, arouses particular controversy. As they cannot benefit from the study, there is no possible trade-off between risk and benefit, other than an altruistic reward. The reliance on such altruism in young children to justify using them as research subjects is controversial, being difficult to prove.

As children cannot benefit from the research and cannot give consent for themselves, nontherapeutic research has, in the past, been prohibited on young children. However, as Alderson (1992) shows, this rule has been relaxed over recent decades so that by 1991 the Medical Research Council guidelines accepted proxy consent by parents for research on children provided that the child did not show an objection. The BPA guidelines (BPA 1992) state that 'a research procedure which is not intended directly to benefit the child subject is not necessarily either unethical or illegal'.

Discussion over the legality of parental, proxy consent for nontherapeutic research arises because of the legal requirement that parents should act in their child's best interests. The question then arises whether participation

in a research project, which cannot benefit the child and which bears some associated risk, can ever be in a child's best interests. This question is usually resolved by the quantification of the risk.

The BPA guidelines (1992) and Nicholson (1986) discuss the complex factors which determine risk and benefit, stressing the importance of the child's personal view as an integral part of the risk/benefit equation; for example, 'a procedure which does not bother one child arouses severe distress in another' (BPA 1992).

Risk has been classified as minimal, low or high (BPA 1992):

(1) Minimal risk – sensitive questioning, observing, measuring, the collection of a single urine sample or using blood from a sample taken as part of treatment.
(2) Low risk – procedures causing brief pain, tenderness, small bruises or scars.
(3) High risk – lung or liver biopsy, arterial puncture and other similar procedures which are not justified for research alone.

'. . . non-therapeutic research on children, regardless of possible benefits, can only be undertaken ethically if the risks of the procedure involved are in the "minimal" category'. (Nicholson 1986)

As has already been implied, the standard for the acceptance or rejection of a pre-autonomous child's consent or assent to nontherapeutic research is more sensitive than that applied in treatment. Guidelines, such as those published by the BPA in 1992, also give a more rigorous standard for the detail of information which must be given to the person (parent) giving consent.

Any action which could be interpreted by the parents or child as coercion to agree to participating in the research, is explicitly forbidden.

Therapeutic research

At first glance one might think that therapeutic research poses fewer ethical problems than nontherapeutic research. This is an illusion. Despite the term therapeutic, there can be no guarantee of benefit for an individual child participating in the research. By its very nature research implies uncertainty, with the relative benefits of treatments unknown. This brings into question the validity of using the term therapeutic research (Alderson 1992).

Another anxiety associated with the notion of therapeutic research is the potential conflict of interests between the demands of the research project and the duty of the doctor to give the child the best care available. For example, the relative benefits of two drugs may become clear before the research study is complete and the required data is assembled. Should the researcher abort the project, taking the risk that the conclusions of the study might be invalidated, in order to give a particular patient the more effective drug?

TRUTH TELLING

Introduction

It ought perhaps to seem strange that, in a discussion about ethics, any doubt should be raised that telling the truth and upholding the ethical principle of veracity is right. One is brought up not to lie. But there is a tradition, as old as the Hippocratic oath, that it may be right to lie to patients. The requirement to do a patient no harm, within the Hippocratic oath, has often been interpreted as justifying deception (Higgs 1985; Gillon 1985). Traditionally this led to a paternalistic approach to telling the truth, permitting health care professionals to lie and deceive. Justifying statements such as 'the truth would kill her' are familiar to many. Although this paternalistic approach is changing to one of greater openness and truth, dilemmas about whether, when and how to tell the truth persist.

In children's nursing the child's parents are normally given comprehensive, truthful information. How they are given information may affect their ability both to come to terms with the information themselves and to help their child to understand. A potential ethical problem may arise if parents wish to prevent or protect their child from learning the truth.

Ethical and legal principles

In any quest for openness it should not be forgotten that truth can harm. A word once spoken can never be retrieved. Great hurt can be caused by thoughtless words. The way in which something is said affects the way it is understood by the listener. The truth can do good (beneficence) and it can do harm (maleficence).

One of the best guides as to whether and when to give information to parents and children is to listen to what they say, either explicitly or implicitly. Remarks or questions often indicate that they wish to know more or, on the contrary, could not cope with more information. Taking such cues from children and their parents respects their autonomy. When caring for children there is a dual and potentially conflicting duty: to respect the autonomous decision of the parents over how much the child should be told, and a respect for a child who is asking questions and seeking knowledge.

An important justification for asserting that telling the truth is beneficial is the need for trust between the health care professional, the child and the parents. The nature of a professional relationship demands that the patient can trust the professional. Trust has to be a casualty of any detected deception. The need for trust and respect for autonomy tends to support telling the truth.

One of the problems inherent in giving truthful information is knowing what the truth is. This is both a philosophical problem over the nature of truth (Higgs 1985) and a practical problem where a diagnosis or prognosis is uncertain. However this should not be used as an excuse for lying. As Higgs explains, the intention should be to tell the truth as far as it is known. The fact that explaining complex medical or nursing details is difficult, or that all the answers are not known, should not prevent professionals from telling the truth, where truth will not harm.

Another impetus towards greater honesty with parents and children is the legal issue of negligence. This may arise where insufficient information has been given, resulting in invalid consent, and where harm has been caused by the procedure.

Truth telling in practice

As has already been suggested, all health care professionals need to show sensitivity when giving information to parents and children. Although it is the doctor's responsibility to give a medical diagnosis and explain treatment, the nurse may be present to support the parents, the child and the doctor, and to enable later reinforcement of the explanation.

Questions such as 'will it hurt?' may be more important to young children than questions concerning their condition. Truthfully answering such questions exemplifies, for children's nurses, the need to tell the truth to earn a child's trust. It takes no great leap of the imagination to understand how children might feel being cared for by nurses who do not answer such straightforward questions truthfully.

The earlier discussion of consent described how quite young children may be able to understand information if this is given to them in an appropriate way. Parents may need explanations about the cognitive ability of children and the mutual advantages of honesty, to help them confidently to allow their child to be told difficult and sad information. A real dilemma is presented when parents want information to be hidden from a child who is asking searching questions. Once again, such a situation can only be resolved by the multidisciplinary team giving time to the family. The advantages and disadvantages of telling the truth and the difficulties experienced by all carers if they cannot truthfully answer a questioning child could be explored.

The parent's views must not be disregarded. Their responsibilities for their child are uniquely important and usually continue long after those of individual professionals have ended.

RESOURCE ALLOCATION AND CHILDREN

Introduction

At first glance it might be supposed that children are in an advantageous position in relation to the allocation of health service resources. Many, if not most people, consider that children's needs should be given priority. On the other hand children have no political power and it can be argued that, in reality, their needs and rights are given little importance by policy and law makers in the UK.

Nurses should not feel themselves impotent to influence decisions. Besides individual political involvement, we can work through professional and parent's organizations to uphold and improve the rights of children.

Decisions about resource allocation are not all on a big scale. In daily practice nurses make resource decisions such as to which patient they should give most time.

Ethical principles

As has already been suggested, the principle of justice or equity is central to the allocation of resources, but, as current experience shows, limited resources may result in the disregard of the individual's wishes or justified needs, with consequent harm and a lack of respect for autonomy.

Aristotle suggested that equity could be achieved when equals were treated equally and unequals unequally in proportion to their relevant inequalities (cited by Gillon 1985). However appealing this dictum appears, Aristotle's application of justice does little to help us in anything but a general manner, other than to remind us that decisions about resources should be made for morally relevant reasons. The fact that someone has green eyes is not a morally relevant reason for awarding resources. Aristotle does little to help resolve conflicting claims as, for example, between a child needing treatment to prevent blindness and another needing treatment to enable them to walk. The problem remains: what reasons are morally relevant to decisions about resources.

Claims can be measured according to medical need or the likelihood of a successful medical outcome, but as Gillon (1985) explains, neither of these criteria necessarily achieve equity. The current debate over the treatment of smokers exemplifies the difficulty of applying such criteria.

A contemporary influence on resource allocation has been the implementation of the White Paper 'Working for Patients' (1989). One of the expressed aims of this paper was to move the level of decision making about health services nearer to the consumer. For better or worse, local health authorities are now making decisions about the health services to be bought for the local community. Each reader will have a view about whether this has been effective in increasing the possibility of choice for individuals. A certain outcome is that health care administrators are involved in assessing the economic worth of services.

A system for judging the worth of giving certain

treatments to certain patients, called quality adjusted life years (QALYs), has been developed by health economists. This formula aims to correlate quality and length of life, thus defining which health care services or treatments are most beneficial. The service giving maximum QALYs at lowest cost is the most efficient, and the one to which, it is suggested, highest priority should be given in resource allocation.

QALYs were greeted with some disapproval by moral philosophers (Harris 1987; Rawls 1989). The system ignores two critical moral principles: that everyone's life is of equal value (equity and justice) and that life itself, even if short, has inherent value. It has been suggested (Harris 1987) that QALYs could be racist, sexist and also ageist with an inherent bias favouring the young. A child who needs an appendectomy would get a high score. However, services for very low birthweight babies, with possible life long morbidity, would achieve a low QALY score.

Contemporary debate over whether very low birthweight babies should be treated exemplifies the dangers of simplifying complex moral arguments. Discussion tends to revolve around the cost of treating each baby and possible long term morbidity, whilst ignoring critical issues: for example, respect for the baby's life, that the life of the handicapped is not of less value than others, and the fact that withholding the full range of medical treatment does not necessarily mean that the baby will die. The withholding of active treatment may mean continuing and worse morbidity rather than mortality.

The moral resolution of conflicting claims to health resources is difficult but the debate demands the involvement of health professionals.

CONCLUSION

Nurses who care for children carry particular responsibilities: towards vulnerable children, for whom the experience of illness may have life-long effects, and towards parents and other family members, in distress for their child. Such responsibilities, which have profound ethical and legal consequences, are best fulfilled working in partnership with the family and within a multidisciplinary team.

The range and complexity of ethical problems facing nurses and other professionals would appear to be increasing. The development of new treatment options through medical technology is but one reason for this. It is easy to fall in with the misguided notion that because one can, one should use a treatment in every case. New treatments may be expensive and the current debate about resources is unlikely to go away.

At the same time as nurses are required to explore the morality of their practice, they must also ensure that they comply with the law. Children's nurses are particularly challenged by the area of child protection. Children are not only harmed within their families. Protecting children from illegal and immoral behaviour by nurses is, unfortunately, one of the most difficult problems which now faces children's nurses.

Although this picture may seem threatening, it is also a picture of opportunity. The opportunity is for children's nurses to participate in debate and thereby contribute to the decisions that are made about the practice of nursing and care for children.

CASES ON WHICH TO REFLECT

Case 1

Peg is eight years old. She was born with a severe cleft lip and palate for which she has had multiple corrective operations. Peg's parents are insistent that she should have further surgery to lift the tip of her nose and improve the outline of her upper lip. They feel that Peg should have the chance to look as 'good' as possible and it is their responsibility as parents to give her this chance. Peg is equally insistent that she is fed up with operations and is quite happy with her appearance as it is.

Case 2

Peter is 11 years old. He has severe cystic fibrosis and the doctors recommend that he should have a heart lung transplant. Peter is intelligent and very independent. He has known other children in hospital who have had a much better life after a transplant and is keen to have one too. Peter's parents are ambivalent about agreeing and a psychosocial assessment suggests that they may be unable to sustain the long term therapy Peter will need.

Case 3

Jo is 10 years old. You are the paediatric community nurse caring for Jo. He contracted HIV during treatment for haemophilia. His parents are extremely protective and insist that Jo is not told about the infection.

Case 4

The manager of a paediatric community nursing service has been asked to accept two new patients. Both will require the same amount of care once discharged home. Providing nursing care for one of these patients will commit all available resources: the team of nurses will have no further available time and there is no money to take on extra staff. Patient one, Sue, is an oxygen-dependent 12 month old baby. Her parents are desperate to take Sue home for the first time, to allow her, their other children and themselves to return to a normal family life. Patient two, Tom, is 12 years old. He is severely physically and mentally disabled. The unit in which Tom has been cared for is closing and the other alternative is 100 miles away. Tom is his parents' only child. They have always been closely involved in his care and now want to take him home.

REFERENCES AND FURTHER READING

Alderson, P. (1990) *Choosing for Children: Parents' Consent to Surgery*, p. 102. Oxford University Press, Oxford.

Alderson, P. (1991) Children's consent to surgery. *Paediatric Nursing*, 3(10), 10–13.

Alderson, P. (1992) Did children change, or the guidelines? *Bulletin of Medical Ethics*, 80, 21–8.

Alderson, P. (1993) *Children's Consent to Surgery*. Open University Press, Buckingham.

Alderson, P., Aylwood, W. & Davidson, R. (1994) A new approach to ethics: demystifying ethics in the care of adolescents. *Child Health*, 1(5), 187–92.

Atherton, T.M. (1994) The rights of the child in health care. In *The Child and Family: Contemporary Issues in Child Health and Care* (ed. B. Lindsay). Bailliere Tindall, London.

Berlin, I. (1969) *Four Essays on Liberty*, pp. 118–72. Oxford University Press, Oxford.

BPA (1992) *Guidelines for the Ethical Conduct of Medical Research Involving Children*. British Paediatric Association, London.

Brazier, M. (1987) *Medicine, Patients and the Law*, p. 53. Penguin Books, Harmondsworth.

Brykczyńska, G. (1989) *Ethics in Paediatric Nursing*. Chapman & Hall, London.

Brykczyńska, G. (1993) Ethical Issues in Paediatric Nursing. In *Advances in Child Health Nursing* (eds E.A. Glasper & A. Tucker). Scutari Press, London.

Charles-Edwards, I (1991) Who Decides. *Paediatric Nursing*, 3(10), 16–18.

Charles-Edwards, I. & Casey, A. (1992) Parental involvement and voluntary consent. *Paediatric Nursing*, 4(1), 16–18.

DoH (1991) *The Children's Act 1989: an Introductory Guide for the NHS*. HMSO, London.

Dimond, B. (1990) *Legal Aspects of Nursing*, p. 28. Prentice Hall, London.

Dworkin, G. (1988) *The Theory and Practice of Autonomy*. Cambridge University Press, Cambridge.

Freeman, M.D.A. (1983) *The Rights and Wrongs of Children*, pp. 244–77. Frances Pinter, London.

Gillon, R. (1985) *Philosophical Medical Ethics*, pp. 14–27, 86–99, 101. John Wiley, Chichester.

Harris, J. (1987) Qualifying the value of life. *Journal of Medical Ethics*, 13, 117–23.

Hendrick, J. (1993) *Child Care Law for Health Professionals*. Radcliffe Medical Press, Oxford.

Higgs, R. (1985) On telling patients the truth. In *Moral Dilemmas in Modern Medicine* (ed. M. Lockwood), pp. 187–202. Oxford University Press, Oxford.

Kennedy, I. (1988) *Treat Me Right*. Clarendon Press, Oxford.

Kennedy, I. & Grubb, A. (1989) *Medical Law: Text and Materials*, p. 226. Butterworths, London.

Kennedy, I. & Grubb, A. (1994) *Medical Law: Text and Materials*, 2nd edn, p. 378. Butterworths, London.

Korgaonkar, G. & Tribe, D. (1993) Children and consent to medical treatment. *British Journal of Nursing*, 2(7), 383–4.

Lee, L. (1991) Ethical issues relating to research involving children. *Journal of Paediatric Oncology Nursing*, 8(1), 24.

Montgomery, J. (1994) The retreat from Gillick. In *Children's Decisions in Health Care and Research*, pp. 7–14. Social Science Research Unit, Institute of Education, London.

Nicholson, R. (ed.) (1986) *Medical Research with Children:*

Ethics, Law and Practice, pp. 76–124. Oxford University Press, Oxford.

Rawls, J. (1989) Castigating quality adjusted life years (QALYs). *Journal of Medical Ethics*, 15, 143–7.

Seedhouse, D. (1988) *Ethics: the Heart of Health Care*. John Wiley, Chichester.

Sutherland, E. & McCall Smith, A. (eds) (1990) *Family Rights: Family Law and Medical Advances*, pp. 4–20. Edinburgh University Press, Edinburgh.

Taylor, J. (1994) Research and Child Care. In *The child and family: contemporary issues in child health and care* (ed. B. Lindsay). Bailliere Tindall, London.

UKCC (1992) *Code of Professional Conduct for the Nurse, Midwife and Health Visitor*, 3rd edn. United Kingdom Central Council, London.

Weithorn, L.A. & Campbell, S.B. (1982) The competency in children and adolescents to make informed treatment decisions. In *Child Development*, 53, pp. 1589–98.

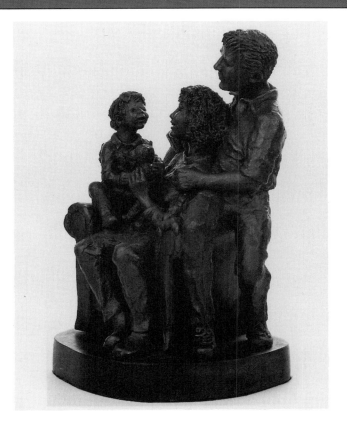

This part provides in-depth material on the key health and ill health issues, such as development, disability and life crises, which affect children and their families.

These issues are complex and interrelated. The division of topics into separate chapters is somewhat artificial or arbitrary since some areas naturally overlap, thus reinforcing both the complexity and comprehensiveness of the knowledge and skills required by the children's nurse. The focus is on the perspective of the child and their family throughout, since this will allow the nurse to appreciate their experiences.

Effective nursing care must be based on an extensive knowledge base that considers the child as a member of a family as well as a member of society in general, and with complex psychosocial as well as physical needs.

Chapter 6

Children, Health and Families

Maggie Wilson

INTRODUCTION

This chapter is concerned with the impact of social pressures on children's health. It will review some of the main changes which have occurred in the lives of children and families during this century and particularly in the last 50 years in the UK. It will also place these issues in context, with some reference to other European countries and to the conditions of children's lives in the less privileged parts of the world.

The family is often seen as the cornerstone of society. Children and their families have adapted to changing circumstances in many creative ways. Yet there is a dark side to family life, and children's health and wellbeing can come under threat within families. This chapter will introduce the reader to some of the ways in which family life can affect children's wellbeing, including variations in material circumstances.

In the wider public sphere, the results of significant improvements in child health care will be outlined. Negative influences on children's health will also be reviewed. Finally, the chapter will include a brief summary of the United Nations Convention on the Rights of the Child and will pose the question as to what extent we are meeting the health needs of children – in their broadest sense – today.

CHANGES IN CHILDHOOD AND FAMILY LIFE

Memories of childhood past

'I knew I was desperate for a baby boy because I'd lost my Jackie. He was our four year old son, and we'd lost him with diphtheria. I was heartbroken about that, but I'd kept going thinking I'd have another boy and he'd be my new Jackie. Well, I went into labour, and it was a long and difficult labour, but eventually the baby came out. It was a boy. But the doctor held him up in front of me and said, "He's useless" and threw him down on the bed. He were dead. He'd been strangled coming out. Of course, I was in a terrible state and they wouldn't let me see my dead baby. My brother came round and wrapped him up in paper and put him in a big margarine box. And because we didn't have any money, he took him on the bus to the grave digger in the cemetery and they put him in a common grave. I don't know where he is to this day. It took me a long time to get over that.' (Humphries, Mack & Perks 1988, pp. 39–40)

This is the testimony of Emma Jones, a young mother in Grimsby in the early years of this century. Such accounts are by no means unusual. At the turn of the century 163 in every 1000 babies died before the age of one and of those who survived babyhood, one in every four did not survive beyond the age of five. The major childhood diseases were whooping cough, measles, diphtheria, scarlet fever and tuberculosis. These took an appalling toll, especially in inner city areas where chronic overcrowding and poor sanitary conditions prevailed. One of the main spurs to the establishment of the School Medical Service in 1907 was the discovery that 40 to 60% of enlisting men were unfit for service in the Boer War (Kurtz & Tomlinson 1991). Life could often be 'nasty, brutish and short' and survival was the key concern in many families. Many children suffered from pneumonia, bronchitis and general undernourishment, while dental decay, headlice, ringworm, ear and eye infections were rife.

Within families, fathers would often rule with a 'rod of iron'. As the main breadwinner, the father would be given the pick of the food on offer and would expect absolute obedience from his children. Under the pre-war National Insurance Scheme, fathers were often the only member of the family entitled to free healthcare. Children were treated with homespun or quack medicines, such as treacle or animal fat. When a new piece of road was being laid, children with bronchial complaints were taken to breathe in tar fumes. With a high birth rate in families, older girls were expected to be 'little mothers' to younger siblings, helping with heavy domestic chores from an early age. At the age of 12 or 13 many entered domestic service. Until the 1920s child labour was rife. Children worked as errand boys and girls, paper sellers, street hawkers or were involved in light assembly work such as making matchboxes or artificial flowers. In rural areas there were numerous tasks to perform to help make the family ends meet. Children would gather and sell watercress or flowers, tend animals or help with the harvests. In some areas they were recruited through agricultural hiring fairs until as late as the 1930s.

Childhood: a golden age?

All this is in marked contrast to popular images of childhood in the 1990s: a time of innocence, dependency, playfulness, set apart from the exigencies of adult life. As this chapter will show, improvements in health care, infant welfare, housing and sanitation have created enormous improvements in the quality of life of children in our society. Within the family, attitudes towards children and relationships between parents and children have changed considerably. Changes in the birth rate and intervals between births have resulted in fewer children being born and consequently a greater sense of investment in children. Children have experienced a gradual removal from the sphere of paid work, and have seen the growth of educational and leisure facilities, alongside the multi-million pound toys industry.

Yet there are still wide differences in the life chances of children from different social backgrounds in the UK, and an even wider gap between these and the fate of many children in Africa, Asia, the Caribbean and Central and South America. In these places an estimated 12.7 million children die under the age of five every year and 35,000 every day, two-thirds of these from pneumonia, diarrhoea and measles (Grant 1993). In the poorer communities of such countries even minor infections, such as coughs and colds, can be lethal when a child's underlying state of health is so poor (Vittachi 1989).

Major immunization programmes have dramatically improved the chances of survival of millions of children, yet children are affected disproportionately in times of global recession. Child welfare programmes are often cut back first and children are more vulnerable to malnutrition than most adults. Estimates of child labour suggest a picture of the exploitation of children, reminiscent of the time of Dickens in Britain.

Reviewing contemporary and historical evidence, some sociologists and historians maintain that in many ways childhood has been 'discovered' in the twentieth century. Where life is a daily struggle for survival, children are often expected to be 'mini-adults'. It is not until a relatively high standard of living has been reached that a recognition of the need for state protection and intervention on behalf of the 'nation's children' emerges. In 1800 the meaning of childhood was still ambiguous but by 1914 a recognizably modern understanding of the term was in place in the UK (Hendrick 1990). The state intervened initially to protect children from cruelty and neglect and to provide a baseline for the physical care of infants and of school-aged children. In the inter-war period the development of child welfare services and child guidance clinics underscored an increasing concern for the individual child and for children's perceived psychological needs. In the post-war period there has been a growing emphasis on the parent–child relationship, concern over the quality of institutional care and debate about the privacy of the family and the state's right to intervene when children are at risk. From the 1970s on there has been an increasing recognition that children are persons with their own right, and are not simply the property of their parents.

This recognition has been manifested in the establishment of such organizations as the Children's Legal Centre, and Childline, and has been expressed at national and international levels in the Children Act 1989 of England and Wales and the 1989 United Nations Convention of the Rights of the Child. The latter defines children as all those under the age of 18, yet for many people in the past and present the end of childhood can occur at different stages in life: on leaving home, on marriage, on leaving school, on entry into paid employment. As compulsory universal education has been extended and as more children stay on at school, so the period of dependency has been extended. Yet more children are also experiencing changes in family patterns, some of which present them with the new problems of the late twentieth century.

CHANGES IN FAMILY SIZE AND STRUCTURE

'We go to see my gran every month. My Scottish gran that is. I've got two English grannies and gramps, but I don't see much of them. My other gran is dead. My dad comes to see us every other weekend. He brings us presents and at birthdays he gets us really big things. It's nice to be a bit spoiled but I think he's trying to sort of buy our love.' (An eleven year old girl in 1993)

Facts and figures

A full population census of the UK is held every ten years, the most recent on 21 April 1991. Data from the census is readily accessible through the government publication *Social Trends*, and this helps to create a fascinating picture of changes in the British family since the 1940s.

There are over 13 million children under 16 in the UK, which represents about 20% of the population. The number of births is expected to peak in 1994 and then to fall, as the large generation born in the 1960s passes its peak child-bearing age. The average age of mothers at the birth of their children has remained similar between 1951 and 1991 at 28.4 and 27.6 years respectively. However, the fertility rate for women born in the UK has dropped from 2.15 to 1.82 children.

As with all averages, such figures mask interesting differences. The percentage of births to mothers aged 15–19 years has nearly doubled over the last 40 years, from 4.3 to 7.6% of all births. The percentage of births to women over 35 fell from 17% in 1941 to 8% in 1981, but had risen again to 9% in 1991, as Table 6.1 illustrates. The birth-rate for women born overseas has also fallen in the last 20 years, though rates for mothers born in India, Pakistan, Bangladesh and Africa remain slightly higher than for those born in the UK. The average interval between marriage and the birth of the first child is now 28 months and between the first and second birth 34 months. Parents from a semi- or unskilled manual background tend to start their families more quickly than those from a professional or managerial background.

The general decline in the average number of children born to mothers in the UK is similar to trends in other European countries, with the exception of the Irish Republic. Another common trend is the proportion of children born outside marriage, although there are wide country by country variations. One in two births in Sweden are outside marriage, one in three in the UK and one in 50 in Greece. The increasing divorce rate in the UK is also part of a European pattern but is high in comparison with other European countries, apart from Scandinavia, at 12.6 per 1000 existing marriages, as Table 6.2 shows. One in three new marriages will end in divorce, if present trends continue, and the divorce rate has doubled between 1971 and 1991 (Social Trends 1993).

Family break-up

An estimated 150 000 children per year experience parental divorce and about a third of all divorcing couples have children under 16. Reasons for the increased rate include increasing legal tolerance of divorce, the secularization of society, financial independence of women, and greater geographical and social mobility. The highest divorce rates are among those who marry at a young age, those who have experienced

Table 6.1 Live births: by age of mother, 1941–1991, Great Britain. (*Source:* Office of Population Censuses and Surveys; General Register Office (Scotland))

	% and thousands					
	1941	1951	1961	1971	1981	1991
Age of mother (years)						
15–19	4.3	4.3	7.2	10.6	9.0	7.6
20–24	25.4	27.6	30.8	36.5	30.9	24.8
25–29	31.1	32.2	30.7	31.4	34.0	35.6
30–34	22.1	20.7	18.8	14.1	19.7	23.0
35–39	12.7	11.5	9.6	5.8	5.3	7.6
40–44	4.2	3.4	2.7	1.5	1.0	1.2
45–49	0.3	0.2	0.2	0.1	0.1	0.1
All births (= 100%) (thousands)	669	768	912	870	704	766

Table 6.2 Marriage and divorce: EC comparison, 1981 and 1990. (Source: Eurostat Demographic Statistics 1993)

	Rates			
	Marriages per 1,000 eligible population		Divorces per 1,000 existing marriages	
	1981	1990	1981	1990
United Kingdom[1]	7.1	6.8	11.9	12.6
Belgium	6.5	6.5	6.1	8.7
Denmark	5.0	6.1	12.1	12.8
France[2]	5.8	5.1	6.8	8.4
Germany (Fed. Rep.)	5.8	6.6	7.2	8.1
Greece	7.3	5.8	2.5	—
Irish Republic	6.0	5.0	0.0	0.0
Italy	5.6	5.4	0.9	2.9
Luxembourg[2]	5.5	6.1	5.9	10.0
Netherlands	6.0	6.4	8.3	8.1
Portugal	7.7	7.3	2.8	—
Spain	5.4	5.5	1.1	—
Eur 12	6.0	6.0	—	—

[1] 1990 column for marriages contains 1989 data and divorce column contains 1987 data.
[2] 1990 column for divorces contains 1989 data.

parental divorce, those whose partners are from different social backgrounds, among unskilled workers, and those whose occupations involve a high degree of travel, separation or work involvement (Joseph 1990). Divorce rates are highest in the 25–29 age group and among those who have been married between five and nine years (Social Trends 1993).

There is conflicting evidence about the effects of divorce on children. If present trends continue, one child in every five born in 1987 will have to cope with divorce by the age of 16, and by the year 2000 only half of all children will spend all their childhood with both natural parents (Bradshaw 1990). The percentage of all dependent children living in lone parent families has more than doubled since 1972 to reach 18% in 1991. Children often blame themselves for their parents' break-up, idealize one parent and vent their anger on the other. Parents may use children as a go-between or overindulge them (Jaques 1987). In terms of the objective measures of educational attainment and delinquent behaviour, living in a single parent family is not a problem in itself. Studies, such as the National Child Development Study which has traced the lives of 17 000 children born in one week in March 1958, suggest that it is where single parenthood is combined with other disadvantages, in particular a low income, that such problems arise (David 1993). Family break-up can also lead to positive changes, such as an absence of conflict, and the majority of children cope well with parental divorce and grow up well adjusted (White & Woollett 1992).

Changing family patterns

However, such statistics have been used to suggest that the 'traditional' family, often contrasted with an idealized vision of the Victorian family, is in decline. Despite these trends, over 80% of children still live in families which contain a married couple. Remarriage is also popular: about a third of all marriages involve one partner getting remarried (Wicks 1989). Many children therefore have to cope with increasingly complex family patterns, including perhaps four sets of grandparents, several aunts and uncles and many cousins in so-called 're-constituted' families. However, the rate of single parenthood is about half that reported in the 1851 census. There are also indications that a high proportion of the children born 'out of wedlock' are born into a stable family situation. Three-quarters of births outside marriage are registered by both parents, and a half by both parents living at the same address (Social Trends 1993).

One further feature of family life in the 1990s which merits attention is the erosion of extended family support networks. In the post-war period onwards, there has been a general assumption that family ties between generations and siblings have loosened, as families move for occupational and other reasons. Yet research has indicated that family support networks are still strong among both middle and working class families, with the telephone increasingly replacing face-to-face contact in times of need. Studies of new mothers show the degree to which they value their own mothers' advice on childcare over and above that of professional health care workers (Mayall 1990; McIntosh 1992). Grandparents often help in cash or kind at the time of childbirth. In addition, family support networks remain strong among many ethnic minority groups in the UK.

The family suffers from more myth-building than many other areas of social life. Few people today would have wanted to live in Victorian families, where marriages were often scarred by poverty, violence and hard drinking or broken by the death of a parent. Although television advertising reinforces an image of family life dominated by the two-parent, two-child model, the majority of people in Britain do not live in such households, as Table 6.3 illustrates. It is probably more accurate to see the family as an institution responding flexibly to external events at different stages in its life cycle in different time periods.

CHANGES IN CHILDCARE PATTERNS

Maternal deprivation?

'I was caught up in the Truby King Mothercraft doctrine. The health visitor prated and bullied; one's baby screamed and tears splashed down one's cheeks while milk gushed through one's jersey. But one must never pick the baby up – it was practically incestuous to enjoy one's baby.' (Humphries *et al.* 1988, p. 58)

Table 6.3 People in households[1]: by type of household and family in which they live, 1961–1991, Great Britain. (Source: Office of Population Censuses and Surveys)

	% and thousands			
	1961	1971	1981	1991
Type of household				
Living alone	3.9	6.3	8.0	10.7
Married couple, no children	17.8	19.3	19.5	23.0
Married couple with dependent children[1]	52.2	51.7	47.4	41.1
Married couple with non-dependent children only	11.6	10.0	10.3	10.8
Lone parent with dependent children[1]	2.5	3.5	5.8	10.0
Other households	12.0	9.2	9.0	4.3
All people in private households[2] (= 100%) (thousands)	49,545	52,347	52,760	24,607

[1] These family types may also include non-dependent children.
[2] 1961, 1971, 1981 Census data. 1991 General Household Survey. 1991 column contains sample size.

This is how a mother describes her experience of child-rearing in the 1940s, when the clock-watching routines advocated by the child care expert, Truby King, were in vogue. This was replaced in popularity by the babycare 'bible' of Benjamin Spock and the writing of John Bowlby in the 1950s. The former stressed affection, intuition and warmth in the upbringing of children. The latter stressed the importance of the emotional bond between mother and child as crucial to the child's later life. Much of Bowlby's work was in fact concerned with children in institutional care, yet his ideas were taken to support the view that children would be emotionally deprived if cared for by anyone other than their mothers in the early years (Rouse 1990; Smith & Cowie 1988).

However, such theories have been challenged by subsequent events. The 1970s onwards saw a huge influx of women into the labour force. Nearly two-thirds of all women of working age are now 'economically active' in the UK. (The rate for women from a Pakistani or Bangladeshi background is considerably less, at about a third of women in these groups.) This rate is the second highest among European Community countries and increasingly includes women with children. Just under a half of women with children under four are working on a full- or part-time basis, while over two-thirds of those with children between five and nine are employed or self-employed. Women in the professional and managerial class are more likely to work at all stages of their children's development (Social Trends 1993).

This trend has had two main consequences. The first is an increasing demand for quality childcare and the recognition of the value of women's contribution to the labour market. The second is a movement towards a greater degree of role sharing within the family, as mothers become equal or main breadwinners.

Childcare and nursery education

There has been an increasing amount of research directed towards policy and practice in early childcare (Moss 1990; Rouse 1990; Hennissey *et al.* 1992; Pugh 1992). Much of this draws unfavourable comparisons of state provision in other European countries with the UK (Moss 1992; Melhuish & Moss 1990; Sommer 1992). Comparisons have to be made with care, as the age of compulsory schooling varies between countries and some provision is only available on a part-time basis.

Nevertheless, the assertion that the UK is near the bottom of the European Community 'league table' of state sponsored provision can still be supported by evidence. In particular, the UK is outstripped by all countries, except for Portugal, in its provision of childcare for children between the age of three and compulsory school-age. In Denmark, public expenditure on childhood services is six times as high as in the UK (Moss 1992). In France the state levies subsidies from industry to pay for childcare and pre-school education and virtually all children attend full-time education between the ages of three and six. Unpaid parental leave is generally available until the child is three years old (Hennessey *et al.* 1992). In Sweden, over 80% of women with pre-school children are in employment and most children are in state funded day-care (Moss 1990). Either parent is entitled to 90 days leave per child per year to cover sickness, to a reduced working day of six hours, and to parental leave of up to 18 months until a child is eight years old. The provision of after school day-care and leisure centres to cater for older children whose parents are at work is also widespread.

In contrast, policy in Britain is underscored by the assumption that childcare is a private concern. The government has supported the development of the pre-school playgroup movement and some 600 000 children attend playgroups. This is often the only service available to parents and the hours do not usually meet the needs of working parents (Moss *et al.* 1992). Public daycare is generally limited to children defined as in need. A government commitment in 1972 to provide nursery places for all three to four year olds was never implemented. Table 6.4 gives figures for the use of childcare services in England. The majority of parents use childminders or relatives to look after young children and there are twice as many places available in private registered nurseries as local authority nurseries. From the age of three to four playgroups remain the main form of provision. A minority of children attend part-time or full-time nursery education at this age, despite the proven benefits of a good early start to education. Twice as many parents from a professional and managerial background use pre-school education as those from an unskilled manual background. Although research stresses the importance of continuity of care, many parents have to piece together a jigsaw of provision. In one study of London families, nearly half of the children in the sample had experienced one change of

Table 6.4   Under fives and pre-school services, 1991. (Source: Early Childhood Unit, National Childrens Bureau)

Total population aged 0–4 years	3,234,900
Under fives as % of total population	6.73
Places with registered childminders per 100 children aged 0–4 years	7.21
Places in local authority day nurseries per 100 children aged 0–4 years	0.84
Places in registered day nurseries per 100 children aged 0–4 years	2.38
Places in playgroups per 100 children aged 3–4 years	33.44
Total children using playgroups as % of 3–4 year olds	60.19
Total children in nursery schools/classes as % of 3–4 year olds	24.81
Total children in infant classes as % of 3–4 year olds	22.30
Total children in independent schools as % of 3–4 year olds	3.54

day-care by the time they had reached three years and a quarter, two or more changes (Brannen & Moss 1991). Day care for children after school hours is rare.

In response to the continued popularity and persistence of Bowlby's attachment theories, research has addressed the questions of whether public childcare is detrimental to the wellbeing of children and whether one form of childcare is better than another. On the first point, no clear link has been established between separation from the mother and subsequent adolescent behavioural problems (Smith & Cowie 1988). Indeed, there is considerable evidence that pre-school education can compensate for disadvantages in a child's home background and can encourage language development, sociability and cognitive skills among all children (Moss, 1990; Hennessey *et al.* 1992). Much depends on the quality of care, which should be stable, responsive to children's needs and sensitive to all aspects of a child's development.

Although parents show a continually expressed preference for nursery schools and day nurseries, research into the quality of different types of childcare warns against making ready judgements. Unregistered childminders received a bad press in the 1980s. At that time many parents were forced to use this form of provision if they worked long or antisocial hours and for low pay (David 1990). This group included a large number of single parents, especially from an Afro-Caribbean background. The Children Act 1989 has established minimum standards of quality and training for childminders, over and above which quality varies as much as within other forms of provision.

One recent study which attempted to compare the development of children in different types of childcare

tested a sample of children at the ages of four months, 18 months and three years (Melhuish & Moss 1990). This found that there were no significant differences in children's behavioural problems attributable to type of childcare used. At the age of 18 months, children at nursery school had developed fewer phrases and word combinations and were more indifferent to strangers than children looked after by relatives or childminders. By the age of three years, parents' own educational background was the strongest factor in promoting children's cognitive and verbal development, a variable which previous research has tended to ignore. More important than the type of childcare used appears to be the levels of affection expressed by carers, how much they talk to children and how many opportunities children have for play, especially fantasy or imaginative play (David 1990).

Childrearing: partnerships and practice

As more women have taken up employment opportunities, there has been a growing assumption that the 'division of labour' within families has correspondingly changed. There is some evidence of this, but research suggests that there is considerable variation according to region or socio-economic background, that major family decisions are usually made by husbands and that only certain tasks are shared. Table 6.5 gives responses to an attitude survey of such issues in 1987. From this it is clear that the majority of married respondents felt that the primary care of children is still the mother's job, although this view was much less strongly supported among unmarried people. In a study of first-time

Table 6.5 Household division of labour: by marital status, 1987 (Great Britain, %). (Source: *British Social Attitudes: The Fifth Report*, Eds Roger Jowell, Sharon Witherspoon & Lindsay Brook, Gower, 1988).

	Married people[1]						Never-married people[2]		
	Actual allocation of tasks			Tasks should be allocated to			Tasks should be allocated to		
	Mainly man	Mainly woman	Shared equally	Mainly man	Mainly woman	Shared equally	Mainly man	Mainly woman	Shared equally
Household tasks (%[3] allocation)									
Washing and ironing	2	88	9	—	72	27	—	57	41
Preparation of evening meal	6	77	17	—	55	42	—	42	55
Household cleaning	4	72	23	1	45	52	1	35	62
Household shopping	7	50	43	1	33	65	—	22	77
Evening dishes	22	39	36	11	18	69	9	14	74
Organization of household money and bills	32	38	30	22	14	62	24	15	59
Repairs of household equipment	82	6	8	74	1	23	64	—	34
Child-rearing (%[3] allocation)									
Looks after the children when they are sick	2	67	30	—	47	51	—	40	58
Teaches the children discipline	13	19	67	10	5	83	17	2	80

[1] 983 married respondents, except for the questions on actual allocation of child-rearing tasks which were answered by 421 respondents with children under 16.
[2] 234 never-married respondents. The table excludes results of the formerly married (widowed, divorced, or separated) respondents.
[3] 'Don't knows' and non-response to the question mean that some categories do not sum to 100 per cent.

parents of children aged 0 to 36 months, in Greater London, similar patterns were found, whether mothers were in employment or not (Brannen & Moss 1991). Over 90% of fathers participated in play with their children, but the majority never saw to their child at night. A minority of fathers were engaged in changing nappies, feeding, bathing and dressing the child on a regular basis, again even when mothers were employed on a full-time basis. Two-thirds of mothers took the decision about whether to take the child to the doctor and took time off work for the child's illness. The majority of women interviewed regarded their husbands as assistants, rather than equal partners, and were reluctant to criticize them. They also felt positive on balance about returning to work, although would have preferred the option of part-time work to being offered full-time or no employment in many cases. However, most reported that they felt concerned and guilty in the face of entrenched attitudes concerning working mothers.

Such attitudes are reflected in a study of the divergence between the views of health-care workers and mothers of babies of 21 months (Mayall & Foster 1989; Mayall 1990). This showed how fathers were marginal to the upbringing of children in the eyes of the professionals, and clinic times reinforced the widely expressed view that mothers of children under two or three should not be at work. Health visitors were strongly influenced by child development theories and stressed the importance of guiding children successfully through stages of development. Mothers took pleasure in watching their children develop as active communicators and learners in the give and take of everyday life and were far less concerned about routines and consciously stimulating children. While mothers valued immunization programmes and clinics as clearing houses for child health problems, they displayed far more ambivalence towards development tests and other advice. Mothers who had arrived in the country relatively recently had more recourse to professional advice and less to the family and friendship networks valued by mothers born in the UK. However, many of the black women interviewed rejected what they perceived as the denigration of paid work and patronizing attitudes of health-care workers. A study of working-class mothers in Glasgow also revealed concern over professional attitudes, seen as intrusive, irrelevant and patronizing. This resulted in a sharp decline in attendance at child health clinics three months after the birth of the first child (McIntosh 1992).

In the Greater London study there was some evidence of a higher degree of shared childcare among parents with higher status occupations (Brannen & Moss 1991). Research in the 1960s showed substantial differences in child-rearing practices according to social class (Newsom & Newsom 1965). Middle-class parents sought more professional advice, punished children according to principles rather than specific acts, participated in play and read to children on a regular basis more often. There were also differences reported concerning the use of dummies, bed times, attitudes towards potty-training and breast-feeding. Research conducted over 30 years later suggests that social class differences in child-rearing practices persist. One more recent study recorded that over twice as many mothers (34.2%) from a professional and managerial background were still breast-feeding babies at three months as mothers from an unskilled manual background (16.4%) (White 1989).

A further study of preschool children reported a wide variation in practices, much of which was related to social class (Davie *et al.* 1988). Such variations concerned attitudes towards early potty-training, a daily wash, the use of dummies and snacks between meals. In 58% of middle-class families and 35% of working-class families children were encouraged to 'dine' with adults. In 33% of working-class and 17% of middle-class families, no 'dining' at table was observed; children generally ate sandwiches or snacks in front of the television. Over a third of parents smacked children, but there was no clear relationship between this and social class. Similarly there was wide variation between families across the social spectrum in the degree of affection shown to children and the degree to which children were allowed to play in front gardens or in the street.

CHILDREN, FAMILIES AND HEALTH

Health gains and losses

'I was six when I went into hospital so my sister must have been just over one year old. I had scarlet fever and I went onto a ward especially for scarlet fever. There were children there from our neighbourhood. I didn't have it very bad, but of course there was the baby at home. To say I couldn't play with the others isn't true because we weren't allowed to play in hospital anyway then. I was completely on my own. We weren't allowed any toys and parents couldn't visit. Not that we had many dolls and things then. We all shared our toys – they weren't just mine. The other thing was when you were ill you had to stay in bed, and that's what I did, all day for six weeks. It seemed a lot longer. I just lay in bed. I wasn't really scared. I just felt ill and strange.'

This was how a little girl experienced serious illness in the 1930s. Since then, enormous improvements have occurred in the treatment of childhood diseases and of children during illness. There has been a dramatic decline in the number of stillbirths and in the perinatal and neonatal mortality rates. In the 1930s 2500 women died per year during pregnancy and childbirth in the UK, as opposed to seven per 100 000 per year in the 1990s (Social Trends 1993). The infant mortality rate has fallen from 150 per 1000 live births in 1901 to 7.4 per 1000 live births in 1991 (Social Trends 1993). This figure is about two-thirds of the rate in 1963 but is still higher than in many comparable European countries, such as France, the Netherlands and Germany (Woodruffe & Glickman 1993).

Life expectancy is another indicator of improvements in standards of health. The average expectation of life at birth is projected to rise to 75 years for a male and 80 years for a female by the year 2001. In 1901 their life expectancies would have been just 46 and 49 years and in 1961 67.9 and 73.8 years respectively (Social Trends 1993). In 1990 the World Health Organisation put forward a global immunization target of 80% of a

Table 6.6 Immunization of children, UK. (Source: Department of Health; Welsh Office; Scottish Health Service, Common Services Agency; Department of Health and Social Services, Northern Ireland)

	Percentage immunized[3]				
	1971[1]	1976	1981	1986	1990–91[2]
Diphtheria	80	73	82	85	93
Whooping cough	78	39	46	66	84
Poliomyelitis	80	73	82	85	92
Tetanus	80	73	82	85	92
Measles	46	45	54	71	89

[1] England and Wales only.
[2] Scotland figures are for 1991.
[3] Children born two years earlier and immunized by the end of the specified year.

nation's children. Table 6.6 shows that the proportion of infants immunized against diphtheria, poliomyelitis and tetanus rose from 73% to 92% between 1976 and 1990–1. The percentage of children now vaccinated against measles and whooping cough also exceeds the WHO target in this country (Social Trends 1992). This has resulted in an overall decline in notifications of the most infectious diseases since the 1950s. Table 6.7 shows the dramatic decline in the incidence of measles and whooping cough and shallow rates of decline in the incidence of tuberculosis and jaundice. Before 1970,

measles epidemics occurred every two years and improvements in this area are attributable to large scale vaccination programmes. However, there is general agreement that improvements in children's and adults' health is essentially due to improvements in social and public health and water quality, sewerage, better housing, less overcrowding, and better family planning, education, nutrition and working conditions, although effective treatment has played its part (Health of the Nation 1992).

Despite these general improvements, there are still

Table 6.7 Notifications of selected infectious diseases, UK. (Source: Office of Population Censuses and Surveys; Scottish Health Service, Common Services Agency; Department of Health and Social Services, Northern Ireland)

	Thousands and number										
	1951	1961	1971	1976	1981	1984	1986	1987	1988	1989	1990
Notifications (thousands)											
Infective jaundice[1]	—	—	17.9	7.6	11.0	7.0	4.3	4.4	6.4	8.3	9.8
Whooping cough	194.9	27.3	19.4	4.4	21.5	6.2	39.9	17.4	5.9	13.6	16.9
Measles	636.2	788.8	155.2	68.4	61.7	67.6	90.2	46.1	90.6	31.0	15.6
Tuberculosis											
Respiratory[2]	—	22.9	10.8	9.1	6.8	5.6	5.4	4.5	4.5	4.6	4.5
Other[2]	—	3.4	3.0	2.6	2.5	1.4	1.5	1.2	1.3	1.4	1.5
Meningococcal meningitis[3]	—	—	0.6	0.7	0.5	0.4	0.9	1.1	1.3	1.3	1.1

[1] Viral hepatitis for Scotland, and for England and Wales from 1989.
[2] From 1984, categories overlap, therefore some cases will be included in respiratory and other tuberculosis.
[3] England and Wales only.

wide variations in the quantity and quality of health care in different parts of the country and in standards of health between social and occupational groups. The gap between the expected health careers of children born to parents of a professional and managerial background and those born to parents of an unskilled manual background is startling. The infant mortality rate in the latter group is about twice as high as in the former, at 12 per 1000 compared with six per 1000. The rate for children born to Afro-Caribbean and Pakistani mothers is still higher, at about 15 per 1000. If rates were similar, about 500 babies per year would be saved (Oppenheim 1993). Children whose parents are of unskilled manual background are twice as likely to die before the age of 15 and four times as likely to die of accidental injury, as the children of professional or managerial parents (Woodruffe & Glickman 1993). More working class infants are lost through gastroenteritis and respiratory diseases. There are also social class differences in the use of antenatal care, of immunization and health care services, breast-feeding rates, and percentage of low birth weight babies (Joseph 1990). These disparities continue into

adulthood, where mortality and sickness rates for all major diseases are lowest in the professional and managerial classes. Even life expectancy varies in this country by social class.

Addictive habits

Overall, smoking levels have declined since the 1970s. There is now considerable evidence of a strong association between parents' smoking habits and children's propensity to smoke, along with peer group pressure. A recent study found that three-quarters of all children surveyed were aware of cigarettes by the age of five (Ferguson & McInlay 1991). This study also found that 17% of boys and 12% of girls had experimented with smoking by the age of 11. By the age of 15, 22% of girls and 17% of boys were regular smokers, boys smoking an average of 35 cigarettes per week and girls an average of 28 cigarettes per week. These figures are in excess of those given in response to a broader government survey of 11–15 year olds, included in Table 6.8. Overall, 30%

Table 6.8   Smoking behaviour of children[1]: by sex, England and Wales. (Source: Office of Population Censuses and Surveys)

	Percentage and numbers			
	1982	1986	1988[2]	1990[2]
Smoking behaviour (percentages)				
Boys				
Regular smokers	11	7	7	9
Occasional smokers	7	5	5	6
Used to smoke	11	10	8	7
Tried smoking once	26	23	23	22
Never smoked	45	55	58	56
Sample size (= 100%) (numbers)	1,460	1,676	1,489	1,643
Girls				
Regular smokers	11	12	9	11
Occasional smokers	9	5	5	6
Used to smoke	10	10	9	7
Tried smoking once	22	19	19	18
Never smoked	49	53	59	58
Sample size (= 100%) (numbers)	1,514	1,508	1,529	1,478

[1] Aged 11–15 years.
[2] England only.

of the population aged over 16 smoke (Social Trends 1993). This figure has declined from 46 percent in 1972 but again includes a wide variation by social class. In 1990 16% of professional men and women smoked, in comparison with 48% of unskilled manual men and 36% of unskilled manual women. Despite a now clearly demonstrated link between smoking and cancer, coronary heart disease, chronic respiratory diseases, low birthweight babies and perinatal mortality, the highest rate of smoking is among 20–24 year olds. There is now also evidence to suggest that passive smoking can cause pneumonia, respiratory problems, asthma and ear, nose and throat problems in children. It has been estimated that the children of smokers inhale the equivalent of 60–150 cigarettes per year (RCP 1992).

A further negative example set by parents concerns alcohol consumption. This is notoriously difficult to measure with any accuracy. Social survey data consistently record less than would be expected from Customs and Excise statistics on alcohol, with the implication that adults do not 'come clean' about their alcohol intake. However, the Health of the Nation survey classified 1.4 million people as heavy drinkers and estimated that one in four men and one in 12 women consumed more than the recommended limits on alcohol consumption (Health of the Nation 1992). The rate of alcohol consumption for women is about a third of the male rate, and gender differences far outweigh those of social class in this area. Despite police evidence of the role of alcohol in road accidents and crimes of violence, there is a need for considerably more research into the effects of adult 'role models' on under-age drinkers. One 1989 survey found that three-quarters of all 13 year olds in England and Wales drank alcohol and that one in fifteen 15-year-old boys and one in ten girls drank above the limits (Bradshaw 1990).

A more recent survey has assessed that 5% of 14–15 year olds could be drinking in excess of safe weekly adult limits. This may underestimate the effects of alcohol on teenagers. Solvent abuse, largely through peer pressure, is also increasing and accounted for 134 deaths in 1988. A nationwide sample of over 20 000 12–16 year olds has found that fifteen percent of 13–14 year olds have tried drugs, most commonly cannabis, and that the percentage of 11 to 14 year olds experimenting with drugs doubled between 1989 and 1992. It is hard to assess whether single acts or regular use are involved but the finding that 13% of 11–12 year old boys and 7% of 11–

12 year old girls had been offered drugs is alarming (Balding 1992).

Changing diets

Dietary habits in families have shown some healthy trends over the last thirty years. There has been a decline in the average consumption of beef and veal, mutton and lamb, white bread, sugar, butter, cakes and biscuits and an increase in consumption of poultry, fresh fruit, brown bread and cheese (Social Trends 1993). However, the decline in the consumption of fish and fresh vegetables can be considered as a less positive trend and the average contribution of fat to diet is still well above the recommended intake (Health of the Nation 1992). In addition, the proportion of obese and overweight adults has risen during the 1980s and shows a strong association with region and social class. The main dietary sources of energy for many school children are now bread, chips, biscuits, sweets, cakes, meat products and milk. School meals account for 30–40% of average calorie intake. The nutritional standards requirements for school meals were abolished in 1980 and there is now broad concern over the quality of school meals on offer as well as the choices which school children make at cafeteria-style school lunches, especially when this is combined with an increasing tendency towards the consumption of snacks and fast foods as meal replacements at home.

Over a quarter of 11–12 year olds have nothing or just a drink for breakfast and about 10% have lunches from a takeaway or shop. School-aged girls tend to drink far less milk than boys because of perceived social pressures to remain slim, and they tend to have lower than adequate iron, riboflavin and calcium intakes. In a 1992 survey, 45.7% of 11–12 year old girls and 55.2% of 14–15 year old girls said that they would like to lose weight. Over a third of girls in this age group have nothing or just a drink for breakfast (Balding 1992).

Since 1988 only families on income support have been entitled to free school meals, milk and vitamins and the proportion of children taking school meals has declined by about a quarter in the last ten years. For the families of the very poor this can have serious consequences, with mothers cutting down on their own food consumption in order to try to give their children adequate diets, or having recourse to cheap, filling, but unhealthy food

(Cohen *et al.* 1992). With sweets used as 'treats' to vary monotonous diets, the incidence of dental decay is twice as high among poorer than well-off families.

Accidents to children

Accidents are the commonest cause of death among all children over the age of five. Road traffic accidents accounted for two-thirds of all fatal accidents among school-aged children in 1991, when 383 children died and 44 500 were involved in such accidents. The greater proportion of these were pedestrian accidents, although there were over 8000 casualties to cyclists in the same year (Road Accidents Great Britain 1992). Most accidents occur at a peak danger time of the journey to and from school. The volume of traffic has virtually doubled in the last twenty years and speed limits in built-up areas are often flouted. A survey of parental responses to this situation showed that three and a half times more children were chauffeured to school in 1990 as in 1971 and the proportion of children allowed to cross roads on their own or to use bicycles on roads had also sharply declined (Hilman *et al.* 1991).

The accident rate shows social class differences as well. The chances of a child of unskilled manual parents being killed in a traffic accident are four times as great as those of a child of professional managerial parents, and for a child of an unemployed head of household they are seven times as great, reflecting a lack of safe play areas or access to private transport in less privileged residential districts (OPCS 1988). 'Stranger danger' or the fear of child abductions has also contributed to the increasing tendency of parents to shepherd children. Such cases represent a tiny fraction of the mortality rate for children, but a real fear for parents. The effect has been a curtailment of the 'licence' for independence among children, and fewer opportunities to learn gradually the responsibilities of road use, walking home alone or making purchases from shops, which were enjoyed by their parents' generation.

Accidental injury at home still continues to be a major concern. The chief cause of fatal accidents among children aged under 15 is fire and there are again strong social class variations in this area. Children in low income families are more likely to live in poorly maintained housing stock, with faulty electrical circuits, and the higher rate of smoking among this group also con-

tributes to the risk of fire. This is especially the case in bed and breakfast accommodation for homeless families, where safety standards are often extremely low (Conway 1988). Low income families are also often unable to afford other child safety equipment items, such as stairgates, cupboard catches or cooker guards, which again results in a higher home accident rate. Boys have a greater home accident rate than girls and twice as many die from accidents overall. One reason for this may be because they are often encouraged to take part in more active situations and to be more actively curious about their environments, which can lead to a greater number of falls or experiments with dangerous household substances.

The standard of maintenance and safety in public playgrounds has also given rise to concern. There were nearly 50 000 playground accidents in 1991, attributable to inadequate supervision, poor design or poor maintenance (Consumer Safety Unit 1992). Children who have little play space at home are particularly vulnerable in this respect. Many public playgrounds effectively debar children with physical disabilities, and children's needs are often not considered in planning the use of public space or amenities.

Other threats to children's health

Improved uptake of ante-natal screening has reduced the number of children born with a congenital abnormality and the number of infant deaths. However, children of the parents of unskilled manual workers are still three times as likely to die of sudden infant death syndrome as those of professional and managerial parents. This accounted for just under half of postnatal deaths in 1990, at a rate of 1.3 per 1,000 babies (Woodruffe & Glickman 1993). A high profile health education campaign has reduced this rate by about a third, but social class differences still pertain. Low birthweights, smoking and bottle feeding may all contribute to these disparities.

Many children experience more private affluence in their families than their grandparents or parents did. Prime time advertising for children encourages wants and 'needs' which would have been exceptional treats thirty years ago and rarely experienced sixty years ago. It is debatable whether this represents an improvement in children's opportunities for play and development, or whether it diminishes creativity and imagination. Whatever the case, the increase in material affluence for the majority contrasts with growing concern over the quality of life in the public sphere. Lead and nitrate levels in the water supply, drift from pesticides in fields, contaminated landfill sites, polluted beaches and car exhaust levels are giving rise to fears that such levels of pollution are detrimental to children's health in the short term and will have unforeseeable consequences in the future. Seven hundred thousand children are now affected by asthma, representing about 8% of under 15 year olds. Respiratory diseases are the most common cause of hospital admissions, after accidental injury, and are increasing. In schools asbestos roofs and pipe lagging, old lead plumbing and poor standards of maintenance have also given rise to concern (Rosenbaum 1993). Safe intake levels of most substances found in the environment are assessed for adults rather than children. A more child-friendly society, it is argued, would make children's health needs a benchmark for all safety and pollution policies.

Worrying as such trends are, it is salutary to place them again in the context of global patterns of health and mortality. In the 'developed' regions of the world, the projected infant mortality rate for 1990–5 is 12 per 1000 births; in the 'developing' world as a whole it is 70 and in Africa 94 per 1000 births. Projected life expectancy is 75 years in Europe, 63 in the 'developing' world and 54 in Africa (Social Trends 1993). If the 1990 World Health Organization goal of 80% immunization was reached, three million children would be saved every year (Grant 1993).

Ninety-seven per cent of child deaths occur in the 'developing' or third world. The risk of a mother dying in childbirth is one in 20 in Africa and one in 10 000 in Northern Europe. The short interval between births can have debilitating effects on many women in the third world, reminiscent of the treadmill of childbirth and childrearing experienced by the mothers of large families in this century in Britain. Three and a half million children still die from pneumonia and the same number from diarrhoea every year. Yet, according to UNICEF estimates, the cost of controlling major childhood diseases, halving childhood malnutrition and making family planning, safe water and sanitation universally available is about a half of European expenditure on cigarettes per year (Grant 1993).

FAMILIES, STRESS AND CHILDREN

Children and poverty

'There was such poverty, you left school at 14 and got a job to help the family. You had to give your wages right up to your mother. My first job when I left school was working in a factory that made cardboard boxes, most unexciting, and I only got eight shillings a week, the equivalent of 40p in today's money. The kids of 14 today are all glamorous and made up, but in them days I still wore lace up sandals and woolly ankle socks, really like a child. My mammy would make my dinner to take with me, well when I say dinner, it was usually just a piece of bread and butter or beef dripping, if we had any.

You don't see kids out now skipping or playing rounders or hopscotch. I was mad about marbles, I'd play for hours rolling marbles in the gutter, there were no cars remember, they were few and far between. We'd throw old buttons against the wall to see who could get the nearest. Up to 12, or 13, or 14 you'd be out playing that is, not hanging round corners like today. I used to love putting a rope round a lamppost and swinging round on it, I used to spend hours spinning round a lamppost. We had to make our own games from what little we had. We never had pocket money in our life, we never got any toys from Father Christmas, now you'll find that hard to believe but it's true. What we'd get, I remember one Christmas, was two great big Jaffa oranges, now that stayed in my mind all my life. We woke up, we had to share beds, so me and my sister Mona, who died, slept together, and I remember waking up, 'Oh Father Christmas has been', and there were two big Jaffa oranges at the end of the bed. We rarely got fruit then. My mother, if she could manage it, would go down Moor Street where you could buy fruit, the little old dears with their black shawls, they'd sit there all day selling fruit, and some of it would be damaged and this'd be what my mother would get. God love her she went through it, trying to feed seven of us on what little money my father gave her. We ate stew mainly, an awful lot of stew, Irish stew, but she'd laugh and say it was more like blind stew than Irish stew. When we could afford a piece of meat, when my dad wasn't drinking so much and we'd have a few extra bob, she'd have enough for the Sunday dinner, then cold next day, she'd put it through the mincer to make a cottage pie, that was like a feast to us.

They were poor days, but happy days, my mother had a rough time, but we didn't realise that till we got older. We weren't the only ones, there was poverty all around, some days you'd feel well off compared to others.'

This is an original testimony of the childhood of May, born in 1928. The poor today are relatively better off, but still at odds with the image of the 'good life' displayed on television. During the 1980s the gap between the richest and poorest section of the community grew wider (Wicks 1989; Bradshaw 1990; Woodruffe & Glickman 1993). Although there is no official definition of poverty in the UK, according to measures commonly used in the European Community, just under a quarter of all children in the UK are living in poverty, a two and a half fold increase since 1979 (Oppenheim 1993). In over half of such families, the head of the household is unemployed and a further 38% are classified as low income families. About three-quarters of the two million children of single parents are at or below income support level.

The majority of single parents would work if good quality, cheap or free childcare were available. One report has estimated that this would bring a half of the under fives affected out of poverty (Cohen 1991). Regional differences mean that poor families tend to be clustered in Northern Ireland and some areas of Scotland and the North of England. Where families contain children with disabilities, the extra costs involved and the more hidden cost of lost potential income adds to the likelihood of such children living in poor circumstances.

A report commissioned by UNICEF in 1990 attributed this increase in poverty to the economic trends of a rise in unemployment and earnings differentials, the demographic trends of increasing divorce and family breakdown, and also to deficiencies in policy concerning taxation, social security benefits and health and social services (Bradshaw 1990). One example of the latter is the move from a grants system for essential household items to a loans system through the social fund. This has

meant, according to one government report, that many families experience problems in buying bedding, nappies, baby and children's clothes, washing machines and cookers (Huby & Dix 1992). Parents try to cope by cutting down on food or fuel or by going further into debt and so adding to this source of stress. The increase in the number of households disconnected from gas, electricity or water supplies has also caused growing concern, especially where there is evidence that the diseases of the past, hepatitis and dysentery, are recurring in families without water (NACAB 1992).

Housing and homelessness

The problems of poverty are often augmented by those of poor housing conditions. A Department of Environment survey in 1993 found 1.3 million homes to be unfit in England alone (DoE 1993). To be classified as unfit, a dwelling must be defective in one of nine areas in terms of such matters as state of repair, ventilation, freedom from damp, facilities for food preparation, drainage, etc. Overall, since 1971, the number of dwellings lacking basic amenities, such as sole use of a bath, an inside wc or central heating, has declined considerably (Social Trends 1993). However, for those who do live in unsatisfactory conditions, the chances of poor health among adults and children are much higher. There is a close association between poor standards of living and asthma, bronchitis, respiratory diseases, pneumonia, infections and stress-related complaints. Children in poor families are also more likely to suffer from eczema, growth problems, bed-wetting, behavioural problems, poor speech and physical coordination, and poor dental health (Spencer 1990; Cohen *et al.* 1992). The National Child Development Study provided evidence of a clear association between poor educational attainment and social disadvantage, which can result in a cycle of poverty between generations. Family stability and parental involvement with children can mitigate this (Davie 1993).

The official figures for homelessness have tripled since 1978. Those families housed in bed and breakfast accommodation experience particular problems in health terms. They are often unable to become registered with a GP or enrol their children at school. In cramped accommodation, there are few opportunities for play or for the preparation of adequate meals. Poor safety standards result in a greater number of accidents to children (burns, scalds, falls, swallowing poisonous substances) than elsewhere. Many such properties are damp, have inadequate sanitation and are pest-ridden (Conway 1988; Bradshaw 1990). The situation of the young homeless on the streets of London and other big cities is also a continuing area of concern. Vulnerable to exploitation and abuse, such youngsters are also more susceptible to depression, drug-related problems and to respiratory conditions.

Three quarters of ethnic minority families in Britain live in the metropolitan areas, and of these a disproportionate number live in inner-city areas of multiple deprivation and in overcrowded conditions (Bradshaw 1990). The infant mortality rate and post neo-natal mortality rates among children born of parents from the New Commonwealth and Pakistan are consistently higher than the average UK rate (Spencer 1990). Among the ethnic minority groups in the UK, the post neo-natal mortality rate is lowest among mothers born of an Indian, Bangladeshi or East African Asian background. Along with the diseases of poverty, the increase of rickets among Asian children and sickle-cell anaemia among Afro-Caribbean children also presents serious problems. The experience of low-income or unemployment among ethnic minority families is often compounded by the stress caused by racial harassment. One report depicted a daily barrage of abuse experienced by black people in the street. One half of black people interviewed had experienced physical abuse and the majority verbal abuse (Gordon 1990).

Children at risk

Other sources of stress on children and parents can cut right across the social spectrum. The incidence of child abuse in families in the past and present is one such area which is gradually coming to light. Child protection registers are still probably a gross underestimate of the incidence of child abuse, and definitions of abuse still vary between cultures. One broad definition is: 'A child is considered to be abused if he or she is treated in a way which is unacceptable in a given culture at a given time' (Meadow 1989). According to this definition, many British parents would be abusers under Swedish law, where all forms of physical punishment of children, including smacking, are illegal.

Tragically for some children normal parental responsibilities and patterns of parenting break down and the child is exposed to actual abuse or the risk of abuse (Douglas 1993). This constitutes a real life crisis for the child and their family. Abuse can be active or passive and can occur in the form of physical, psychological and sexual harm. Although the incidence of reported child abuse has been increasing since the mid 1970s there has been a narrowing of the gap between actual and reported cases.

In the UK, over 45 000 children in 1991 were registered on the official child protection register as cases 'of grave concern'. At least one child per year per 1000 under the age of four suffers from severe physical abuse and four children per week will die as a result of neglect or physical abuse (Meadow 1989). Media 'moral panics' have highlighted certain forms of abuse above others, especially since the discovery of the 'battered baby' syndrome in the 1960s. Sexual abuse of children accounted for 11% of official child protection cases in 1991, a proportion exceeded by cases of neglect and physical abuse. A small proportion (6%) were registered because of emotional abuse (Social Trends 1993). NSPCC publicity literature gives the case of a three year old girl who thought that her name was 'Oi' because this was how she had been addressed up to that point. Emotional abuse – threats, shouting, taunting – can arguably harm children as much as the use of excessive force – shaking, squeezing, hitting children. Cases of neglect, where children are confined in unheated rooms, without lighting, adequate clothes, food or human company, can be as poignant. All kinds of abuse show the destructive use of adult power, where children are regarded as the property of their parents (White & Wollett 1992).

There are a few clear-cut patterns to abuse. It can sometimes last for short periods of crisis and can sometimes be a permanent feature of life. However, it is often related to other forms of family stress from external factors, such as unemployment or poverty, or internal factors, such as unsatisfactory relationships. Whatever the case, the increasing recognition of this century-old phenomenon raises questions about the commonsense benign view of the child's best place in the family. At present the long-time effects of child-abuse or the links between being abused and becoming an abuser are not absolutely clear. As more victims of child abuse 'come out' and tell their stories, greater knowledge and understanding may aid prevention and treatment.

Abuse is a contentious subject and one which engenders a range of feelings, which the health care professional needs to recognise (RCN 1994b). Children have the right to a life free from abuse (United Nations 1992, article 19) and all nurses have a role in prevention of abuse through the provision of education and support to the parents, and in identifying families under stress. Additionally, by highlighting to children and young people their right to personal safety, children can be made more knowledgeable. The identification of child abuse is fraught with difficulties; a multidisciplinary approach is vital and nurses should be aware of the indicators of child abuse. The RCN document *Protecting Children* (1994b) highlights four important points to remember (Table 6.9).

Table 6.9 Important points to remember (RCN 1994).

- The child's welfare must always come first.
- Children have the right to live a life free from abuse.
- Nurses have the responsibility to uphold the rights of children and to ensure they are protected from abuse.
- Your local area child protection committee handout contains precise instructions which you should follow if you suspect a child is being abused.

Nurses are responsible for both understanding and being able to use the child protection system and for knowing who the designated health professional is who co-ordinates child protection work. Additionally the RCN (1994a) recommends that 'all nurses who work with children and young people should have access to, and quality time with, designated senior nurses.'

Nurses are also responsible for providing support and care for the child's psychological and emotional needs.

The issue of bullying has likewise received increased media attention in recent years. Like child abuse, estimates of its incidence are extremely difficult to verify. Bullying can represent a range of behaviour from name-calling and taunting to sexual or physical harassment. Whatever the definition, its effects on children's psychological and physical wellbeing can be disturbing, as one sixteen year old expressed:

'I have been picked on. People think I am nothing and say anything they want to me. Every day I feel rejected. It's not that people use violence much but I feel I am treated like a dustbin' (Mellor 1991).

During the first three and a half years of the existence of the children's helpline, Childline, 91 000 phone calls and several thousand letters were received. In a sample of 4000 children surveyed in 1986–7, 38% claimed to have been bullied or badly frightened, and bullying started at a very young age (Roland & Munthe 1989; La Fontaine 1991). Most incidents occurred at school, although the most serious were often on the way to or from school. Bullying could last for a year and was often underestimated by teachers. Evidence is mixed but it appears that boys are more likely to be both bullies and victims. Boys are also more prone to violent aggression and girls to taunting. No type of school is immune, although active school policies can have a dramatic effect. For bullied children, the experience can be nightmarish, involving feelings of powerlessness and rejection and resulting in a range of disorders: bed-wetting, stammering, headaches, crying themselves to sleep, withdrawal, truancy and, in extreme cases, suicide.

Bullying is often the result of the experience of violence or discord in families but the prime movers usually galvanize a group to cheer on their acts. The victim can be singled out because of a difference in appearance, size, accent or other personal attribute. Frequently, this difference is based on race. In a study conducted in Manchester primary and secondary schools, after the playground murder of a 13-year-old Asian boy, 79% of children of an Afro-Caribbean and 76% of an Asian background reported that they had been picked on in fights, while the majority had been called names which made them 'angry or miserable' (Kelly & Cohn 1988). A small-scale observational study of 10–11 year olds showed racial taunting to be a daily experience for many children at school, in shops, and in their neighbourhood. The authors concluded that this has contributed cumulatively to 'an insidious atmosphere of racial harassment and intimidation' and described several observed incidents of children crying and shaking in reaction (Troyna & Hatcher 1992).

Children and employment

With increasing pressures on all children to 'spend,

spend, spend', there is evidence of a growing number of children in employment in the UK. For many, this is a positive experience and gives the child or young person a sense of responsibility and growing independence. For some, their earnings, however small, represent a necessary direct or indirect contribution to family income. However, a great number are employed illegally and constitute a casual unprotected workforce. A survey published in 1991 estimated that two million children are employed and about three-quarters of these illegally (Pond & Searle 1991). The study, conducted in Birmingham, found that over 40% of children between the ages of 10 and 16 had some kind of job, a finding in line with an earlier study conducted in 1985 in London, Luton and Bedfordshire (MacLennan *et al.* 1985). This figure excluded babysitting and running errands and included paper rounds, shop work, cleaning, decorating, modelling, clerical work and working in garages, farms, street markets, catering services and for removal firms. In both surveys, hourly earnings were very low and accident rates high. Over 30% of children had been involved in accidents, from falls or slipping to accidents involving dangerous weights or machinery. The Birmingham study found that a quarter of those employed were under the age of 13 and the earlier study reported that a third of all working children suffered from fatigue. Where long or antisocial hours were worked, school performance suffered. The issue of child labour cannot be disassociated from homelessness among teenagers, some of whom turn to prostitution in order to survive (Fyfe 1989).

While employment can affect the welfare and health of children in all European countries and in North America, it is salutary to place it in a wider context. It is impossible to establish the incidence of child labour in developing countries with any accuracy. One United Nations estimate was of 150 million child labourers in Asia alone (Vittachi 1989). From the ages of five or six children are often denied the right to play, learn or enjoy what many would consider to be a normal childhood. In rural areas children draw water, tend animals, weed fields. Girls undertake heavy domestic duties. Children are drawn into the cash economy through home-working or sweatshop industries, with no legal protection. In India, children are bonded to small factories to pay off debts. Here, conditions are reminiscent of those under early industrialization in Britain:

'They were made to work in a carpet factory 18 to 20 hours a day. Whenever they made a mistake, weaving, they were beaten up, poked and wounded. Whenever any of these children fell down out of exhaustion and fatigue, they were branded with a hot iron. Whenever anyone tried to escape or run away, he was caught hold of and hung upside down from a jack fruit tree and dropped on the ground.' (Lee-Wright 1990, pp. 53–4.)

In Thailand, children become prostitutes, often to Western tourists, from the age of 12 or 13 for the sake of their families. In Brazil, street children live off their wits and are regularly abused or murdered. Child labourers can develop postural deformities, hearing and eyesight problems; they are exposed to toxic substances, such as glue and pesticides; they are more susceptible to infections diseases through fatigue and anaemia; and they are exposed to accidents, drugs and sexually transmitted diseases. They have less access to educational and medical services (Fyfe 1989).

CONCLUSION: CHILDREN'S RIGHTS – MYTH OR REALITY?

The United Nations and the Rights of the Child

- Children are defined as those under the age of 18, unless national laws fix an earlier age of majority.
- Every child has the inherent right to life, and States shall ensure to the maximum child survival and development.
- Every child has the right to a name and nationality from birth.
- When court, welfare institutions or administrative authorities deal with children, the child's best interests shall be a primary consideration. The child's opinions shall be given careful consideration.
- States shall ensure that each child enjoys full rights without discrimination or distinctions of any kind.
- Parents have the primary responsibility for a child's upbringing, but States shall provide them with appropriate assistance and develop childcare institutions.

- Disabled children shall have the right to special treatment, education and care.
- The child is entitled to the highest attainable standard of health. States shall ensure that health care is provided to all children, placing emphasis on preventive measures, health education and reduction of infant mortality.
- Primary education shall be free and compulsory as early as possible; discipline should respect the child's dignity. Education should prepare the child for life in a spirit of understanding, peace and tolerance.
- Children shall have time to rest and play and equal opportunities for cultural and artistic activities.
- States shall protect the child from economic exploitation and work that may interfere with education or be harmful to health and wellbeing.
- States shall protect children from the illegal use of drugs and involvement in drug production or trafficking.
- Children who have suffered maltreatment, neglect or detention should receive appropriate treatment or training for recovery and rehabilitation. (Taken from Vittachi 1989.)

This is an extract from a summary of the 1989 United Nations Convention on the Rights of the Child, ratified in 1991 by the UK. It was intended to provide a benchmark for the treatment of children worldwide, providing a minimum package of rights and legitimacy to such issues. Critics have pointed out that it was more concerned with child protection than with giving young people political rights, and that it is inappropriate to place all 'children' under the age of 18 in the same category (Franklin 1989). However, it is important in establishing the right to a minimum standard of health, education, physical care, family life, play and recreation; and the right to be protected from discrimination, abuse, exploitation, substance abuse, injustice or conflict; and the right to be consulted and to challenge decisions. In the UK, the Children Act 1989 also strengthened the principle that children's wishes and feelings should be taken into account when decisions are made on their behalf and that the child's welfare should be paramount in all legal cases concerning their welfare (Riches 1991).

The preceding sections have shown that we are still a long way away from attaining such standards. In 'developing' countries, children are still dying on a massive scale from preventable diseases and malnutri-

tion. If the world of childhood has largely been 'invented' in the twentieth century in Europe and North America, it has not yet reached children in many parts of the world. Of course children the world over will play with minimal equipment. Many traditional games, using simple sticks and stones, are to be found across cultures. Children learn a huge amount from each other, irrespective of formal education. They can be remarkably resilient in the face of adversity. In less fragmented communities than those evident in the cities of the West, children are often seen as a common responsibility and can expect both protection and discipline from their extended families and wider society. Yet even the most loving families can be forced to submit their children to harsh conditions of employment through poverty. Where the necessary infrastructure for public health – clean water, sanitation, good access to medical care – is lacking, mass immunization programmes can only have a limited effect.

Is the right to good health attainable?

We have seen that the chances of attaining a good standard of health in the UK have increased remarkably over this century and particularly in the post-war period. More children survive birth and infancy, enjoy healthy lives, have good access to health care and can expect to live longer than their grandparents. Public awareness of healthy eating habits, the dangers of smoking and alcohol, the importance of dental care, ante-natal screening, immunization and child development tests has increased. Health education is a recognized cross-curricular theme in the national curriculum of England and Wales. Yet the right to a good standard of health is enjoyed to a greater degree by some sections of the community than others. Disabled children are still marginalized from many mainstream services. Children from ethnic minority groups are more likely to be living in conditions adverse to health. Children in homeless or poverty-stricken families suffer from a higher accident rate and have poorer health records than the rest of the population. Health can still be seen as a privilege for certain groups of children. Access to opportunities for self-development through play is likewise unevenly spread. Poorer children are more likely to live near industrial sites and busy roads and are less likely to have opportunities for safe play indoors or outdoors. Poor housing conditions and homelessness also undermine the health of many children.

Although standards of public provision in this country have contributed to the improvement in children's health, increasing levels of pollution may have a counter-effect. The decline of the school meals service and the use of schools to counterbalance deficiencies in family diets affects a large number of children. Insufficient levels of publicly funded childcare have led to a variation in the quality of childcare and exclude many single parents from the job opportunities which would significantly improve their family income. Children in this country, as elsewhere, are still engaging in work which may be harmful to their health and wellbeing. Some are exposed to the illegal use of drugs. More are using the socially accepted drugs of tobacco and alcohol under the legal age or are exposed to passive smoking. At school, children's wellbeing can be undermined by bullying or a sense of failure. Within families, children can be exposed to the problems of marital breakdown or to abuse.

Through the United Nations convention and the Children Act 1989 the integrity of the child underscores the principles outlined. The child is entitled to an identity, to be consulted, to have access to information, freedom of speech and opinion, and to challenge decisions made on his or her behalf. The child's best interests are placed at the heart of the matter. To what extent our schools, social services, courts, hospitals, childcare clinics, GP practices, advertising agencies, television and so on follow this code is open to question.

Acknowledgement

I would particularly like to acknowledge the assistance of the Children's Rights Development Unit, London.

REFERENCES AND FURTHER READING

Balding, J. (1992) *Young People in 1992.* Schools Health Education Unit, University of Exeter.

Bradshaw, J. (1990) *Child Poverty and Deprivation in the UK.* National Children's Bureau, London.

Brannen, J. & Moss. P. (1991) *Managing Mothers: Dual Earner Households after Maternity Leave.* Allen & Unwin, London.

Cohen, B. (1991) *Childcare in a Modern System: Towards a New National Policy.* Institute for Public Policy Research, London.

Cohen, R., Coxall, J., Craig, G. & Sadiq-Sangster, A. (1992) *Hardship Britain: Being Poor in the 1990s.* Child Poverty Action Group, London.

Consumer Safety Unit (1992) *Home and Accident Research.* 1990 Data, Department of Trade and Industry. HMSO, London.

Conway, J. (1988) *Prescription for Poor Health: the Crisis for Homeless Families.* Shelter, London.

David, T. (1990) *Under Five – Under Educated?* Open University Press, Milton Keynes.

Davie, R. (1993) The impact of the National Child Development Study, *Children and Society,* 7(1), 20–36.

Davie, C.E., Hunt, S.J., Vincent, E. & Mason, M. (1988) Essential Child-Rearing Practices. In *Early Education: the Pre-School Years* (eds A. Cohen & L. Cohen.) Paul Chapman, London.

DoE (1993) *English House Conditions Survey 1991 – Preliminary Report on Unfit Dwellings.* Department of the Environment, HMSO, London.

Douglas, J. (1993) *Psychology and Nursing Children.* Macmillan, BPS books, Basingstoke.

Ferguson, A. & McInlay, I. (1991) Adolescent Smoking. *Childcare, Health and Development,* 17(3), 213–24.

Franklin, B. (1989) Children's rights: developments and prospects. *Children and Society,* 3(1), 50–66.

Fyfe, A. (1989) *Child Labour.* Polity Press, Oxford.

Gordon, P. (1990) *Racial Violence and Harassment.* Runnymede Trust, London.

Grant, J. (ed.) (1993) *The State of the World's Children.* UNICEF. Oxford University Press, Oxford.

Health of the Nation (1992) *Health of the Nation: A Strategy for Health in England.* HMSO, London.

Hendrick, H. (1990) Constructions and reconstructions of British childhood: an interpretative survey. 1800 to the present. In *Constructing and Reconstructing Childhood* (eds A. James & A. Prout). Falmer, Basingstoke.

Hennissey, E., Martin, S., Moss, P. & Melhuish, E. (1992) *Children and Day Care: Lessons from Research.* Paul Chapman, Liverpool.

Hilman, M., Adams, J. & Whitelegg, J. (1991) *One False Move … a Study of Children's Independent Mobility.* PSI Publishing, London.

Huby, M. & Dix, G. (1992) *Evaluating the Social Fund.* DSS Research Report No. 9. HMSO, London.

Humphries, S., Mack, J. & Perks, R. (1988) *A Century of Childhood,* pp. 39–40, 56. Sidgewick & Jackson, London.

Jaques, P. (1987) *Understanding Children's Problems – Helping Families to Help Themselves.* Unwin Hyman Ltd, London.

Joseph, M. (1990) *Sociology for Everyone.* Polity Press/Basil Blackwell, Cambridge.

Kelly, E. & Cohn, T. (1988) *Racism in Schools – New Research Evidence*. Trentham Books, Stoke-on-Trent.

Kurtz, L. & Tomlinson, J. (1991) How do we value our children today, as reflected by children's health, health care and policy? *Children and Society*, 5(3), 207–22.

La Fontaine, J. (1991) *Bullying: the Child's View*. Caloustie Gulbenkian Foundation, London.

Lee-Wright, P. (1990) *Child Slaves*, pp. 53–4. Anti-Slavery Society, London.

McIntosh, J. (1992) The perception and use of child health clinics in a sample of working class families. *Childcare, Health and Development*, 18(3), 133–50.

MacLennan, E., Fitz, J. & Sullivan, J. (1985) *Working Children*. Low Pay Unit, London.

Mayall, B. (1990) A joy or a hassle: child health care in a multi-ethnic society. *Children and Society*, 4(2), 197–223.

Mayall, B., & Foster, M.C. (1989) *Child Health Care, Living with Children, Working with Children*. Heinemann, Oxford.

Meadow, R. (ed.) (1989) *ABC of Child Abuse*, p. 1. British Medical Journal, London.

Melhuish, E. & Moss, P. (1990) *Day Care for Young Children: International Perspectives*. Routledge, London.

Mellor, A. (1991) Helping victims. In *Bullying: a Practical Guide for Coping in Schools* (ed. M. Elliott), p. 93. Longman/Kidscape, Harlow.

Moss, P. (1990) Work, family and the care of children: equality and responsibility. *Children and Society*, 4(2), 145–65.

Moss, P. (1992) Perspectives from Europe. In *Contemporary Issues in the Early Years: Working Collaboratively with Children* (ed. G. Pugh). Paul Chapman Publishing, London.

Moss, P., Brophy, J. & Statham, J. (1992) Parental involvement through playgroups. *Children and Society*, 6(4), 297–316.

NACAB (1992) *High and Dry: CAB Evidence on Water Charges, Debts and Disconnections*. National Association of Citizen's Advice Bureaux, London.

Newsom, J. & Newsom, E. (1965) *Patterns of Infant Care in an Urban Community*. Penguin, Harmondsworth.

OPCS (1988) *Occupational Mortality, England and Wales – Childhood Supplement*. Office of Population Censuses and Surveys. HMSO, London.

Oppenheim, C. (1993) *Poverty: the Facts*. Child Poverty Action Group, London.

Pond, C. & Searle, A. (1991) *The Hidden Army: Children at Work in the 1990s*. Low Pay Unit, London.

Pringle, M.K. (1980) *A Fairer Future for Children*. National Children's Bureau, London.

Pugh, G. (ed.) (1992) *Contemporary Issues in the Early Years: Working Collaboratively with Children*. Paul Chapman Publishing in association with the National Children's Bureau, London.

RCN (1994a) *Nursing and Child Protection: an RCN survey*. Royal College of Nursing, London.

RCN (1994b) *Protecting Children: an RCN guide for nurses*. Royal College of Nursing, London.

RCP (1992) *Smoking and the Young*. Royal College of Physicians, London.

Riches, P. (1991) The New Children Act: an Overview. *Children and Society*, 5(1), 3–10.

Road Accidents: Great Britain (1991, 1992). HMSO, London.

Roland, E. & Munthe, E. (1989) *Bullying: an International Perspective*. David Fulton, London.

Rosenbaum, M. (1993) *Children and the Environment*. National Children's Bureau, London.

Rouse, D. (ed.) (1990) *Babies and Toddlers: Carers and Educators. Quality for the Under Threes*. National Children's Bureau, London.

Smith, P.K. & Cowie, H. (1988) *Understanding Children's Development*. Basil Blackwell, Oxford.

Social Trends (1992). HMSO, London.

Social Trends (1993). HMSO, London.

Sommer, D. (1992) A child's place in society: new challenges for the family and day care. *Children and Society*, 6(4), 317–35.

Spencer, N.J. (1990) Poverty and child health: an annotation. *Children and Society*, 4(4), 352–64.

Troyna, B. & Hatcher, R. (1992) *Racism in Children's Lives: A Study of Mainly White Primary Schools*. Routeledge, London.

Vittachi, A. (1989) *Stolen Childhoods*. Polity Press/Basil Blackwell, Cambridge.

White, A. (1989) Early infant feeding practice: socio-economic factors and health visiting support. *Childcare, Health and Development*, 15(2), 129–36.

White, D. & Woolett, A. (1992) *Families: a Context for Development*. Falmer, London.

Wicks, M. (1989) Family trends, insecurities and social policy. *Children and Society*, 3(1), 67–79.

Woodruffe, C. & Glickman, M. (1993) Trends in health care. *Children and Society*, 17(1), 49–61.

Chapter 7

The Impact of Illness on the Child and Family

Kathy Bird and Annette K. Dearmun

INTRODUCTION

This chapter has two main aims: to give an overview of some of the psychological and social impacts, influences or effects of illness on the child and their family, and to identify some strategies which may be used to minimize some of the potentially negative responses associated with illness and, in some situations, admission to hospital.

The emphasis in this chapter will be upon the British context although it is recognized that rich and diverse literature pertaining to this topic has been generated by authors and researchers in the United States of America.

An awareness of the impact of illness (Fig 7.1) is important to the children's nurse when planning health promotion strategies and comprehensive care, taking into account individual psychological and social needs. The first section offers some overall strategies to minimize the impact of illness. Sections two to five explore perspectives on development, culture, the family, siblings and child in hospital respectively.

OVERALL STRATEGIES TO MINIMIZE THE IMPACT OF ILLNESS

It could be argued that there are several overall strategies which may reduce the impact of illness and potential disruption to family life.

First, as 'parents are primarily responsible for the health and care of their children as well as recognizing signs of illness and seeking appropriate help and advice' (Murphy 1990), by encouraging parents to utilize health promotion opportunities, many illnesses may be prevented; for example, accident prevention programmes (Levene 1992) or immunization schemes.

Adequate education may also reduce the number of inappropriate attendances in the accident and emergency department (Bolton & Storrie 1991) and nurses can create opportunities to address primary health education (Philpott 1994). By drawing on the skills of a community nursing service it is possible to keep children out of hospital and in their own homes (Burr 1991). By reviewing the time the child spends in hospital and introducing, for example, day surgery (Thornes 1991; Coleman 1993) and innovations in outpatient depart-

ments (Stower 1993) and procedures, the amount of time spent in hospital will be reduced.

The environments in which children are nursed should be monitored to ensure that they are child oriented. This includes the accident and emergency department which may be the first point of contact with the health services (Gay 1991; Powell 1991), or the outpatient or X-ray areas (Stower 1993).

Finally, members of the multiprofessional team should have the appropriate knowledge and skills to work with children.

It could be argued that all these aspects will be addressed if health professionals subscribe to a philosophy of children's care that embraces the psychosocial needs of the child. These have been identified by many authors including Shelley (1993) and Swanwick & Barlow (1993).

DEVELOPMENTAL PERSPECTIVES

Illness and development can be seen to be interrelated. For example, the way in which illness is perceived may be affected by development, and illness may have an impact on developmental progress. Some illnesses are more prevalent in certain age groups; examples of these include accidents in the under fives and diabetes in the over fives.

The child's perception of health and illness

The impact of an event is largely unique to the individual and their reactions will often depend upon current circumstances, previous experience and their interpretations.

> 'Children at every stage of development are attempting to form mental constructs of the world around them in order to understand it' (Swanwick 1990a).

Therefore the nurse needs to have an appreciation of a child's understanding of illness as their cognitive development may influence their reactions and interpretation of illness. Several authors (Bibace & Walsh 1980; Swanwick 1990a, b; Eiser 1991a) have drawn on the work of developmental theorists, generally domi-

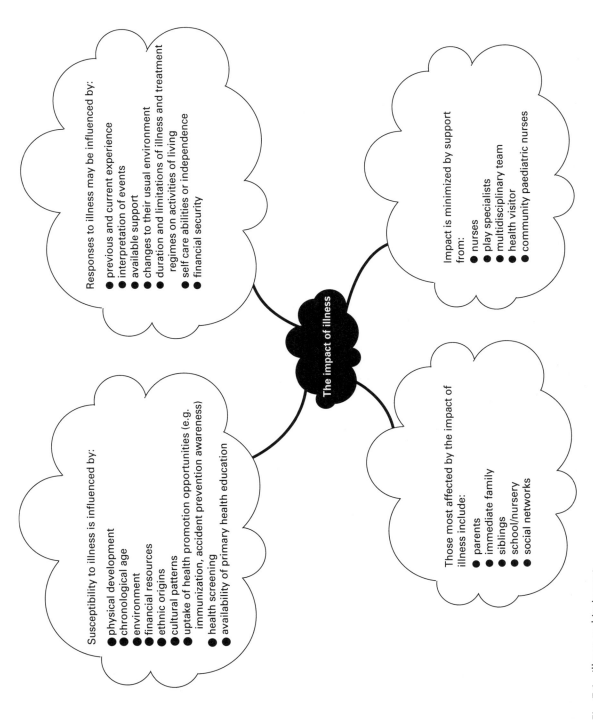

Responses to illness may be influenced by:

- previous and current experience
- interpretation of events
- available support
- changes to their usual environment
- duration and limitations of illness and treatment regimes on activities of living
- self care abilities or independence
- financial security

Impact is minimized by support from:

- nurses
- play specialists
- multidisciplinary team
- health visitor
- community paediatric nurses

Susceptibility to illness is influenced by:

- physical development
- chronological age
- environment
- financial resources
- ethnic origins
- cultural patterns
- uptake of health promotion opportunities (e.g. immunization, accident prevention awareness)
- health screening
- availability of primary health education

Those most affected by the impact of illness include:

- parents
- immediate family
- siblings
- school/nursery
- social networks

The impact of illness

Fig. 7.1   Illness and its impact.

nated by the Piagetian perspective, to provide a framework within which to discuss these issues. Other perspectives are offered by Vygotsky (1978, cited in Rushforth 1994) who emphasized the nature of the social and cultural context, and by Eiser (1989).

Bibace and Walsh (1980) offered a framework, drawing on the theory generated by Piaget. They interviewed children at various ages in order to understand their concepts of illness. Swanwick (1990a) applied a similar approach to the understanding of children's concepts of illness and suggested ways in which this knowledge could be used by nurses to offer meaningful explanations about care and treatment. Swanwick (1990b) in another study took a different perspective and considered the theory put forward by Erikson in order to identify particular developmental needs of chronically sick children.

There is considerable evidence to suggest that a child's belief of health and illness develops in a systematic and predictable sequence (Eiser 1985) and for this reason the discussion will take a chronological focus.

Some of the particular features at each age will now be discussed, together with some of the relevant nursing interventions which may be used to enhance children's own coping mechanisms if they are admitted to hospital.

From 0–2 years

The child of 0–2 years is described as being in the sensory motor stage, as babies are thought to learn mainly through their senses and by activity. During this stage the baby gains information from objects around them by sucking, kicking, crying and smiling. Babies may have feelings associated with pleasure, discomfort or pain but probably will not understand the reasons for these. Their actions generate responses for both objects and other humans. Familiar objects and people may begin to give them a feeling of security, especially when they receive positive attention.

A baby who is crying will often respond to a cuddle from their parents (consistent carers), particularly when the baby feels hungry, in discomfort or unwell, and the consistent carer will usually be able to interpret and meet the child's needs. It is particularly important that security and comfort are maintained during illness and the parents are in a prime position to achieve this. This is one of major reasons given in support of the inclusion of parents in the care of their children in hospital.

Bowlby (1952) identified a series of behavioural

reactions displayed by toddlers when left in an unfamiliar environment; these came to be known as protest, despair and regression. Further research into this area, related to children in hospital, was undertaken by Robertson (1958) and the results began to influence child care and the nursing of ill children. This historical progression has received considerable attention in the literature, for example Cleary (1992), Nethercott (1993) and While (1992).

The nurse with knowledge of the potential effects of separation is able to help parents in making decisions about staying in hospital. It is important to consider the parents' perspective and to support their decisions so that value judgements are not made about those parents who have their own reasons for not staying in hospital if, for example, they have a fear or dislike of hospitals or have other siblings at home requiring their attention. Some parents perceive that if they are unable to be resident, visiting their child will be detrimental. The following quote from a mother may illustrate this:

'He cried when I got here and doesn't want to know, I can't do anything with him . . .'

In this situation the nurse who can interpret these reactions will be able to explain them to parents, thereby supporting them through this difficult experience.

If parents are not able to be present, nursing can be organised to enhance consistency by using primary, team or named nursing systems (Grahan and Rogers 1993).

From 2–7 years

During 2–7 years the child enters the pre operational or pre-logical stage. As children pass from infancy into the toddler stage they appear to develop independence and an increasing ability to help themselves, to become more able to make their desires known and to begin to experience a sense of autonomy. This autonomy may depend upon the maintenance of security, routine and rituals. Medical procedures, even a noninvasive medical examination, taking of temperature or applying EMLA cream, may threaten this security and limit autonomy, resulting in a display of negative reactions such as anger and forceful resistance.

Children of this age group appear to be egocentric, thinking mostly of themselves. To the parent or nurse looking on their thought processes probably seem illogical and they may engage in magical thinking. For example Bibace & Walsh (1980) found that some children thought 'that people got colds from trees'. Other writers have reported that children associate hospital with punishment for wrong doing (Brewster (1982) or that 'you go into hospital healthy and became ill whilst you are there'. Both these examples indicate that children may perceive illness as external or remote and that they have limited understanding of their bodily functions. The key question is do these misconceptions demonstrate developmental immaturity or merely the child making sense of their world on the basis of limited information. There is evidence from American based studies to suggest that understanding can be significantly enhanced by education (Bessinger & Stevens 1991), a factor not congruent with a Piagetian perspective; this should be borne in mind when explaining procedures or illness.

A toddler's memory and attention span can be short and they seem to move from one activity to another. Since they are very active in exploring their environment this can lead to hazards both in the hospital and home environment. The nurse who is aware of these features will plan play opportunities and preparation schemes to provide a variety of stimuli, and will recognize the need to ensure the child's safety.

From 7–11 years

The child of 7–11 years is within the concrete operational stage. During this time understanding and reasoning abilities are becoming more refined and sophisticated. Often children still perceive the cause of illness to be external, constructed in terms of physical contact with harmful agents for example 'germs' (Brewster 1982). The Piagetian view would contend that children of this age do not fully comprehend the mechanisms of illness and see their bodies on the surface, rarely speculating upon what goes on inside. Later in this stage their reasoning becomes more developed and they may begin to make connections between, for example, eating something and experiencing tummy ache (Perrin & Gerrity 1981). But again, many of the more recent theorists refute these notions.

The lack of understanding may have more to do with knowledge than developmental maturity, especially as it appears that the child is able to apply knowledge from lessons at school, to name internal organs and begin to realize where they are situated, and to recognize that illness may be prevented by eating good food or not smoking.

Sometimes the child may have difficulties in vocaliz-

ing their emotions and may use defences such as adopting an air of bravado in order to cope or 'contend with' their feelings of stress (Jennings 1992b).

Enforced immobility, for example as a result of trauma, may be a particular challenge in this age group as they are generally used to being active and lack of opportunity to utilize energy may create frustration for the child and parents.

Young adults

When considering the young adult it may be difficult to view the thought processes in isolation from the rapid physical growth and change at this time, because the physical development has emotional and social implications and they are thus interrelated. At the formal operation stage, young adults can usually reason and think more logically. They may be increasingly aware of the many causes of illness, seeing it in terms of non-functioning body processes. As they become increasingly independent from their parents, they may become susceptible to peer pressure to experiment with practices that may be harmful to their health (Murphy 1990b). In some cases their knowledge may be incomplete and they may have particular anxieties about the future.

Body image and self esteem are especially important (Price 1993) and illness which results in changes in appearance, for example leukaemia or growth hormone insufficiency, are particularly distressing. Evans (1993) identifies some of these challenges in respect to the young adult with cancer.

The issue of the needs of the young adult as a distinct group is currently high on the agenda and has received increasing interest in the literature (Burr 1993; Shelley 1993).

Overall development

Overall, although it may be particularly useful to use the Piagetian framework in order to structure a discussion about the child's perception of illness, the limitations of this approach should be acknowledged. Piaget's methodology has been criticized (Vessey 1988; Bird & Podmore 1990; Hergenrather & Rabinowitch 1991). It makes little reference to cultural or social influences, there is no account of the transition of one stage to another, no recognition of different experiences, and minimal integration of the social and emotional implications of physical development. It also assumes that observed behaviour identifies the limitations of a child's ability, and it gives limited credence to the potential to enhance understanding by instruction.

Knowledge of development is important for the children's nurse but more as a base upon which to determine the appropriateness of preparation or educational programmes, rather than as a demonstration of the child's optimum level of understanding.

Swanwick (1990b) identified the extent to which chronic illness can influence developmental progress and suggested that the impact of chronic illness can depend upon several factors including:

- The type of illness;
- Iatrogenic effects of medication.
- Subsequent limitations or disruptions to life.
- Differences in the individual.
- Family dynamics.
- Attitudes of peers and siblings.

Many illnesses bring about temporary or permanent changes in appearance. Although this is a generally under-researched area, Price (1993) offers several case studies in order to explore the impact that this has upon a child's body image. It is suggested that:

'the aesthetic qualities of a splint or brace, the choice of hat during alopecia or ways of handling feelings about insulin injections or dependence upon medications, may depend upon how these additions make the child feel about their body during these times of change' (Price 1993).

Although various theories are put forward to explain ways in which children develop these images about themselves, again their reactions to this aspect of their illness may be unique.

The impact of restrictions or treatment regimes

Children who have a long term or disabling illness are often given limited opportunities to explore their environment and are restricted in play; this may hinder their development. For example, in both hospital and home settings, the neonate with multiple problems may have their developmental needs overshadowed by the technical and medical needs of their care (Horsley 1990). Nurses planning the care of vulnerable babies need to

take into account sensory, motor and intellectual stimulation of these babies, who may be in a restricted environment, and to initiate programmes of care that will promote motor, cognitive, social and emotional development (Sparshott 1991).

Technological advances, especially in neonatology, have created a population of neonates who have extended hospital stays. Ludman (1992), a research psychologist, recognized that there were few longitudinal studies which explored the potential impact of this on the infant's social and emotional wellbeing, therefore he undertook experimental research comparing the development of healthy new born babies with that of babies admitted for intensive care. When followed up over time the results showed that play and behavioural patterns were similar, although the play in the intensive care group was less advanced and more passive, and behaviour was less active and social.

Ludman (1992) concluded that it should not be assumed that parental presence alone will prevent emotional damage to the child in hospital; in addition lengthy periods in hospital may interfere with parenting. This study may emphasize the importance of the nurse's role in promoting positive developmental outcomes for the ill child, by attempting to minimize the negative effects of technology on development and by educating the parents of critically ill babies to enable them to seek opportunities to provide additional stimulation and to develop their child's independence.

A developmental plan can be incorporated into nursing activities; for example, talking to them whilst checking the intravenous infusion, playing peek-a-boo whilst changing a nappy, or encouraging water play during a bath.

The nurse who has knowledge of developmental principles will be able to assess the child's needs, and by liaison with the play specialist, community groups, toy libraries and opportunity play groups will continue the development of appropriate milestones.

It has been suggested that parents who experience guilt may become over protective and thus inhibit the child's attempts to attain independence. They may fear that socialising with peers or a return to school may expose the child to the risk of infection; this may be particularly true of the child who is on immunosuppressant or steroid therapy. Such parents need to be given the opportunity to discuss their fears, and given help, encouragement and information, they may be able to put the risks into perspective and to be aware of appropriate action to take if their fears are realized. If this is achieved it will be more likely that they will allow the child to participate in activities with their peers, and thus maximize the child's social development.

Education may be disrupted by absence from school due to frequent illness, the unpleasant effects of medication and admission to hospital (Wilson 1993). Home tuition can be offered, together with liaison with the nursery and school to encourage the child's integration in educational activities.

If nurses have knowledge of the personal and social tasks commensurate with optimal health during the life span of an individual, they will be in a prime position to support the child and family through the concerns and conflicts unique to each stage. Swanwick (1990b) maintains that the nurse needs to consider all aspects of development in order to assess the extent to which the child's illness or management may be imposing limitations. It is important to make an appraisal of whether the needs associated with the management of the illness are taking priority over the needs for stimulation, socialization and education.

Both the effects of the child's cognitive development upon their understanding of illness and the effect of the illness on their development have been discussed; however, there are other factors which influence the impact of illness on the child and family, including cultural aspects, and the responses and reactions of parents, siblings and peers.

CULTURAL PERSPECTIVES

This section will address the cultural perspective on the impact of illness. Culture and illness may be seen to overlap. A definition of culture is offered by Linton (1940, cited in Weller 1994) as 'the knowledge, attitudes and habitual behaviour patterns shared and transmitted by a particular society'. Dodson (1983) suggests that culture should be viewed as dynamic as well as socially inherited. Richardson (1993) suggests that cultural issues 'have been gaining popularity among British nurses as a topic worthy of study'. However, to date the cultural dimension of children's nursing care appears to have been given scant overt attention in the British nursing literature.

Some illnesses are culturally linked, for example thalassaemia or sickle cell anaemia. Reactions to illness can be influenced by cultural and religious beliefs because individuals from different cultures have different value systems and personality characteristics. Indeed, illness in the family may induce an examination of religious beliefs or cultural practice in an attempt to rationalize or discover the reasons for the illness (Robertshaw, 1987). Some treatments associated with illness may create dilemmas, for example the child in a Jehovah's Witness family who requires blood products, or the Jewish child who requires animal insulin.

There may be food preferences which influence adherence with treatment; for example, there is a Chinese philosophy which considers that certain foods are not compatible with certain medical conditions (Slater 1993), so parents may not feel comfortable in adhering to dietary advice. Pain may be manifest depending upon the 'cultural differences in acceptable external behaviour' (Weller 1994). Child rearing practices, family dynamics and the position of women may differ between different societies. This latter point may have implications when identifying the most appropriate family member to keep informed of care and changes in a child's condition.

It can be seen that there are several reasons why it is important for the children's nurse to consider the cultural perspective on the impact of illness. Weller (1994) suggests that there is essentially an 'ethnocentric orientation' to health care provision and this has not shifted fundamentally since 1948. So when one cultural perspective, commonly the Western perspective, is perceived as the 'best' or 'correct' way to behave, this often leads to the development of value judgements according to this criteria.

When discussing culture it may also be important to consider language. If a child and family do not feel confident communicating in the English language, this may lead to challenges in communication, leading to additional stress. Slater (1993) described parents' feelings of frustration because of difficulties in communication and the associated humiliation and embarrassment of not being able to understand. If nurses are aware of the local interpreting arrangements they can support these families by providing access to interpreters.

Nurses should consider the differences between cultural groups and reflect upon these influences on the child and family. During assessment, cultural needs, the influence of culture and the subsequent beliefs and expectations of health care, should be explored with the family. The importance of respecting an individual's values and beliefs is recognized in the UKCC Code of Professional Conduct (1992), clause 7:

> 'Recognize and respect the uniqueness and dignity of each patient, client, and respond to their need for care irrespective of their ethnic origin, religious beliefs, personal attributes, the nature of their health problem or any other factor.'

THE FAMILY'S PERSPECTIVE

Whilst examining parents' responses to illness it is important to emphasize the positive roles they can play in protecting their child from illness, in managing common disorders as well as complex treatment regimes, and in helping children to cope with their problems. Effective performance in these aspects of care may reduce the impact of illness by enabling the child to stay at home.

Whenever a child is sick parents will worry. This level of concern may be heightened if the child is admitted to hospital, and it will vary depending on whether the illness is acute and short lasting or chronic and long term. In any event, parents will have to make arrangements for the care of other children and reorganize family routines. Parents also have to divide their loyalties to cope with maintaining the normality of life for the rest of the family, and to make decisions and prioritize their time in order to give care to the child who is sick.

Murphy (1990) suggested that 'health for children will depend upon the physical, emotional, sociocultural, political and economic environment into which they are born and raised'. It could be argued that response to illness and ability to cope may depend largely upon the same factors, as well as how the event is perceived. Some families seem realistic in their outlook and may have more supportive family networks and resources at their disposal. Other families, particularly if they are financially disadvantaged, may be more pessimistic. The Black Report (DHSS 1980) found that different social groups responded to illness in different ways. The nurse is in a position to maximize the coping abilities and

parenting skills of parents by offering support and providing access to a range of resources (Bishop 1992).

Cox (1992) examines the parental role in critical care and discusses the parents' perceptions of stress and the coping strategies developed by the families in order to deal with them. Cox identifies these as role changes, financial concerns, isolation from the family and loss.

The response of the family to the diagnosis of chronic illness has been described in various ways (Whyte 1990; Canam 1993). These range from shock and disbelief through to adjustment and final acceptance of the situation. Canam (1993) identified the adaptive tasks facing parents of children with chronic illness. These seem to relate to those focused on the child, those centred around the family, and those involving others; for example, accepting and managing the child's condition; meeting the developmental needs of the whole family as well as the ill child; and establishing support systems and educating others about the child's condition. The range of activities demonstrates the enormity of the tasks facing these families.

Whyte (1990) used a family profile to demonstrate a progression through various stages, including rejection and eventual adaptation to the child's problems. This study illustrated the coping mechanisms employed and ways in which each individual is affected in a unique way. An appreciation of some of the responses and coping mechanisms used by families when faced with the illness of a child may enable nurses to help them understand these feelings, as nurses are ideally placed to recognize coping strategies and to intervene appropriately (Cox 1992).

When offered a diagnosis parents often describe feelings of great relief. The following example illustrates this:

> '... the not knowing is awful; although it is still upsetting to know what he has, at least I know what I am up against.'

However this relief of 'putting a label' on the child's illness can also be associated with feelings of disbelief and shock. Timely, accurate information at the appropriate level may help parents to accept the situation (Muller *et al.* 1992).

It is important for the child's nurse to be with the parents and the medical staff when 'bad news' is broken, as the nurse can provide time afterwards to sit with the family whilst they assimilate the information they have been given. Whyte (1990, cited in Jennings 1992a) suggested that if the nurse intervenes early, at the critical point, this is likely to be more effective than trying to alter maladaptive responses. Although it may feel more comfortable to be able to reassure the parents that 'it will be alright . . .', 'it's OK, they are easily controlled by drugs these days and can carry on a normal life' or 'no of course he is not going to die', it is important not to offer complacent responses as this may inhibit parents in exploring their feelings and asking further questions.

Shock and disbelief may become denial and parents and family may appear to distance themselves from the emotional impact of the diagnosis by making unrealistic plans for the future or refusing to discuss the illness; sometimes they may become critical of care or may insist upon another medical opinion. Guilt is another common response of families (Jennings 1992b), and this may also be felt by siblings (Hewitt 1990). If the illness is of genetic origin or the child is disabled as the result of a preventable accident, these feelings and expressions of guilt are likely to be heightened.

If the child is severely disabled and unable to achieve the potential to which the parents aspire, there may be intense feelings of love combined with loathing. The following illustrates this point: '. . . I didn't want her or the trouble she was causing. I wanted to wheel her pram into a shop and leave her there . . .'

On other occasions this mother said: 'Some days I love her so much, and if I don't and don't protect her, who will?'

A frequent issue for parents is the physical, emotional and financial cost relative to the positive outcomes of treatment regimes, especially when they do not guarantee success. If treatment regimes are realistic and take into account the family lifestyle they are more likely to be seen as part of life rather than the life revolving around the illness.

Sometimes voluntary temporary or permanent unemployment is the only option for the parent who has to look after the ill child. This can lead to loss of independence and identity, may create further isolation, and may have other negative consequences for the family in addition to the loss of income.

There may be effects on the parents' personal relationships. If they become preoccupied by the child's problems and the child's needs become paramount, they may have less time for each other, fewer opportunities to socialize, and be unable to offer practical, social, emotional or sexual support to each other. This may increase the tension in the relationship. A comment from a father is illuminating:

'To arrange to go out needed organization; it was difficult to tell how she would be a day ahead, let alone a week ahead, and the uncertainty rather dulled the anticipation and enthusiasm of planning.'

Although Jennings (1992b) found that the divorce rate in such families may be higher than average, it was also acknowledged that some parents actually became closer during the child's illness:

'. . . He [the partner] gave me endless support; he is placid and resolute, he helped to keep me on an even keel . . . he was at home in the evenings as early as possible, prepared supper most evenings and allowed me to lie in on Sunday morning by taking over the care.'

Nurses should be aware of the range of specialist information or resources, for example, support groups, written information which should be current, accurate and clear, and access to a named health professional or 'befrienders' (Jennings 1992b). Jennings undertook a study into the way in which parents cope with a child with a life threatening or terminal illness. It seems that many parents experienced strong feelings of anger and aggression which they felt were largely unrecognized by the professionals. Other negative feelings were highlighted, including guilt or self blame. They also reported 'taking things day by day' and many turned to religion or prayer for support, taking a 'mental' rather than physical approach to coping.

Perhaps the ultimate impact of illness is the death of a child and Brenkley (1991) discusses the stages of grief and suggests ways in which support may be given. In essence again, reactions are variable, and Kubler Ross (1974), Parkes (1974) and Warder (1982), all cited in Brenkley (1991), identify these and they suggest that sometimes resolution of them takes years.

THE SIBLINGS' PERSPECTIVE

It is relevant to explore the impact of illness upon siblings as this is likely to be the longest relationship that is shared with another human being; they spend lengthy periods together during childhood and share many experiences. They experience life through each other and learn from each other (Dunn 1983, cited in Hewitt 1990). They share, compete, compromise and co-operate with one another and develop a close attachment bond; any alteration to this relationship may evoke negative responses or reactions. Studies related to this area tend to centre on the effects of chronic illness, cancer (Mikklelsen 1993) or children with learning disabilities rather than acute illness.

Sometimes siblings are concerned that some action of theirs has caused the illness. Reactions vary and many factors will influence their behaviour, for example when the sick child becomes the focus of attention it may evoke feelings of jealousy and brothers or sisters may exhibit negative behaviour (Ferrari 1984), leading to disruptions in relationships at school or to psychosomatic problems.

Although the focus tends to be on negative reactions, siblings may become caring and protective towards the sick child. Hewitt (1990) conducted interviews to study this aspect; although the limitations of the study are acknowledged, there were several relevant findings.

First, siblings displayed several concerns, related to the child being ill, separation from the ill child and the need to be able to visit. This last aspect seemed particularly significant as it gave them reassurance. Interestingly they showed neither a negative nor positive response to the fact that their brother or sister was in hospital.

Second, commonly siblings were called upon to take on a caring role and accept responsibility for younger members of the family; they therefore experienced role disruption themselves. This may be minimized if nurses are aware of the potential impact of illness, discuss the likely reactions with parents in advance and involve siblings in care, providing them with comprehensive information (Martinson *et al.* 1990).

Dominic (1993) explores the anxieties and coping mechanisms demonstrated by siblings of children with cancer, and draws upon Walker's taxonomy of coping (Walker 1988, cited in Dominic 1993) to show the diversity of coping mechanisms that these children use to meet their own needs. They can be helped to adapt to potentially stressful situations by the use of education, distraction and opportunities to communicate.

THE CHILD'S PERSPECTIVE OF A HOSPITAL EXPERIENCE

Many children are still admitted to hospital during their childhood and many of these admissions will occur during the first five years of life (NAWCH 1987; Cleary 1992). As suggested earlier, children of differing ages respond to being in hospital in different ways. Their reaction will largely depend on previous experiences of separation and the nature of any preparation for admission and treatment.

Cross (1990) studied children aged two to seven years following discharge from hospital and identified nervousness about separation, demanding behaviour and disturbed sleeping patterns. It was discovered, however, that children over the age of five settled more easily.

Apart from the overall strategies to minimize the impact of illness, as mentioned in the introduction to this chapter, other aspects of care which should be given further consideration are avoiding separation, parental participation, attention to the environment, and the related aspects of play and preparation for events.

The value of parental involvement in care is given considerable attention in the literature and there is evidence that a parent's presence in hospital makes a major contribution to a child's welfare, not least by reducing separation. Furthermore, Taylor & O'Connor (1989) suggested that length of stay may be reduced if the parent is resident with their child. Many areas are explored in the literature, including the role or contribution of parents to care giving (Cleary (1992); Dearmun (1992)), involvement during particular critical events, for example in the anaesthetic room (Glasper 1991) or in pain assessment and management (Dearmun 1993), and analysis of the concept of family centred care (Campbell & Summergill 1993; Campbell *et al.* 1993).

It is generally accepted that providing information and offering emotional support reduces parents' anxiety and this in turn lessens the child's distress (Visintainer & Wolfer 1975). Misunderstanding may occur if the nurse and parent do not have clear common goals (Casey & Mobbs 1988). It is important to negotiate involvement so parents do not feel that 'they are just left to get on with it' (Callery & Smith 1991).

Separation anxiety may be further minimized if organizational strategies are devised to provide continuity of care by named nursing, team or primary

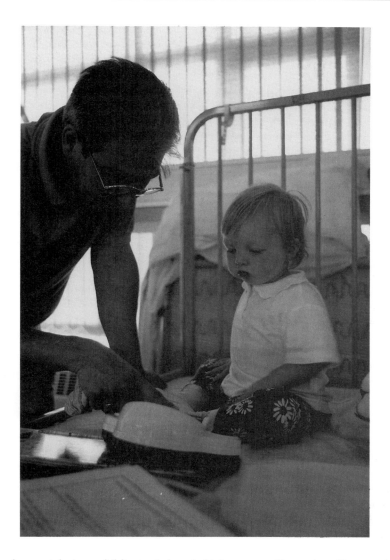

Fig. 7.2   Family involvement during a child's stay in hospital is important. *(Reproduced by permission of Jon Sparks.)*

nursing (Gahan & Rogers 1993). This relationship can enable the nurse to develop rapport with the child and gain knowledge from the parents of the child's reactions and coping strategies in strange environments.

Doverty (1992) offers a comprehensive appraisal of the therapeutic use of play in hospital. He suggests that:

'play provides a child with learning opportunities in self mastery, skills in environmental experience, reality testing, co-ordination versus passivity, wish fulfilment and most importantly spontaneous free fun.'

It may be seen that the ability to play may be affected by the limitations of illness, for example lethargy associated with anaemia or immobility due to trauma, but also may be used to help a child to make sense of their situation. Therefore it is relevant to explore ways in which play may be used to minimize the impact of illness. Many articles are available on this topic and they discuss the positive effects of play in reducing anxiety (Peterson 1989), promoting normality in an alien environment (Save the Children Fund 1989), generally helping the child to understand and cope with hospital procedures

(Whiting 1993), and meeting special developmental needs (Honeyman 1994).

The Save the Children Fund (1989a) reported on play schemes and emphasized the role of the play specialist. The combined efforts of the nurse and play specialist can pool resources, offer suitable play materials and provide a catalyst for play. Hospital play specialists (Table 7.1) are educated to identify the child's current level of understanding and can initiate play that can be diversional and interesting. The Play in Hospital Liaison Committee in 1990 defined the need for play to be provided as a service distinct from the nursing function.

Table 7.1 The role of the play specialist.

- Providing the impetus for sick children to play at all.
- Reducing children's fears and anxieties during the day.
- Helping to prepare children undergoing surgery and other treatments.
- Contributing to developmental assessments.
- Involving parents in the play scheme and teaching them about play.
- Contributing to the education of other hospital staff.

As mentioned earlier, if children do not understand what is happening they may engage in fantasy and expect discomfort and pain. The importance of preparation has been widely discussed in the literature, for example Rodin (1983), Glasper & Stradling (1989), Eiser & Hanson (1991), Price (1991), Acharya (1992) and Collier & MacKinlay (1993). There are various methods used, from booklets sent out in advance of the child's admission, to pre-admission programmes where children have an opportunity to engage in preparatory play and visit the relevant departments (Whiting 1993) or visits to schools (Eisner & Hanson 1991) and road-shows (Leslie 1990).

CONCLUSION

Over the last thirty years the care for sick children seems to have changed profoundly. The philosophy of child-care has gradually moved away from a preoccupation with treating the illness to a focus on treating the child within the context of the family. This adoption of different approaches has largely been driven by recognition of the potentially negative impact of illness on the child and family.

This chapter has provided an overview of some of the aspects to consider when reflecting on the impact of illness. The issues mentioned are not exhaustive and there are other aspects that could be explored. For example, the impact of illness on travelling families or those in inner city environments, and the effects of illness on nutritional status, relationships and future employment opportunities.

Although there are many theories on development or coping, and the use of these may be helpful on one level to predict and determine the impact of illness on the child and family, they should only be used as a guide. Each individual should be individually assessed and it is inadvisable to attempt to fit the individual into the theory.

REFERENCES AND FURTHER READING

Acharya, S. (1992) Assessing the need for pre admission visits. *Paediatric Nursing*, 4(8), 20–22.

Ainsworth, H. (1989) And the guinea pig came too. *Nursing Times*, 85(39), 54–6.

Bessinger, B. & Stevens, C. (1991) Lessons of the heart: expanding practice. *Maternal and Child Health Care Nursing*, 16, September/October, 241–6.

Bibace, R. & Walsh, M.E. (1980) Development of children's concepts of illness. *Paediatrics*, 66, 913–17.

Birch, E. (1993) The key to real partnership: the importance of parent information. *Child Health*, 1(1), 25–8.

Bird, J. & Podmore, V. (1990) Children's understanding of health and illness. *Psychology and Health*, 4, 175–85.

Bishop, J. (1992) Aspects of Parenting. *Paediatric Nursing*, 4(10), 12–14.

Bolton, K. & Storrie, C. (1991) Inappropriate attendances to A&E. *Paediatric Nursing*, 3(2), 22–4.

Bowlby, J. (1952) *Maternal Care and Mental Health*. World Health Organisation, Geneva.

Brenkley, W. (1991) Understanding bereavement. *Paediatric Nursing*, 3(1), 18–21.

Brewster, A.B. (1982) Chronically ill children's concepts of their illness. *Paediatrics*, 69, 355–62.

Burr, S. (1991) The wider view. *Paediatric Nursing*, 3(5), 9–10.

Burr, S. (1993) Adolescents and the ward environment. *Paediatric Nursing*, 5(91), 10–13.

Callery, P. & Smith, L. (1991) A study of role negotiation between nurses and the parents of hospitalised children. *Journal of Advanced Nursing*, 16, 772–81.

Campbell, S. & Summergill, P. (1993) Keeping it in the family: defining and developing family centred care. *Child Health*, 1(1), 17–20.

Campbell, S., Kelly, P. & Summergill, P. (1993) Putting the family first: interpreting a framework for family centred care. *Child Health*, 1(2), 59–63.

Canam, C. (1993) Common adaptive tasks facing parents of children with chronic conditions. *Journal of Advanced Nursing*, 18, 46–53.

Casey, A. & Mobbs, S. (1988) Partnership in Practice. *Nursing Times*, 84(44), 67–8.

Cleary, J. (1992) *Caring for Children in Hospital: Parents and Nurses in Partnership*. Scutari Press, London.

Coleman, D. (1993) The value of day surgery. *Paediatric Nursing*, 5(6), 8–11.

Collier, J. & MacKinlay (1993) Play at work: play preparation guidelines for the multi-disciplinary team. *Child Health*, 1(3), 123–5.

Cox, P. (1992) Children in critical care: how parents cope. *British Journal of Nursing*, 1(15), 764–8.

Croft, M. (1991) Sibling helping children with cerebral palsy. *Nursing Times*, 87, 3 April, 50–51.

Cross, C. (1990) Home from Hospital – A CPQS Project. *Nursery World*, 90, 30 August, 22–3.

Dearmun, A.K. (1992) Perceptions on parental participation. *Paediatric Nursing*, 4(7), 6–9.

Dearmun, A.K. (1993) Towards a partnership in pain management. *Paediatric Nursing*, 5(5), 8–10.

DHSS (1980) *Report of the Working Group on Inequalities in Health* (Black Report). HMSO, London.

Dodson, S. (1983) Bringing culture into care. *Nursing Times*, 9 February, 53–7.

DoH (1991) *Welfare of Children and Young People in Hospital*. HMSO, London.

Dominic, K. (1993) Left out in the cold. *Paediatric Nursing*, 5(3), 28–9.

Doverty, N. (1992) Therapeutic use of play in hospital. *British Journal of Nursing*, 1(2), 77–81.

Eiser, C. (1985) *The Psychology of Childhood Illness*. Springer-Verlag, New York.

Eiser, C. (1989) Towards an alternative to the stage approach. *Psychology and Health*, 3, 93–101.

Eiser, C. (1991a) What children think about hospitals and illness. In *Child Care: Nursing Perspectives* (ed. A. Glasper), pp. 211–14. Wolfe Publishing, London.

Eiser, C. (1991b) Its OK having asthma . . . young children's beliefs about illness. In *Child Care: Nursing Perspectives*. (ed. A. Glasper), pp. 203–10. Wolfe Publishing, London.

Eiser, C. & Hanson, L. (1991) Preparing children for hospital: a school based intervention. In *Child Care: Nursing Perspectives* (ed. A. Glasper), pp. 215–9. Wolfe Publishing, London.

Evans, M. (1993) Teenagers and Cancer. *Paediatric Nursing*, 5(1), 14–17.

Ferrari, M. (1984) Chronic illnesses: psychological effects on siblings. *Journal of Child Psychology and Psychiatry*, 25, 459–76.

Frude, N. (1990) *Understanding Family Problems, A Psychological Approach*. Wiley & Sons Ltd, Chicester.

Gahan, B. & Rogers, M. (1993). Primary nursing in a general paediatric medical ward. In *Recent Advances in Child Health Nursing* (eds E.A. Glasper & A. Tucker), pp. 91–105. Scutari Press, London.

Gay, J. (1991) Caring for children in A & E. *Paediatric Nursing*, 3(7), 21–3.

Gear, P. (1991) The terminally ill child. *Paediatric Nursing*, 3(4), 22–3.

Gills, A.J. (1990) Nurses' knowledge of growth and developmental principles in meeting the psycho-social needs of hospitalised children. *Journal of Paediatric Nursing*, 5(2), 78–87.

Glasper, A. (1991) Parents in the anaesthetic room: a blessing or a curse. In *Child Care: Nursing Perspectives* (ed. A. Glasper), pp. 238–43. Wolfe Publishing, London.

Glasper, A. & Stradling, P. (1989) Preparing children for admission. *Paediatric Nursing*, 1(5), 18–21.

Hawthorn, P.J. (1974) *Nurse, I want my Mummy*. Royal College of Nursing, London.

Hergenrather, J.R. & Rabinowitch, M. (1991) Age related differences in the organisation of children's knowledge of illness. *Developmental Psychology*, 27(6), 952–9.

Hewitt, J. (1990). The sibling response to hospitalisation. *Paediatric Nursing*, 2(9), 12–13.

Hogg, C. (1990) *Quality Management for Children's Play in Hospital*. Save the Children, London.

Hogg (1990) Standards for Play. *Paediatric Nursing Standards*, 2(8), 6

Honeyman, L. (1994) Play for children with special needs. *Paediatric Nursing*, 6(3), 18–19.

Horsley, A. (1990) The neonatal environment. *Paediatric Nursing*, 2(1), 17–19.

Jennings, P. (1992a) Coping strategies for mother. *Paediatric Nursing*, 4(9), 24–6.

Jennings, P. (1992b) Coping mechanisms. *Paediatric Nursing*, 4(8), 13–15.

Jolly, J. (1989) The child's adaptation to hospital admission. *Nursing*, 3(34), 40–42.

Jolly, J. (1988) Meeting the special needs of children in hospital. *Senior Nurse*, 8(4), 6–9.

Leslie, O. (1990) Paediatric roadshows. *Paediatric Nursing*, 2(9), 8.

Levene, S. (1992) Preventing accidental injury to children. *Paediatric Nursing*, 4(9), 12–14.

Ludman, L. (1992) Emotional development after major neonatal surgery. *Paediatric Nursing*, 4(4), 20–22.

Martinson, I.M., Gilliss, C., Colaizzo, D.C., Freeman, M. & Bossert, E. (1990) Impact of childhood cancer on health of school-age siblings. *Cancer Nursing*, 13(3), 183–90.

Mayall, B. (1990) A joy or a hassle: child health in a multi-ethnic society. *Children and Society*, 4(2), 197–224.

Mikkelsen, J. (1993) Sibling Care. In *Advances in Child Health Nursing* (eds E.A. Glasper & A. Tucker), pp. 141–53. Scutari Press, London.

MoH (1959) *Report of the Committee on the Welfare of Children in Hospital* (Platt Report). HMSO, London.

Müller, D.J., Harris, P.J., Wattby, L. & Taylor, J.D. (1992) *Nursing Children: Psychology, Research and Practice*. Chapman and Hall, London.

Murphy G. (1990a) Promoting Child Health. *Paediatric Nursing*, 2(3), 24–25.

Murphy, G. (1990b) Promoting Child Health. *Paediatric Nursing*, 2(5), 24–5.

NAWCH (1987) *Caring for Children in the Health Services. Group report from NAWCH (now ASC), Royal College of Nursing, British Paediatric Association and National Association of Health Authorities and Trusts.* National Association for the Welfare of Children in Hospital (now ASC), London.

NAWCH (1991) Caring for Children in the Health Services: *Just for the Day*. National Association for the Welfare of Children in Hospital (now ASC), London.

Nethercott, S. (1993) A concept for all the family. Family centred care: a concept analysis. *Professional Nurse*, September, 794–7.

Parmar (1985) Family care and ethnic minorities. *Nursing*, 36, 1068–71.

Penfold, J. It's not all fun and games. *Nursery World*, 90(16), 15–17.

Perrin, E.C. & Gerrity, P.S. (1981) There's a demon in your belly: children's understanding of illness. *Paediatrics*, 67, 841–9.

Peterson, G. (1989) Let the children play. *Nursing*, 3(41), 22–5.

Powell, C. (1991) A better service. *Paediatric Nursing*, 3(7), 18–20.

Philpott, B. (1994) Our responsibility for health. *Paediatric Nursing*, 6(2), 28–9.

Powell, C. (1991) A better service. *Paediatric Nursing*, 3(7), 18–20.

Price, B. (1993) Disease and altered body image in children. *Paediatric Nursing*, 5(6), 18–21.

Price, S. (1991) Preparing Children for Admission to hospital. *Nursing Times*, 87(9), 46–9.

Richardson, J. (1993) Transcultural Aspects of Paediatric Nursing. In *Recent Advances in Child Health Nursing* (eds E.A. Glasper & A. Tucker), pp. 79–89. Scutari Press, London.

Robertshaw, D.M. (1987) Multicultural and multiracial aspects of the care of children in hospital. *Nursing*, 23, 876–80.

Robertson, J. (1958) *Young Children in Hospital*. Tavistock Publications, London.

Robertson, J. & Robertson, J. (1989) *Separation and the Very Young*. Free Association Books, London.

Rodin, J. (1983) *Will this hurt?* Royal College of Nursing, London.

Rushforth, H.E. (1994) *A study to investigate some nurses' knowledge base and reported practice with respect to children's understanding of concepts of illness.* Unpublished BA nursing education dissertation, University of Portsmouth.

Sadler, C. (1991) Child's Play. *Nursing Times*, 86, 14 March, 16–17.

Save the Children Fund (1989a) *Hospital: A deprived environment for children? The case for hospital playschemes*. Save the Children Fund, London.

Save the Children Fund (1989b) Play provision in hospitals. *Paediatric Nursing*, 1(3), 19–20.

Scott, G. (1992) Professional Play. *Nursing Standard*, 18, November, 22–23.

Shelley, H. (1993) Adolescent needs in hospital. *Paediatric Nursing*, 5(9), 16–18.

Shelley, P. (1993) Giving children a voice. *Child Health*, 1(1), 21–4.

Slater, M. (1993) *Health for All our Children*. Achieving appropriate health care for black and minority ethnic children and their families. Action for Sick Children, London.

Sparshott, M. (1991) Creating a home for babies in hospital. *Paediatric Nursing*, 3(8), 20–22.

Stone, M. (1993) Lending an ear to the unheard: the role of support groups for siblings of children with cancer. *Child Health*, 1(2), 54–6.

Stower, S. (1993) Innovative practice in the outpatient setting. In *Recent Advances in Child Health Nursing* (eds E.A. Glasper & A. Tucker), pp. 42–51. Scutari Press, London.

Swanwick, M. (1990a) Knowledge and control. *Paediatric Nursing*, 2(5), 18–20.

Swanwick, M. (1990b) Development and chronic illness. *Nursing*, 4(16), 24–7.

Swanwick, M. & Barlow, S. (1993) Defining quality care for paediatric nursing. *Child Health*, 1(4), 137–41.

Taylor, M. & O'Connor, P. (1989) Resident parents and short hospital stays. *Archives of Disease in Childhood*, 64, 274–6.

Vessey, J. (1988) Comparison of teaching methods on children's knowledge of their internal bodies. *Nursing Research*, 37(5), 262–7.

Visintainer, M.A. & Wolfer, J.A. (1975) Psychological pre-paration for surgical patients: the effects on children's and parents' stress responses and adjustment. *Paediatrics*, 56, 187–202.

Vygotsky, L.S. (1962) *Thought and Language*. Wiley, New York.

Vygotsky, L.S. (1978) In Review of the literature: Mind in Society (M. Schwebel). *American Journal of Orthopsychiatry* (1979), 49(4), 530–6.

Weller, B. (1994) Cultural aspects of children's health and illness. In *The Child and Family: Contemporary Nursing Issues in Child Health and Care*, pp. 96–107. Bailliere Tindall, London.

While, A. (1992) The contribution of nurses to children's well-bring in hospital: a selective review of the literature. *Journal of Clinical Nursing*, 1, 117–21.

Whiting, M. (1993) Play and surgical patients. *Paediatric Nursing*, 5(6), 11–13.

Whyte, D. (1990) The family with a chronically ill child. *Paediatric Nursing*, 2(8), 20–23.

Wilson, K. (1993) Education and the hospitalised child. *Paediatric Nursing*, 5(4), 24–5.

Chapter 8

Life Crises for Children and Their Families

Carolyn J. White

INTRODUCTION

This chapter aims to examine the effect of life crises on the child and their family and the role which children's nurses may take to ameliorate the traumatic effect, both in the short and long term.

What are life crises? For most children the normal events that form part of growing up will provide their life crises – starting school, moving house, losing a friend. For a few there will be critical incidents such as severe illness, accidents, alteration in body image, and death. These are events which are generally unplanned for, that rock the foundation of the family unit. These life crises pose a threat to the security of normal routine and often, in the case of ill health, alter the focus of attention to one family member.

It is not the purpose of this chapter to give explanations of what to do and what not to do when faced with difficult situations; there are no hard and fast rules. The aim has been to identify some of the pitfalls and common mistakes, to highlight and share other people's experiences and coping mechanisms, and to encourage the readers to explore their own beliefs and attitudes.

Nurses play a unique part in many people's lives, particularly at times of crisis. There is no doubt that other professionals are available to offer support, information and care. However, nurses are often the only ones available constantly, and as such they hold a privileged position, meeting the needs of families when they are at their most vulnerable. Nurses must make themselves available to families so that those families feel comfortable about sharing their fears and concerns with nurses, and in return nurses must offer a guarantee of openness and, above all, honesty.

COGNITIVE DEVELOPMENT – A CHILD'S ABILITY TO COPE WITH CRISIS

Children's ability to cope with a traumatic event in their lives depends on the developmental milestones they have reached, both physically and psychologically. Piaget (1958) wrote comprehensively on cognitive development in childhood. In essence his theory suggests that children attempt to analyse new experiences by matching them to previous experiences. When new events do not fit neatly to those experiences the child tries to mould or adapt them to similar and familiar experiences, so gradually building on life's events. It is therefore understandable that where children are exposed to events which are alien to them, such as trauma, severe illness or death, they may have difficulty in coming to terms with the complexities of the situation and may choose to dismiss or ignore the issue, or display what might, to adults, appear to be inappropriate behaviour. In the child's mind they are doing neither, they are simply coping the best way they know with a strange situation.

Piaget hypothesized that children pass through four stages to maturity, each stage being related to age and cognitive development.

- Sensorimotor (0–2 years).
- Pre-operational (2–7 years).
- Concrete (7–12 years).
- Formal operational (12 years).

It is important that children's nurses have an awareness of these developmental stages when trying to help a child come to terms with a negative aspect of life. This understanding enables the nurse to provide an explanation to the child at a level they will understand. This knowledge is also helpful when sharing information with parents who are working through a difficult situation with their child.

Considering Piaget's stages of cognitive development in more detail allows the nurse to understand what influences children's interpretations of their life crises.

Babies are wholly dependent on their family, spending much of their time in the comfort of the arms of those who love them. Babies are easily affected by the emotional state of their parents and will quickly sense when a parent is tense or distressed. This may result in the baby becoming unsettled, having disturbed sleep or feeding poorly.

Toddlers respond to the emotional environment they are in. A young child can burst into tears simply because another child in the room is crying. Similarly toddlers will respond to adults who appear to be sad or angry, often mimicking emotions. Toddlers have little sense of permanence and can be easily distracted. So on the one hand they may appear to be in tune with the situation if those around are upset, and on the other hand they will want to engage in play or some other activity totally unrelated to the former. This at times can be beneficial, for example when trying to distract a toddler from an unpleasant intervention, but can be confusing for grieving parents whose young child appears suddenly to have forgotten about a sibling, demanding attention only for themselves. When under stress toddlers may exhibit regressive behaviour in toilet training, speech or sleep patterns, and may demonstrate their own feelings of insecurity by demanding more attention and refusing to be left alone with strangers.

Children enjoy being the centre of attention. They believe in their own thoughts, actions and wishes, and view the world through their own eyes and experiences, believing in their own ability to influence what is around them. Fantasy games feature as a large part of their play (Lovell 1987), and may include home and hospital role play, combat games such as cowboys and indians, and soldiers. Weapons of all descriptions, both real and imaginary, appear on a regular basis. Television and radio play a significant part in the lives of many young children and serve to confuse them with regard to injury and death as permanent concepts, as heroes often recover magically, always having a 'happy ever after' ending.

Children have problems coping with the permanence of severe injury, disablement or death, and may repeatedly ask 'When will they get better?' or 'When will they come back?' when referring to a sick or dead relative. This is often confusing and distressing for parents who have to go over the same information time and time again. It is important that adults avoid ambiguity of speech when talking to children. Phrases such as 'We have lost your sister' are likely to be met with 'Well, let's go and look for her then'.

As children move towards adolescence, they develop concerns related to personal relationships. Any major event affecting an individual's ability to keep up with their peers is likely to cause concern and a lowering of self esteem. This is particularly relevant when considering any change of physical appearance and may lead to demonstrations of anger, denial, frustration and withdrawal.

It is likely that adolescents will have experienced some loss by the time they reach that age (Furnivall & Wilson 1991), possibly an older family member or perhaps a pet. They are able to understand the permanence of death and cope with its abstract nature.

However, emotionally they may still be immature and may require reassurance and open demonstrations of love and security. Adolescents are more likely to try to protect their parents from distress by hiding their own feelings and avoiding talking about their own fears and concerns. Often they choose to share these special thoughts with other relatives, family friends, staff or other children, or they share them indirectly through drawings, poetry or diaries.

Social development

The basis of healthy social and emotional development is a positive self image and good self-esteem (O'Hagan & Smith 1993). From an early age babies participate in social interactions, reaching out, smiling and babbling. Much of what they learn is through observation of their family and repetition of actions. As the child develops it learns what is acceptable within the family social code. This will be influenced by the family's culture, religion, environment and attitude to others. The older the child gets, the greater the influences. Nursery, school, friends and the media will all play a part in the social development of the child. Adults play an important role in developing self-confidence and self-esteem in children by providing a secure and happy environment for them to grow in, by praising and encouraging their achievements, no matter how small, and by acting as a positive role model.

Children can also be socialized into accepting values which may conflict with society's values as a whole. Examples include discrimination on the basis of skin colour or religion. Prejudices of influential family members such as parents will be positively reinforced on a regular basis, causing the child to develop stereotypical views of certain groups of people.

Part of learning social skills for children is through the development of relationships with other children. From about three years of age children begin to interact with each other in play and to understand the concept of sharing. From four years onwards children develop friendships and co-operate when playing with each other. If at this stage in their development children are impeded by a physical or learning disability, it may affect their ability to develop friendships and may result in them withdrawing into themselves, or conversely becoming outwardly aggressive to gain attention

(Rathus 1988). Peer influence becomes increasingly more important with age and children who are unattractive, less friendly or aggressive will be less popular and may find themselves isolated from social groups.

Health and education professionals play a great role in destroying the barriers of stereotyping and help children appreciate the value of individuals regardless of their background. Children who have problems must be supported and helped to integrate. Carers should act as positive role models by recognizing and rewarding achievements and not by criticizing attitudes.

Erikson (1965) described eight stages through which an individual passes, each stage outlining life crises the individual might face as part of normal development (Table 8.1). These experiences in turn enable the individual to learn and prepare for the future. The individual's physical maturity and relationships with others determine the characteristics and experiences at each stage. Traumatic events such as ill health or bereavement may hinder an individual's ability to achieve the developmental tasks at any stage.

Body image

Johnson (1990) defined body image as 'the constantly changing mental picture of one's body', indicating that

Table 8.1 Stages of development (Erikson 1965).

Age		Life crises	Developmental task
Stage I	0–1 years	Trust versus mistrust.	Learning to trust mother and the environment. Security. Association of surroundings with feelings of inner goodness.
Stage II	2–3 years	Autonomy versus shame and doubt.	Developing the wish to make choices and self-control to exercise choice. It is important that the child is supported in exercising self-control and not forced to demonstrate it through feelings of doubt or shame.
Stage III	4–5 years	Initiative versus guilt.	Adding, planning and goal setting to influence choice. Becoming more assertive.
Stage IV	6–12 years	Industry versus inferiority.	Learning skills and tasks which enable achievement. A sense of inferiority may hinder a child's attempts to acquire new skills and to compete with peers.
Stage V	Adolescence	Identity versus role diffusion.	Development of identity. Formation of career objectives.
Stage VI	Young adulthood	Intimacy versus isolation.	Formation of intimate relationships and lasting friendships.
Stage VII	Middle adulthood	Generativity versus stagnation.	A period of procreativity, productivity and creativity.
Stage VIII	Late adulthood	Integrity versus despair.	Achievement of wisdom and dignity. Acceptance of the limits of own lifespan.

it is a dynamic thought process which is not necessarily linked to a physical change. The importance of socialization and the need for children to participate in activities with friends have already been emphasized. It stands to reason therefore that anything influencing a child's ability to participate in group activities or which makes them stand out from the crowd may influence their own body image and self-esteem. Race, religion, cultural background all play an important role in a child's development, both socially and morally. The attitude of others will influence the child's own self-view and self-value. Fig. 8.1 broadly outlines areas that may influence a child's own self-image and that of its peers.

Physical attractiveness in an individual, looks and physique, are important factors for acceptance in peer groups during childhood. Children who are, for example, overweight and not able to participate easily in sport and play, are less likely to be accepted. Skevington *et al.* (1987) described a study regarding the perceptions of attractiveness in young people with

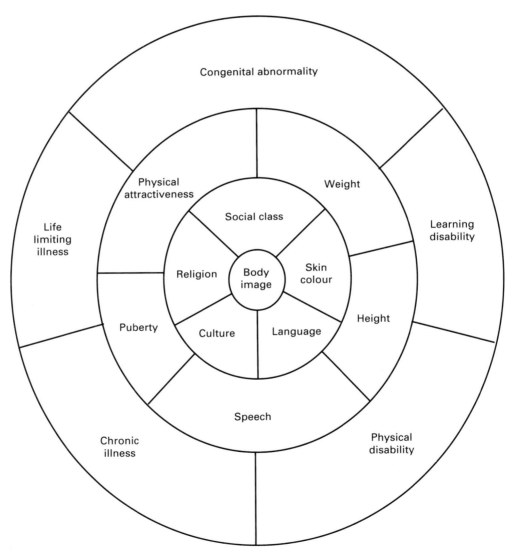

Fig. 8.1   Factors influencing body image.

rheumatoid arthritis and the negative effect this had on their self-esteem.

Adolescents become ever more aware of their own maturing bodies. Peer pressure and the need to promote a sense of individuality result in adolescents trying to control their own body image through diet, fashion and exercise. Anorexia nervosa is most commonly diagnosed in pubescent females and it is accepted that there is a strong link between anorexia and an effort by the girl to remain in the pre-pubescent stage of her development. Severe anorexia not only results in gross weight loss, but hinders physical development in the individual's body such as breast development and the onset of menstruation. This weight phobia may be a direct response to society's view that the ideal female form is a slender, waif-like figure.

Effect of chronic illness on body image

For many children ill health is a way of life. Children with chronic illnesses such as cystic fibrosis, asthma and epilepsy will almost certainly have to comply to therapeutic regimes which impinge on their lifestyle. The severity of their illness will dictate the frequency of their periods of hospitalization and hence their absence from school.

When a child is newly diagnosed as having life-long illness it is a devastating fact for the child and family to come to terms with. The child may feel as though they have lost control over their own body. The natural reaction for the parents is to protect their offspring. For the child this can feel oppressive and it immediately singles them out as different. Initially, adherence with treatment will seem the only option to a child who feels unwell and who is perhaps being cared for in a strange environment. This may reinforce their feeling of loss of self-control. Where treatment regimes and physical disabilities interfere with a child's ability to participate with peers, it is likely that the child will exhibit feelings of anger and frustration. A natural reaction for children faced with these threats, and the restrictions imposed by their illness, may be nonadherence with treatment and disregarding advice given to them by adults. It is important therefore that right from the start the child and family learn that the illness is now part of their normal daily lives. Where it is necessary to make adaptations to their lifestyle, the involvement of other

families who have undergone a similar experience, or the recruitment of voluntary support agencies, may be of help.

As health care professionals we have an important role in:

- Helping the child learn about their illness.
- Assisting teachers and other children or families to understand their illness.
- Promoting the health of the child to minimize absence from school.

Being informed

It is crucial that the child and family are fully informed about the illness and it is explained to them in a way they understand. By informing the child about their illness the nurse gives them the means to participate in making decisions about their own future. This is particularly important for older children as it indicates to them that they are mature enough to be responsible for their own care, thus allowing them to regain control over their own bodies. By the same token it is important that all those involved with the child are well informed so that they can continue to support the child in reaching their full potential. Health professionals such as paediatric community nurses, health visitors and school nurses play a key role in educating parents, families, youth leaders, school teachers and other pupils about the individual child's disease in order that prejudices and fears can be overcome and the child can participate as fully as possible in all activities.

For some children going back into mainstream school will mean having to cope not only with the challenges of growing up and peer group pressure, but also with treatments as part of their normal school day. The school nurse, supported by specialist staff, has an essential role in ensuring the child is afforded privacy and dignity in carrying out whatever needs to be undertaken, be it the administration of medication or the changing of peritoneal dialysis fluid. Hospital and community staff must work closely together to ensure that treatments can be timed so as not to interfere with classroom activities. Failure to do this could further isolate children from their peers and jeopardize their development. In addition the school nurse will have an ongoing role in monitoring the child's health and perhaps acting as a friend and confidante.

Physical deformity

For some children the effect of their illness may be more obvious. Physical scarring or deformity will often be the cause of great curiosity, and will attract staring and, in some cases, blatant criticism from the general public (Carlisle 1991). For these children and their families it is crucial that professional help is given to help them adjust to their impaired appearance. Hillbeuf & Porter (1984) suggest that age plays an extremely important part in adjustment to physical scarring, with junior high school years being especially traumatic. The child with a physical deformity must therefore be supported and encouraged to develop a positive self-image. Emphasis should be placed on the child's positive attributes, and efforts focused on helping them to develop their other competencies. As part of the adaptation to their deformity, health carers should try to identify any areas of concern that the child has. Rosenstein (1987) describes a school re-entry programme designed for children following burn injury who had identified physical therapy as a concern. The study describes how this need was identified and met and how it might be transferred to other children with chronic illness.

Individuals working with children can do a great deal to help them promote a positive self-image. The reactions of carers are very important to the child and it is essential therefore that realistic goals are set for the child and their achievements are recognized and rewarded. The Warnock Report (DES 1978) emphasized the need for children with disabilities to be integrated with peers for education wherever possible. This philosophy should be developed one stage further to allow children with special needs to participate in all activities to a level that they feel comfortable with. Children with special needs should abide by the same rules of discipline and conduct; to treat them differently singles them out. Above all, each child must be considered as an individual.

PARENTS AS PARTNERS IN CARE

When a child first becomes ill, their parents will almost certainly feel vulnerable. They, like their child, will be unsure of what the future holds. They will not feel in control of what is happening to their child and often will not feel in a position to make informed decisions. It is therefore very important from the outset that parents are made to feel part of the team. They should be encouraged to participate in care if they wish, and time should be taken to explain in detail what is wrong with their child. A detailed plan of care and treatment for their child should be discussed and agreed with them. Where there is doubt regarding the diagnosis, this should be explained and an outline of proposed investigations discussed. It is only by involving and informing parents and making them feel part of the team of care, that confidences and a foundation of trust can be established. It is important that parents feel secure in order that they relax and instil confidence into their child.

Parents may ask the same questions time and time again. The nurse must be patient and answer them openly and honestly. If the nurse does not know the answer, they should tell the parents and try to find someone who can help them.

Care of the dying child

The care of the dying child is one of the most challenging, stressful, yet rewarding roles a children's nurse can undertake. In these days of high technology care and good health, the death of a child is a relatively rare event in the western world (Hindmarsh 1993). This lack of exposure to death and dying in childhood makes it all the more difficult to cope with when it does occur. Nurses working within general paediatric units may have limited experience of caring for dying children and their experience may seem inadequate or non-transferable to the situations they are confronted with. There are no right or wrong ways to deal with these situations – indeed it would be wrong to lay down rules as this would detract from the nurse's prime concern in treating each child and every family as individuals.

Good nursing practice should form the basis of caring for a child with a potentially life-limiting illness. A primary nurse who has the necessary experience should be allocated to support the child and family in making decisions about their care. The nurse must be someone who has the confidence to include the child and family in decision-making and who has the ability to work as a member of a multidisciplinary team. The nurse has a vital role in co-ordinating care and ensuring continuity and consistency of treatment and information. Comprehensive history taking and care planning will guarantee that the child's individual needs are taken into consideration and the child and family should be encouraged to take an active part in this process.

When caring for any sick child the nurse is not merely challenged with meeting their physical needs, but also with assessing and dealing with their psychological needs. This is particularly important when caring for a dying child.

Including the dying child

Whether children are being cared for at home, in hospital, or in another caring environment, they have the right to participate in decisions about their care. By allowing choice, the nurse allows and encourages the child to exert some control over their situation. This has to be managed within a disciplined framework. Choice does not mean allowing them to do what they want, when they want, as this can be destructive. Part of a child's security stems from the rules and codes of conduct a family imposes. Where appropriate these can be relaxed, but to disregard them altogether may lead to manipulative behaviour or a loss of sense of security. The same rules should apply to siblings to avoid feelings of jealousy towards a sick child who might be seen to be receiving preferential treatment.

Talking about a child's illness with them may be difficult, particularly if it involves talking about dying and death. Parents should be encouraged to talk to their child about their illness and answer any questions truthfully. Skirting around difficult issues or avoidance of the truth may lead to feelings of guilt for parents after the death of their child. If a child senses that parents, nurses or other carers are not telling the truth, mistrust and feelings of frustration may develop.

Children sometimes avoid talking about death with parents in an effort to protect them from the hurt and distress they know it will cause. This does not mean they do not have a need to express their fears and concerns. Staff must be sensitive to these needs and facilitate the sharing of them. Children may exhibit signs of anger and frustration directed at others and occasionally at themselves and their failing body. It is important that they are able to work through these complex emotions. Creative art is a useful medium and the role of the play therapist should not be underestimated (O'Hagan & Smith 1993). By encouraging children to share their feelings through painting, writing or play, it is possible to explore fears or concerns and to help them come to terms with issues that are troubling them.

When faced with death, children can be very blunt and carers should be prepared for questions such as 'Am I going to die?' or 'What will happen when I die and where will I go?'. Answers should be truthful, straightforward and easy to understand. It is important that ambiguous statements such as 'You'll have a long sleep' are not used, as the child may then be afraid to sleep. Simple statements such as 'Your body will stop working' often suffice. It is useful to ask the child to describe what they think will happen and to use books, videos and other aids specifically designed to help children understand the concept of death (Hemmings 1990). Drawing on experiences the child may have had in relation to death, such as the death of an older relative or family pet, can help the nurse explore different ideas with the child and correct any misconceptions they have.

SHARING BAD NEWS

When bad news has to be shared with parents, it should be undertaken in a private and quiet area. If the news is to be given by a doctor, it is helpful to have present a member of the nursing staff known to the parents, so that they are able to clarify issues after the doctor has left and can ensure colleagues are kept up to date with developments in the child's management. Parents are sometimes so shocked they cannot immediately think of the things they want to ask. It may be necessary to arrange for the doctor to return to go over specific information. Parents should be encouraged to write down questions as they think of them to ensure that they understand all aspects of their child's management.

Reactions to bad news will vary. Anger, despair, physical illness, denial are all common and it is important that as much time as necessary is given to parents to help them come to terms with the information they have been given. Isabelle tells of her feelings when told her daughter was going to die:

'When they told us that Kelly was going to die, it was as if I had been kicked hard in the stomach. I felt sick. I didn't cry. I could hear the doctor's voice but his words didn't go in. I remember everything about the room. The empty coffee mugs, the teddy bear badge on the nurse's uniform, the picture on the wall, but I couldn't hear what he was saying.'

Parents may want help to decide what to tell their child and other family members. They should be encouraged to be truthful and explain things in a way that their child will understand and which will not frighten the child. Parents may choose to do this on their own, in their own time, or may ask that someone supports them. Time must always be available to the child who wishes to ask questions or clarify issues. Parents should be reassured that it is not wrong for their child to see them cry and that expressing sadness reinforces the important place that the child has within their family.

Grief is a normal and natural reaction to loss. It is not surprising therefore that parents and other family members will exhibit behaviour more commonly associated with bereavement when faced with the potential loss of their child. Parents may describe feelings of helplessness, guilt, disbelief, not being able to concentrate, and feeling as if they are going mad. In searching for a reason why, parents may focus their frustration and anger on others, perhaps hospital staff or a GP (Lishman *et al.* 1990). Some will try to blame themselves: 'If only I had...'. It is vital that those involved with caring for the family help them to rationalize these feelings, talking them through it and helping them come to terms with the situation without having to apportion blame.

THE DEATH OF A CHILD

For many parents the death of their child will be their first experience of death and because of this they may be harbouring fears that it will be violent or distressing. It often helps to verbalize these fears and to talk about them, reassuring parents that they will be able to hold and cuddle their child after death. It is important to warn them of the physical changes that will occur in their child's temperature and colour and to explain what happens to their child's body. Where death is suspected to be imminent, parents and family should have the choice of being with their child, and where possible, of

holding and cuddling them. Some parents may wish to lie alongside their child in bed, or simply to hold their hand. Staff should seek clarification as to whether the family wish them to be present or not, reassuring them that whatever their decision is, they will be near at hand.

Following the death the family should be allowed as much time as they want with their child (Sumner *et al.* 1991). They may want to take responsibility for washing and dressing their child, or assisting the nursing staff in this final act of caring. The choice of clothing is often important to parents (Dominica 1987). Perhaps a favourite playsuit, football strip or pyjamas. Parents may request that a favourite toy be left with their child. When a child dies in hospital, it is essential that these special requests are communicated to the mortuary staff and funeral directors. For some parents mementos, such as a lock of hair or the footprint of a baby, will be important. Others may choose to remember their child from memories and photographs of happier times. It is essential that the family is given as much time as they wish with their child after death, to say their goodbyes.

After the death of a child people often find it difficult to know what to say, although it is not always necessary to say anything. Touch often means more than talk (Walker 1986). The nurse's presence and the fact that they are showing support are enough to show how much they care. Many health professionals are taught that it is wrong to cry. For many parents the shedding of tears by staff indicates just how much they are hurting (Walker 1986). Jane Davies (1979), a mother of a six year old child who died of a Wilms tumour, spoke of her experience at a conference of the Royal College of Physicians:

'I know all about any display of emotion being unprofessional, but it can help parents, it really can. If your child is going to die, it becomes vitally important that that child dies as a person, as an individual, not as yet another patient and another statistic.'

Nurses should share their fears; there is no shame in feeling sad, although an awareness that they should be supporting the family is vital. If the nurse is not able to control emotions, they may not be able to provide the support the family needs. If the nurse becomes overwhelmed, they need to ask someone to step in in order to regain composure and help the family through their ordeal.

When a child dies in hospital, parents are often

concerned about what happens to their child's body when they leave. This should be explained truthfully to them. Parents may wish to accompany or carry their child to the mortuary and they should be prepared for what to expect. As a staff nurse, the writer was asked by a father if he might carry his little boy to the mortuary. The initial reaction was horror and concern about his reaction when he saw the refrigerators. Dissuasion did not work due to his insistence, and appropriate arrangements were made. The father went about the task very calmly and on return to the ward, he expressed his thanks saying: 'It is important I can always imagine where he is. At least I know he is not on his own.' The latter was reference to the body of a tiny baby lying next to his son.

Many parents do not realise that they can have the body of their child at home with them until the funeral. As long as a postmortem examination is not required, this should be explained to the parents and the necessary arrangements made if requested.

Practical information for parents is very important and should be given to them in written form for reference at a later date. It should include details on how to obtain a death certificate, how to register the death, and how to arrange a funeral. Arrangements for the family to visit the body of their child should be confirmed. Ideally this will be on an open access basis although the nurse might request that the parents telephone the hospital first so that arrangements can be made for a nurse familiar to them to escort them.

Jennings (1992) undertook a study into the way in which parents cope with a child with a life threatening disorder. She identified a difference in perception between the professional and parents with regard to coping strategies. Parents experienced strong feelings of aggression which were largely unrecognized. They reported 'taking things day by day' and many turned to religion or prayer for support, taking a 'mental' rather than physical approach to coping. Negative feelings were highlighted, in particular guilt or self blame.

Siblings

All too often siblings are left out of the hubbub surrounding the care of the sick child. Parents naturally focus their attention on the sick child, passing the care of other children to family or friends. Jonathon, aged 9, explains what happened when his sister became ill:

'When Nicola went into hospital, Mummy and Daddy went with her and stayed there all the time. I went to stay with Nanny and had to go to school every day. I went to see Nicola at the weekends but only for a short time because she was very poorly. Nobody asked me what I wanted to do, or really told me what was going on. They all said she would get better soon, but she didn't.'

It is important that brothers and sisters share in the care of their sick sibling as, if the outcome is death, it helps them to adjust to their loss (Malcolm 1985). Depending on their age and maturity, their ability to understand and cope will vary.

It is not unusual for a terminally ill child to be showered with gifts and treats, for bad behaviour to be ignored and routine disregarded. It is hardly surprising that often siblings react to this, making extra demands on parents and trying to draw the focus of attention to themselves. Some children become fearful that they may become ill and die themselves and they may become clingy, not letting parents out of their sight. Some children blame themselves for what has happened to their sibling because of a fight they had or because they wished the other dead over a silly incident. It is important that parents recognize their fears and give their other children time with them and their sick brother or sister. Many parents express concern that their other children will be frightened by the trappings of the hospital. Often they are only expressing their own fears, and they need to be supported and encouraged to allow their other children to visit. It is important, particularly for older brothers and sisters, that they have private times with their sick sibling, time to settle accounts and time to say goodbye.

Siblings have been described as the forgotten mourners (Hindmarsh 1993) as too often they are excluded and shielded from what is going on. Parents overwhelmed by their own grief sometimes forget that their other children have lost a friend and companion too. Cohen (1994) describes how siblings can be helped to come to terms with the death of their brother or sister through attending a child bereavement group. The need for children to talk about their loss is identified and the group setting is seen to be a safe environment in which to express their feelings. Riley (1993) offers some practical ideas to suggest to parents how to cope with bereaved children (Table 8.2).

As health care professionals caring for dying children we assume an enormous responsibility. Everything we

Table 8.2 Practical ideas for parents on how to cope with bereaved children.

- Many children will respond to physical comfort:
  (1) Give special foods; soft foods can be reassuring and are a reminder of earlier, easier times.
  (2) Children respond to snuggling against a warm, soft surface so let them sleep between flannelette sheets or have a blanket on top of them.
  (3) Extra clothes in the daytime help to reduce the coldness of shock and instil a feeling of being lovingly wrapped and protected against possible harm.
- If the child has difficulty in settling to sleep for relaxation, allow a radio tape or television to play softly.
- If they fear the dark, use a night light.
- Children need physical play; try not to cut this time down, even if the child is getting behind with his school work because of an inability to concentrate.
- Grief is tiring so alternate a child's passive and active play, arrange a quiet time in the afternoon and plan an early bedtime.
- If a child is having difficulty in following directions, make lists out for them. These can be done in the form of pictures for the very young.
- Treat the child to a special outing, a treat, a present or new colourful clothes. These can bring comfort and help to create a feeling of security.
- If the child is overeating, serve the food on individual plates. You could suggest a cuddle instead of something else they want to eat.
- Offer small nourishing meals to those who lose an interest in eating.
- For both overeating and undereating, it may help to teach the child to cook.
- Love and cuddles are essential.

do, however great or small, will be remembered by the parents of the child we have cared for, sealed together with the other precious memories they hold. Our inadequacies, presumptions and complacencies will be matched against our honesty, compassion and caring. It is the needs of the child and family that must be our prime concern. In assessing those needs, we should remember that parents know their child far better than we do. As stated by the Compassionate Friends (a voluntary organization offering bereavement support and counselling to families):

'there is no death as sad as that of a child and perhaps no death so hard to come to terms with.'

The following case history provides one degree of insight into the needs of the dying child and their family. The interview is a profound and moving account of a father's feelings about his son, Christopher, who was terminally ill. Christopher was a normal, happy, fun loving teenager who particularly enjoyed fishing and playing football. His father shares with us his feelings when Christopher became ill.

'When Christopher was first admitted to hospital, no one knew what the problem was. It was thought that he had glandular fever. Once his paediatrician began to realise that there was more to it, he contacted a specialist and was told that there would appear to be a malignancy involved. His mum and I were asked to go to talk to the specialist and were told the likelihood of the malignancy and that we should prepare ourselves. When we returned to the side ward Christopher was in, we were met by the nursing staff in full gowns, masks and gloves. Both of us were horrified to see the look of terror on Christopher's face. Why could they not wait for our return so that we could explain to Christopher what was going on? The damage had been done and Christopher remained frightened until we were transferred to the next hospital about 24 hours later.

After our transfer information was slow in coming. In fact the most frustrating thing we had to face was a long wait for two weeks while they were coming up with the diagnosis. The specialist told us right from the start that we were looking at six to twelve months, which was the length of time that they expected him to live. We had to be told this information again and again. The staff would pass on all the information that they had, but you needed to arrange an appointment to see the specialist to have the definitive answers to all the questions.

We were given daily tasks to do such as cleaning the side ward Chris was in, being actively involved in keeping a record of all Chris' blood test results and being asked if we noticed an improvement in Chris' general condition. The consultant sat on the side of Chris' bed and talked to all of us as a family, asking for Chris' ideas as to the amount of help he could give to help in his treatment. Christopher visibly improved the more the doctor talked to him. We were totally involved with the decision making about Chris' treatment and future. The only thing that was kept away from Chris and his sister was the fact that Chris might die. The nursing staff would let us all become involved at the level we wished. This was also true of the other parents in the ward. One of the frustrating things was that I could not do a lot physically to help; it was just being there for Christopher when he needed me.

It seemed as though Chris was not like the others on the ward. We were seen as being different, but this could just have been me. The other parents had all spent many months coming to and from the hospital knowing each other well. I felt we were looked on as the new faces, with nothing to relate to, until we had a handle on Christopher's condition.

Physically it was draining to rush after work to be with Chris each day, but once at his side, it all seemed to fade away. The staff would always give a warm welcome to us, even when they had been having a bad day, and for that I will always remain grateful. Once back at home, some days it was hard to get off to sleep as I wanted to be with Chris. He wanted to be grown up and to be left at night-time once he began to feel sleepy, happy in the knowledge we would return the next day. Emotionally I swung from being happy and optimistic to a feeling of total despair and unable to cope.

Christopher's sister began to feel out of it and wanted some time spending with her. She would say that I never had time for her and Chris was taking up my time, while at the same time she knew why I was with Chris, but she too needed a hug and reassurance. Normally if anyone was hurt I could pick them up and make them feel better, but this was out of my hands and I could no longer make it OK again. That was the hardest thing to come to terms with. I found that in work all I wanted to do was get the day over so I could be with Chris. All other things took second place, but once with Chris I needed to let him know that I was still involved with all the things I did before. Sometimes I got it right, and sometimes wrong, but you can't plan for something like this.

One day I was walking our dog and the wind was blowing hard from behind me. The clouds in the sky were all going at a great rate of knots. It was as if they were all running away from me and this feeling of helplessness came over me. I could not control what was going on with the clouds as I could not help Chris. I felt totally useless.

Chris appeared to cope better than us. Once he got over his initial fear from the first hospital, he had total faith in the doctors and nurses. His ability rubbed off on us too and he would make us feel at ease with the situation. He had a number of low days when he knew that he was going for more bone marrow tests, or he was to be put on a nightly antibiotic drip. He accepted all that was given to him and any questions he asked, I would answer, giving him all the information. He never asked if he was going to die, but I did tell him when the nurse from the St David's Trust arrived at the house that she dealt with children with life threatening diseases. I noticed that as I said that he changed, so I reiterated the fact. He began to cry and get upset. He said, could we not say that, but say it was serious. We all agreed to use this term, but that I would not hide anything from him.

When he was at home, Chris had his friends around most evenings so he was kept up to date with all that was going on at school. He never wanted to be different from all his friends and when people began to raise money for him, he could not understand why, but he did enjoy spending it on presents for others and, of course, himself. When things became too much for him, he would change and become more child-like, looking for quiet talking with reassurance that we would be there if he wanted. During the moments at home, he would just give a look to me and come and sit next to me, no need to talk, just sitting with my arm around him.

On Christmas Eve the nursing staff allowed his sister to sleep on a put-you-up bed next to Chris. On Boxing Day we were transferred to another hospital as Christopher needed dialysis as his kidneys were packing up and he was in some distress with his breathing. After he had been on the kidney machine and settled back into his bed, at 2AM on 27 December, Chris went off to sleep with him telling me to go home and to return in the morning. When we arrived back in the morning, he looked a lot happier but was in some pain and he was being given some painkillers. We had a talk with our specialist, the consultant from the renal unit, the doctor on the ward and the sister about what we wanted for Christopher. The choice was for him to be put onto a life support machine in the intensive care unit, or for him to be kept pain free on the ward and able to talk to us. The decision we felt was right was to keep Christopher out of pain and the medical staff agreed to do this.

After the meeting we walked back to Christopher's bed. When I was asked what I would say if Chris asked if he was going to die, it was like having a hard slap that made me literally take a step back. But I knew Chris would never ask; plus, when I returned to Chris with tears in my eyes, he must have known. From that moment on I did feel that it was important that Christopher had time alone with each of us to say whatever he wanted. He said his goodbyes to his mother and sister, and for myself I was told not to be sad when he had to go. The nursing staff let us come and go inside his side ward, never making us feel that we were in the way, but at times we must have been. We all had time alone with Chris. If the nursing staff noticed that Chris was talking, they just left us alone (or it appeared to be like that). They called us by our christian names and attempted to normalize the situation. How they remembered our names, I don't know, but it was nice.'

The input of the nursing staff can't be over-emphasised. As the doctors have to treat so many and can't get too involved, it is left to the nursing staff to fill the very big gap of talking to the parents and trying to help them come to terms with the child that is going to die. All I would say is to be patient with the parents as they never expect their child to die. You expect your parents to die first, but never your child. Listen to them, don't judge them, just help them come to terms in their own way. Be honest with the whole family, remembering that they will have to be told things more than just the once. Help them understand that each child is unique and you are there

to help the child and the family come to terms with this devastating situation. There can't be a correct course of action, so let the child and family decide the way they want to handle the situation. You, the nurse, will be needed for support more than you will ever know.

MULTI-CULTURAL/SPIRITUAL NEEDS

Britain is a multi-cultural society and each group has its own special customs, rituals and beliefs. Many families coping with a dying child seek the support and comfort of their religion. It is important that nurses consider the religious needs of the children and their families and offer them the opportunity and privacy to practise their religion freely. Staff faced with a religion unfamiliar to them are often worried about doing the right thing, or conversely doing the wrong thing. Support and advice should be sought from religious leaders; the hospital chaplain will often prove to be a good point of contact for relevant people. The nurse must remember that religion is personal and although a family has indicated a religious following, this does not mean they are actively practising. They should be allowed the opportunity to make their own arrangements. The rituals surrounding death vary greatly from one religion to another and nurses caring for families from different faiths should be familiar with them in order that spiritual and cultural needs can be assessed and met. Neuberger (1987) and the Lisa Sainsbury Foundation provide a wealth of material that can help the nurse to understand the family's needs and give them advice on how to provide support.

CONCLUSION

Children's nurses are well trained to meet the physical needs of young patients but when faced with a major change in children's health, they must also be prepared to accept the challenge of meeting their increased emotional and psychological needs. Nurses can only do this by recognizing each child as a unique individual and understand that their ability to cope will be based on their life's experiences.

For the family their child's serious illness, hospitalization and continued care in the community will be a frightening ordeal and they will often turn to the child's nurse for advice, understanding and support. Such expectations place an enormous burden and privilege on nursing staff. They demand the willingness and ability to take on board parents' feelings of frustration, anger, despair, and perhaps sorrow. Distancing oneself from such agony and grief may accord with professional objectivity but makes for a cold and unsupportive relationship. In meeting the needs of the child and family, nurses must be aware of their own tolerance level for emotional self-survival and those managing services must provide effective support mechanisms.

Support group

Compassionate Friends
6 Denmark Street
Bristol
BS1 5DQ
Tel: 01272 292778

REFERENCES

Carlisle, D. (1991) The scars of childhood. *Nursing Times*, 87(42), 31.

Cohen, P. (1994) The Loss Adjusters. *Nursing Times*, 90(9), 14–15.

Davies, J. (1979) Death of a child. *World Medicine*, Nov, 23–6.

DES (1978) *Special Educational Needs*. Report of the committee of enquiry into the education of handicapped children and young people (Warnock Report). HMSO, London.

Dominica, F. (1987) Reflections on death in childhood. *British Medical Journal*, 294, 108–110.

Erikson, E.H. (1965) *Childhood and Society*. Penguin, Harmondsworth.

Furnivall, J. & Wilson, P. (1991) Coping with loss in childhood. *Medical Monitor*, Nov, 56–62.

Hemmings, P. (1990) Dealing with death. *Community Care*, April, 16–17.

Hillbeuf, A. & Porter, J.D. (1984) Children Coping with Impaired Appearance: Social and Psychologic Influences. *General Hospital Psychiatry*, 6(4), 294–301.

Hindmarsh, C. (1993) *On the Death of a Child*. Radcliffe Medical Press, Oxford.

Jennings, P. (1992) Coping Mechanisms. *Paediatric Nursing*, 4(8), 13–15.

Johnson, B.H.(1990) Children's drawings on a projective technique. *Paediatric Nursing*, 16(1), 1–7.

Lishman, J., McIntosh, L. & McIntosh, B. (1990) A Child Dies. *Practice*, 3 & 4, 271–84.

Lovell, B. (1987) Sharing the death of a parent. *Nursing Times*, 83(42), 36–9.

Malcolm, D. (1985) Letting Alan Go. *Nursing Times*, July, 30–31.

Neuberger, J. (1987) *Caring for Dying People of Different Faiths*. Austen Cornish, London.

O'Hagan, M. & Smith, M. (1993) *Special Issues in Childcare*. Bailliere Tindall, London.

Piaget, J. (1958) *The Child's Construction of Reality*. Routledge & Kegan Paul, London.

Rathus, S.A. (1988) *Understanding Child Development*. Holt, Rinehart and Winston, Orlando, Florida.

Riley, M. (1993) *Coping with Children and their Families in Death*. A Teaching Package, Royal Hull Hospitals NHS Trust.

Rosenstein, D.L. (1987) A school re-entry programme for burned children part 1: development and implementation of a school re-entry programme. *Journal of Burn Care and Rehabilitation*, 8(4), 319–22.

Skevington, S.M., Blackwell, F. & Britton, N.F. (1987) Self esteem and perception of attractiveness: an investigation of early rheumatoid arthritis. *British Journal of Medical Psychology*, 60, 45–52.

Sumner, M., Dinwiddie, Matthew, D.J. Skuse, D.H. (1991) Loss on a paediatric intensive care unit: parental reactions. *Care of the Critically Ill*, 7(2), 64–6.

Walker, K.L. (1986) Easing the Pain of Bereaved Patients. *Nursing*, April, 49–50.

Chapter 9

Children's Development

Angela Hobsbaum

INTRODUCTION

As children get older they change in many ways, some obvious and some more discreet. Before embarking on a discussion of children's development it may be useful to distinguish the process known as development from other terms which also refer to changes, such as growth, maturation and learning. Growth generally refers to physical incremental processes; maturation refers to changes which seem to be hardly affected by environmental conditions or experience, while learning refers to changes in behaviour which have been brought about through the experience of events. Development refers to changes which make behaviour more mature, advanced or sophisticated, brought about by age and experience.

Some aspects of development are universal, occurring to all children regardless of their environment, while others are affected by the child's surroundings and experience. Developmental psychologists have tried to set out the general changes which occur as children grow older, and have attempted to explore the influence of the environment on these general developmental processes, to unravel the contribution of nurture to nature. Within the general features of cognitive change will be the individual features which characterize the intellect of a particular child.

Understanding of children's development has passed through a number of phases or fashions. Some of the earliest workers were concerned to establish developmental norms which showed the effect of maturation on various processes; Gesell (1928) described the stages of locomotion from crawling to walking to running, hopping and climbing stairs, and claimed that the developing skills were due to the maturation of the nervous system which was unaffected by individual experiences such as practice or stimulation. Similarly Piaget's (1968a) account of children's cognitive development ignores the role of particular experiences such as schooling or family lifestyle. In his view cognitive development will progress through the same stages and take the same form in the transition from immature to mature logical thought regardless of individual experiences.

Yet psychologists have also been preoccupied with issues of continuity and discontinuity, with the prediction of later behaviour from earlier experiences This has been the special concern of those interested in emotional development and the formation of feelings, attachments and relationships. Ever since Freud claimed that unresolved conflicts in early life led to later problem behaviours, psychologists have endeavoured to explore the extent to which early life events can influence later outcomes and have been particularly interested in the precursors of deviant, delinquent or aggressive behaviour.

However, as our understanding of child development has increased, it is clear that the influences are more complex than had originally been imagined. Development is seldom determined by a single event but is the product of many interactions between whatever the child is biologically equipped with and its surroundings. This chapter will present a description of the general changes which take place from infancy to adolescence, focusing upon perception, cognition, and social and emotional aspects of development.

Stages of development

It is common when talking about development to talk of different stages. A stage is generally defined by a collection of features which make it qualitatively distinct. A stage theory asserts that:

(1) Stages are acquired in a fixed order.
(2) Stages are cumulative, one stage building on the previous one.

More controversial is the question of whether the transition from one stage to the next is gradual or abrupt and whether the change occurs simultaneously in all aspects of behaviour. Freud's theory of emotional development and Piaget's theory of cognitive development are both examples of stage theories; however, in Freudian theory regression was possible, that is the child could move backwards to a less mature stage. In his later work, Piaget (1972) acknowledged that some areas of thinking might be more advanced than others.

Models of development

Descriptions of development are not explanations of it. Theories of development seek answers to questions. For example: 'Why does the child behave in this way?' and 'Why does behaviour change?'. In the process of trying to address such questions, psychologists have developed different models of development; currently one of the most popular is the constructivist model. In this model children's ideas, concepts and understanding are constructed in response to experience; they are not passively absorbed or learnt but emerge through the interaction between the child's existing processes and new demands or information presented from the world outside. Children are active, generating hypotheses and seeking information to confirm their ideas about the world. The view of children as active both in constructing their own views of the world and in influencing the environment in which they live, is widely held.

The question about what drives development receives more diverse answers. Some theorists, such as Piaget (1968b), stress internal mechanisms which propel the child's development given sufficient environmental input; others, like Vygotsky (1978) or Bruner (1964, 1974), feel that social interaction provides the essential stimulus for development. Social interactionists emphasize the fact that meanings are socially constructed, not inherent in the stimulus, and the child's understanding both of self and the world depends on this social significance. In the course of growing up children interact with more competent and mature members of their culture, who pass on their expert understanding.

INFANCY

This early period of life has attracted a disproportionate amount of interest from psychologists because it seems to offer the possibility of answering some fundamental questions about the baseline from which subsequent development occurs, about the nature/nurture controversy and about the kinds of competences that are in-built or 'wired-in' to the human brain. Although demonstrating the existence of capabilities in early infancy does not prove they are innate, since experience of some kind has always been present, researchers now are concerned to discover how far cognitive or perceptual processes seem to be invariant and in that sense must be innate, part of the way in which all humans process information about their world.

Exploring the world: reaching, touching and moving

At birth the infant has little postural control (Fig. 9.1); the newborn cannot support head or body unaided and it will be two to three months before the baby can lift its head from the floor to look around. But at birth the baby has a repertoire of reflexes whose purpose and evolution have been debated. The newborn will grasp if the palm of the hand is stimulated and will 'step' if held over a surface with pressure under the foot. However, these reflexes seem to disappear or be replaced by other movements in the early months, although Zelazo (1976) showed that if the stepping reflex is exercised it can be maintained (Bremner 1988). It has been suggested that these reflexes are remnants of earlier behaviours which had an evolutionary adaptive significance; it is also argued that the maturing cortex inhibits the functions of the lower brain which controlled the reflexes, and this accounts for their diminution with age.

By six months the infant should be able to sit without assistance, using just the hands for support; by ten months to one year the baby should be creeping and crawling, able to move from one place to another. This improvement in posture and voluntary control of the limbs enables the baby to look at the world and reach out and explore as he or she gets older.

Newborn infants appear to be uncoordinated, as though their eyes and limbs are not under their control. But appearances may be deceptive; careful examination under optimal conditions when the head and torso are supported reveals that infants younger than one month track objects with their eyes and will reach towards objects too with their arms. However, experiments with infants, even studies which only require observation of their responses, must be especially sensitive because newborn babies do not spend long in the state of quiet arousal which experimenters need in order to collect accurate data.

The infant's state of arousal can be classified along dimensions of activity and wakefulness as well as mood; a positive, active, wakeful state may change rapidly into a negative one as a baby becomes fretful and cries. Initially after birth, the transitions from one state to another are rapid and may seem to the bewildered parent to be unpredictable. Since the baby is faced with a completely new environment at birth, it is not sur-

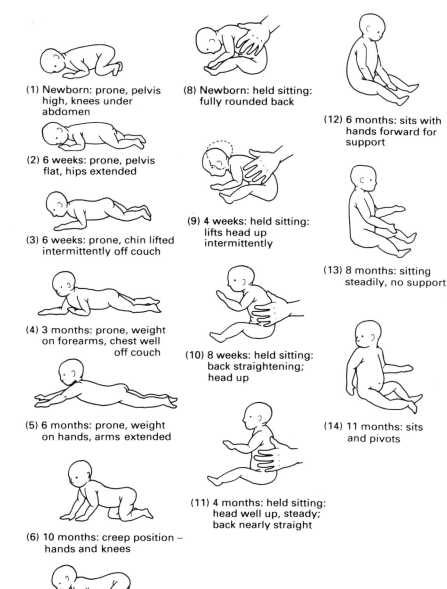

(1) **Newborn:** prone, pelvis high, knees under abdomen

(2) **6 weeks:** prone, pelvis flat, hips extended

(3) **6 weeks:** prone, chin lifted intermittently off couch

(4) **3 months:** prone, weight on forearms, chest well off couch

(5) **6 months:** prone, weight on hands, arms extended

(6) **10 months:** creep position – hands and knees

(7) **1 year:** walking like a bear on soles of feet and hands

(8) **Newborn:** held sitting: fully rounded back

(9) **4 weeks:** held sitting: lifts head up intermittently

(10) **8 weeks:** held sitting: back straightening; head up

(11) **4 months:** held sitting: head well up, steady; back nearly straight

(12) **6 months:** sits with hands forward for support

(13) **8 months:** sitting steadily, no support

(14) **11 months:** sits and pivots

Fig. 9.1 Chart showing development of postural control during infancy (From Illingworth, 1973).

prising that the infant's system takes time to adjust to a stable rhythm, especially as the experience of feeding will be quite novel and will produce unaccustomed sensations.

Perceptual development in infants

Research on infancy over the past forty years has continued to reveal the unexpected competence of the very young child. Far from babies being unable to make sense of the world, it now seems that they are well-equipped to perceive sights and sounds and to begin to make sense of their surroundings from the moment of birth. Because their response capabilities are more limited, it has been difficult for investigators to detect what the baby is able to see, hear or discriminate. But by using new indicators of awareness they have been able to monitor babies' perceptual capacities in many different areas.

An example of such a technique is the use of habituation to explore babies' ability to discriminate. When shown a stimulus, the baby will show interest in it; if the same stimulus, whether a sound or rhythm, a pattern or picture, is shown repeatedly, the baby will get bored and cease to pay attention to it; this is called habituation. The heart rate changes and the baby may stop looking at or showing interest in the stimulus. If the stimulus is then changed the baby's interest is aroused again and heart rate drops. These subtle indicators of attention can show whether the baby can tell the difference between two stimuli or can remember from one presentation to the next.

Through such techniques it has been possible to show that soon after birth babies can see, hear, taste and smell. During the first month their ability to scan patterns improves as they are able to see more clearly and fixate better; they tend to scan contours and contrasts to obtain visual information. Their visual system seems to develop rapidly so that by three months of age they can focus on near and far objects, see colours in much the same way as adults do, distinguish between face-like patterns and jumbled patterns, tell the difference between a familiar and an unfamiliar face and between various shapes, and are beginning to show shape and size constancy. They can discriminate between their mother's voice and that of a stranger and can tell the difference between different phonemes or speech sounds (such as 'p' and 'b').

Research cannot prove that infants are innately equipped with these capacities as all babies have benefited from experience even before birth and researchers can never be sure how much has developed through interaction with the environment, whether pre-natally or since birth. However, these studies demonstrate that babies are far more competent perceptually than had been believed and that insofar as these skills emerge regardless of different surroundings, babies' ways of perceiving the world appear to be inbuilt.

More than forty years ago Piaget (1955) claimed that infants perceived the world as a succession of images and that they had no understanding that objects continued to exist even when they were no longer in view. He suggested that until about eight or nine months of age, the object and the action the child makes to reach, suck or shake it are fused; the object does not have a separate existence. Gradually during the first year the child realizes that objects can be associated with different actions and have an independent existence even if they are out of sight; Piaget called this achievement 'object permanence', by which he meant the understanding that objects are solid and have an independent existence. On the basis of observations he made of his own children when they were babies, Piaget came to the conclusion that infants did not develop mental representations of objects until around a year. If an object was hidden under a cover or a blanket, babies did not seem to search for it but seemed to treat the disappearance as meaning that the object no longer existed. Piaget suggested that their world was a series of evanescent events as people and objects came into view and then faded out.

Other researchers have suggested that Piaget's interpretations of the baby's view of the world, based on the act of reaching or searching for toys, may be misleading. In Piaget's task, the baby had to pull aside the cloth covering the toy and then reach for it. But the baby may be unable to co-ordinate these actions into an organized search towards a hidden goal. Other reactions, such as showing surprise, may offer a more sensitive window on to the baby's understanding. For example, Baillargeon (1987) has used habituation techniques in experiments to show that babies as young as three months are surprised when a screen appears to pass right through an object, suggesting that they already understand that objects are solid and continue to occupy space even when they are hidden by a screen.

Experiments indicate that babies' ideas about the world may develop earlier than had been supposed; the experiments don't show that babies are innately equipped with these ideas, but that they emerge both earlier and more gradually than had been first thought. Every discovery poses fresh challenges: if four month old babies expect objects to be solid and tangible, it is interesting that they are delayed in showing the co-ordinated search behaviour which, as Piaget noted, does not appear until approximately eight months.

Bradley (1989) points out that much depends on how scientists interpret the babies' behaviour. From the scientist's point of view, since the solidity and existence of objects is an irrefutable fact, the babies' looking behaviour must mean that they too show an understanding of this. But Bradley warns that the scientist must be wary of concluding that the babies' response means that their thought processes are similar to the scientist's.

Experimenters trying to investigate perceptual development have to try to see the world through the baby's eyes, but as the baby explores the world and becomes more mobile, perceptual understanding also changes. Gibson & Walk (1960) investigated children's perception of depth in a classic experiment in which babies were encouraged to crawl towards their mothers over a glass panel; under one half of the panel was a patterned surface but under the other half the pattern was set some distance below the glass. Gibson was curious to see whether the babies would be willing to crawl across the 'visual cliff'. Most babies from six months of age avoided the apparent drop. Subsequent work has shown that babies perceive depth from around two months of age; however, it is only once they begin to crawl that they show fear of a drop.

Social development in infancy

Talking about perceptual development as though the world consisted only of objects, no matter how bright, colourful and noisy they may be, is to ignore the importance of the social environment in which the child grows up. The baby is born into a social world where people, usually a few special people, provide a recurring source of stimulation. Experiments have been undertaken to discover whether babies react to people in the same way that they react to pictures, and whether they can tell the difference between human and inanimate

objects; also at what age they can distinguish one person from another.

Babies seem to react more obviously to real faces than to pictures of faces or to the schematic black and white face-like patterns which have been utilized by experimenters. Real faces are more complex, have shadows and generally move and change; in real life people don't just look at babies but they talk to them as well, thus offering more and different stimuli. Babies less than a week old seem able to distinguish their mother's face from that of a stranger (Field *et al.* 1984), which shows how salient human faces must be for them if they learn about them so quickly. It is likely that at first babies recognize features such as hairline rather than facial features because they tend to scan the edges of the face.

Familiar voices too are recognized in the first week; since babies can hear even in the womb, it is likely that the characteristics of the mother's voice can be learned pre-natally. By two weeks of age, babies are more likely to stop crying to listen to a parent's voice than to a stranger's (Hulsebus 1975).

The smile is often taken by adults to demonstrate the social awareness of the baby; parents certainly feel delighted when the baby seems to smile at them and they respond enthusiastically. But this may not mean that the baby identifies them as significant social beings. Early smiles only seem to involve the mouth, whereas a mature smile includes the eyes, which wrinkle up; perhaps early smiles should not be called smiles at all since they seem to occur spontaneously rather than in response to particular stimuli. But by about a month the human voice begins to elicit smiles and soon the human face will do the same. However, the face stimulus need not be a real face; babies will smile as readily at a portrait photograph, especially where the eyes are emphasized. Further evidence that the smile is not necessarily a social event is provided by observations that babies will smile and coo when they learn to control a mobile by pulling a string, or when they learn to produce an effect on an inanimate object, so the smile may be a signal of their internal state of satisfaction rather than a specifically social response to the outside world.

Bowlby (1969) has proposed an influential theory of the development of social relationships in infancy. In his view, babies are born equipped with behaviours such as crying, clinging, sucking, smiling and making eye-to-eye contact, which provoke a protective response from adults. This ensures that babies are kept close to their caregivers for the first months of life and are given comfort and protection from cold and hunger to ensure their survival. Through this proximity, they are able to develop a stable preference to a few people. Thus there is an initial stage, which Bowlby calls one of indiscriminate attachments, when the baby will respond to and can be soothed by anyone; from about seven to nine months of age the baby becomes increasingly selective and will be wary of strangers. This phenomenon of stranger anxiety has been shown to occur in many societies but its intensity and duration seem to be affected by other circumstances of the child's life. For instance, in groups where few strangers are seen the reaction may be powerful, while in other groups where the infant may have had more familiarity with a greater diversity of people it may be less marked (Super & Harkness 1982).

Bradley (1989) argues that the development of focused attachments may not stem from an emotional bond such as love but from a need to establish more predictable reactions from adults, which will enable babies to begin to have some control over their otherwise unpredictable and unstable surroundings. Again, the problem is how to interpret the baby's behaviour; adults regard smiling as affectionate behaviour indicating an emotional response, but they cannot be sure what the baby feels.

As the baby comes to be able to distinguish between one face and another and to prefer the familiar face to a stranger's, other behaviours become associated with the familiar person. The baby will tend to smile more readily at the familiar caregiver and will be more easily soothed by them too. This pattern of preference is termed attachment, and all babies seem to develop these social relationships by six months. Usually the person who does most of the caregiving will be the preferred focus of attachment, but this need not always be the case (Schaffer & Emerson 1964).

Bell (1970) showed that babies demonstrated 'person permanence', in the sense of understanding that their mothers continued to exist even when not in view, about a month before they manifested object permanence in the Piagetian task of searching for a hidden toy. This may be due to the development of an emotional relationship with the mother which underpins the baby's sense of security. Or perhaps social stimuli are more memorable than inanimate objects.

There has been considerable debate on the role played by adults in the establishment of social preferences and attachments. While some work has focused on the baby's increasing ability to discriminate a familiar figure from a stranger, other work has suggested that the adult's response to the baby is critical. For example, Bell & Ainsworth (1972) carried out a longitudinal study of 26 mothers and babies over the first year of life; every three months they observed them for a whole day at home. They recorded how often the babies cried and how quickly their mothers responded. Their conclusion was that the mothers who responded quickly to their crying babies had babies who cried less by the end of the year than the babies of mothers who had been slower to respond.

This work has certainly been influential in shaping ideas about mothering and child-rearing. It fuelled the argument about whether babies should be 'left to cry' or not. Babycare manuals in the 1970s cited this study as evidence that babies should be picked up as soon as they cried. However, the work has been quite properly criticized on methodological grounds; the researchers did not distinguish between 'fussing' and 'screaming' and thus failed to note potentially important differences between the babies to which the mothers themselves were reacting. It may be helpful to pick up an easily-soothed baby, but just frustrating to pick up an irritable and fussy baby who is not readily calmed. While Bell and Ainsworth interpret the differences in the amount of crying as a result of the mothers' behaviour, other work suggests that babies differ in their fussiness and irritability from early life. It seems likely, however, that the growth of attachment is not due either to the caregiver's sensitivity or the baby's developing discriminations alone, but to a more complex interaction between the baby's characteristics and the caregiver's expectations and skill.

Another example of the view that mothers are especially important in the infant's early life is the idea of bonding. While the term attachment refers to the relationship which the infant develops towards the adult caregiver, the term bonding refers to the reciprocal relationship, from the mother to the infant. Klaus & Kennell (1976) suggested that, by analogy with some animal species such as sheep, immediately after birth the mother experiences a 'sensitive period' when she is most susceptible to develop a deep and lasting relationship with her baby. In order for this bond to develop, Klaus and Kennell argued that the mother needed time and opportunity to be close to the baby, to hold and nurse it.

While their research has no doubt been persuasive in introducing more human hospital practices in post-natal wards, allowing mothers to spend time with their babies rather than whisking the babies off to separate nurseries, other research has not shown clear-cut evidence that mothers who hold their babies straight after birth and are allowed more contact with them in the following days, are more likely subsequently to be more responsive, to talk to them more or to handle them more sensitively than mothers who do not have this opportunity. And the idea of a single, time-limited opportunity to develop such a bond between mother and child has some awkward sequelae. Some mothers, for example of premature or sick babies, cannot handle them after birth; where babies are adopted, the adoptive mother has of course missed this opportunity to develop a bond. But this may not necessarily mean that such relationships will be forever vulnerable or inadequate. It is now felt that while the establishment of affectionate ties between mother and baby is important, it is unlikely to occur only during a brief post-natal period; such ties may take time and may be influenced by a number of factors (Sluckin *et al.* 1983).

Although most research on social development has concentrated on the baby's relationships with adults, recent work by Dunn (1984) has recognized the significant role played by siblings in the young child's life. These relationships are often characterized by demonstrations of intense emotions which reveal much about the growing understanding of what others feel. Dunn's observations show that even one year olds know how to comfort, tease and annoy their older siblings.

The development of communication

The term 'infancy' literally refers to the stage before the child learns to speak and a major achievement of the first year is laying the foundations of this important skill, culminating in the ability to say the first words. Becoming vocal is a process which starts in the earliest months when babies are involved in social interactions with those around them.

Trevarthen (1979) and Newson (1979) note how in western culture mothers tend to make eye contact with their babies, talking to them in a particular high-pitched voice with a slightly exaggerated intonation, holding a conversation even though all the baby can do is gurgle in the pauses. These proto-conversations have many of the characteristics of real dialogue: the participants appear to be taking turns and they seem to listen and attend to each other's contributions even though the baby has not yet mastered language. But the adult will frequently interpret the baby's noises as though they were meaningful and will attribute intentions to the baby's burps, yawns and cries. Thus from the first months the baby is encouraged to enjoy this kind of social dialogue. Other playful social rituals extend the repertoire of pleasurable interactions; peek-a-boo and repetitive actions like tickling games and give-and-take exchanges. The adult at first plays both roles but gradually the baby takes part in the exchange, joining in with 'ta' or 'atishoo!' on cue. Thus the structure of dialogue is developed before much content is conveyed.

Words are not merely sounds but are one aspect of symbolic development; the baby is developing the understanding that symbols can represent things. Objects and people have names; pointing to things is one way to draw attention to them but naming them can be even better. The first words tend to refer to people, objects and events which matter to the baby; early words may accompany actions and indicate needs and wants, like 'more' or 'da' (for 'that', meaning 'I want that'). Different meanings can be expressed by different intonation; 'milk' can mean 'I want some milk' or (with a shake of the head and a falling intonation) 'no more milk'. Once babies have learnt that words can have a powerful effect on others, they will learn more and more, so that an average two year old might say 200 words and understand many more.

Language development is not simply the acquisition of words; it involves putting them together into more complex structures. Generally by two years old the baby will be putting two words together to make simple utterances, like 'big doggie', 'go-way doggie', 'nice doggie'. These early word combinations lack grammatical finesse – plurals or tense endings will be missing, for example – but they allow the baby to express a far greater range of meanings and they mark an important stage of language development. At this stage the baby will stretch the words he or she knows to cover events or objects which have some similarity; thus 'ball' may be used to refer to a ball, the moon, or anything round.

The achievements of infancy

To summarize, by the end of infancy babies will be able to control posture and limb movements with increasing skill, although finer co-ordination has not yet developed. They will be able to act within the environment not merely physically but also indirectly, controlling others by making known their own wants and needs. They will have a stable set of preferences for people around them and will be attached to some familiar adults more than to others. They will have learnt simple cause-and-effect relations and will have developed expectations about their world.

THE PRESCHOOL YEARS

As children get older, their world, both animate and inanimate, expands; they come into contact with more people and are expected to perform different tasks and roles. They need to communicate with a wider audience and make themselves more clearly understood, to behave more maturely and to begin to conform to greater social demands. No longer a baby, and now able to move independently, amuse themselves, make friends and create games of endless fascination with make-believe and a few playthings, for them the preschool period offers new excitement to a mind ready to grasp them.

Motor development

The muscle control which allows the preschool child to gain bowel and bladder control also gives the co-ordination to manage things like getting dressed and putting shoes on, although buttons and zips are still a challenge initially. Hand–eye co-ordination enables the development of drawing and the enjoyment of making marks on paper which will eventually become writing.

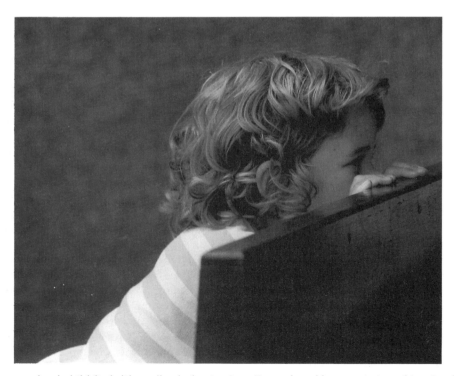

Fig. 9.2   The preschool child finds life endlessly fascinating. *(Reproduced by permission of Jon Sparks.)*

The gross motor skills of hopping, skipping and jumping are practised in everyday activities and, given a diet which provides enough energy, there is ample enthusiasm for physical exercise, which improves co-ordination and balance.

Representation and symbolic development

Growing up in a culture where pictures of objects and two-dimensional representations of the world abound, provides opportunities for the child to learn how to perceive these artificial representations of reality. Children learn informally, through sharing books and talking about illustrations, to 'see' and understand the conventions which are used to show depth and solidity on a flat page. Indeed it may be taken for granted that children will interpret these images in the same way as adults, although in cultures where pictures are not used even adults have difficulty at first in making sense of them. Even in western society, children may at first misunderstand the conventions of diagrams, enlargements or cut-away pictures; but learning both how to see and how to draw pictures usually takes place incidentally and without deliberate teaching. In a culture where symbols are widespread, this is a fundamental step in representing ideas about the world.

Language development

During the preschool period, the language system becomes more powerful in a number of ways; not only does it become structurally more complicated but the purposes for which language can be used become more sophisticated. By the end of infancy, the baby will be using single words and holophrases – units like 'all-gone' and 'do-it' – together with expressive intonation to communicate wants and needs. During the preschool years the child shows an impressive ability to build up a structured system. Early structures will omit function words and word-endings but retain the important content words; thus the child will say 'There my shoe' rather than 'There are my shoes', but no one misunderstands.

The developing system shows regularities in that words are not put together in random order but according to an emerging and changing 'grammar'; for instance initially the child may use 'no' at the beginning of a sentence, and then use 'not' inserted in the middle. What is significant is that the child's system is constrained by memory and information-load so that it is quite resistant to adult tutoring. Correcting the grammar is not helpful and may be frustrating for the child who is trying to communicate a message.

Over-generalization also appears; the child will produce forms which have not been copied from adult speech, like 'mouses' as a plural and 'goed' as a past tense, by analogy with the regular forms. This kind of error demonstrates that children have worked out the regular principles from the speech addressed to them.

The sequence of language development has been investigated in different ways. Some experimenters have taken a longitudinal approach, following a few children over a period of time; often their own children are the most accessible and linguists' offspring are well-documented. More recently a large-scale research project directed by Wells in Bristol used a more representative sample of 128 children who were tape-recorded in their own environment every three months for two and a half years, using a small radio-microphone (Wells 1985). Half the children were recorded from the age of 15 to 42 months and the other half from 39 to 60 months. This study produced considerable data from the conversations between children and their mothers at home, and has been comprehensively analysed to show not only general patterns of language development but also factors associated with different rates of development such as social class or the extent of language addressed to the child.

Wells (1985) was able to show that increasingly complex structures emerged in an ordered sequence, and also that being able to express meaning preceded the ability to articulate it in an appropriate grammatical form. For example, from an early stage children can express want with a single word, making full use of intonation and gesture, but can only later produce utterances like 'want teddy' or 'want go car'. The rate at which children proceed through the stages varies widely, some taking less than three years while others take more than five years, with the average being about four; the sequence of development, however, was generally similar. Despite a widespread view that girls develop language more quickly than boys, there were no consistent sex differences in rate of language acquisition although there were some differences in the contexts and kinds of conversations that boys and girls had with their mothers at home.

While family background variables were associated with the rate of language development at three and a half years, Wells emphasizes that the influence of social class should not be exaggerated; it is likely that the strength of the correlation found in his study was affected by the over-representation of families from both ends of the social class range. Other factors have almost as strong an effect on rate of language development, such as whether or not the parents read to the child, the amount of speech addressed to the child, and whether the child's speech is corrected (this is negatively related to the child's language development, i.e. it slows it down).

Many studies have explored the role of the adult's speech and its relation to the child's language development; it is clear that it is not merely the amount of input which is important but the quality with which the adult builds up and sustains the dialogue. In the process of communicating with the child, the adult must be aware of what the child can understand, which will be in advance of what can be expressed. In trying to maintain a conversation the adult will fine-tune the message so that the child can contribute, and will expand the meanings which the child is struggling to express. Wells' books offer many examples of how adults clarify and amplify the child's utterance; for example Gerald (aged 18 months) has found teddy's bed empty:

> Gerald: 'Teddy!'
> Mother: 'Where's teddy? I think Teddy's downstairs. I think we took him downstairs with us.'

The child's single word elicits a long and full reply. By contrast, children whose rate of language development was slower seemed to have adults around them who were less interested in responding to the child's attempts or who spoke to them less.

Becoming a person: learning gender roles

During the preschool years parents begin to demand more adherence to socially acceptable behaviour. Some of the rules concern politeness, like saying please and thank you or waiting your turn, while others involve conformity to social rules, such as showing gender-appropriate behaviour.

Research has shown that parents react differently to boys and girls even from birth (Rubin *et al.* 1974) and during the preschool years this differentiation becomes more obvious when boys and girls may be encouraged to play at different activities with different toys (Rheingold & Cook 1975). Their conceptions of themselves as having a gender also develops; by three most children can correctly label themselves and others as boys or girls, and by five they understand that gender does not change with age: once a boy, always a boy. Initially they tend to think that gender depends on physical characteristics like hair or clothes and only later will they appreciate that it is based on genital characteristics.

Children growing up in most societies are made aware of what is sex-appropriate behaviour by the adults around them. In western culture they receive messages from the media and from books as well as from the behaviour they observe. These messages may not always be consistent and the adults they meet may not conform to the stereotypes. Nevertheless, by around three years of age children will know what the social expectations are, for example, the toys and clothes right for a boy and those right for a girl and the most appropriate occupations. Children whose mothers are employed outside the home may show less conventional sex-stereotyped attitudes, although some studies suggest that the general stereotypes are still powerful (Cordua *et al.*, 1979).

Becoming sociable: friendship and playmates

One of the most misleading terms which has been used to describe young children is to refer to them as egocentric. The term was used by Piaget (1926) to refer to young children's tendency to carry on long monologues in their play, and was then extended to cover the child's difficulty in co-ordinating perspectives. However, subsequent observers have failed to find a preponderance of egocentric monologues of the kind which Piaget thought were typical at this age; indeed, this period seems notable for the child's sociability. Hay (1994) suggests that children are at their most prosocial during infancy, when they will spontaneously offer toys to another, while during the second and third year of life they become more aware of social norms and conventions and will regulate their behaviour to comply with adult requests or prohibitions.

Parents and teachers encourage social relations by suggesting that children should share toys and not hurt each other; it has been suggested that this can be most effective when exhortations stress not only the social desirability but also offer a reasoned explanation for the behaviour. Dunn suggested that mothers who talked about the new baby's feelings and needs to the older sibling encouraged more positive interactions between them (Dunn & Kendrick 1982).

Play is a feature of the preschool period which our culture encourages (Fig 9.3); while its educational value is still debated, it has been elevated to a position of importance because of the role which children occupy in our society. Protected from having to contribute to the domestic economy, with a prolonged childhood and no longer at risk from disease or starvation, children have time to play. Today's emphasis on play must therefore be seen as part of the cultural niche which society has constructed for children, rather than as an inherent part of the preschool child's repertoire. As Tizard (1977) has pointed out, children are now provided with special toys and are expected to occupy themselves rather than being encouraged to assist with household chores.

Cross-cultural studies show that children elsewhere may be expected to take care of younger siblings, weed crops or tend animals, while those from a western culture may be playing with dolls or cars. The difference between play and other activities is that play has no extrinsic goal; it is done for its own sake or for the pleasure it gives. The consequences of pulling out the 'wrong' weeds may be serious, but if the child drops a pretend cake they can just retrieve it! Functional behaviours and non-functional play may be equally helpful in providing opportunities to develop new skills.

During the preschool years children's play undergoes some important changes. One of these is the ability to use one thing to stand for another, which is at the heart of much imaginative play. At first children need realistic props, but gradually they use less realistic substitutes. Another important feature is the ability to sustain an invented story, developing the plot to incorporate characters and events as necessary. Sociodramatic play increases during the preschool period, when children will act out roles together, being mummy and daddy, teacher and pupil or doctor and patient. These tend to be stereotyped caricatures and their behaviour may seem rigidly predictable. Mummies stay home and cook meals while daddies go out to work; doctors (who are boys) give injections while nurses (who are girls) tuck patients up in bed and comfort them. Teachers are strict and children misbehave. These roles seem pervasive and widespread, despite the child's own experience.

Another common type of play is rough-and-tumble play, which may involve chasing and wrestling and is

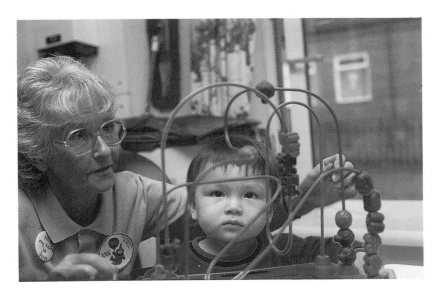

Fig. 9.3 Promoting play to maintain optimal development. (*Reproduced by permission of Jon Sparks.*)

quite distinct from serious fighting. This is pre-dominantly boys' activity. Perhaps it is a prelude to later team games like football.

Whether play promotes development is not an easy question to answer. For one thing, in a society in which all children are encouraged to play it is difficult to deprive them of this experience. Experimental studies have compared short sessions in which children were allowed to play, with sessions in which they were taught to do something, thus giving both groups equal amounts of adult involvement or novel experience. Such artificial studies seldom show much effect (Smith & Simon 1984). Longer-term studies, which have fostered sociodramatic play over a school term, have shown some effects but these studies too suffer from other methodological weaknesses which mean that it is not clear which aspects of play are effective. It may well be the adult's interaction which is beneficial. It has been claimed that structured play of the kind advocated by the High/Scope programme (Hohmann *et al.* 1979) in nursery classes, provides greater benefits for both academic and social gains than free play does. In the High/Scope nursery, children regularly plan their activities with adult assistance and review their achievements daily (Smith *et al.* 1987).

Play can also be used for therapeutic purposes. When therapeutic play provides a safe environment for children to explore fantasies and fears with a sensitive adult who can understand and interpret the child's behaviour, it can be beneficial. For example, it may help children who experience abuse or those children admitted to hospital to become familiar with equipment and rehearse roles and practise procedures on themselves or on an inanimate object, thus minimising fear or apprehension. In such contexts play has been demonstrated to be helpful in reducing stress and enabling children to cope (Cassell 1965; Schwarz *et al.* 1983).

Becoming a thinker

Piaget's description of cognitive development (Inhelder & Piaget 1964) still provides the most coherent account of development at this stage, although more recent work has shown that he seriously underestimated children's abilities in many respects. Children's thinking at this stage is heavily influenced by the appearance of things and by the child's own viewpoint; the child cannot

understand complementary and inclusive relations because these involve reversibility (see the dialogue with Gerald earlier in this chapter). Examples of the child's limited reasoning are shown in the dialogue with Jane aged 3.

> Adult: 'Have you any brothers or sisters?'
> Child: 'Yes, a sister.'
> Adult: 'What's your sister's name?'
> Child: 'Kate.'
> Adult: 'Has Kate got a sister?'
> Child: 'No.'

The child fails to see the reciprocal relationship. An example of the inability to cope with inclusive relations is shown in this exchange when the adult shows the child a picture of daisies and buttercups. The child seems limited to coping with one relationship at a time:

> Adult: 'Are the daisies flowers?'
> Child: 'Yes.'
> Adult: 'Are the buttercups flowers?'
> Child: 'Yes.'
> Adult: 'If I take away all the daisies, will there be any
>   flowers left?'
> Child: 'No.'

Another of the tasks which Piaget used to demonstrate the pre-operational child's limited reasoning ability was that of seriation (Inhelder & Piaget 1964). When asked to arrange a series of sticks of various lengths in ascending order, children at this stage find it difficult to do consistently. However, Bryant & Trabasso (1971) have shown that provided the child can remember all the necessary information, this task can be completed. They trained children using different coloured sticks until they had learnt which was longer/shorter out of each pair; they were then able to arrange the whole series of six sticks correctly.

More recently, Pears & Bryant (1990) successfully demonstrated that children as young as four are able to make an inference when given other information. Piaget had argued that children in the pre-operational stage were unable to make transitive inferences, but it now appears that his method was insensitive to children's developing reasoning skills.

Donaldson (1978) argues that the child brings to all situations a strong set of expectations based on everyday experiences about the ways in which adults usually behave. If the adult repeats a question, the child infers that this must be because the previous answer was wrong. If the adult changes some aspect of a test display, the child interprets this as a meaningful change which should be attended to. However, if the test situation is made more sensible or realistic from the child's viewpoint, the child produces more 'advanced' answers.

Instead of asking children to predict views of mountains from different viewpoints, as Piaget had done, Hughes (1978) asked children to hide a doll from a toy policeman in various 'rooms' in a layout; most preschool children were able to do this, demonstrating, so Hughes claims, that they were able to see things from another's viewpoint and were not cognitively egocentric. Donaldson (1978) and Hughes (1978) both believe that when children are tested in situations which make sense to them in terms of their everyday life, and when care is taken to remove ambiguity from the wording of instructions, they will demonstrate more advanced reasoning skills. However, there is still a ceiling on their understanding and psychologists are still working to develop a clearer picture of what preschool children can achieve.

THE SCHOOL YEARS

Clearly the precise definitions of the preschool and school periods are arbitrary and change according to local customs. In Sweden children are 'preschoolers' until they are seven, although most are in kindergarten from five years old. In England the age of school entry is variable too, some children starting full-time school soon after their fourth birthday and others not until a year later. Those who oppose early entry to school generally cite developmental arguments to support their case: that children of four are not yet 'ready' for school tasks and cannot cope with either the academic demands of the classroom or the social demands of the playground. It is recognized that the characteristics of the school years are not acquired instantly on crossing the threshold; there are gradual changes which occur some time between six and twelve years of age.

Of more particular interest to psychologists is the effect of an institution like school on the child's developing intellect. One way to think of the relationship is to assume that the child's level of understanding influences what can be taught and how it is learnt; an alternative view would suggest that the experience of being at school may affect the kinds of cognitive skills which are developed in response to the learning demands of the classroom. As Wood (1986) points out, schooling is a comparatively recent introduction, and learning in school differs significantly from learning which occurs informally in everyday settings.

Whether the source of the change in the child comes from receiving the school curriculum, or whether it stems from the child's growing ability to understand more abstract concepts, a key feature of the child's development during this period is the ability to think, reason and understand about decontextualized things. Donaldson (1978) shows how school tasks require children to deal with general principles and abstract relations rather than the specifics of particular events in real life. School tasks require the ability to set aside common sense and ignore the inferences which are appropriate in real life. Thus learning what is required in school learning is itself a challenge.

Cognitive development

According to Piaget (Piaget & Inhelder 1969, 1974), the important feature of cognitive development at this stage is the ability to reason mentally, without being affected by irrelevant perceptual features. This achievement enables the child to grasp that appearances can be deceptive and that underlying logical relations can be manipulated independently. The tasks which Piaget used to demonstrate this have now become well known as measures of conservation; in these situations the child is asked to compare two quantities and to agree that they remain the same despite changes in shape. So for number conservation, a child must agree that the number of objects in a row remains the same whether they are spread out or condensed; for the conservation of length, that a string is the same length whether it is straight or curled up; for the conservation of quantity, the child must know that two lumps of modelling clay remain the same amount even if one is rolled out thin or flattened; for liquids, conservation of quantity requires the child to maintain equivalence when the contents of a tall thin glass are poured into a short, wide glass.

In these tasks children must be able to justify their answers and Piaget regarded the reason given as important evidence that the child had grasped the underlying principles. The child who understands conservation may say 'They're the same because you didn't add any or take any away', or 'It was long and thin and now it's short and fat, but if you poured it back you'd have the same amount'. The child who has not yet grasped conservation seems to think that when the appearance changes the amount changes too. Children take time to develop this understanding, and conservation of number is generally appreciated before conservation of quantity, weight or volume. But the achievement is not an all-or-nothing event; children will generally perform best when familiar materials are used, suggesting that in the early stages this ability is still dependent on the knowledge derived from everyday life about how objects behave. Only later can the principles be abstracted and manipulated regardless of the physical embodiment of the task.

Not only is the attainment of conservation a gradual process but even adults may be deceived by appearance and behave like nonconservers. Although adults *know* that there is the same amount of milk in a carton as in a bottle, they may still feel that the bottle looks as though it has more. And the packaging industry is determined to make shoppers buy the packet which looks bigger, although the small print may prove that it actually contains less. Although adults possess the reasoning ability to deal with these situations logically, they do not always do so!

Once the importance of this mental achievement was recognized, many psychologists were fascinated by the possibility that children's cognitive development might be accelerated by teaching them conservation at an earlier age. A veritable industry of training studies grew up in America and England in the 1960s and 1970s to see whether children, given appropriate experience or assistance, would show advanced development. The outcome in general was negative. Just as children cannot be taught more advanced grammar than they have developed for themselves, so they cannot be trained to acquire concepts before they have the necessary understanding to grasp them. Beilin (1971, 1978) has reviewed these training studies; while they were not always successful in training children to grasp conservation earlier, they provided much understanding of the role of a number of factors, such as allowing children to handle the material themselves or the kinds of questions asked by the experimenter. Some of this work

has led to substantial critiques of Piaget and re-evaluations of his theory (Sutherland 1992).

This ability to reason logically affects not only the child's understanding of the physical world but also the social and moral world; this will be considered later.

Developing memory strategies

The ability to reason is not the only factor which determines how a child will think or learn; the ability to remember is also important. In school tasks, recall may be especially important. Changes in memory do not depend on increasing storage capacity but on memory activities which children carry out. Memory is 'a series of interlocking activities which eventually become automatic and often seemingly effortless, but which in reality take years of learning and practice to develop' (Wood 1988).

Examples of these activities are attending to, rehearsing and organizing the material to be memorized. Young children are less able to focus selectively on the important elements, to exclude irrelevant material and to concentrate on the important parts. This may be because they don't know what is important or because they cannot maintain their concentration. Research suggests that younger children have difficulty in attending only to specific features and are prone to distraction. They are also inefficient in using rehearsal strategies which will help their recall. Older children and adults know that strategies like writing lists, repeating, rehearsing and making associations between elements all improve recall. Children under school age seldom use these strategies spontaneously, although if reminded they will carry them out (Keeney *et al.* 1967). They are also unrealistic about their own memory skills and will overestimate their ability to recall items. Because they are poor at monitoring their own memory they do not focus on the 'difficult' items or material which they did not get right on the first attempt, whereas older children and adults will devote more attention to the things they got wrong before.

Remembering is an invisible activity, like knowing and forgetting. It refers to mental processes which are not directly observable; there is no overt behaviour to be copied. Not surprisingly, young children have difficulty knowing what they are meant to do when told to 'remember' and will stare at a list without knowing how to ensure that the material is remembered. If shown how to group items together or to organize them in some way, by someone older and more competent, the younger child can literally 'see what is meant' and will eventually internalize these strategies and be able to use them appropriately at a later date.

Learning by heart and learning by doing

In western society where all children go to school, being able to remember effectively is a demand which all children routinely encounter. That children and adults discover ways to do this is an example of how their mental processes are moulded by their cultural experience. In non-schooled cultures where adults do not need to remember such arbitrary information remote from everyday life, such memorization strategies are not used. Children and adults learn through imitating and practising the necessary skills. What is sometimes taken for granted as an essential achievement is in fact a response to a cultural demand for the acquisition of more and more information which needs to be stored until needed.

Becoming literate

Although there is a tendency to think that children learn to read and write at school, as of course many do, the precursors of literacy are laid in the preschool years and the achievement is a gradual process. By the time they go to school, children will know that print conveys messages. Many will have shared stories and books with parents or carers and will know the difference between the print and the pictures, and where to start reading a book and how to turn the pages as the story unfolds. Most children start writing by copying the letters of their own name, and even before they produce distinguishable letters they will produce 'play-writing' which is quite different from drawing. Bissex (1980) describes her own child's progress in writing before school, and Ferreiro & Teberosky (1982) provide many examples of the developing writing process.

There is evidence that it is not merely an acquaintance with print which is necessary for children to learn to read. Learning to read involves the ability to split words up into their constituent sounds and to relate these sounds to the marks on the page. This phonological

awareness has its roots in the preschool years; at this age young children will show by their word-play that they appreciate sounds, when they make up words which rhyme with their own names. Bryant & Bradley (1985) tested a group of four and five year olds who could not yet read and found differences in how well they could identify the odd one out in a set of words with similar sounds (bun *hut* gun sun, or *hug* pig wig dig). When the same children were eight or nine years old they were given a standardized reading test; the correlations between their ability to categorize sounds and their subsequent reading levels were higher than the correlations with either memory or vocabulary.

Writing is not just speech written down. While speech succeeds in face-to-face communication, the conventions of print ensure that the message is conveyed across time and space to an unseen audience. The individuality of a speaker's voice is lost but the text can be read by anyone who understands the language. To do this, writing has to be more explicit and the writer must anticipate what the reader needs to know. In a conversation the meaning is jointly negotiated, but in writing the writer must take responsibility for ensuring that the reader understands. As children become literate they learn about different uses of language; as speakers they use language to get others to do things, to narrate events and to convey feelings, but as readers and writers they will use language not only to convey information but to present an argument logically and persuasively, to lecture or debate. In becoming literate they extend their use of language for many different purposes.

This is not the place to argue the merits of different methods of teaching reading; the key point is that learning to read is not merely the acquisition of skills but also involves cognitive challenges in focusing on language as the medium for the message. So many school subjects require literacy that learning to read well is a passport to learning history, geography, science and many other things; they all involve reading and writing and each one uses language in a distinctive way. So the child who does not find these skills easy is likely to find the handicap far larger.

Making friends

In the preschool years, friendship becomes an important dimension of the child's social life and during the school years the role of the peer group increases in terms of widening the opportunities for different kinds of emotions and interactions beyond the family. Children who are popular are generally seen as helpful, friendly children who play by the rules in interactions; unpopular children tend to be aggressive or unpredictable children who are unhelpful or disruptive (Coie, Dodge & Kupersmidt 1990). But children who are unpopular at one age may not always be so; at younger ages rejection seems less stable than at older ages, but it is not clear what factors lead to more permanent unpopularity. It is clear, however, that there are different kinds of unpopularity; some unpopular children are aggressive, others tend to be shy and passive, while others seem to withdraw from social contact. It may be interesting to consider whether children who are withdrawn have been rejected by their peer group or whether children who are rejected become withdrawn. Only longitudinal studies can indicate the direction of causality and as yet the available information is limited and unclear.

Research on children's peer relations has applications to practical issues such as bullying. Recent work by Olweus (1991) in Norway suggests that bullies are quite secure but are aggressive individuals who target weak, unassertive peers. Applied research focuses on strategies which empower the victim as well as trying to change the aggressor's behaviour.

It is not yet clear whether children's difficulties in peer-group relations arise from problems in their understanding of others' intentions or from social cues.

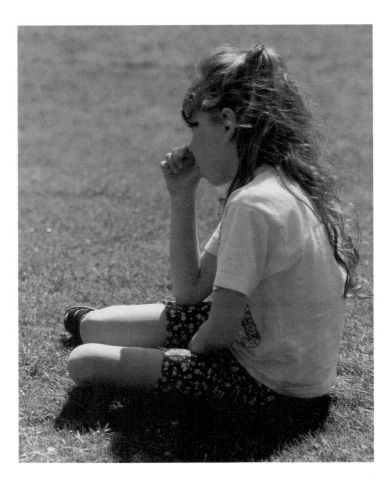

Fig. 9.4 Some children may withdraw from social contact. *(Reproduced by permission of Jon Sparks.)*

Some research has found differences in the way that popular and unpopular children interpret ambiguous actions, but again the direction of effect is inconclusive (Dodge & Feldman 1990).

Developing ideas about right and wrong

Children do not just think about school problems or what makes things work; they think about people and what makes them behave. Their ability to think in more complex ways and to take account of different factors also enables them to develop more sophisticated understanding about right and wrong. This does not mean that their behaviour will necessarily improve; the factors which govern why people behave as they do are not the same as those which influence their reasoning. Moral judgements are not the same as moral behaviour.

Piaget (1932) studied children's understanding of rules in the context of games, and he identified three stages. Initially, up to the preschool period, children recognize no rules at all and simply do what they want to do. Gradually they come to accept that rules are laid down by others and cannot be changed. There is a black-and-white view of rules: things are either completely right or totally wrong and the intention of the person cannot be taken into consideration. Thus if someone causes damage accidentally, the child views the damage caused as more important than the aim. In this heteronomous stage of moral reasoning, the child will argue that the greater the damage the bigger the wrong-doing.

During the school years, children's ideas undergo further transformation as they come to understand that rules are made by society and that these may be changed or adapted to fit particular circumstances. Intentions are taken into account and punishment is not automatic but should suit the situation.

During adolescence the ability to reason more abstractly enables deeper consideration of right and wrong as principles. Rules are internalized rather than imposed and a more coherent system of values is developed.

Piaget's original investigations (1932) were considerably extended by Kohlberg (1976); he explored children's moral reasoning by presenting them with a series of moral dilemmas and analysing their responses. His research has been applied to school settings where training studies to improve children's understanding of right and wrong have been devised. His work has also been criticized, partly on methodological grounds and partly because his studies originally only involved boys. Gilligan (1982) argues that girls and women develop a different view of moral behaviour which is more 'person-centred', giving more weight to feelings and a concern for responsibility.

ADOLESCENCE

This stage has a reputation for being one of dramatic transition, frequently accompanied by turmoil. But these impressions of upheaval and unease in the quest for identity were the legacy of psychoanalytic views which are less dominant today. The notion that adolescence is inevitably accompanied by storm and stress has not been borne out by close scrutiny.

Puberty

The physical changes of puberty provide a clear marker for the start of the transition into adolescence (Fig. 9.5), although for both sexes the process takes some years to complete. In general, girls reach physical maturity earlier than boys. For girls the first manifestation of approaching maturity is increasing height, starting around 11 and lasting until about 14 years. For boys the development of the testes is the first indicator, followed by the height spurt which lasts from 12 to 16 years.

Height changes are accompanied by other changes in body shape and proportions, and the hormones which regulate the development of sexual maturity are also responsible for less welcome changes such as increased sebaceous gland activity producing spots and blackheads. The whole process takes a few years to complete but to the teenager concerned the changes may seem sudden and unexpected. In western societies, where masculinity is associated with muscularity, boys may welcome the gains in their height and weight; girls, on the other hand, may be less pleased with their increasing fat and may respond by dieting. Rutter & Rutter (1992) found that 'by late adolescence, about half of all girls in the UK and USA have dieted – usually unsuccessfully!' Although girls reach sexual maturity earlier than boys, their sexual behaviour tends, in western societies, to be

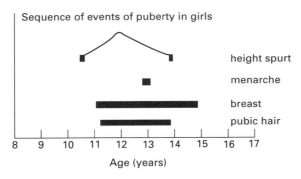

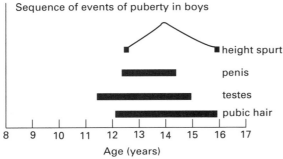

Fig. 9.5 Sequence of events of puberty in girls and boys.

later; more boys than girls are likely to report that they had their first sexual experience before the age of 15, although there are also large differences between socioeconomic and cultural subgroups in the kinds of sexual activity undertaken.

While adolescents may report feeling more moody and depressed, attempts to demonstrate a clear-cut relationship between mood and hormone levels have been less successful. Susman *et al.* (1987) studied the level of sex hormones and ratings of mood in a sample of children aged 9–14. For boys, higher levels of adrenal androgens were related to feeling low and rebellious, but no relation was found for girls. It has been suggested that for girls the effect may depend on changes in hormone production rather than absolute oestrogen level. For both sexes, the size of the relationship is quite small.

Family relations

There is a common view that living with adolescents involves conflict. But more systematic research, looking

at population samples rather than at clinical groups, indicates that only a minority of families is affected seriously by these (Hill 1987). However, while deteriorating relationships may not affect most families, many will experience a change in the quality of interactions. Some research suggests that there may be frequent quarrels, usually sparked off by disagreements about dress, tidiness, hygiene or the adolescent's contribution to household tasks. While these may seem trivial issues, they are invested with an importance which ensures that to the adolescent they become a focus from which he or she defends the right to decide. Parents who had grown used to amenable children may find these conflicts distressing and the fact that the issues are perceived so differently by the participants means they may be difficult to resolve to everyone's satisfaction.

Decisions, for example, about hairstyles and sexual behaviour relate to the larger issues of independence and autonomy. It is generally agreed that the main task of adolescence is to become autonomous, although this term can be interpreted in a number of different ways. It may mean detachment, independence from parental control, self-confidence or the ability to resist peer pressure. Steinberg & Silverberg (1986) suggest that over the age-range 10 to 16, different aspects develop at different rates: while emotional self-reliance shows a gradual increase over this period, ability to resist peer pressure lessens during the 11–13 period and then increases slowly. Thus as teenagers become less dependent on parental authority, they seem to become more susceptible to peer influence.

Ryan & Lynch (1989) studied a wider age-range and suggested that in early adolescence teenagers who reported feelings of emotional autonomy also felt rejected by their parents and made less use of parental support; those who felt more attached to their parents also showed closer relationships with friends.

Monck (1991) studied 15–20 year old young women in London and showed that the majority of them had close and confiding relationships with other women. Boyfriends were also cited by half of the oldest girls as sources of support if they had financial problems or trouble with authority, but fathers and brothers were seldom mentioned. There is no comparable sample of young men which would indicate whether they derive support from fathers and brothers. However, close relationships with mother and a same-sex friend were also reported in a study carried out with high school students in Turkey (Hortacsu 1989). Hill (1993) concludes that as adolescents get older they extend their networks of social and emotional relationships and, rather than the peer group supplanting parents, the adolescent develops complementary and differentiated relationships for different purposes.

Thinking in adolescence

Piaget (1972) proposed that during adolescence the concrete-operational mode of reasoning would be superseded by the highest stage of logical thought: that of formal operations. A main feature of this stage is the ability to reason in terms of verbally stated hypotheses, without recourse to concrete objects or images. Piaget regards this ability to extend reasoning beyond the realms of reality to the realms of possibility, as an important expansion of the scope of thinking. Piaget saw that this would enable thinkers to go beyond their own experience, not only when considering abstract ideas but also when involved in reasoning about social issues such as justice or political ideology (Piaget 1972).

Piaget's original experimental work involved mathematical and scientific problems such as working out the factors involved in the amplitude of a pendulum swing or the displacement of water by sinking objects. Certainly the ability of children to solve these problems increases with age and from about 11 years they begin to show the hallmarks of formal logical reasoning; they think systematically through all the possibilities and their ability to consider logical implication increases.

Piaget (1972) claimed that this development was universal, that all adults would achieve this level of reasoning ability. However, attempts to demonstrate formal reasoning in settings other than the elite Genevan schools in which Piaget worked, immediately began to highlight problems; in other societies adolescents and even adults did not seem to show the expected progression towards formal logic. Piaget's response to this was to admit the role of the environment in providing intellectual stimulation and challenge, although not 'teaching' in the narrow sense. He also recognized that as children get older their intellectual development diversifies and they may show advanced development in some spheres – artistic, literary or scientific – but not in all; so the achievement of formal operations may occur at different rates in these different spheres and may be

affected by the kind of working knowledge the young adult is developing, whether in practical tasks or in educational settings.

While Piaget maintained that 'It is quite true that one of the essential characteristics of formal thought appears to be the independence of its form from its reality content' (Piaget 1972), he acknowledged that when investigating formal thought it was necessary to capture the interest and curiosity of the adolescent in order to probe their most advanced thought. It is this acknowledgement of the role of context and the influence of everyday reasoning which has led to the widespread scepticism about the Piagetian account.

Keating & Clark (1980) looked at the relation between young adolescents' reasoning on physical tasks and their reasoning about interpersonal situations. They found that one-third of 16 year olds did not show formal reasoning on either physical or interpersonal tasks, although the tendency to use formal reasoning increased from the age of 12. They also found that more advanced interpersonal reasoning was achieved later than formal reasoning on the physical tasks, and many children who could use formal reasoning on the physical tasks did not show it when faced with the interpersonal problems. Similar problems with the Piagetian stage of formal operations have arisen when other investigators have tried to demonstrate it. Yet clearly, thinking does become more powerful as children get older and if these changes are not to be described in terms of cognitive stages, other frameworks to explore alterations in thought patterns need to be sought.

Children's thinking skills develop in a number of ways during adolescence. They become more able to direct their attention efficiently, both to focus it and to divide it between two tasks, such as doing homework while watching television. They become able to remember better and to monitor their own mental strategies. Adolescents develop an understanding that knowledge is relative rather than absolute and they tend to reason in abstract rather than concrete terms (Keating 1990). As a consequence there is a tendency to feel that everything is relative and they frequently respond with a 'can't tell' answer to logical problems even when in fact a conclusion can be drawn. Keating suggests that as they become aware of uncertainty and relativism this may extend to a fatalistic position where they believe that no knowledge is reliable and no firm conclusions can ever be drawn.

During early adolescence, specialized abilities and skills emerge and become more differentiated. These skills become channelled through the educational and vocational system so that by mid-teens the adolescent may have a clear view of him or herself as being strong at sciences, weak in the arts or having a good practical approach. This pattern of development has given rise to the domain-specific view, that instead of general cognitive skills which underpin all abilities, abilities are specific to particular content areas and will not necessarily transfer to other contexts.

The importance of unravelling the ways in which adolescents reason and make decisions applies not just to education generally but more specifically to those areas of adolescent decision-making where the penalties of poor judgement are most serious, such as health behaviour, alcohol use and drug-taking. However, in these areas decisions are strongly affected not just by reasoning skills but by social and cultural influences. As adolescents get older they become more able to consider alternative possibilities, to look at situations from a variety of perspectives, to evaluate evidence and anticipate consequences. Some health education programmes have sought to harness these skills and to offer practice in simulated contexts. Providing information does not ensure that appropriate decisions from an adult's perspective will always ensue, but at least it encourages an awareness of the complexity of the situation and may allow more thoughtful rather than impulsive behaviour. Society cannot protect the adolescent from difficult decisions but in seeking to regulate adolescent behaviour, by setting a legal age for drinking or sexual activity, it seeks to postpone them. It may be important to provide information early enough for it to be influential.

Personal development

The search for personal identity was regarded by Erikson (1969) as the main developmental task of adolescence, a task which is assisted by the adolescent's increasing intellectual powers and wider knowledge of the world. But as the adolescent develops a greater awareness of relativism and uncertainty and a capacity for reflection, this can affect their awareness of themselves. The definition of self shifts from concrete characteristics – for example, I'm tall or I like sports – to one which comprises traits, attitudes and values – for example, I care passionately about animal rights or I want to become a nurse so I can help people. This is often accompanied by an uncomfortable awareness of the gap between the ideal self and the reality.

Hill (1993) suggests that current views and research on the process and models of identity achievement are becoming more sophisticated and earlier views which had as a goal a unitary construct of identity may require revision. Perhaps because of the position of adolescents in western industrialized societies, constrained by a protracted education and often uncertain vocational future yet targeted in the media as consumers, adolescent identity may show many facets which evolve at different rates. Sexual, vocational, racial, religious and political identities may emerge independently and may not be achieved until later in life.

While most adolescents cope with everyday demands adequately, if not perfectly, the increase in psychiatric disorders shows that for some adolescents this is a time associated with particular challenge. Rutter & Rutter (1992) note that some disorders such as anorexia nervosa and schizophrenia usually start or become most frequent during adolescence, and clinical depression becomes more marked. There may be reasons why adolescents are more prone to depression. Rutter & Rutter consider it unlikely that hormonal changes directly cause depression although they concede that 'it could be that hormones provide a sensitizing vulnerability factor of some kind, even if they do not precipitate the onset of depression as such'. However, some adolescents may be more vulnerable to stress because their abilities to anticipate consequences may lead to a feeling of overwhelming hopelessness about the future.

This account of adolescence has tried to stress the continuity with other processes of development which occur throughout the lifespan. While the focus of this chapter is on children's development, psychologists have become increasingly aware that many changes occur during adulthood and it may be limiting to perceive that adolescence represents some end-point, after which change becomes either slower or more difficult to achieve. In their recent book, Rutter & Rutter (1992) include chapters on adulthood, mid-life transitions and old age, which reflect the increasing understanding of development as a life-long process.

CULTURAL DIFFERENCES

While it may be relatively easy to investigate differences between children which are due to obvious differences in their backgrounds or experiences, it is more of a challenge to investigate the effects of more pervasive cultural influences. Yet these factors may be equally influential on the developing child. For example, in western cultures quite young babies are expected to be able to put up with long intervals between feeds with minimal contact from adults, without being held or rocked, and to stay quiet and tranquil despite being left alone. These expectations are not necessarily related to how babies 'naturally' develop. The environment is artificial and makes particular demands on children which in other cultures they would not have to face. This is not to suggest that any social context is inherently more 'natural' than any other, but simply to emphasize that what may be taken for granted is highly contrived.

Here are some ways in which the world constructed for babies affects their development. Super & Harkness (1982) studied the early development of Kipsigis babies born in Kokwet in the western highlands of Kenya. In their first month, Kipsigis babies are rarely out of reach of the mother; they are almost always held in very close proximity and they are not put into a separate cot or room specially darkened for sleep. In fact there are no special sleeping arrangements for the infant; the baby will nap and doze as the mother goes about her usual routine. There is thus no pressure on the baby to develop the sustained sleeping pattern, which western mothers value, of a long night-time sleep. Super and Harkness found that at four months the average Kipsigis baby sleeps for 12 hours in contrast to 15 hours for an average American baby, and that their longest sleep episode is about four and a half hours, while Western babies may achieve eight hours.

Similar contrasts can be found in feeding patterns. Where babies are breast fed and are constantly carried around by their mothers, feeding the baby need not disrupt ongoing activity and the mother can respond easily to what she feels the baby needs. Thus among the !Kung San bushmen a baby may feed several times an hour; such a frequency would be regarded as indicative of a 'problem' in a western baby. Confined to their cots, often out of sight and almost out of ear-shot, western babies have to signal their hunger or discomfort by

crying !Kung babies, however, only have to become restless for the mother to respond to their needs, so they rarely cry and when they do, it signals real distress and is never ignored. It takes on average six seconds to respond to the cry of a !Kung baby, while in western cultures babies may be allowed to cry for anything from five to thirty minutes (Konner 1991). Western babies too signal their growing hunger by snuffling and moving and becoming fretful; however, as the average western mother is preoccupied with other activities she is unaware of these signs until she hears her baby cry.

In England and America babies are not expected to share their parents' beds and health visitors and baby-care manuals offer varied advice on how to encourage babies to sleep alone or to discourage them from sleeping with their parents. The reasons given for this range from possible smothering or sexual over-stimulation to disturbing the parents' sleep; but as Morelli *et al.* (1992) argue:

'Folk wisdom in the United States considers the early night-time separation of infants from their parents as essential for the infants' healthy psychological development.'

Thus parents who find this hard to achieve may worry about whether they are harming their baby in some way. Yet this practice, which is regarded as common sense in America and England, is quite uncommon elsewhere in the world. In most societies babies sleep with their mother at least until they are weaned and they may often share a room, if not a bed, after that.

A recent study by Morelli *et al.* (1992) compared the sleeping arrangements of a group of Mayan families in Guatemala with a group of American families with toddlers, and interviewed the parents to explore their attitudes towards their practices in this area. By three months of age over half the American babies were sleeping in a separate room, and by six months 80% of them were. By contrast, all the Mayan mothers shared a bed with their infants throughout the first year of life; even by two years none of the babies slept in a bed or room alone. Giving night feeds was no problem for the Mayan mothers, who said they did not have to wake up but just turned over to make the breast accessible. American mothers had to get up and stay awake during night feeds which, in most cases, lasted until the baby was over six months old. Thus American mothers aimed to reduce night feeds at the earliest opportunity since these disturbed their own sleep patterns.

Most interesting, however, was the Mayan mothers' reactions to the typical American pattern:

> 'Invariably, the idea that toddlers are put to sleep in a separate room was met with shock, disapproval and pity ... they regarded the practice of having infants and toddlers sleep in separate rooms as tantamount to child neglect.' (Morelli *et al.* 1992)

Mayan babies have to give up a place in their mother's bed only when another sibling is born; Mayan mothers try to prepare for this by moving the toddler in to sleep with another member of the family, but still in close proximity to the mother. Some psychologists have speculated that sharing a bed with the mother provides the kind of gentle stimulation required to enable the baby to regulate its breathing and thus avoid cot deaths (McKenna 1986).

Regardless of the actual or potential benefits, of more interest are the ways in which such practices become part of the culture's view of childrearing. Thus Americans see babies as dependent at birth and needing to become independent, while the Mayans see the encouragement of interdependence as vital. The Japanese, too, apparently regard the mother and child sleeping together as one way in which interdependence can be fostered (Caudill & Plath 1966), and they may regard the infant as still intimately part of the mother at a young age. Americans construct elaborate bedtime routines to ease the transition from being with others to being alone, and they recognize that this is stressful for the child so they encourage the infant to take a favourite toy or blanket to bed, while Mayan babies have no special sleeping clothes or bedtime rituals. In another study of 60 nine year olds in a Mayan community, only 8% were in a separate bed and none in a separate room (Rogoff 1977). As Morelli puts it: 'sleeping alone is considered a hardship'.

While childrearing practices may be influenced by many practical, physical aspects of the environment – Japanese households may have less space than American ones for example – what is of interest is the way in which they become embedded in a set of cultural values which include what it means to be a child and what the goals of adulthood are. It may be important to bear in mind that what is often assumed to be part of 'natural' development is in fact an adaptation to a particular set of environmental pressures. Other circumstances may produce other patterns of adjustment; styles of behaving and responding which may appear in one culture to be well-adjusted are maladaptive in another. Most knowledge about child development has been based on research carried out in western industrialized societies, but as more is learnt about children in other parts of the world there may be a realization that what was assumed to be universal may actually be typical only of the societies which have been studied.

It is important to remember that cultural practices are dynamic and constantly changing and in culturally diverse societies like our own, the ways in which families raise children change from one generation to the next, not simply with child health views which spawn new babycare manuals, but as families move and adapt to different circumstances. Awareness of cultural influences should encourage a broader view of development, seeing it as a result not merely of personal history but influenced by family circumstances and expectations and the wider cultural demands.

CONCLUSION

This chapter has presented a general description of the main features of development. While this account may apply to all children it has not attempted to capture the individual features which make each person unique. In describing the general changes which take place, two points should be stressed:

(1) Development is not a process of gradual accretion in which new items are added to old ones; it has periods of rapid change and reorganization interspersed with phases of slower change and consolidation. The epochs which have been labelled here as infancy, the preschool period, the school years and adolescence, are periods which culminate in marked cognitive reorganization, but changes occur within these periods and at different rates in different children.

(2) The child does not respond passively to surrounding stimuli but is an active contributor to the environment; this view of children as constructing their own worlds has two meanings

    (a) Individual differences which may be innate, such as temperament, affect the reaction of parents and carers to the child and so each one will experience a unique environment and a child's input cannot be ignored.

(b) In developing understanding about the world, the child is an active information-seeker and hypothesis generator, not a passive absorber of knowledge.

Early theories of child development ascribed considerable power to early events; this view had both positive and negative implications. On the positive side, if early experience was crucial then it was vital to make the first years of a child's life as beneficial as possible; while on the negative side if early experiences were irreversible then a child who had encountered adversity was likely to be 'scarred for life'. Such ideas have been prevalent from Greek philosophers to more recent theorists such as Freud and Bowlby. Clarke & Clarke (1976) redressed the balance in a comprehensive review of evidence that behaviour was not determined by early experience but that children were often far more resilient than had previously been thought. Early adversity did not inevitably lead to poor outcome; single events in particular were not good predictors, and continuity of experience and concurrent conditions were often more important.

Understanding of the complexity of the influences of different factors has increased in the last ten years. In 1988 Professor Michael Rutter, a leading child psychiatrist, gave a lecture entitled 'Pathways from Childhood to Adult Life' in which he demonstrated the many unpredictable routes that people take as they negotiate the transitions of growing up. He stressed that 'transitions need to be considered in personal terms' (Rutter 1989) and that what may be a stressful event for one person may be insignificant for another. Such an appreciation of the complexity of developmental outcomes has come about through careful longitudinal studies which have enabled psychologists to understand how events are perceived and how they influence outcomes. In trying to explain why people react differently, psychologists now use the term 'coping strategies' to explain how children respond to different events.

Research on children's development is not confined to scientific laboratories insulated from the outside world; the findings of research are constantly being applied to try to improve the conditions of children's lives. Theories of attachment have led to studies of the effects of day care and of separation in hospital; studies to accelerate

concept acquisition have led to new curricula designed to enhance children's learning, plus strategies to assist children in dealing with health care interventions, for example preparation for events in hospital or invasive procedures. Schaffer (1990) points out that care should be taken when applying knowledge derived from research to practical situations and problems, but he emphasizes that the careful use of research can expand upon opinion and beliefs and allow a more objective view of the situation. His book demonstrates ways in which research can encourage more informed decisions about children's welfare.

While research on children's development in western societies has been applied to improving the conditions of life for families and children, research on children elsewhere has enlarged an understanding of the role of cultural demands and should lead to a re-evaluation of notions of appropriate outcomes or desirable goals. Nunes *et al.* (1993) shows how street children develop mathematical skills which are ignored in a formal school context. Nunes (1994) stresses that society's, parent's and children's goals are not always identical and that interventions may fail if they are not sensitive to the complex cultural context in which they take place. Richman (1993), referring to children affected by war and growing up in situations of political violence, suggests that:

'It is frequently said that we need to make programmes ... culturally appropriate, but in practice this is not easily attained because western psychological paradigms are so powerful'.

The account of development which this chapter has presented has been largely drawn from western psychology with its highly individualistic goals in which autonomy and independence are valued. Therefore a critical appraisal of the research should precede its application.

REFERENCES AND FURTHER READING

Baillargeon, R. (1987) Object permanence in 3½ and 4½ month old infants. *Developmental Psychology*, 23(5), 655–4.

Beilin, H. (1971) The training and acquisition of logical operations. In *Piagetian Cognitive-developmental Research and*

Mathematical Education (eds M.F. Rosskopf, L.P. Steffe & S. Toback). National Council of Teachers of Mathematics, Washington, D.C.

Beilin, H. (1978) Inducing conservation through training. In *Psychology of the 20th century* (ed. G. Steiner) vol. 7, Piaget and beyond. Kindler, Zurich.

Bell, S.M. (1970) The development of the concept of object as related to infant–mother attachment. *Child Development*, 41, 291–311.

Bell, S.M. & Ainsworth, M.D.S. (1972) Infant crying and maternal responsiveness. *Child Development*, 43, 1171–90.

Bissex, G. (1980) *GNYS AT WRK: a child learns to write and read.* Harvard University Press, Cambridge, Mass.

Bowlby, J. (1969) *Attachment and Loss*, Vol. I, Attachment. Hogarth Press, London.

Bradley, B.S. (1989) *Visions of Infancy: a Critical Introduction to Child Psychology.* Polity Press, Cambridge.

Bremner, J.G. (1988) *Infancy.* Blackwell Publishers, Oxford.

Bruner, J.S. (1964) The Course of Cognitive Growth. *American Psychologist*, 19, 1–15.

Bruner, J.S. (1974) *Beyond the Information Given: Studies in the Psychology of Knowing.* George Allen and Unwin, London.

Bryant, P.E. & Bradley, L. (1985) *Children's Reading Problems.* Blackwell Publishers, Oxford.

Bryant, P.E. & Trabasso, T. (1971) Transitive inferences and memory in young children. *Nature*, 232, 456–8.

Cassell, S. (1965) Effect of brief puppet therapy upon the emotional responses of children undergoing cardiac catheterization. *Journal of Consulting Psychology*, 29(1), 1–8.

Caudill, W. & Plath, D. (1966) Who sleeps by whom? Parent–child involvement in urban Japanese families. *Psychiatry*, 29, 344–66.

Clarke, A.M. & Clarke, A.D.B. (eds) (1976) *Early Experience: Myth and Evidence.* Open Books, London.

Coie, J.D., Dodge, K.A. & Kupersmidt, J.B. (1990) Peer group behaviour and social status. In *Peer Rejection in Childhood* (eds S.R. Asher & J.D. Coie). Cambridge University Press, Cambridge.

Cordua, G.D., McGraw, K.O. & Drabman, R.S. (1979) Doctor or nurse: children's perceptions of sex typed occupations. *Child Development*, 50, 590–93.

Dodge, K.A. & Feldman, E. (1990) Issues in social cognition and sociometric status. In *Peer Rejection in Childhood* (eds S.R. Asher & J.D. Coie). Cambridge University Press, Cambridge.

Donaldson, M. (1978) *Children's Minds.* Fontana, London.

Dunn, J. (1984) *Sisters and Brothers.* Fontana, London.

Dunn, J. & Kendrick, C. (1982) *Siblings: Love, Envy and Understanding.* Harvard University Press, Cambridge, Mass.

Erikson, E. (1968) *Identity, Youth and Crisis.* Norton, New York.

Ferreiro, E. & Teberosky, A. (1982) *Literacy before Schooling.* Heinemann, London.

Field, T., Cohen, D., Garcia, R. & Greenberg, R. (1984) Mother–stranger face discrimination by the newborn. *Infant Behaviour and Development*, 7, 19–26.

Gesell, A. (1928) *Infancy and Human Growth.* Macmillan, New York.

Gibson, E.J. & Walk, R. (1960) The 'visual cliff'. *Scientific American*, 202, 64–71.

Gilligan, C. (1982) *In a Different Voice: Psychological Theory and Women's Development.* Harvard University Press, Cambridge, Mass.

Hay, D.F. (1994) Prosocial development. *Journal of Child Psychology & Psychiatry*, 35(1), 29–71.

Hill, J.P. (1987) Research on adolescents and their families: past and prospect. In *Adolescent Social Behaviour and Health* (ed. C.E. Irwin). Jossey-Bass, San Francisco.

Hill, P. (1993) Recent Advances in Selected Aspects of Adolescent Development. *Journal of Child Psychology and Psychiatry*, 34(1), 69–99.

Hohmann, M., Banet, B. & Weikart, D.P. (1979) *Young Children in Action: a manual for preschool educators.* High/Scope Press, Ypsilanti, Michigan.

Hortacsu, N. (1989) Targets of communication during adolescence. *Journal of Adolescence*, 12, 253–63.

Hughes, M. (1978) Selecting pictures of another person's view. *British Journal of Educational Psychology*, 48, 210–19.

Hulsebus, R.C. (1975) *Latency of Crying Cessation: Measuring Infants' Discrimination of Mothers' Voices.* Paper presented at the meeting of the American Psychological Association, Chicago, (cited by Bremner 1988).

Illingworth, R.S. (1973) *Basic Developmental Screening.* Blackwell Science, Oxford.

Inhelder, B. & Piaget, J. (1964) *The Early Growth of Logic in the Child: Classification and Seriation.* Routledge & Kegan Paul, London.

Keating, D.P. (1990) Adolescent Thinking. In *At the Threshold: The Developing Adolescent* (eds S.S. Feldman & G.R. Elliott). Harvard University Press, Cambridge, Mass.

Keating, D.P. & Clark, L.V. (1980) Development of physical and social reasoning in adolescence. *Developmental Psychology*, 16(1), 23–30.

Keeney, J.T., Cannizzo, S.R. & Flavell, J.H. (1967). Spontaneous and induced verbal rehearsal in a recall task. *Child Development*, 38, 953–66.

Klaus, M. & Kennell, J. (1976) *Maternal–Infant Bonding.* Mosby, St. Louis.

Kohlberg, L. (1976) Moral stages and moralization: the cognitive-developmental approach. In *Moral development and behaviour* (ed. T. Lickona). Holt, Rinehart, Winston, New York.

Konner, M. (1991) *Childhood.* Little, Brown and Co, Boston.

McKenna, J. (1986) An anthropological perspective on the sudden infant death syndrome (SIDS): the role of parental breathing cues and speech breathing adaptations. *Medical Anthropology*, **10**, 9–92.

Monck, E. (1991) Patterns of confiding relationships among adolescent girls. *Journal of Child Psychology and Psychiatry*, 32, 333–45.

Morelli, G.A., Rogoff, B., Oppenheim, D. & Goldsmith, D. (1992) Cultural variation in infants' sleeping arrangements: questions of independence. *Developmental Psychology*, **28**(4), 604–13.

Newson, J. (1979) The growth of shared understandings between infant and caregiver. In *Before Speech: the Beginning of Interpersonal Communication* (ed. M. Bullowa). Cambridge University Press, Cambridge.

Nunes, T. (1994) *The Environment of the Child*. Bernard van Leer Foundation, The Hague.

Nunes, T. Schliemann, A.D. & Carraher, D. (1993) *Street Mathematics and School Mathematics*. Cambridge University Press, New York.

Olweus, D. (1991) Bully/victim problems among schoolchildren: basic facts and effects of a school-based intervention program. In *The development and treatment of aggression* (eds D. Pepler & K.H. Rubin). Erlbaum, Hillsdale, N.J.

Pears, R. & Bryant, P. (1990) Transitive-inferences by young children about spatial position. *British Journal of Psychology*, 81, 497–510.

Piaget, J. (1926) *The Language and Thought of the Child*. Harcourt Brace, New York.

Piaget, J. (1932) *The Moral Judgement of the Child*. Penguin, Harmondsworth.

Piaget, J. (1955) *The Child's Construction of Reality*. Routledge & Kean Paul, London.

Piaget, J. (1968a) A Theory of Development. *International Encyclopedia of the Social Sciences*. Crowell Collier Macmillan, New York.

Piaget, J. (1968b) *Six Psychological Studies*. University of London Press, London.

Piaget, J. (1972) Intellectual evolution from adolescence to adulthood. *Human Development*, 15, 1–12.

Piaget, J. & Inhelder, B. (1969) *The Psychology of the Child*. Routledge & Kegan Paul, London.

Piaget, J. & Inhelder, B. (1974) *The Child's Construction of Quantities: Conservation and Atomism*. Routledge & Kegan Paul, London.

Rheingold, H. & Cook, K. (1975) The content of boys' and girls' rooms as an index of parent behaviour. *Child Development*, 46, 459–63.

Richman, N. (1993) Children in situations of political violence. *Journal of Child Psychology and Psychiatry*, 34(8), 1286–1302.

Rogoff, B. (1977) *A Portrait of Memory in Cultural Context*. Unpublished doctoral dissertation. Harvard University, Harvard.

Rubin, J.Z. Provenzano, F.J. & Luria, Z. (1974) The eye of the beholder: parents' views on sex of newborns. *American Journal of Orthopsychiatry*, 44, 512–19.

Rutter, M. (1989) Pathways from childhood to adult life. *Journal of Child Psychology and Psychiatry*, **30**(1), 23–51.

Rutter, M. & Rutter, M. (1992) *Developing Minds: Challenge and Continuity across the Life Span*. Penguin Books, London.

Ryan, R.M. & Lynch, J.H. (1989) Emotional autonomy versus detachment: revisiting the vicissitudes of adolescence and young adulthood. *Child Development*, 60, 340–56.

Schaffer, H.R. (1990) *Making Decisions about Children*. Blackwell Publishers, Oxford.

Schaffer, H.R. & Emerson, P.E. (1964) The development of social attachments in infancy. *Monographs of the Society for Research on Child Development*, 29, 1–77.

Schwarz, H.B., Albino, J.E. & Tedesco, L.A. (1983) Effects of psychological preparation on children hospitalized for dental operations. *Journal of Paediatrics*, **102**, 634–8.

Sluckin, W., Herbert, M. & Sluckin, A. (1983) *Maternal Bonding*. Blackwell Publishers, Oxford.

Smith, P.K. & Simon, T. (1984) Object play, problem solving and creativity in children. In *Play in Animals and Humans* (ed. P.K. Smith). Blackwell Publishers, Oxford.

Smith, T., Moore, E. & Sylva, K. (1987) *The High/Scope Approach to Early Years*. OMEP Update 22, OMEP (UK) [World Organisation for Early Childhood Education].

Steinberg, L. & Silverberg, S.B. (1986) The vicissitudes of autonomy in early adolescence. *Child Development*, 57, 841–51.

Super, C.M. & Harkness, S. (1982) The Development of Affect in Infancy and Early Childhood. In *Cultural Perspectives on Child Development* (eds D.A. Wagner & H.W. Stevenson). W.H. Freeman, San Francisco.

Susman, E.J., Inoff-Germain, G., Nottelmann, E.D., Loriaux, D.L., Cutler, D.B. & Chrousos, G.P. (1987) Hormones, emotional dispositions and aggressive attributes in young adolescents. *Child Development*, 58, 1114–34.

Sutherland, P. (1992) *Cognitive Development Today: Piaget and his critics*. Paul Chapman Publishing, London.

Tanner, J.M. (1973) Growing up. *Scientific American*, 229, 34–43.

Tizard, B. (1977) Play: The Child's Way of Learning? In *Biology of Play* (eds B. Tizard & D. Harvey). Heinemann, London.

Trevarthen, C. (1979) Communication and co-operation in early infancy: a description of primary intersubjectivity. In *Before Speech: the Beginning of Interpersonal Communication* (ed. M. Bullowa). Cambridge University Press, Cambridge.

Vygotsky, L.S. (1978) *Mind in Society*. Harvard University Press, Harvard.

Wells, G. (1985) *Language development in the preschool years*. Cambridge University Press, Cambridge.

Wood, D. (1986) Aspects of teaching and learning. In *Children of Social Worlds* (eds M. Richards & P. Light). Polity Press, Cambridge.

Wood, D. (1988) *How Children Think and Learn*, Blackwell Publishers, Oxford.

Zelazo, P.R. (1976) From reflexive to instrumental behaviour. In *Developmental Psychobiology: the significance of infancy* (ed. L.P. Lipsitt). Lawrence Erlbaum, Hillsdale, NJ.

Chapter 10

Learning Disabilities, Children and their Families

Sue Hooton

DISABILITY AND LEARNING DIFFICULTY – THE SOCIAL CONTEXT

Childhood disability presents many challenges and this chapter is written with the intention of promoting an understanding of them. The opportunities for developing care provision are presented through exploration of needs arising from physical, social, educational and emotional child and family experiences.

Disability is used as an umbrella term to describe the full range of childhood physical disabilities. Learning difficulties which might arise from intellectual or sensory disability are also discussed. Further classifications used are mild, moderate and severe learning difficulty and multiple disability. However, a word of warning about such terminology; universal terms do little to explain individual abilities or characteristics. Disability is all too often in the eye of the beholder.

Dalley (1991) discussed the effects of group labelling when criticizing socially constructed models which represent an able bodied definition of disability. She suggested that such models gave little insight into explanations of the true disabled situation, often being based upon medical criteria most suited to the purpose of administration. Professional labelling is a power-laden process (Illich 1976) and when used it should be remembered that the way in which disabled children see and hear themselves described will do much to affect their self-image, as well as determining parental and professional attitudes and expectations.

Changes in care provision

The majority of disabled children always have been and will continue to be cared for by their natural parents, in their own homes. For families who feel unable or unwilling to fulfil such a role, alternatives must be provided. Traditionally, care received in large institutions has been the predominant alternative care model, especially for children with severe learning difficulties and multiple physical disabilities. However, growing concern regarding institutional standards of care is described by Locker (1983) who portrays images of dehumanizing and depersonalized approaches to care, with individual needs being seen as secondary to organizational regimes.

The Care in the Community Act 1988 has directly affected such alternative care provision for disabled children, as it has prompted the closure of the large institutions. The care in the community concept has its foundations in the principles of family care within an environment conducive to social valorization. This concept is based upon social integration and acceptance of children and adults with learning difficulties and disabilities, directly opposing segregated, institutionalized care provision. The subsequent change to care in the community schemes, favouring family care or small group living models of accommodation, has received support from most professional and voluntary groups (Dalley 1991; Thompson & Mathias 1992).

However, such changes have inevitably resulted in some families finding themselves without the care choices historically available to them. As a result many more multiply disabled children are now expected to live with their natural families or may be placed with foster families, both situations requiring the carers to be engaged in long term 'informal caring' roles. Informal carers are usually relatives, friends or neighbours, who provide long term care without payment. It can be argued that most parents care without payment. However, Pitkeathley (1989) defends the 'plight' of informal carers, explaining the role in terms of 'restriction' arising from the 'duty' of being responsible for the care of another on a permanent basis. There is also a great deal of evidence as to the poorer physical and emotional health of informal carers, which can be directly attributed to the informal caring role (Miles 1992; General Household Survey 1985; Pitkeathley 1989). Dalley (1991) provides a detailed analysis of the wider effects of informally caring for a disabled relative.

The way in which the community care model has been implemented has received much criticism. This includes the ongoing dilemma surrounding total social integration of disabled individuals (Topliss 1982), and resource issues such as inconsistent and inadequate health/local authority funding (Ham 1988), along with professional issues such as staff education and monitoring of standards. Attention to such issues is of utmost importance if the prospect of creating myriad mini-institutions is to be avoided. Clearly, quality community care provision cannot be seen as a cheap option to large scale residential care.

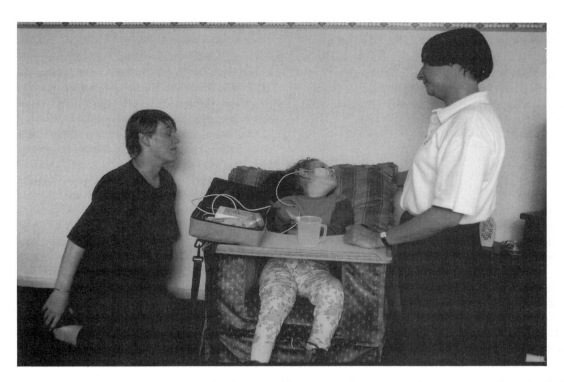

Fig. 10.1   Professional carers can support family centred home care. *(Reproduced by permission of Jon Sparks.)*

Societal attitudes

The ultimate fulfilment of a care in the community philosophy depends largely upon an accepting, caring community. Unfortunately social attitudes towards disability, particularly when associated with severe learning difficulties, are historically negative (Thompson & Mathias 1992). Children do, however, tend to face fewer problems than their adult contemporaries in terms of social acceptance.

As a result of community care legislation, many multiply disabled children and young adults now live in local authority or multiagency small group living accommodation such as Barnardos or Mencap. These houses are run on an 'ordinary life' principle (Oswin 1981) based upon a philosophy of social 'normality' and rights of citizenship.

It is envisaged that such community living models which involve day to day sharing of community facilities, will consolidate the social integration process. However, feelings of fear and suspicion which have been perpetuated by historical approaches to segregated care provision, cannot be changed overnight. They can, however, be considerably improved by a policy of 'determined sensitivity', which involves continuous integration by full use of public facilities, where the real pleasures and nonthreatening challenges of sharing everyday experiences together can be fully realized. After all, fear arising from the prospect of social integration is not exclusive to the nondisabled community.

Rights of the disabled child

All children have rights. The disabled child, due to the potentially limiting nature of disability, has particular rights to the provision of a range of essential services, that help to support the child and family. Hendrick (1993) states that in Great Britain there are 'approximately 360 000 children under sixteen with one or more disabilities, representing 3% of all children'. Clearly, identifying and meeting the individual needs of these children requires a rigorous and well co-ordinated support system.

The Children Act (1989) is a major piece of legislation which aims to secure the rights of all children, irrespective of ability. Part III of the Children Act describes disabled children as being 'in need'. It states:

> 'For the purposes of this part, a child is disabled if he is blind, deaf or dumb or suffers from mental disorder of any kind or is substantially and permanently handicapped by illness, injury or congenital deformity or such other disability as may be prescribed.'

The Children Act aims to identify and promote the well-being of children in need, by identifying family support mechanisms. Under the Act local authorities are responsible for:

- Identification of children in need.
- Maintenance of registers of children in need.
- Assessment of need.
- Provision of suitable accommodation and family support.
- Maintenance of family relationships, with special consideration to racial background.

Such issues must be considered when providing care for disabled children, irrespective of the caring context. Hendrick (1993) provides a comprehensive overview of The Children Act related to childhood disability.

Also under the Children Act, the Foster Placement (Children) Regulations 1991 have responded to the increased trends in foster care and respite provision, by effecting clearer guidelines for carers. They state that regular reviews must be held to assess the suitability of all foster and respite care placements. All foster/respite family members are expected to attend the regularly held reviews. Following review meetings, contracts are drawn up between the foster/respite carers and the child care agency, clearly indicating the agreed responsibilities of both parties.

Each child will also have statutory reviews, which are usually held at the child's school. The child's individual care plan is discussed and amended in the presence of the full caring team, which includes, of course, the child's permanent carers.

Educational provision

A disabled child with learning difficulties may attend school from the age of 2 to 19 years (Education Act 1981). For the majority of children, school is a vitally important socialization process which provides the first experiences of social contacts outside the home.

The Warnock Report (DES 1978) has been the major influence on the provision of education to meet identified, special educational needs. This early report emphasized the need for individualized assessment and the need to meet any special educational needs from pre-school to adolescence. It promoted the concept of integrated education, with shared learning between mainstream school children and children with learning difficulties and/or physical disabilities.

The Education Act 1981 gave legislative force to some of Warnock's recommendations, amending the previous Education Act of 1944. It made it the duty of the local health authorities to inform parents and local education authorities of the particular special needs of their children. In addition, it made local education authorities responsible for assessing and meeting special educational needs provision. The need for early educational intervention was also emphasized, with nursery provision being available for two year olds and, in certain cases, for children under two.

However, the Warnock Report did not adopt a wholly integrationist education strategy. It forecast a distinct need, although much reduced, for 'special schooling' (Robson 1989).

Since the 1981 Education Act, 90% of children identified as having special educational needs are educated in ordinary schools with appropriate 'within class' support (DES 1990). Different approaches have been used to support disabled children, such as designated specialist teachers, progressive use of information technology, and specialist teaching groups. At its most successful, integrated education offers 'normality' through children not being segregated and therefore being less likely to be ostracized by their peers. It also affords opportunities for large groups of children to learn about disability in a nonthreatening way.

Annual school population returns to the Department of Education and Science (DES 1990) have shown that the most marked reduction in special education attendance has been in the moderate learning difficulty group. This has resulted in the current trend towards smaller, special needs schools, which have a higher concentration of children with severe learning difficulties, often associated with multiple disabilities, and children with challenging behaviour.

Any decision concerning integrated services for children with disabilities and learning difficulties must take into account a number of principles (Table 10.1).

Table 10.1 Principles on which to base integrated service decisions.

> ■ Decisions must be based on an individual assessment of need.
> ■ The child and carers must be fully involved in the decision making process.
> ■ The benefits of the chosen system must be considered by the caring team to be in the child's best interests.

The advantages of specialist school services often include expensive specialized equipment, professional support and opportunities to establish friendships with children and carers who face similar problems. Such advantages should be considered against the stigma that might arise from socially isolating activities. For many children and their families, different types of activity and provision will suit them at different stages of the child's development, suggesting an ongoing need for pluralist service provision (Table 10.2).

DISABILITY AND LEARNING DIFFICULTY – THE FAMILY CONTEXT

The majority of disabled children receive long term care from their natural parents within the family home. Foster care is the most frequently used permanent child care alternative, as it has the potential to provide an environment which nurtures stability and caring attachments (Brazelton 1981). Other groups of children receive long term care in local authority or voluntary agency small group living accommodation.

It has been suggested that a family with a disabled child becomes a 'disabled family' (Singhi 1990) since few family members will escape the long term effects of caring for a disabled child. Whatever the caring context, families will face all of the usual joys and demands encountered in child-rearing, along with the challenge of facing the particular needs arising from the child's disability.

Prevention and identification of disability

Many disabilities can be prevented through measures such as screening and immunization. Some disabilities are identified before birth through procedures such as ultrasound scanning and amniocentesis. Many other disabilities are identified at birth, or during the routine health checks in infancy, or by parents identifying some developmental delay. Educational personnel such as nursery nurses and school teachers are often instrumental in realizing a child has some form of learning

Table 10.2 Overview of changes in the social experiences of disabled children.

Traditional focus	Current focus
■ Community segregation.	■ Community integration.
■ Special educational provision.	■ Integrated education.
■ Institutionalized care.	■ Family focused care.
■ Medical care model.	■ Holistic care model.
■ Group identity.	■ Individual identity.
■ Social invisibility.	■ Social valorization.
■ Negative attitudes to disability.	■ Positive, challenging attitudes.
■ Professional decision making.	■ Individual decision making.

difficulty in their early years. All professionals working with children should have a basic knowledge and understanding of child development in order to be able to identify children in need of extra support.

Over the years, improved national antenatal and infant screening programmes have led to a reduction in the number of babies born with disabling conditions such as spina bifida, Down's syndrome, hypothyroidism and phenylketonuria. Improved immunization uptake has effected a reduction in the number of babies born with rubella related disabilities, along with chronically disabling conditions resulting from serious childhood illnesses, such as whooping cough, measles and meningitis.

The problems of accurately recording such trends in infant/childhood disability are great and depend upon factors such as accurate diagnosis and recording (Topliss 1982). Once a disability or learning difficulty has been identified, the child may be entered onto the disability register. This is a live record of the local incidence of childhood disability, and is useful in predicting future service provision. However, entry onto the register is at the discretion of the child's parents and certain children such as children of homeless or travelling families who may not settle in any place for long, or who might experience problems registering with health services, can often remain undetected. Therefore the disability register can only give an estimate of the real incidence of childhood disability.

Overall, the incidence of childhood disability and learning difficulty remains unnecessarily high, being mainly due to the continued incidence of children whose development is seriously affected as a result of anoxia at birth. Another contributing trend is the increased amount of intensive neonatal intervention which may result in residual learning difficulties (Wariyar & Richmond 1991). The ethics of intervention at very early stages of gestation, which might result in future disability, is a topic receiving much contemporary nursing and medical ethical attention. Kuhse & Singer (1990) provide a detailed discussion of the issues related to early intervention.

Parental reactions to the birth of a disabled child

Parents are rarely prepared for the birth of a baby who is disabled. They will have most likely endured months of waiting and planning, full of expectation for a healthy, fully developed infant. They may well experience extreme, unexpected emotions when they realize that their baby has some form of disability.

Such reactions have been described in terms of 'loss', that is, an overwhelming sense of loss for the baby and child that the parents had expected. The stages of the grief/loss process have been described as shock, denial, anger, bargaining, depression, and acceptance (Kubler-Ross 1969). The stage of acceptance is characterized by signs of 'positive adjustment' which indicate a move towards acceptance of the new family member.

However, some families may never fully accept their child's disabilities; they may demonstrate signs of 'pathological grief', which is a desperate situation where the parent seems unable to progress through the recognized grieving process.

Other parents may feel that the demands that are placed upon them in this altered caring role will be too much to bear and they may prefer their baby to be fostered. At a time of such mixed emotions, the family must be handled extremely sensitively and must be supported and respected in making their own informed choices. Alternative care arrangements should respect the family background and offer contact with the natural parents. The arrangements should be flexible and able to accommodate future choices should family adjustments lead to a desire to provide future care. The short and longer term care arrangements should predominantly make the child's welfare a priority (Children Act 1989).

Counselling services can provide a great deal of support at the time of, and in the years following, the birth of a disabled child. It is often nursing staff who are in direct contact with families in the immediate postnatal period when support and information are important influences in formulating parental reactions to and expectations of their child. The parents may not know of the existence of support services, therefore the ward environment should be one that provides a range of accessible information, including details of local organizations which provide counselling and support services, such as parent support groups and help lines.

Unfortunately, parental accounts reveal that emotional support is not always available. Nurses and doctors can appear too busy or reluctant to talk openly and honestly (therapeutically) when the parents most need to talk and ask questions. It has been suggested that such behaviours are characteristic of professional coping (Menzies 1970). However, the repeated accounts of parents discharged from hospitals without knowing their child's exact diagnosis or prognosis, or the nature of the available support, call for health professionals to communicate more effectively with families (Failla & Jones 1991).

It is vital for health professionals to understand the factors that might influence the way in which a family reacts and adapts after the birth of a disabled infant. Factors that affect family adaptation to this new situation include any previous experience of disability, the presence of supportive relationships, and existing family coping mechanisms. Cultural attitudes to disability, family size and social class may also affect the adaptation process. Professional skills and attitudes at the time of and immediately following the birth, opportunities for parent/infant bonding, and family support networks, are all important extrinsic determinants which can affect the way in which families react. It is important to remember that there is no universal parental reaction following the birth of a disabled child – feelings are intense and unpredictable.

Health professionals can greatly lessen the impact of such an event by considering the emotional needs of family members. In creating opportunities for 'therapeutic dialogue' and nurturing positive attitudes towards childhood disability, messages of hope and realistic expectation are projected, providing an essential foundation for family adjustment and acceptance.

Family dynamics

The number of informal carers is increasing and will continue to increase due to the community focus of care provision for children and young adults with chronic illnesses and disabilities (Pitkeathley 1989). Long-term family caring roles are most often undertaken by women. Anderson & Elfert (1989) go so far as to describe informal caring as 'care by women'. As such, women are particularly at risk of jeopardizing their own health as a direct result of their informal caring role (Graham 1993). Continuous lifting, inadequate aids or appliances and constant stress and social isolation are common sources of caring-related ill health (Hicks 1988; Pitkeathley 1989).

Tension resulting from exhaustion and anxiety is

likely to affect the standard of care of the disabled child and the quality of relationships with other family members. The realization that the carer is not performing to everyone's requirements is likely to cause further tension and anxiety. Such factors are often the causative elements in the typical family crises that arise from informal caring. Resulting feelings of guilt at not fulfilling the established role within the family may emerge. Guilt is also commonly experienced in cases where the child's disability is hereditary in nature, or if it is suspected that the cause of the disability could possibly be attributed to maternal behaviour during pregnancy.

Siblings may be particularly affected by the birth of a disabled child. Life usually changes quite drastically following the birth of a new baby, particularly for the first born child, but in the case of the birth of a disabled baby, overwhelming feelings of resentment and of being second priority may prevail. Feelings of embarrassment are often experienced by siblings, arising from the perceived social stigma of disability and having a brother or sister who is 'different' and who may behave oddly. Such feelings may result in the siblings not inviting friends to the family home and not wishing to accompany the family on outings.

Seligman (1987) describes the different responsibilities shouldered by siblings of disabled children, who often find their own childhood being sacrificed as they are expected to fulfil adult-like responsibilities within the family. In some instances the primary carer can appear almost 'obsessed' with meeting the needs of the disabled child and maintaining the child's caring programme, to the detriment of the rest of the family (Harrison 1977). Whatever the family circumstances, family life will change following the birth of a disabled child and families will react in their own unique way.

Health professionals' awareness of the particular difficulties arising from parenting a disabled child can only help in providing effective, family centred care.

The costs of caring for a disabled child

The socio-economic status of the family may change following the birth of a disabled child, as one parent often has to give up work to fulfil the full time caring role. This predicament can be especially devastating for single parent families, who may find themselves particularly disadvantaged (Oppenheim 1993). Smyth & Robus (1989) report that families with disabled children have typically lower incomes than other families, whilst having to spend more time in meeting the particular needs of their children. Such economic factors can also place families with a disabled child at considerable social disadvantage.

Extra costs incurred in caring for a disabled child often include extra heating, laundry bills, special dietary requirements, specialist play equipment, shoes and clothing. The following extract from an interview with a parent of a disabled child may give some added insight into the difficulties encountered by many families.

| Interviewer: | 'Do you experience any particular financial difficulties in providing care for your son?' |
| Mother: | 'Yes, we have an old van that keeps on breaking down and I find getting the bus with the children and D in his wheelchair an awful experience. Transport is such a terrible subject, because if I don't get out then I think I will go mad, but I tend to spend all our mortgage money on taxis and that causes terrible problems between me and my husband.' |

This conversation reveals family tensions relating to the practical and financial problems that arise in making transport arrangements for a family which includes three young children, the youngest of whom is disabled. The conversation was laden with maternal guilt for not being able to financially contribute to the house, along with feelings of remorse at spending what little mortgage money was available to prevent social isolation for herself and her children. This situation is by no means unique for parents with disabled children who are too young to qualify for mobility allowance.

Extra costs, such as wheelchairs and the need for house adaptations such as shower rooms and bedroom extensions, will follow children throughout their development. Grants are available for some of this necessary work but, as discussed by Topliss (1982), they rarely cover the total cost of the work.

A nursing commitment to family-centred care must include a family needs analysis. Carers who are anxious

and exhausted and caring in inadequate conditions, cannot competently fulfil their demanding caring role. Nurses as 'front line' carers are able to form relationships with carers, assess need and liaise with other professionals allied to nursing, in order to provide an effective support network (Meyer 1990; Hooton 1991). An innovative and creative approach to formulating and testing models of nursing that more accurately facilitate implementation of an holistic caring philosophy, will enable nurses to meet such caring challenges.

Respite care

Most families welcome a well deserved break from their demanding caring routine and there is a wide range of respite care provision available for disabled children. Few people would disagree that there is a growing need for expansion of respite care provision, especially for older disabled children and young adults.

Traditionally, respite care has been provided by children's wards in hospitals and this has been a much valued and well used source of respite care in the past. It has, however, been criticized for being potentially harmful to children, who in receiving respite care are often introduced to infection and may find themselves 'nursed' alongside very ill children.

Hospital based respite care is thankfully being replaced with more desirable alternatives. There has been a growth in the amount of respite care organized and provided by local authorities and children's agencies, particularly Barnados. This family based respite care involves a slow process of child/family introductions and befriending, along with some basic training for the respite carers. It is based on a 'home from home' principle and can be mutually rewarding and stimulating to the child and respite carers, thereby giving the permanent carers a guilt-free break.

Other sources of respite provision are religious organizations, voluntary groups, neighbourhood schemes, and parental support groups. Whatever the source, respite care should aim to offer the child a stimulating break away from home, built upon the security derived from loving, caring and familiar relationships with carers who are able to meet the child's individual needs within a homely, flexible routine.

Perhaps the most important and little recognized form of daily respite available to carers is the child's attendance at school. So much so, that many schools/ local authorities run summer play schemes to help bridge the summer break for both the child and the carers.

EARLY LEARNING AND INTERACTION

Preschool provision

Early education is believed to be an essential element of every disabled child's development (DES 1978; Brimblecombe 1984; Young 1990). Unfortunately, there is little concrete evidence to confirm its beneficial effects.

Some disabled preschool children will attend a special needs nursery from the age of two years, but as places are extremely limited, carers are forced to look for alternative solutions. Ordinary nursery provision is a well used alternative, encouraging integration from the earliest age, but good nursery provision is expensive and many carers feel that there is a lack of specialist developmental input.

Other alternatives such as peripatetic teaching systems are available, which involve specialist teachers working with infants and young children in the family home. The aim of peripatetic teaching is to promote early interaction, thereby preventing problems that frequently arise from visual and auditory impairment, which can seriously affect the developing parent/child relationship (Blau 1986). Another well used approach to early learning and stimulation is the Portage home teaching system, a system in which many carers will participate in the preschool years.

Home based assessment and structured learning

The Portage system is based upon the principle of family teaching and stimulation for any child with learning difficulties. It has been particularly useful for carers wanting to do something positive towards their child's preschool development. Portage teachers are from multidisciplinary backgrounds; they visit families in their own homes and assess the disabled child with the carers, against extensive preset criteria in the form of 'can do' checklists. They then advise the carers on the recommended form of instructional activity. This is designed to help teach the child to achieve the next, carefully sequenced, developmental skill. Many carers find that this approach bridges the service provision gap, and if motivated and empowered with teaching skills and knowledge, they often make the most committed teachers.

Such approaches to criterion-based assessment have been criticized as being constructed without adequate knowledge of how the development of children with disabilities differs from patterns of 'normal' child development (Sailor & Guess 1983). They do not include, for example, any indication of the interrelationship of skills, rather portraying behaviours as occurring independently. They also tend to imply that development occurs in a predictable, orderly manner, without any indication of the individual capabilities or environmental limitations that different children experience. Carer/child interactions should be filled with the spontaneous pleasure that can be derived from play and activity. As such, overzealous use of instructional activities, involving contact which is only established in the desire for the child to achieve, should be avoided.

Developmental assessment which avoids the 'snapshot phenomenon' and which is compiled in a familiar environment by parents and professionals who best know the child's individual abilities, is an essential basis for educational need analysis and the future development of realistically sequenced teaching programmes. Such teaching programmes form an essential part of the child's individual intervention/care plan. They are reviewed regularly, and are regarded as the focus of multiprofessional interventions.

Play and communication

The need and desire for play and communication is universal to all children. These are necessary processes for cognitive, social and physical development. Due to restricted mobility, impaired vision and communication difficulties, many disabled children experience difficulties in initiating play and interaction.

Carers seeking to involve disabled children in play activities are faced with the challenge of being imaginative and creative in their choice of tools for play and range of play activities. Usual toys and games may hold little interest for the disabled child, necessitating play activities which are geared to the individual abilities and preferences of each child. Caring activities such as bathing, feeding and dressing can incorporate an element of play and communication, whilst activities involving rough and tumble play, involving close physical contact, are also enjoyed by most children.

Activities designed to promote sensory stimulation can be enjoyable and provide rich learning opportunities. The use of objects which are visually stimulating and have different textures, aromas and sounds can add interesting dimensions to most play situations and may provide the child with a great deal of environmental information. Wind chimes and pot pourri can be used to provide sensory room demarcations where verbal communications may be ineffective.

For total sensory experiences Snoezelan rooms are very popular and can be of great benefit. They aim to provide a range of sensory experiences geared to the individual preferences of each child, within a purpose built, comforting environment.

Structured play activities do not necessarily have to involve expensive, specialist equipment. Basic play activities can be built around the simple pleasures of holding a child closely, thereby promoting feelings of familiarity and trust. Social play is denied to many disabled children and children with learning difficulties, and can be arranged by grouping children within close proximity to each other, or enabling children to roll around a play mat together. The stimulation of touching other children's hair, limbs, etc. and being touched in return, along with experiencing spontaneous noises such as gasps and laughter, can be great fun. Such activity can be an awakening experience for children who are so often deprived of close contact.

Stimulation through play promotes increased awareness and verbal activity, whilst preventing the particularly harmful behaviours that might arise from understimulation, such as head banging and other self-injurious behaviour. Attention to safety must be emphasized, as the disabled child is particularly dependent upon the carer to provide a safe play environment.

THE HOSPITAL EXPERIENCE OF THE DISABLED CHILD

Proving quality care for the disabled child and their family during a period of hospitalization presents particular challenges to the children's nurse. Most disabled children will be familiar with hospital outpatients departments or child development centres, but they may never have experienced a stay in hospital. Hospitalization may be necessary due to health deficits directly associated with the child's disability, or a spontaneous, unexpected illness which might befall any child. For a few children frequent hospital admissions will be the norm, the child and family becoming familiar with the ward staff and hospital routine. Many disabled children and children with learning difficulties find hospitalization an isolating experience. Disabled children who appear noisy or hyperactive may find themselves classed as 'disruptive'. They are often 'cubicalized' to avoid 'disturbing the other children', a situation which should be avoided wherever possible, as it promotes feelings of isolation and stigma for the child and carers.

The disabled child and family will experience the same effects of hospitalization as any other family and should be afforded the same rights and opportunities as outlined in *The Welfare of Young People and Children in Hospital* (DOH 1991). The principles of care shown in Table 10.3 may be helpful in providing a caring charter for children with disabilities, helping this vulnerable group of patients to overcome the adverse effects of hospitalization.

Facing the future

Most parents worry about who will care for their children in the future. The inevitability of a change in future care provision is realized as children grow heavier and carers grow older. Families need support and information when preparing for future caring arrangements.

Richardson & Ritchie (1989) discuss the dilemma facing families at this difficult time. They explain that over the years the whole family routine may well have evolved around the care routine of the disabled child/adolescent, leaving a future prospect of empty, disordered family life. They also describe the carer's feelings of guilt and anxiety that arise from usual, teenage 'stay/

Table 10.3 Principles of care – a caring charter for the disabled child in hospital.

- Care is individualized, based on an ability model rather than one of disability.
- The child's wishes and choices are encouraged in the care programme.
- Continuity of multidisciplinary teaching programmes is effected.
- Nursing goals must be complementary to the child's overall multidisciplinary intervention programme.
- Care is empowering, encouraging independence in self caring skills.
- The care environment should be as homely as possible.
- The child's rights and dignity are respected at all times.
- Natural bonds/friendships are encouraged and nurtured.
- Nurses act as advocates for disabled children.
- Aids and appliances that support independent activity should accompany the child into hospital.
- The family support network should be assessed prior to discharge.
- Carers support groups and contact between carers should be facilitated.

leave home' decisions becoming 'keep/send away' decisions.

Informed families can be introduced to care services designed to make the break from home as natural as possible. This can be facilitated by introductions and short term visits to the new care setting, to establish familiarity and trust, in readiness for the caring exchange. Such initiatives facilitate the usual break from family ties that most young adults experience, whilst providing support for families no longer able to cope.

At a time when informal caring is increasing, it is a sad reflection on services that many carers feel that professional support is often unavailable or is misdirected. The lack of emotional support for carers is well documented (Maclaughlin *et al.* 1986; Cleary 1988; Pitkeathley 1989), along with general dissatisfaction at the availability of information regarding family support services.

CONCLUSION

Professional awareness and understanding of the demands experienced by carers of disabled children and children with learning difficulties is vital. The themes developed in this chapter aim to have enhanced professional insight. It takes professional carers who are committed and knowledgeable to effectively meet the many challenges presented by childhood disability.

REFERENCES AND FURTHER READING

Anderson, J. & Elfert, H. (1989) Managing chronic illness in the family: women as caretakers. *Journal of Advanced Nursing*, 14, 735–43.

Blau, P. (1986) *Exchange and Power in Social Life*. Transaction Books, New Brunswick.

Brazelton, T.B. (1981) *On Becoming a Family; the Growth of Attachment*. Dell Publishing Co. Inc., New York.

Brimblecome, F. (1984) The needs of young handicapped children living at home. In *Stress and Disability in Childhood – The Longterm Problems*. (eds N. Butler and B. Gomer), p. 187. Wright, Bristol.

Cleary, J. (1988) The needs of children in the community. i*Senior Nurse*, 8, 17–19.

Dalley, G. (ed.) (1991) *Disability and Social Policy*. Policy Studies Institute, London.

DES (1978) *Special Educational Needs*. Report of the committee of enquiry into the education of handicapped children and young people (Warnock Report). Department of Education and Science. HMSO, London.

DES (1990) *Special Needs Issue* – a survey by H.M. Inspectorate. Department of Education and Science. HMSO, London.

DES (1983) Department of Education and Science & DHSS Assessments and Statements of Special needs (Circular 1/83). HMSO, London.

DoH (1991) *The Welfare of Children and Young People in Hospital*. HMSO, London.

Failla & Jones (1991) Families of children with developmental disabilities. *Research in Nursing and in Health*, 14(1), 41–50.

General Household Survey (1985) HMSO, London.

Graham, H. (1993) *Hardship and Health in Women's Lives*. Harvester Wheatsheaf, Hemel Hempstead.

Ham, C. (1988) *Health Policy in Britain*. 2nd edn. Macmillan Education, London.

Harrison, S. (1977) *Families in Stress*. Royal College of Nursing, London.

Hendrick, J. (1993) *Child Care Law for Health Professionals.* Chapter 11. Radcliffe Medical Press, Oxford.

Hicks, C. (1988) *Who Cares: Looking after People at Home.* Virago Press, London.

Hooton, S. (1991) *Life After Discharge.* An analysis of children's nurses' understanding of the psychosocial domains of informal caring for children with severe learning difficulties. Unpublished thesis, Manchester Met. University.

Illich, I. (1976) *Limits to Medicine – Medical Nemesis; the exploitation of health.* Penguin, Harmondsworth.

Kubler-Ross (1969) *On Death and Dying.* Macmillan, New York.

Kuhse, H. & Singer, P. (1985) *Should the Baby Live?* Oxford University Press.

Kuhse, H. & Singer, P. (1990) The quality/quantity of life distinction and its moral importance for nurses. *International Journal of Nursing Studies,* 26(3), 203–12.

Locker, D. (1983) *Disability And Disadvantage; The Consequences of Chronic Illness.* Tavistock Publications, London.

Maclaughlin, M. et al (1986) The need to understand the family. *Parents Voice.* Winter, p. 12–15. MENCAP, London.

Menzies, I. (1970) *The Functioning of Social Systems as a Defence Against Anxiety.* Tavistock Institute, London.

Meyer, G. (1990) Who knows best? *Paediatric Nursing,* May, 14.

Miles, A. (1992) *Women, Health and Medicine.* Open University Press, Buckingham.

Oppenheim, C. (1993) *Poverty – The Facts.* Child Poverty Action Group, London.

Oswin, M. (1981) *Issues and Principles in the Development of Short-term Care for Mentally Handicapped Children.* Kings Fund Centre, London.

Pitkeathley, J. (1989) *It's My Duty, Isn't It? The Plight of Carers in our Society.* Souvenir Press, London.

Richardson, A. & Ritchie, J. (1989) *Developing Friendships.* Policy Studies Institute, London.

Robson, B. (1989) *Special Needs in Ordinary Schools.* Cassell Education, London.

Sailor, W. & Guess, D. (1983) *Severely Handicapped Students: An Instructional Design.* Houghton Mifflin Co, Dallas.

Seligman, M. (1987) Adaptation of children to a chronically ill or mentally handicapped sibling. *Canadian Medical Association Journal,* 136(12), 1249–52.

Singhi, P. (1990) Psychosocial problems in families of disabled children. *British Journal of Medical Psychology,* 63, 173–82.

Smyth, M. & Robus, N. (1989) *The Financial Circumstances of Families Living with Disabled children Living in Private Households.* OPCS Surveys of Disability in Great Britain, Report 5. HMSO, London.

Thompson, T. & Mathias, P. (1992) *Standards and Mental Handicap Keys to Competence.* Bailliere Tindall, London.

Topliss, E. (1982) *Social Responses to Handicap.* Longman, Harlow.

Young, C. (1990) *Standing Still or Getting Worse?* King's Fund Carelink No. 13 Autumn. King's Fund Centre, London.

Wariyar, U. & Richmond, S. (1991) Increased survival rate in very low birth weight infants: incidence of handicaps. *Journal of Paediatrics,* 118(2), 322–3.

Chapter 11

Mental Health, Children and Their Families

Della Wait

INTRODUCTION

Children and adolescents have mental health needs and if these are not met health problems can arise. Their emotional and behavioural problems can arise alongside and as a result of other medical problems. Some children's mental health problems may require a period of hospitalization, whilst others receiving professional support can continue/maintain their lives in their home community. Children with a mental health problem need support, security and understanding (as does every child) and appropriate intervention and management strategies. The nurse needs to be able to appreciate the factors that have contributed to the child's problems and appreciate that:

> 'The problem child is invariably trying to solve a problem rather than be one. His methods are crude and his conception of his problem may be faulty.' (Senn 1959)

The non specialist nurse's role lies in communicating with the child and their family, assessing the problems and needs, and where appropriate referring the child on and/or liaising with the specialist team. Not all the problems that children present with may seem major to the nurse, even though a behavioural problem such as soiling can still have an immense impact on the family.

Although the physical and emotional needs of children have been considered unique and worthy of special note for some years, children's mental health has received relatively little attention. This is perhaps partly due to the assumption that children simply do not get mental health problems. Additionally the services to meet children's mental health needs have not had a high profile.

This chapter aims to explore the development of children's mental health services as this provides contextual material for understanding the present position of service provision. The chapter will also examine the causes of mental health breakdown in children; by doing so the multifactorial nature of mental ill health can be illuminated. The theoretical basis for mental health care, as well as the epidemiology of mental health problems, will be discussed to provide the reader with information on the nature and extent of the problem. Finally treatment approaches and preventative measures will be examined to complete the discussion of the area.

THE EARLY ROOTS OF CHILD PSYCHIATRY

Child and adolescent mental health/illness is a comparatively new concept. Until the twentieth century there was little evidence that children were acknowledged to be the unique, developing and special individuals that they are seen as today. The concept of childhood did not really exist and therefore as such children's health needs, both physical and emotional/mental, were not generally considered. The importance of childhood as the foundation of lifelong patterns of behaviour was often overlooked. Children, once past the stage of infancy and total dependence, were viewed as young adults and were expected to accept a level of responsibility in the adult world (Aries 1960). Children's psychological, emotional, intellectual or spiritual development needs received minimal attention from professionals.

However, during the nineteenth century some recognition of the importance of childhood as a period of development and preparation for adulthood began to develop when Charles Darwin and Stanley Hall instigated investigations which were to become the foundation of developmental psychology. In 1867 Henry Maudsley described the development of insanity in early life. Management strategies of the time were often harsh: disturbed children were often beaten and kept in solitary confinement. This treatment was thought to be appropriate as even disturbed children were held morally responsible for their behaviour. There was much controversy as to the cause of psychiatric disturbance in childhood, and organic causes such as brain deterioration were commonly considered to blame.

By the twentieth century the importance of the concept of children's mental health was evolving. Services were developed based upon a philosophy that recognized children as being unique and having individual differences and characteristics. Freud's studies of disturbed adults had pointed to early childhood experiences as the root of their problems and difficulties. It was the prediction that adult psychiatric disturbance could be reduced or prevented by intervening and treating children showing signs of deviant/disturbed behaviour that brought about the development of child psychiatric services.

Other initiatives aimed at promoting child mental

health included the streaming of classes in schools and the development of educational testing aimed to facilitate the individual maturation of children whose attendance at school was now compulsory. Special classes were developed to cater for those unable to profit from teaching in the general education system. School medical services were established in 1907 with a new body of school doctors entering an unexplored area of medicosociological work concerned with defects and disorders of all kinds (Kelynack 1915).

In the 1920s Piaget's work on intellectual development became an important influence on child psychology. Teachers were encouraged to be involved in identifying children who had emotional or social problems. Parent–teacher organisations developed with their aims including working together to improve the school environment and the development of their children (Wickman, cited in Connell 1985). Increasingly, professionals saw the importance of understanding the factors which could influence the child's mental health status. The need to try and understand the conflicts underlying their disturbance was recognized, and appropriate strategies were developed in order to meet the child's needs and help the child and family resolve them.

Anna Freud (1928) and Melanie Klein (1932) pioneered the use of play as a means of communication and emotional release, and play therapy was described by Lowenfield (1935). Play therapy offered a treatment approach for young children who would otherwise have difficulties in communicating. Gradually the climate for the development of a child-focused service became more favourable; attitudes to the whole question of children's mental health were changing and at the same time appropriate research and studies were being undertaken, published and disseminated that gave a theoretical underpinning to professional practice.

An important breakthrough came in the 1920s when the Child Guidance Movement was established, initially in the USA (Parry-Jones 1989). From this movement came the model of inter-disciplinary collaboration by psychologists psychiatric social workers and psychiatrists. The Child Guidance Clinics in the UK developed in response to the American movement. The first of these clinics to be established in the UK was founded by the Jewish Health Organisation and was opened in the East End of London in 1927. The honorary director was the psychiatrist Emanuel Miller who worked with an American trained social worker and a psychologist (Renton 1978).

Child guidance clinics saw their role primarily as one of helping the growing individual to adjust to their own immediate environment, rather than having a curative role in respect to mental illness or in treating the mentally ill (Keir 1952). This approach/philosophy could account for both their popularity and the reason they spread so rapidly. By 1948 and the advent of the NHS there were child guidance services in most health districts, although the services offered were relatively unsophisticated. According to Black (1987) these clinics were often geographically isolated away from other health facilities, resulting in the child psychiatrists becoming alienated from their colleagues. The other team members, such as the social worker and psychologist, were in a similar position.

Isolation from other professionals in hospitals and local authorities appears to have resulted in a relative decline in new ideas and developments. Additionally time available for teaching and research was curtailed due to the high workloads and pressures that the child psychiatrists carried. This combination of pressures also placed some limits on the opportunities for campaigning for more resources to support the hard pressed services; thus expansion did not occur. Recruitment problems resulted as potential candidates saw the speciality as an unattractive option. Without the input of new blood to challenge established practice and the principles upon which it was based, the service in some clinics was ineffective and nonprogressive. The importance of developing preventative services along with undertaking research and improving treatment strategies was somewhat overlooked (Brunel Institute 1976; Sampson 1980; Black 1987).

Coinciding with the opening of the child guidance clinics more attention was devoted to publishing texts on the functional nervous disorders in childhood. Psychiatrists and paediatricians began to forge links and work more harmoniously, and in the 1930s the first steps were made to organize an outpatient clinical service (Kanner 1959). The term 'child psychiatry' was first introduced in 1933 (Kanner 1960) and Kanner chose this as the title for the first text about psychiatric illness in childhood, published in 1935. A separate child psychiatry section of the Royal Medico-Psychological Association was founded in 1946 and the subspeciality began to develop slowly within the NHS from 1948.

There was a rapid growth of hospital based outpatient clinics following World War II. The child guidance clinics continued to be run by local education authorities, under the leadership of either a psychologist or psychiatrist. However there were increasing levels of uncertainty and disagreement concerning the optimum method for service delivery.

The child guidance clinics were only addressing a small proportion of the children needing help. Less than 1% of the total child population was actually receiving care (Kolvin 1973), when Rutter *et al.* (1970) had identified between 7–20% of children as suffering from a definite and functionally handicapping child psychiatric disorder. Inpatient services were slow to develop (Wardle 1991). It was only in the late 1960s that the need for separate services for adolescents, following concerns about teenagers being nursed with the adult mentally ill, was more universally accepted. This brought about the development of inpatient units for adolescents on a regional basis (Parry-Jones 1984).

Academic departments of child psychiatry did not open in England until the 1970s, the first being headed by Professor Michael Rutter at the Maudsley Hospital in 1972. The momentum for this could have been the establishment of the Royal College of Psychiatrists in 1971, which created a speciality within psychiatry and a framework for the development of academic standards, the facilitation of research and the monitoring of training (Black *et al.* 1990). The opening of such departments enabled child psychiatric research to become established; however, growth in this area has remained slow. Some of the early work is currently frequently quoted and utilised and is seen to act as benchmarks in the history of child psychiatry (Table 11.1). By the 1970s child psychiatry was deemed to be flourishing (Graham 1976) with appropriate practice-based developments occurring.

ORGANIZATION OF SERVICES

A series of studies in the 1970s and 1980s found difficulties with continuing to organize the child guidance services in their present form, since they identified a lack of clear leadership and a very unclear management structure which led to insurmountable problems in some clinics (Brunel Institute 1976; Royal College of

Table 11.1 Landmark research within child psychiatry.

- Delineation of the new syndrome 'infantile autism' (Kanner 1943), although the first description of an autistic child was made by Haslam in 1799 (Walk 1964).
- Effects of the hospital environment on children (Robertson 1952, 1958).
- Attachment and loss (Bowlby 1969, 1973, 1980).
- Concept of 'good enough mothering' and the attention paid to the mother/child relationship (Winnicott 1965).
- Epidemiology of Child Mental Health (Rutter *et al.* 1970).
- Assessment of treatment strategies (Kolvin *et al*, 1981).

Psychiatrists 1978, 1986; Interdisciplinary Standing Committee 1981). The 1970s were characterized by a number of Governmental changes which resulted in changes in the administrative structure of the service. However, these changes in policy and administration resulted in little in the way of results of progress within service provision and practice. The advent of the general management in 1983 was expected to give opportunities for each locality to provide a tailor-made service to meet the actual and perceived needs of its defined population. However, this was in reality restricted by budget constraints and the savings targets which had been set. This, along with a difficulty in generating coherent management strategies, meant that most districts only responded to outside pressure or internal crises, which were usually brought about by overspending. Thus very little development and only slow progress resulted.

Modern practice needs to be both proactive and very flexible. The services of a much wider variety of people need to be brought together, including child psychotherapists, psychiatric nurses (including those holding children's registration and with the ENB 603), teachers, dieticians, and occupational, art and music therapists to name but a few. The Government White Paper 1989 and the Children Act 1989 supplied an ideal opportunity for the development of new-style district specialist services for child and adolescent psychiatry. According to Donald Brooksbank, Senior Medical Officer for the Department of Health (1990): 'It will be essential for the District Director of Public Health to receive advice on how to obtain good quality epidemiological data on child mental health.'

This suggests that once the needs of the local districts have been identified they can be addressed, and that the service partners (that is the family health services authority, local authority and user groups) can undertake an annual reassessment of need and service provision which in an ideal world would ensure that the service provided meets the needs of the users.

However, this concept of market forces may create an immediate problem in child and adolescent psychiatry. The customers looking for treatment in the marketplace are not usually the children themselves. In some cases it may not even be the parents and when it is, there can be a conflict of interests between the parent and child, for example, some reports from the USA cite adolescents being admitted to units because their behaviour has failed to meet with parental expectation (Gath 1990).

Epidemiological studies are important but need to take local features into account as well as social factors. It is not useful to say that 20% of the child population is in potential need of child and adolescent psychiatric services, without considering the likelihood of them using the service if it were available. A crucial factor here may be whether need does equal demand. It may be easier to provide a service where these coincide. Needs that are not acknowledged by those with them can result in a limited service being available since the current marketplace philosophy of health provision does not recognize the demand, or alternatively if the service is offered the user may not be amenable to it. The need for appropriate services to be available was identified in *Caring for People* (1989) which in para 7.3 gave some prominence to psychiatric services for children and adolescents:

'The main components of a proper locally based service are: provision for children and adolescents with psychological problems. This should be primarily community based ... with easy access to a range of professional support and to hospital services (including inpatient treatment if necessary).'

It may be interesting to consider this statement in relation to the recent widespread destruction of the community based child guidance clinics, as it could be argued that there is some level of dissonance between

messages from the government and actions at grass root level.

One implication associated with allowing districts to draw up their own plans regarding the type of service may be the recent reduction of some inpatient provision. This service is seen to be expensive and less cost effective, with the reduction of funding and the pressure to be cost effective.

In this period of transition it is probably too early to assess the actual effects and whether or not there has been an improvement in the way that children with psychiatric problems are managed and child psychiatric services are delivered. Perhaps if future services are to be cost effective this may mean a more flexible approach to staffing structure. Services in the past have tended to be influenced by theory and ideology, whereas one of the goals should be to evaluate and then develop practice in the clinical arena itself (Kolvin 1990).

It is possible that other professional groups can become more acutely involved in offering and delivering a more cost effective service. Community psychiatric nurses (CPNs), for example, may receive early referrals from general practitioners. Psychologists should be able to offer their services for a variety of conditions. Child and adolescent psychiatrists are a very valuable but expensive resource because they not only have to have a full undergraduate medical training but also a minimum of eight years post graduate experience prior to appointment. It is postulated that their services may be better utilized in caring and treating 'special' or 'extreme' cases referred up from the other professionals.

The future remains uncertain. The changes in care provision usually reflect the political climate and are associated with rapid change, which is often a challenge. However it is encouraging that child and adolescent mental health does appear to be on the government's agenda.

CAUSES OF MENTAL HEALTH BREAKDOWN IN CHILDHOOD

Childhood is a complex period of physical and psychosocial development. The child's mental health develops in response to many factors including love, attention, security and confidence with their surroundings.

Children are dependent upon the adults around them (parents, relatives, teachers and so on) and society at large to create and to maintain an optimal environment in which they can maximize their potential and develop a sense of fulfilment and integrity as they travel the road to adulthood.

It may be a rather simplistic assumption that today's society with its ever changing values and external pressures is solely responsible for mental health breakdown. Many children seem to cope well enough with these demands. Therefore it is interesting to explore the differences in children who do not cope so well. There is as yet no easy answer. Further understanding of brain development and function, of the ways in which the brain influences behaviour and of the interaction between constitution and environment, is needed in order to address such a complex question.

Little is also known about the ways in which aetiological factors combine to produce symptoms and clinical syndromes. Two children from seemingly similar backgrounds and with similar aetiological factors may present in markedly different ways. One child may be very disturbed and the other show no signs of disorder. Likewise two children with identical signs and symptoms may be found to have completely different aetiological factors that contribute to their condition. A feasible reason for this being so is that each child is born with innate characteristics which in turn interact with environmental influences from birth (and possibly before) to produce a particular pattern of development, thereby explaining that children within the same family and surrounding milieu actually experience environments differently due to differing responses to *their* individual character.

Other contributing factors

Other contributing factors can be identified which are of value when considering the different ways in which aetiological factors may impinge on the child (Table 11.2). These factors should be considered in a cyclical pattern and not a linear one. It is not as simple as A + B = C. Often a family's past or present attempts to solve a problem have not only acted as failed solutions but have even served to provoke further problems, as shown in this case study.

Table 11.2   Factors contributing to child mental health problems.

Predisposing factors	Those factors which make some children more vulnerable to the disorder in the first place.
Precipitating factors	Those which may trigger the disorder to start.
Perpetuating factors	Those which will maintain the disorder symptoms long after the precipitating factor has disappeared or been resolved.

Lynn is twelve years old and has experienced feelings of loneliness and rejection since her mother remarried 12 months ago. Since her stepsister, Jane, was born her mother now has even less time and her distress starts to show when she starts to steal from her mother's purse and truant from school. Her mother finds the situation increasingly difficult to cope with and finds Lynn impossible to handle. She therefore ignores her daughter even more as she does not know what to say or how to handle her. Lynn's feelings are therefore those of loneliness and rejection.

After one incident her mother sends her to her room and tells her stepfather to deal with her. The stepfather has little experience of dealing with adolescents and when he starts to tell her off Lynn's response is to cry, tell him to go away and say she wants her mother. He retorts that her mother cannot cope with her, and does not want Lynn because she has been so bad. Lynn responds by saying that she does not want him anyway because he is not even her dad and that she does not care what he thinks. He retaliates stating, 'That's fine by me, 'cos I don't care what you think or do 'cos I don't love you either.'

This scenario highlights a number of issues. Lynn's underlying unhappiness has not been acknowledged and their response to her bad behaviour is in many ways inappropriate. The responses about being bad, not wanted or not loved, whilst perhaps said by her stepfather in the heat of the moment, are all too real for Lynn. She is unlikely to be able to take them in context and this will compound her initial feelings of rejection and distress.

Table 11.3 Factors that can affect the child's mental health status.

Individual	Family	Social
gender	attachment	schools
IQ	separations	social misfortune
physical attributes	marital discord	unemployment
predisposition to physical illness	life events	financial hardship
temperament	family structure	
	family size	
	parenting style	
	parental mental illness	

An alternative means of dividing aetiological factors is to consider them as those concerning the individual child and those resulting from the child's environment (Table 11.3).

Individual factors

These are those innate factors with which the child enters the world, such as temperament, gender, IQ, physical attributes or deficits, and predisposition to physical illness. All of these will influence the child's individual characteristics, which in turn will affect the way they interact with their surroundings and external stimuli, which will affect in consequence the way in which significant others will react/interact with the child.

Family

The family will have a major influence on the child's development, although it should be remembered that the same family may rear totally different individual children. There is, however, some evidence to suggest that dysfunctional families are likely to contain children with psychiatric disorders, although not all dysfunctional families have children with psychiatric disorders and not all disordered children come from families which are dysfunctional. However, there are some potential factors worthy of consideration including:

■ Early attachment (Bowlby 1958; Bretherton & Waters 1985).
■ Brief separations (Quinton & Rutter 1976).
■ Marital discord/divorce (Emery 1982).

■ Life events (Goodyer *et al.* 1985) e.g. bereavement (Van Eerdewegh *et al.* 1985).
■ Arrival of new baby (Dunn 1988).
■ Family structure (Jenkins & Smith 1990).
■ Family size (Davie *et al.* 1972).
■ Parenting style (Tizard & Hughes 1984).
■ Parental mental illness (Rutter & Quinton 1984).

Society

Schools have been shown to influence children's social and behavioural development as well as their education in theory (Rutter *et al.* 1979). Whilst social class alone appears not to be associated with psychiatric disorder, social misfortune certainly is. Financial hardship (Richman *et al.* 1982) and unemployment (Warr & Jackson 1985) are linked with psychiatric disorder in children and their parents.

THEORETICAL PERSPECTIVES OF MENTAL HEALTH BREAKDOWN IN CHILDHOOD

There is as yet no unifying theory to explain the causes of mental health breakdown in childhood. There are, however, theories which account for some of the observations in this area of work (Table 11.4) but it is doubtful if any of them encompass all the answers.

The scope of this chapter does not allow for these to be described in detail and although they all have merits it is generally recognised that an eclectic or integrated

Table 11.4 Theoretical perspectives of mental health breakdown in childhood.

- Learning theories (Berger 1985)
- Cognitive theory (Beck & Emery 1985)
- Developmental theories (Shaffer & Dunn 1979)
- Psychodynamic theories (Dare 1985)
- Systems theory (Lewis *et al.* 1976)
- Biological theory (medical model)

approach should be developed when addressing individual clients to ensure that the best possible help is offered following a holistic assessment. It can therefore be seen that although there are many ideas about what can cause mental health breakdown in children there is no grand, universal, unifying theory to provide an ultimate explanation. It still remains difficult to explain why A + B does not always = C. Why some children develop quite disturbing disorders, whilst others who appear to have the exact same ingredients do not. Obviously only further research into the underlying processes of why some children and families blossom in adverse conditions and others wilt can answer these questions.

Prevalence rates of mental health breakdown in childhood

Despite the fact that since the 1970s a number of epidemiological surveys of prevalence rates have been published, it is extremely difficult to conduct an accurate assessment. Children cannot refer themselves, so some disturbed children may fail to be referred. Some children are referred but their behaviour may be a symptom of a disturbed family; they themselves may or may not be disturbed.

Criteria for disturbance vary, which can affect the statistics in two ways. One family will refer a child displaying the exact same behaviour that another family will accept as 'normal'. Additionally, the admission criteria either as outpatient or inpatient may differ from one unit to another depending on staff beliefs, demands, finances available and priorities.

Also it is necessary to bear in mind certain key issues when reading studies and the statistics that they generate: who undertook the study, for what purposes, the profile of the target population and sample, what methodology was used, and the reliability and validity of the study. Using a critical eye when reading research may go some way to help explain the many different findings that are available. Even within the same study there can be conflicting statistics (Rutter *et al.* 1970). Parent and teacher screening questionnaires were obtained on 2334 children; of these the parent and teachers identified a similar proportion of children with deviant behavioural scores but only 19 out of the 271 were identified by both groups. This emphasizes the need for multiple sources of data collection and a wariness when analysing studies. However, there are some commonly quoted statistics which are presented in the next section.

Prevalence in the pre-school group

Some of the most commonly quoted studies state that behavioural and emotional disorders are common in the general population. It is said that 22% of the preschool age children in the UK suffer significant behavioural problems; of these 22%, 7% were said to be severe enough to require specialist assessment, with the other 15% claimed to be mild–moderate behaviour problems (Richman *et al.* 1982). There was no significant difference between the sexes. The most frequent clinical picture was of a restless attention-seeking child who, although they did not appear to be anxious or unhappy, were difficult to manage. Some common behaviour difficulties have been identified (Fig. 11.1).

There appears to be a connection between language and behavioural disorders in that children with an expressive language disorder are far more likely than children in the general population to have a behavioural disorder – 59% to 14% respectively.

Prevalence in middle childhood

Most surveys identify a larger percentage of children with a disturbance than are being treated. Rutter *et al.* (1970) for example, in stage 2 of their study, identify 6.8% of the children in the survey as having a psychiatric disorder. In most cases they found this disorder had been present for at least three years and yet only

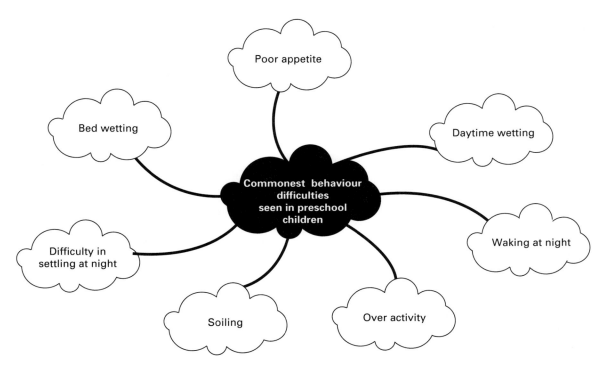

Fig. 11.1   Common types of behaviour difficulties in pre-school children.

10% of those affected had attended a psychiatric clinic. In the Offord *et al.* (1987) study only 16% of the boys and 9% of the girls with a disorder had used mental health or social services in the preceding six months, although half had consulted a physician during that time. In this age group boys seem to be affected more than girls on a ratio of 1.9:1. It would appear that those living in big cities are more likely to be affected than those in small towns – 25% to 12.5% respectively (Rutter *et al.* 1975).

Adolescence

All studies appear to identify larger numbers of disturbed adolescents if the adolescents themselves are interviewed rather than the data being gained from interviews with parents/teachers (Leslie 1974; Rutter *et al.* 1976; McGee *et al.* 1990). Depending on which survey or method or population is used, statistics vary but they suggest that between 10% and 20% of adolescents in the general population suffer a psychiatric

disorder. For example, in the Rutter *et al.* (1976) study, diagnosis based on corroborating sources of information gave an 8% prevalence rate for psychiatric disorder, rising to 13% based solely on parental interview but rocketing to 21% on taking account of individuals. Many adolescents expressed considerable anxiety, misery and other feelings not evident to parents or teachers. There appears to be good evidence that findings in the UK have similar rates to those found in other economically developed areas, especially Europe (Verhulst *et al.* 1986), North America (Offord *et al.* 1989), Australia (Anderson *et al.* 1986), South East Asia (Luk *et al.* 1988), America (Brandenberg *et al.* 1990) and New Zealand (McGee *et al.* 1990).

Prevalence rates in primary care

Children are estimated to occupy 25–33% of GPs' time (Weiselberg 1993). According to a study by Campion & Gabriel (1984) 'behaviour disorder' is the third commonest reason for children to be brought to the attention of the GP. In a study undertaken in the north of England, Garralda & Bailey (1986) found that 23% of 7–12 year old children attending the GP had a psychiatric disorder. Similar results were obtained in the USA by Costello *et al.* (1988).

Association with physical illness

When a child or adolescent has a chronic physical illness of any kind, such as asthma, epilepsy, diabetes and cerebral palsy, there is a potential susceptibility to develop a psychiatric disorder. This does not mean that every child/adolescent with a chronic physical illness will automatically develop a psychiatric disorder. However, they are more vulnerable and therefore the caring profession needs to be aware of and more receptive to possible cues.

Illnesses that do not involve the central nervous system are associated with double the base rate of psychiatric disorder, and idiopathic epilepsy with triple the base rate (Rutter *et al.* (1970). This increased vulnerability was also reflected in a study by Cadman *et al.* (1987) in Ontario. Disability on top of chronic illness further increased the risk to 3.4 times the base rate. This can also work in reverse where a child may use a physical

ailment as an excuse to avoid doing something they find uncomfortable, or it may even be an unconscious thing where a child has a 'genuine' pain leading them to miss out on activities, and no known cause or diagnosis can be found (Faull & Nicol 1986).

Prevalence rates of individual/specific disorders have been researched and provide useful information on the disorder (Table 11.5).

Classification of mental health breakdown in childhood

Classification of disorders ensures meaningful communication can occur between professionals. It also enhances research and provides a means of ordering information and setting it into context. As yet there is no entirely satisfactory classification for child psychiatric disorders. There is always the potential of labelling the child rather than the disorder – which may lead to a plethora of negative effects (Fig. 11.2).

However, caution aired, there are two main types or groups of classification, the commonest appearing to be categorical and which require the professional to make a selection from a list of diagnoses each consisting of identifiable behavioural symptoms. The International

Table 11.5 Studies related to prevalence rates by disorder.

Anorexia nervosa	Szmuckler (1985); Whitaker *et al.* (1990)
Anxiety	Rutter *et al.* (1970); Offord *et al.* (1987)
Autism	Wing (1980); Tsai *et al.* (1981); Lord *et al.* (1982); Steffenburg & Gillberg (1986)
Bulimia	Fosson *et al.* (1987); Whitaker *et al.* (1990)
Conduct disorder	Rutter *et al.* (1975); Offord *et al.* (1989)
Depression	Rutter *et al.* (1976); Garrison *et al.* (1989); Fleming & Offord (1990)
Elective mutism	Kolvin & Fundudis (1981)
Encopresis	Bellman (1966); Rutter *et al.* (1970)
Enuresis	Richman *et al.* (1982); Butler & Golding (1985)
Hyperkinetic syndromes	Prendergast (1988); Taylor *et al.* (1991)
Obesity	Lloyd & Wolff (1976)
Obsessional disorders	Flament *et al.* (1988)
Phobias	Anderson *et al.* (1986)
Psychosis	Gilberg *et al.* (1986)
School refusal	Rutter *et al.* (1976); Waller & Eisenberg (1980)
Substance abuse	Swadi (1988)
Suicidal attempts	Hawton & Goldacre (1982)
Suicide	McClure (1986, 1988)
Tics	Lapouse & Monk (1968); Rutter *et al.* (1970)

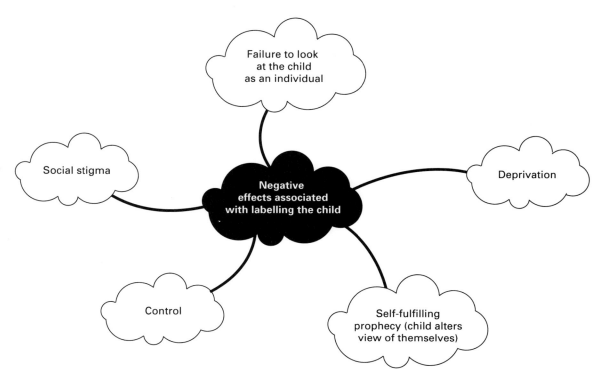

Fig. 11.2   Negative effects associated with labelling the child.

Classification of Disease (10th version) (ICD-10) (WHO 1992) is the one used by most countries and the Diagnostic and Statistical Manual (DSM IVR) (APA 1994) is a very similar system used in America, Canada, and Australia.

The other form of classification is derived by the dimensional approach from the use of multivariate statistical techniques to measure the tendency of specific types of behaviour to occur together in characteristic patterns. This tends to rely on the use of assessment instruments that can be scored. This method of classification is cumbersome, and more importantly statistically significant dimensions may not always be clinically or conceptually meaningful.

TREATMENTS USED IN CHILD/ ADOLESCENT MENTAL DISORDER

There is a plethora of treatment methods available in this area, but because it is a relatively new branch of medicine they are not as well established and researched as in most other branches.

Child and adolescent mental disorders are usually multidimensional and for this reason it is often necessary to employ more than one method of treatment. Knowledge concerning the effectiveness of different types of treatment, or treatment combinations for particular disorders, is often uncertain. So it is not surprising that methods vary immensely from unit to unit and consultant to consultant. Changes have occurred in line with general psychiatry. The development of adult psychopharmacology is reflected by increasing knowledge of the use of medication in children.

As in all areas of childcare, it is extremely important to involve and care for the family as well as the patient. They often suffer along with their child: they may blame themselves and have feelings of guilt, shame and worst of all failure. This is often expressed in seemingly strange ways such as in anger directed towards the professionals. Staff need to be aware of the parents' use of mental defence mechanisms and to listen to them. It is, however, also crucially important for the child to have a voice and to feel that their point of view is heard, understood and truly valued.

It is not possible within this chapter to consider the vast array of treatment methods and options available (Table 11.6), their abuses and effectiveness. Indeed very few practitioners appear to use the therapies in their text book form; most appear to use an eclectic approach or a modified variation.

Where should children be treated?

Before the children can be cared for or treated they need to be identified. As stated previously, 25–33% of a GP's time is taken up by work with children, and although most are presented by their guardian with a physical ailment, the third commonest reason is a behavioural disorder. Yet many family practitioners and primary

Table 11.6 Treatments used in childhood mental disorder.

Behaviour therapy	Yule (1985); Gelfand & Hartmann (1984); Werry & Wollersheim (1989)
Individual psychotherapy	Reisman (1973); Wilson & Hersov (1985); Campion (1991)
Family therapy	Jenkins (1990); Barker (1986); Gorrell Barnes (1985); Lask (1987)
Group therapy	Yalom (1975); Kolvin *et al.* (1988)
Parent counselling	Kraemer (1987); Bywater (1984)
Cognitive therapy	Kendall (1991); Lochman *et al.* (1991)
Hypnotherapy	Olness (1989); Brown & Fromm (1986); Zeltzer & Le Baron (1983)
Dietary therapy	Kaplan *et al.* (1989); Egger *et al.* (1985)
Electroconvulsive therapy (ECT)	This is so rarely used except in life threatening cases that the author has been unable to find any references regarding ECT specifically in child and adolescent treatment.

Drug therapy

Drugs are used sparingly in child and adolescent psychiatry compared with adult psychiatry. There are several research articles which question the usefulness of drug therapy and emphasize the need for caution (Aman & Werry 1982; Puig-Antich *et al.* 1987).

The potential danger of prescribing drugs to children is not only that they suppress the symptoms but also that they mask the underlying problems. They also give the child a message that the problem lies with them and that it is a medical one. Hence not only the child themselves but also those concerned with the care of that child may take an unrealistic view of the problem(s) and stop working on the other areas of concern, feeling that the medication will 'cure all'. Drug treatment is focused on in most child and adolescent mental health text books (e.g. Taylor 1985).

care paediatricians have difficulty in identifying appropriate children for referral (Dulcan *et al.* 1990). Thus there is an obvious dearth in training of doctors in primary care in respect of the psychosocial aspects of their work; the same could arguably be said about children's nurses. It is also important to emphasize that, whilst regular health surveillance of children's hearing, vision, and developmental milestones occurs, time is not set aside to identify potential behavioural and/or emotional problems (Hall 1989) despite the fact that there are checklists developed for this very purpose (Richman *et al.* 1982).

Once a mental health problem/need is identified, a choice of the most appropriate avenue of care and treatment must be made. Care can be provided through outpatient clinics, inpatient units and day units. Each provides a differing type of service to the child and their family, and careful consideration must be made of the best route for care delivery.

Outpatient clinic

Outpatient clinics may be situated in a health centre or education authority premises, or may be part of the local hospital service either attached to a children's or psychiatric hospital. They usually take referrals from a wide range of professionals and will accept children/adolescents for assessment and/or treatment. A large proportion of their work is also educative and advisory, and spent liaising and communicating with other professionals such as teachers and social workers (Black *et al.* 1974).

Day units

Day units allow a more in-depth assessment and a more intense treatment programme to take place, without admitting a child for whom continued home care is practicable and desirable. They also do not interfere too intrusively with the child's usual education and social network, as they can be brought in on a sessional basis, individually designed to cause the least disruption. They also allow for the assessment/treatment of younger children when they are considered too young to be separated from their parents. They often involve the parents more in the care programme at an intervention level, yet at the same time giving the parents opportunity for breathing space which in itself may enable them to cope better, preventing the need for inpatient treatment. Richman *et al.* (1983) claims there is a lack of evidence about the effectiveness of day-care centres in terms of symptom improvement, but they have an important and valuable assessment function and can accelerate delayed development (Cohen *et al.* 1987).

Inpatient units

The popularity of inpatient treatment is on the decline, not just because of the financial cost but also due to the emotional cost to the child and/or family. Parents often feel guilty, ashamed, totally inadequate and deskilled. Children frequently feel abandoned, isolated and scapegoated. Except in extreme cases where emergency admission is necessary, such as when the child/adolescent becomes a danger to themselves or others, inpatient treatment usually follows an unsuccessful attempt at outpatient and/or day care treatment. Inpatient facilities vary immensely in their age range, treatment and assessment philosophy, staffing numbers and skill mix.

Issues about consent to treatment

The same ethical standards apply as in all other branches of medicine. Parents have legally bound responsibilities and it is their duty to exercise these (Children Act 1989). Children under the age of 16 are normally classed as minors and parental consent is legally necessary to carry out any medical procedure, to admit the child to hospital or to administer medication. It is considered good practice in the majority of cases to involve the parents in all such decisions involving their children. However, when a parent refuses to give consent to treatment that is thought beneficial to that child's wellbeing, application can be made for a court order. In the interim period emergency treatment may be undertaken.

The position regarding 'consent to/refusal of' in the older child is more complex. When a child is thought to be capable of forming a mature judgement and refuses treatment, their parents cannot override their wishes. In these circumstances it may be necessary to invoke the Mental Health Act 1983 if the safety of the child or others is at risk. To ensure that these systems are not abused, children and adolescents in the 'system' are overseen by a range of interested bodies such as independent advocates, social service inspectorate, the health advisory service, child protection board and the Mental Health Act Commission.

Prognosis

Although knowledge of prognosis may be seen to be desirable it is not always easy to obtain. There is rarely a simple continuity of the childhood disorder except, for example, in schizophrenia which will generally persist relatively unchanged into adult life. Often there is a 'mix and blend' situation; most children with conduct disorders, for example, will grow out of them, but a few will continue to have problems in adult life, that are likely to be a mixture of an aggressive conduct disorder and affective disorders (Quinton *et al.* 1990). Some problems will transform; for example, children with hyperkinetic syndrome or attention deficit hyperactivity disorder often show conduct disorders in adult life. Generally children grow out of emotional disorders and do not have an increased tendency to be disordered adults (Robins 1966), although Quinton *et al.* (1990)

found that children with emotional disorders whose parents had suffered mental illness themselves, did have a raised rate of affective disorders in adult life. Even behaviour problems appearing in the preschool age years can predict later problems. Stevenson *et al.* (1985) followed up 535 children from three to eight years and found that behaviour patterns at three years were strongly related to deviant behaviour at eight years, especially in boys.

PREVENTION

It is desirable to prevent child mental illness disorders rather than to treat them. Despite the fact that prevention is thought to be more appropriate than cure, it seems to gain less attention than treatment.

Prevention takes three main directions: primary, secondary and tertiary (Caplan 1964). Primary prevention occurs when action is taken to prevent the disorder developing in the first place by removing the cause.

Secondary prevention results from action taken to identify the disorder as soon as it develops and then to minimize its impact. Finally, tertiary prevention results from action taken once the disorder is established to limit the disability it causes (Caplan 1964).

A number of public policy issues have been researched in respect to the effect they have on children's mental health (Table 11.7).

Preventative measure – health and other professionals

Birth to school years

Preventative measures can be used prior to actually becoming a parent; this could include genetic counselling and screening, identifying and reducing the number of pregnancy risk factors, and providing adequate antenatal care. These measures are part of the way in which the risk of birth complications and subsequent brain damage and learning difficulties can be reduced (Newton 1988). Good communication between mother

Table 11.7 Public policy measures which could prevent/allieviate problems.

Alleviation of poverty	This is vital as poverty prediposes to a variety of family difficulties, including family breakdown which in turn has strong links with childhood mental disorder (Rutter & Madge 1976).
Housing	This is an important consideration as children need space to grow up in. Cramped conditions can lead to behaviour problems (Bassum & Rosenberg 1990).
Employment	Adequate work opportunities and good employment prospects would almost certainly reduce the rate of maternal depression and teenage affective disorders (Banks & Jackson 1982).
Child protection	Legislation and social policy to prevent child abuse and neglect is important. It is equally important to protect children from exposure to violence, both that experienced at first hand but also via the television and video, and to protect them from illicit drugs.
Education	Preschool education helps to prevent mild mental retardation and aids socialization and later separation anxiety.
Marital counselling	This should be offered and available from professionals as marital disharmony results in family disharmony and increases the risk of childhood mental disorder.
Neighbourliness	Support from good neighbours would help provide emotional support and reduce stress and tension (Haggerty 1980).

and birth attendant will aid a positive attitude towards the baby (Klaus *et al.* 1986). Parent craft sessions may raise the awareness of risk and help to prevent accidents which can lead to neurological and other injuries, which in turn may cause psychiatric disorder. Regular screening of the child and discussion with the parents with regard to a child centred approach to child rearing may reduce the later development of behavioural problems (Gutelius *et al.* 1977).

Effective observation of parent–child interaction can reveal causes for concern, although it is important not to make assumptions which lead to erroneous conclusions. Preschool programmes for disadvantaged children, with a focus on development, can improve their mental health outcome (Berrueta-Clement *et al.* 1984).

Middle childhood

There are many stressors and challenges associated with middle childhood. Several initiatives have been developed in an attempt to alleviate these, for example problem solving techniques to help children relate to their peers and adults in more satisfying ways (Spivack *et al.* 1976) and strategies to reduce bullying (Olweus 1989). The teacher may have a major role in identifying initial problems and liaising with appropriate professionals to ensure that these early problems are minimized.

Adolescent age group

Providing counselling opportunities for adolescents may enable them to discuss life problems before these lead to adverse psychiatric disorders. This may reduce episodes of self harm or suicidal activity. Programmes are available in the USA but there are few such facilities in the UK. By promoting nonacademic activity such as sport and craft for less academically able adolescents, these programmes appear to reduce the risk of antisocial behaviour (Offord 1987).

Other areas for consideration would be:

- Ensuring that the services available were more user friendly and consumer centred. This would reduce the confusion that often exists, which prevents individuals attending appointments and making initial presentations.
- Reducing the stigma of mental disorder, so that people are more likely to accept that they have a problem and present for treatment.

- Education of society at large, so that parents, teachers, and other responsible adults involved with children know the early signs and warning signals to look for – and what to do about them.
- Education of GPs and general paediatricians and nurses so that they can communicate effectively and highlight the root of the problem when children present with a 'hidden agenda'.
- Education of children themselves to be more alert to signs in themselves and to be more receptive and understanding and aware of avenues they can go down.
- Putting more emphasis and importance on fostering a healthy mental development throughout childhood. All the research has shown the likelihood of later damage as a result of early childhood disorder, so it is surely in our interest to prevent it in the first place.

THE ROLE OF THE NURSE

The role of the nurse in meeting the mental health needs of the child is difficult to define, especially since increasingly children with mental health problems are cared for by nonnurses in the social services. However, it is vital that nurses are aware of their responsibility in respect of the prevention, identification/assessment and management of mental health problems in children in their care.

All children need to be nurtured so that they can gradually learn to become independent human beings and live their life to its full potential. Children need love, security, approval, protection and friendship if they are to grow up liking themselves and being able to return love, affection and support to others in their lives.

Children need carers whom they can look up to and who will be their role model, advocate, protector and guardian, and who will provide an education for them. Children need security, a feeling of love and belonging as well as food, warmth and a safe environment (Maslow 1954) – environments which are safe and stimulating and in which they feel encouraged and motivated to explore and be themselves. In order to facilitate these needs, nurses must be aware of their own beliefs, values and attitudes and must appreciate how they have been shaped by, and respond to, their own environment. By understanding themselves the nurse can start to appreciate the difficulties that a child with mental health needs may be experiencing. Empathy is an important part of being ready to participate in a true therapeutic relationship.

In order to be able to identify mental health needs the nurse must have a number of skills; perhaps the most important of these lies in interaction. Interaction involves assessing a situation holistically (this involves considering the person, their environment, their communications and so on) as well as approaching the child's needs in an appropriate way. The nurse then must be able to respond appropriately and at the same time to be able to cue into the child's feelings. Knowing when to intervene is a matter of skill and judgement which is often based on personal experience and fine judgement of a situation; sensitivity and consideration of the child's

needs are crucial, especially if the nurse is to become accepted by the child. Empathy with the child's needs and problems is vital if progress is to be made within a therapeutic relationship. Effective communication is another essential way in which the nurse can help the child and their family, and this is based on a knowledge and understanding of the child's development. Consideration of their physical, social, emotional, cognitive, and psychological development must be made so that appropriate and effective communication can be established.

In a therapeutic relationship the nurse must ensure that the child feels they are valued and are listened to. They need to know that their feelings and values are respected and that they have the opportunity to confide in the nurse. All interventions should be based on trust and honesty and on realistic expectations of the child

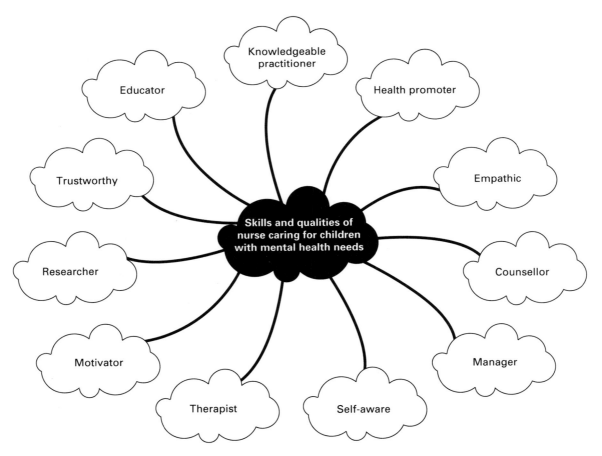

Fig. 11.3 Skills and qualities required by nurse caring for children with mental health care needs.

and the family. The family will, almost always, be central to any programme of care, and parental casework is the traditional form of supportive counselling (Rutter 1975). Here the nurse's role revolves around helping the parents to manage their child's problems. This approach often involves identifying areas of parental behaviour that need to be changed or modified in some way in order to facilitate positive change within the family/child. If the child is admitted to an inpatient unit the implicit message to the patient or carer is that they have, in some way, failed their child. Guilt is often experienced along with this feeling of failure, and some parents become angry and hostile. Again therapy is based on establishing a trusting relationship with both the child and their parents. A non-judgemental approach is important when caring for the whole family.

The qualities and skills needed by the nurse caring for the child with mental health care needs are many and varied; some relate to what may be seen as personal qualities (trust, self-awareness), whereas others can more easily be seen to be practice based (health promoter, therapist and counsellor) (Fig. 11.3). The skilled practitioner is able to draw on skills, knowledge, experience and intuition in order to develop an effective therapeutic relationship with the child/adolescent receiving their care.

CONCLUSION

It is not unreasonable to expect adults to take on the responsibility for ensuring that their children are nurtured through childhood so that they grow and develop physically, psychologically, emotionally, intellectually and socially. The child should be encouraged to develop their potential and become a self-actualised individual. It is equally the role and responsibility of every nurse, regardless of the speciality/environment they are working in, to act as an advocate for the children and adolescents in their care. Nurses must appreciate that children are vulnerable to psychological damage, and nursing care should be consistent in its determination to avoid damage and to identify problems that the child is or has been experiencing. Holistic approaches to care are often discussed and at the centre of this approach is the need to respect the child's psychological/mental health needs; the nurse working as part of a multidisciplinary

team is able to offer a wide range of support to the child and their family.

REFERENCES AND FURTHER READING

Alport, G.W. (1961) Patterns and Growth in Personality. In *Introduction to Psychology* (1983, 8th edn) (eds Hilgard, Atkinson & Atkinson). Churchill Livingstone, Edinburgh.

Aman, M.G. & Werry, J.S. (1982) Methyphenidate and diazepam in severe reading retardation. *Journal of the American Academy of Child & Adolescent Psychiatry*, 21, 31–7.

Anderson, J.C., Williams, S., McGee, R. & Silva, P.A. (1986) DSM-111 disorders in pre adolescent children prevalence in a large sample from the general population. *Archives of General Psychiatry*, 44, 69–76.

APA (1994) *Diagnostic and Statistical Manual of Mental Disorders* (DSM-IV) (3rd Edn). American Psychiatric Association, Washington DC.

Aries, P. (1960) *Centuries of Childhood*. Penguin Books, Harmondsworth.

Aspin, C. (1969) *Lancashire, the First Industrial Society*. United Printing Services, Preston.

Banks, M. & Jackson, P. (1982) Unemployment and risk of minor psychiatric disorder in young people: cross sectional and longitudinal evidence. *Psychological Medicine*, 12, 789–98.

Barker, P. (1986) *Basic Family Therapy* (2nd edn). Blackwell Science, Oxford.

Bassum, E.K. & Rosenberg, L. (1990) Psychological characteristics of homeless children and children with homes. *Paediatrics*, 85, 257–61.

Beck, A.T. & Emery, G. (1985) *Anxiety Disorders and Phobias*. Basic Books, New York.

Bellman, M. (1966) Studies on encopresis. *Acta Paediatrica Scandanavica* (Suppl 170). In *Child and Adolescent Psychiatry* (1993) (eds D. Black & D. Cottrell). Royal College of Psychiatrists, London.

Berger, M. (1985) Learning theories, development and childhood disorders. In *Child & Adolescent Psychiatry: Modern Approaches* (eds M. Rutter & L. Hersov). Blackwell Science, Oxford.

Berreuta-Clement, J.R., Schweinhart, L.J., Barnett, W.S., Epstein, A.S. & Weikart, D.P. (1984) *Changed Lives, the Effects of the Perry Pre-school Programme of Youth through Age 19*. The High Scope Press, Ypsilanti, Michigan. In *Child Psychiatry: A Developmental Approach* (2nd edn, 1986) (P. Graham). Oxford Medical Publications, Oxford.

Black, D. (1987) The future of child guidance. In *Progress in*

Child Health, Vol. 3, (ed. McFarlane). Churchill Livingstone, Edinburgh.

Black, D., Black, M. & Martin, F. (1974) A pilot study of the use of consultant time in psychiatry. *British Journal of Psychiatry*, Supplement news & notes, Sept., p. 3–5. In *Child Psychiatry: A Developmental Approach* (2nd edn, 1986) (P. Graham). Oxford Medical Publications, Oxford.

Black, D., McFadyen, A. & Broster, G. (1990) Development of a psychiatric liaison service. *Archives of Diseases in Childhood*, 65, 1373–5.

Bowlby, J. (1958) The nature of the child tie to his mother. *International Journal of Pyscho-analysis*, 39, 350–73.

Bowlby, J. (1969, 1973, 1980) *Attachment and Loss* (3 vols). Hogarth Press, London.

Brandenberg, N., Friedman, R. & Silver, S. (1990) The epidemiology of childhood psychiatric disorders: prevalence findings from recent studies. *Journal of the American Academy of Child and Adolescent Psychiatry*, 29, 76–83.

Bretherton, I. & Waters, E. (1985) Growing points of attachment theory and research. *Monographs of the Society for Research in Child Development*, 209(50), 1–2.

Brooksbank, D. (1990) In *Child and Adolescent Psychiatry: Into the 1990s*. Occasional paper OP8. Royal College of Psychiatrists, London.

Brown, B.D. & Fromm, E. (1986) *Hypnotherapy and Hypnoanalysis*. Hillsdale, New Jersey. Cited in *Basic Child Psychiatry* (5th edn, 1971) (P. Barker). Blackwell Science, Oxford.

Brunel Institute of Organisation & Social Service (1976) *Future Organisation in Child Guidance and Allied Work*. Working Paper HS1. Brunel University, Uxbridge. Cited in *Child & Adolescent Psychiatry* (1993) (eds D. Black & D. Cottrell). Royal College of Psychiatrists, London.

Butler, N. & Golding, J. (1985) *From Birth to 5: A Study of the Health & Behaviour of Britain's 5 year olds*. Pergamon, Oxford.

Bywater, M. (1984) Coping with a life threatening illness: an experiment in parents' groups. *British Journal of Social Work*, 14, 117–27.

Cadman, D., Boyle, M. & Szatmari, P. (1987) Chronic illness disability and mental social wellbeing: findings of the Ontario Child health study. *Pediatrics*, 79, 805–13.

Campion, J. (1991) *Counselling Children*. Whiting and Birch, London.

Campion, P. & Gabriel, J. (1984) Child consultation patterns in general practice comparing 'high' and 'low' consulting families. *British Medical Journal*, 288, 1426–8.

Caplan, G. (1964) *Principles of Preventive Psychiatry*. Basic Books, New York.

Caring for People (1989) *Community Care in the Next Decade and Beyond*. HMSO, London.

Cohen, N.J., Bradley, S. & Kolers, N. (1987) Outcome evaluation of a therapeutic day treatment program for delayed and disturbed pre schoolers. *Journal of American Academy of Child Psychiatry*, 26, 687–93.

Connell, H.M. (1985) *Essentials of Child Psychiatry*. Blackwell Science, Oxford.

Costello, E.J., Costello, A., Edelbrock, C., Burns, B.J., Dulcan, M.K., Brent, D. & Janiszewski, S. (1988) DSM-III Disorders in paediatric primary care: prevalence and risk factors. *Archives of General Practice*, 45, 1107–16.

Dare, C. (1985) Psychonalytic theories of development. In *Child & Adolescent Psychiatry: Modern Approaches* (eds M. Rutter & L. Hersov). Blackwell Science, Oxford.

Davie, R., Butler, N. & Goldstein, H. (1972) *From Birth to Seven*. Report of the National Child Development Study. Longman, London.

DoH (1989) Preservation Retention and Destruction of Records. Responsibilities of Health Authorities under the Public Records Acts. *Health Circular*, (89), 20.

Dulcan, M.K., Costello, E.J., Costello, A.J., Edelbrock, C., Brent, D. & Janiszewski, S. (1990) The paediatrician as gatekeeper to mental healthcare for children; do parents' concerns open the gate? *Journal of the American Academy of Child & Adolescent Psychiatry*, 29, 453–8.

Dunn, J. (1988) Sibling influence and child development. *Journal of Child Psychology & Psychiatry*, 29, 119–28.

Egger, J., Carter, C. & Graham, P. (1985) Controlled trial of oligoantigenic treatment in the hyperkinetic syndrome. *Lancet*, i, 540–5.

Emery, R.E. (1982) Interparental conflict and the children of discord and divorce. *Psychological Bulletin*, 92, 310–30.

Faull, C. & Nicol, A. (1986) Abdominal pain in 6 year olds: an epidemiological study in a new town. *Journal of Child Psychology and Psychiatry*, 27, 251–60.

Flament, M. Whitaker, A. & Rapoport, J. (1988) Obsessive compulsive disorder in adolescence: an epidemiological study. *Journal of American Academy of Child & Adolescent Psychiatry*, 27, 764–71.

Fleming, J. & Offord, D. (1990) Epidemiology of childhood depressive disorders: a critical view. *Journal of the American Academy of Child Psychiatry*, 29, 571–80.

Fosson, A., Knibbs, J. & Bryant-Waugh, R. (1987) Early onset anorexia nervosa. *Archives of Diseases in Childhood*, 62, 114–18.

Freud, A. (1928) *Introduction to the Technique of Child Analysis*. Nervous & Mental Disease Publishing, New York. Cited in P. Graham *Child Psychiatry: A Developmental Approach* (2nd edn, 1986). Oxford Medical Publications, Oxford.

Garralda, M. & Bailey, D. (1986) Children with psychiatric disorders in primary care. *Journal of Child Psychology & Psychiatry*, 27, 611–24.

Garrison, C.Z., Schluchter, M.D., Schoenback, V.J. & Kaplan, B.H. (1989) Epidemiology of depressive symptoms in young adolescents. *Journal of the American Academy of Child &*

Adolescent Psychiatry, 28, 343–51.

Gath, A. (1990) *Child and Adolescent Psychiatry after the White Papers*. Occasional Paper OP8, Sept, p. 107–9. The Royal College of Psychiatrists, London.

Gelfand, D.M. & Hartmann, D.P. (1984) *Child Behaviour Analysis and Therapy* (2nd edn). Pergamon, Oxford.

Gillberg, C., Wahlstrom, A. & Forsman, A. (1986) Teenage psychoses – epidemiology, classification and reduced optimality in the pre, peri and neonatal periods. *Journal of Child Psychology & Psychiatry*, 27, 87–98.

Goodyer, I., Kolvin, I. & Gatzanis, S. (1985) Recent undesirable life events and psychiatric disorders in childhood and adolescence. *British Journal of Psychiatry*, 147, 517–723.

Gorrell Barnes, G. (1985) Systems theory and family therapy. In *Child & Adolescent Psychiatry: Modern Approaches* (eds M. Rutter & L. Hersov). Blackwell Science, Oxford.

Graham, P. (1976) Management in child psychiatry recent trends. *British Journal of Psychiatry*, 129, 97–108.

Gutelious, M.F., Kirsch, A.D., MacDonald, S., Brook, M.R. & McErlean, T. (1977) Controlled study of child health supervision; behavioural results. *Paediatrics*, 60, 294–304.

Haggerty, R.J. (1980) Life stress, illness and social support. *Developmental & Child Neurology*, 22, 391–400.

Hall, D.M.B. (1989) *Health for all children*. Oxford Medical Publications, Oxford.

Hawton, K. & Goldacre, M. (1982) Hospital admissions for adverse effects of medicinal agents amongst adolescents in the Oxford region. *British Journal of Psychiatry*, 141, 166–70.

Interdisciplinary Standing Committee (1981) Interdisciplinary Work in Child Guidance. Child Guidance Trust, London. Cited in *Child & Adolescent Psychiatry* (1993) (eds D. Black & D. Cottrell). Royal College of Psychiatrists, London.

Jenkins, H. (1990) Family therapy – developments in thinking and practice. *Journal of Child Psychology & Psychiatry*, 31, 1015–26.

Jenkins, J.M. & Smith, M.A. (1990) Factors protecting children living in disharmonious homes: maternal reports. *Journal of the American Academy of Child & Adolescent Psychiatry*, 29, 60–69.

Kanner, L. (1943) Autistic disturbance of affective contact. *Nervous Child*, 2, 217–50.

Kanner, L. (1959) The 33rd Maudsley Lecture: Trends in Child Psychiatry. *Journal of Mental Science*, 105, 581–93.

Kanner, L. (1960) Child psychiatry: retrospect and prospect. *American Journal of Psychiatry*, 117, 15–22.

Kaplan, B.J., McNichol, J., Conte, R.A. & Moghamadam, W.K. (1989) Dietary replacement in pre-school age hyperactive boys. *Paediatrics*, 83, 7–17.

Keir, G. (1952) Symposium on psychologists and psychiatrists in the child guidance service 111. A history of child guidance. *British Journal of Educational Psychology*, 22, 5–29.

Kelynack, T.N. (1915) *Defective Children*. John Bales & Son & Danielsson, London. Cited in The history of child and adolescent psychiatry: its present day relevance (W.L. Parry-Jones 1989). *Journal of Child Psychology & Psychiatry*, 30. 3–11.

Kendall, P.C. (1991) *Child and Adolescent Therapy: Cognitive-Behavioural Procedures*. Guilford Press, New York.

Klaus, M.H., Kennell, J.H., Robertson, S.S. & Soso, R. (1986) Effects of social support during parturition on maternal and infant morbidity. *British Medical Journal*, 293, 585–7.

Klein, M. (1932) *The Psychoanalysis of Children*. Hogarth Press, London.

Kolvin, I. (1973) Evaluation of psychiatric services for children in England and Wales. In *Roots of Evaluation* (eds J.K. Wing & J. Hafner). Oxford University Press. Cited in *Child and Adolescent Psychiatry* (1993, D. Black & D. Cottrell). Royal College of Psychiatrists, London.

Kolvin, I. (1990) *Child & Adolescent Psychiatry into the 1990s*. Occasional Paper 8, Sept, Chapter 16, 113–16. Royal College of Psychiatrists, London.

Kolvin, I. & Fundudis, T. (1981) Elective mute children: psychological development and background factors. *Journal of Child Psychology & Psychiatry*, 22, 219–32.

Kolvin, I., MacKeith, R.C. & Meadow, S.R. (1973) *Bladder Control and Enuresis*. Heinemann, London.

Kolvin, I., Garside, R. & Nicol, A.R. (1981) *Help Starts Here: The Maladjusted Child in the Ordinary School*. Tavistock, London.

Kolvin, I., MacMillan, A. & Nicol, A.R. (1988) Psychotherapy is effective. *Journal of the Royal Society of Medicine*, 18, 261–6.

Kraemer, S. (1987) Working with parents: casework or psychotherapy? *Journal of Child Psychology & Psychiatry*, 28, 207–14.

Lapouse, R. & Monk, M.A. (1968) An epidemiological study of behaviour characteristics in children. Cited in *Child Psychiatry: A Developmental Approach* (2nd edn, 1986) (P. Graham). Oxford Medical Publications, Oxford.

Lask, B. (1987) Family Therapy. *British Medical Journal*, 294, 203–4.

Leslie, S. (1974) Psychiatric disorders in the young adolescents of an industrial town. *British Journal of Psychiatry*, 125, 113–24.

Lewis, J. Beavers, W.R. & Gossett, J.T. (1976) No Single Thread: Psychological Health in Family Systems. Brunel/Mazel, New York. Cited in *Child & Adolescent Psychiatry* (1993) (eds D. Black & D. Cottrell). Royal College of Psychiatrists, London.

Lloyd, J.K. & Wolff, O.H. (1976) Obesity. In *Recent Advances in Paediatrics* (ed. D. Hull). Churchill Livingstone, Edinburgh.

Lochman, J.E., White, K.J. & Wayland, K.K. (1991) Cognitive behavioural assessment and treatment with aggressive children. In *Child & Adolescent Therapy: Cognitive Behavioural Procedures* (ed. P.C. Kendall). New York Press.

Lord, C. Schopler, E. & Revick, D. (1982) Sex differences in autism. *Journal of Autism and Developmental Disorders*, 12, 317–30.

Lowenfield, M. (1935) *Play in Childhood*. Gollancz, London. Cited in *Child & Adolescent Psychiatry* (1993) (eds D. Black & D. Cottrell). Royal College of Psychiatrists, London.

Luk, S.L., Leung, P.W.L. & Lee, P.L.M. (1988) Conners teacher rating scale in Chinese children in Hong Kong. *Journal of Child Psychology & Psychiatry*, 29, 165–74.

Maslow, A.H. (1954) *Motivation and Personality*. Harper & Row, London.

McClure, G. (1986) Recent changes in suicide among adolescents in England and Wales. *Journal of Adolescence*, 9, 135–43.

McClure, G. (1988) Suicide in children in England and Wales. *Journal of Child Psychology & Psychiatry*, 29, 345–9.

McGee, R., Feehan, M. & Williams, S. (1990) DSM-111 disorders in a large sample of adolescents. *Journal of the American Academy of Child & Adolescent Psychiatry*, 29, 611–19.

Newton, R.W. (1988) Psychosocial aspects of pregnancy: the scope for intervention. *Journal of Reproductive and Infant Psychology*, 6, 23–39.

NHS Review (1989) *Working for patients*. HMSO, London.

Offord, D.R. (1987) Prevention of behavioural and emotional disorders in children. *Journal of Child Psychology & Psychiatry*, 28, 9–20.

Offord, D., Boyle, M. & Szatmari, P. (1987) Ontario child health study II. Six month prevalence of disorder and rates of service utilization. *Archives of General Psychiatry*, 44, 832–6.

Offord, D., Boyle, M.H. & Racine, Y. (1989) Ontario Child Health Study: correlates of disorder. *Journal of the American Academy of Child & Adolescent Psychiatry*, 28, 856–60.

Olness, K. (1989) Hypnotherapy: a cyberphysiologic strategy in pain management. *Paediatric Clinics of North America*, 36, pp. 873–84. Cited in *Child Psychiatry* (2nd edn, 1986) (P. Graham). Oxford Medical Publications, Oxford.

Olweus, D. (1989) Bully/victim problems among school children: basic facts and effects of a school based intervention program. Cited in *Child Psychiatry* (2nd edn, 1986) (P. Graham). Oxford Medical Publications, Oxford.

Parry-Jones, W.L. (1984) Adolescent psychiatry in Britain – a personal view of its development and present position. *Bulletin of the Royal College of Psychiatrists*, 8, 230–33.

Parry-Jones, W.L. (1989) Annotation. The history of child and adolescent psychiatry: its present day relevance. *Journal of Child Psychology & Psychiatry*, 30, 3–11.

Prendergast, M. (1988) The diagnosis of childhood hyperactivity: a UK–US cross national study. *Journal of Child*

Psychology & Psychiatry, 29, 289–300.

Puig-Antich, J., Perel, J. & Lupatkin, W. (1987) Imipramine in major prepubertal depressive disorders. *Journal of the American Academy of Child and Adolescent Psychiatry*, 44, 81–9.

Quinton, D. & Rutter, M. (1976) Early hospital admissions and later disturbances of behaviour: an attempted replication of Douglas' findings. *Developmental Medicine and Child Neurology*, 18, 447–59.

Quinton, D., Rutter, M. & Gulliver, L. (1990) Continuities in psychiatric disorders from childhood to adulthood in the children of psychiatric patients. In *Straight and deviant pathways from childhood to adulthood* (eds L. Robins & M. Rutter). Cambridge University Press.

Reisman, J.M. (1973) *Principles of Psychotherapy with Children*. John Wiley, New York.

Renton, G. (1978) The East London Child Guidance Clinic. *Journal of Child Psychology & Psychiatry*, 19, 309–12.

Richman, N., Stevenson, J. & Graham, P. (1982) *Pre-school to School: A Behavioural Study*. Academic Press, London.

Richman, N., Graham, P. & Stevenson, J. (1983) Long term effects of treatment in a pre school day centre. *British Journal of Psychiatry*, 142, 71–7.

Robertson, J. (1952) *A 2-year old Goes to Hospital* (film). Concord Films Council, Ipswich.

Robertson, J. (1958) *Going to Hospital with Mother* (film). Concord Films Council, Ipswich.

Robins, L. (1966) *Deviant Children Grown Up*. Williams & Wilkins, Baltimore.

Royal College of Psychiatrists (1978) *The Role & Responsibilities and Work of the Child & Adolescent Psychiatrists*. Bulletin 2 and (1986) Bulletin 10. Royal College of Psychiatrists, London.

Rutter, M. (1975) *Helping Troubled Children*. Penguin Books, Harmondsworth.

Rutter, M. (1979) Invulnerability and why some children are not damaged by stress. In *New Directions in Children's Mental Health* (ed. Shamsie). SP Medical & Scientific Books, New York.

Rutter, M. (1986) Child psychiatry: looking 30 years ahead. *Journal of Child Psychology & Psychiatry*, 27, 803–41.

Rutter, M. & Madge, N. (1976) *Cycles of Disadvantage*. Heinemann, London.

Rutter, M. & Quinton, D. (1984) Parental psychiatric disorder: effects on children. *Psychological Medicine*, 14, 835–80.

Rutter, M. Tizard, J. & Whitmore, K. (1970) *Education, Health & Behaviour*. Longman, London.

Rutter, M., Cox, A. & Tupling, C. (1975) Attainment and adjustment in two geographical areas: the prevalence of psychiatric disorder. *British Journal of Psychiatry*, 126, 493–509.

Rutter, M., Graham, P. & Chadwick, O. (1976) Adolescent

turmoil: fact or fiction? *Journal of Child Psychology & Psychiatry*, 17, 35–56.

Rutter, M., Maughan, B., Mortimor, P., Ouston, J. & Smith, A. (1979) *Fifteen Thousand Hours: Secondary Schools and their Effects on Children*. Open Books, London/Harvard University Press. Cited in *Child and Adolescent Psychiatry: Modern Approach* (1994 3rd edn) (eds M. Rutter & L. Hersov). Blackwell Science, Oxford.

Sampson, O.C. (1980) *Child Guidance – its History, Provenance and Future*. British Psychological Society, Leicester.

Senn, M.J.E. (1959) Conduct disorders. Cited in *Behavioural Treatment of Childhood Problems* (1981) (Martin Herbert). Academic Press, London.

Shaffer, D. & Dunn, J. (1979) *The First Year of Life: Psychological and Medical Implications of Early Experience*. Wiley, Chichester.

Spivak, G., Platt, J.J. & Shure, M.B. (1976) *The Problem Solving Approach to Adjustment*. Jossey Bass, San Francisco.

Steffenburg, S. & Gilberg, C. (1986) Autism and autistic-like conditions in Swedish rural and urban areas: a population study. *British Journal of Psychiatry*, 149, 81–7.

Stevenson, J., Richman, N. & Graham, P. (1985) Behaviour problems and language abilities at 3 years and behavioural deviance at 8 years. *Journal of Child Psychology & Psychiatry*, 26, 215–30.

Swadi, H. (1988) Drug and substance abuse among 3333 London adolescents. *British Journal of Addiction*, 83, 935–42.

Szmuckler, G. (1985) Review: the epidemiology of anorexia nervosa and bulimia. *Journal of Psychiatric Research*, 19, 143–53.

Taylor, E.A. (1985) Syndromes of overactivity and attention deficit. In *Child & Adolescent Psychiatry – Modern Approaches* (eds M. Rutter & L. Hersov). Blackwell Science, Oxford.

Taylor, E., Sandberg, S. & Thornley, G. (1991) *The Epidemiology of Childhood Hyperactivity*. Institute of Psychiatry Maudsley Monographs, Oxford University Press.

Tizard, B. & Hughes, B. (1984) *Young Children Learning*. Fontana, London.

Tsai, L., Stewart, M.A. & August, G. (1981) Implications of sex differences in the familial transmission of infantile autism. *Journal of Autism and Developmental Disorder*, 11, 165–73. Cited in *Basic Child Psychiatry* (1971) (P. Barker). Blackwell Science, Oxford.

Van Eerdewegh, M.M., Clayton, P.J. & Van Eerdewegh (1985) The bereaved child: variables in influencing early psychopathology. *British Journal of Psychiatry*, 147, 188–94.

Verhulst, F.C., Berden, G.F.M. & Sanders Woudstra, J. (1986) Mental health in Dutch children II. The prevalence of psychiatric disorder and relationship between measures. Cited in *Child Psychiatry* (1986) (P. Graham). Oxford Medical Publications.

Walk, A. (1964) The pre-history of child psychiatry. *British Journal of Psychiatry*, 110, 754–67.

Waller, D. & Eisenberg, L. (1980) School refusal in childhood – a psychiatric paediatric perspective. In *Out of School – Modern Perspectives in School Refusal and Truancy* (eds L. Hersov & I. Berg). Wiley, Chichester.

Wardle, C. (1991) Twentieth century influences on the development in Britain of services for child and adolescent psychiatry. *British Journal of Psychiatry*, 159, 53–68.

Warr, P. & Jackson, P. (1985) Factors influencing the psychological impact of prolonged unemployment and of re-employment. *Psychological Medicine*, 15, 795–807.

Weiselberg, M. (1993) Classifications and epidemiology. In *Child and Adolescent Psychiatry* (eds D. Black & D. Cottrell), Chapter 5, 54–74. Royal College of Psychiatrists, London.

Werry, J.S. & Wollersheim, J.P. (1989) Behaviour therapy with children and adolescents: a 20 year overview. *Journal of the American Academy of Child and Adolescent Psychiatry*, 28, 1–18.

Whitaker, A., Johnson, J. & Shaffer, D. (1990) Uncommon troubles in young people in prevalence of selected psychiatric disorders in a non-referred adolescent population. *Archives of General Psychiatry*, 47, 487–96.

WHO (1992) *The ICD-10 Classification of Mental and Behavioural Disorders: Clinical Descriptions and Diagnostic Guidelines*. World Health Organisation, Geneva.

Wilson, P. & Hersov, L. (1985) Individual and group psychiatry. In *Child and Adolescent Psychiatry* (eds M. Rutter & L. Hersov) (2nd edn). Blackwell Science, Oxford.

Wing, L. (1980) Childhood autism and social class: a question of selection? *British Journal of Psychiatry*, 137, 410–17.

Winnicott, D. (1965) *The Family and Individual Development*. Tavistock, London.

Yalom, I. (1975) *The Theory and Practice of Group Psychotherapy* (2nd edn). Basic Books, New York.

Yule, W. (1985) Behavioural approaches. In *Child and Adolescent Psychiatry* (M. Rutter & L. Hersov) (2nd edn). Blackwell Science, Oxford.

Zeltzer, L. & Le Baron, S. (1983) Behavioural intervention for children and adolescents with cancer. *Behavioural Medicine Update* 5, 17–22.

Part 3
Dimensions of Nursing Care

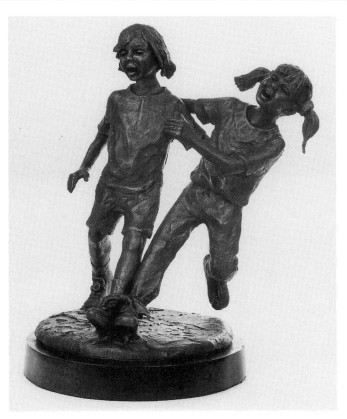

Part 3 examines how the children's nurse can support and meet the needs of sick children and the families in their care. A deliberate attempt has been made to present the roles of the nurse in terms of providing support for the child and their family. The philosophy of children's nursing pervades each chapter and the notion of partnership is implicit.

Principles of care, rather than prescriptions for care, are presented and discussed and not every situation or condition that the children's nurse will meet is explored. A systems approach has been adopted to help frame care and, although this may be criticized as mirroring the medical model, the emphasis is on nursing assessment and interventions.

The importance of the child's diagnosis is seen in relation to how the nurse can provide care, resolve problems and meet needs. Basic knowledge, such as anatomy and physiology, is assumed and specific physiological information will only be introduced where it is deemed vital. Where possible the authors have drawn on British research to provide the rationale for practice, although the relative paucity of paediatric research in some areas of care such as wound management, is evident.

The children's nurse has a diverse range of roles including adviser, health promoter and educator, teacher, friend and playmate, direct care giver and co-ordinator. Each of these roles is explored in the following chapters and provides insight into the dimensions of care. The reader is encouraged to read and reflect upon the issues raised, and consider their application within their own professional practice area.

INTRODUCTION

Pain is one of the most common symptoms which nurses and other health care professionals have to deal with and yet until the 1980s it received little attention. Details about assessing and managing pain are now more widely recognized because of increasing amounts of pain related research. Most paediatric pain research and literature is American, although worldwide, including Canada, Australia and Britain, there is a growing body of health professionals with a special interest in the different aspects of assessing and managing children's pain. The literature to date suggests that children's pain is undertreated and that misconceptions about pain contribute to inadequate relief because healthcare workers have limited knowledge about assessing and managing pain (Burke & Jerret 1989; Carter 1990; Eland 1990; Lloyd-Thomas 1990; RCS & CA 1990; Wilson *et al.* 1992; Burrows & Berde 1993). It is important to include research findings and incorporate them into practice in order to ensure that children do not suffer pain unnecessarily.

Traditionally healthcare workers have had little or no training specifically about pain, although it is covered in broad terms in nursing and medical curricula. The fact that practice is still based upon misbeliefs, and that research findings are not readily put into practice, make a clear argument for making all literature about pain available to healthcare professionals to improve its recognition and treatment. Specific training about pain for all health professionals has been recommended repeatedly (Dilworth & McKellar 1987; Pilowski 1988; Holm *et al.* 1989; Alder 1990; Fields 1991).

This chapter will provide an overview of the growing body of knowledge about children's pain and will demonstrate the importance of recognizing and treating pain effectively. The information will not be prescriptive because there are many methods to, for example, assess pain, and because every child's situation is different depending on issues such as the cause of pain. Consequently the information may be related to hospital and community settings, and unless stated otherwise will apply to both. The following issues will be addressed:

- What is pain?
- Types of pain.
- Misconceptions about pain.

- Why treat pain?
- The assessment of pain.
- The management of pain.

WHAT IS PAIN?

Pain is a highly complex issue which has many causes, e.g. illness, trauma or surgery. Type and cause of pain are discussed in the next section, but before they can be addressed the question 'What is pain?' should be examined. Pain is difficult to define because of co-existing physical and emotional components and also because of influences such as upbringing, culture, environment and gender, any of which cause people to react differently when experiencing pain. However, the International Association for the Study of Pain has defined pain as:

> 'an unpleasant sensory and emotional experience associated with actual or potential tissue damage, or described in terms of such damage.' (Merksey 1979)

Physical pain is a sensation which is perceived as unpleasant. There are several different theories about the physiology of pain (Fordham 1986; Nie *et al.* 1989; McCready *et al.* 1991) but the one which is most commonly subscribed to is the gate control theory, first described by Melzack & Wall (1965) and since refined (Wall 1978; Wall & Melzack 1989). Simply, this theory argues that pain is felt when nerve endings pick up impulses from tissue; these impulses are transmitted along pain pathways via the spinal cord to the hypothalamus in the brain. A return signal is then transmitted via descending fibres in the spinal cord, resulting in the sensation of pain. This theory also proposes that because the hypothalamus is also the emotional centre of the brain, the descending fibres may modify the pain signals thereby allowing a link between physical and emotional pain (Nie *et al.* 1989).

Emotional pain may be felt in terms of mood; however it may also intensify perceived physical pain. Psychological reaction to pain accounts for differences in pain perception between (adult) individuals (Nie *et al.* 1989). In general, anxious people tolerate pain less well than relaxed individuals. Where children are concerned, anxiety or fear both influence children's experience of pain by making the pain worse (Bielby 1984; Beales

1986; Williams 1987a); for example, children as young as two years are afraid of needles (Gureno & Reisinger 1991).

It must be remembered that the transfer of anxiety from parents to their children is a well-recognized phenomenon and that reduced parental anxiety is likely to help to reduce a child's anxiety (Glasper 1990). Most children are less disturbed when a parent is present; however, it is possible that a few may become more disturbed if the parent is extremely anxious. This transferred anxiety between parent and child may increase children's anxiety and consequently their pain. The inevitable vicious circle results when children are labelled as 'difficult' because of their behaviour and their pain is neither recognized nor treated.

TYPES OF PAIN

The type of pain experienced is based on its cause. Both have to be considered but this cannot be done separately because type and cause are interlinked. Pain may be either acute (intense, short, reversible) or chronic (long-standing, less intense). Examples are given in Tables 12.1 and 12.2. Acute pain may be caused by illness, surgery or at the time of an injury, and is resolved within a relatively short time-span. Surgery and invasive procedures are major causes of acute pain in hospitals, while in the community both acute and chronic pain will be managed because of the increase in day surgery and the emphasis on community care.

Chronic pain may be caused by either malignant disease or non-malignant illness such as juvenile rheumatoid arthritis, and can be difficult to treat (Thomson *et al.* 1987; Varni & Walco 1988). Acute and chronic pain can be difficult to distinguish; for example, cancer may cause chronic pain over the long term but secondary disease may cause acute pain in addition. Psychologically, acute pain and anxiety are often related, the pain causing children's behaviour to change quickly, whereas chronic pain is more likely to be associated with depression (Gauvain-Piquard *et al.* 1987; Varni & Walco 1988; Page 1991).

A child with chronic pain is used to living with pain because it is constant, and consequently their appreciation of it is less (Nie *et al.* 1989). On the other hand, a child with acute pain is in an unfamiliar situation and is

Table 12.1 Examples of acute pain.

Cause	Example
Illness	appendicitis earache
Surgery	minor – herniotomy major – nephrectomy
Injury	fracture

Table 12.2 Examples of chronic pain.

Cause	Example
Disease	juvenile rheumatoid arthritis
Injury	fracture
Neurological	back pain in myelomeningocele

more aware of the altered sensation which is being experienced. Children with chronic pain tolerate their pain more than children with acute pain. In other words, if a child with a chronic illness which causes long-term pain, complains of pain, it is likely that by the time they do complain, their pain is considerable. It must always be remembered that the child with chronic pain may be in pain even though he is not complaining. It is highly unlikely that a child without pain will complain unless something is wrong, and so any child who does complain of pain should be taken seriously.

Hayward (1987) found that carefully given information preoperatively reduced the requirement for postoperative analgesia in adults, i.e. in circumstances where there is acute pain. It is also known that children are less anxious when given an understandable explanation about why they have pain and how it can be relieved, e.g. before an invasive procedure or surgery, and as a result they may experience less pain (Bielby 1984; Pakoulas *et al.* 1984).

WHY TREAT PAIN?

There are various theories about why pain should be treated. One is that pain sensation is essential for survival because it warns about tissue damage, e.g. when touching a hot iron or from sunburn (Nie *et al.* 1989). With the first of these there is an immediate reaction but with the second, sunburn, the skin is burned by the time the pain is felt. McGrath (1989) suggests that experience of chronic or recurrent pain leads to modified future behaviour. This may be beneficial in a situation where a young child is burned by touching a hot iron; by doing so the child learns not to touch a hot iron again. However, if a young child experiences pain repeatedly because of illness or invasive procedures, e.g. injections, this could influence his/her future behaviour by creating a fear of injections.

A second theory is that experiencing pain is character building and should not be prevented (Adams 1989). This may be based on cultural or peer pressure and may be one reason why adolescents appear to be in greater control than children when they are in pain.

In situations where nurses have to deal with pain, i.e. where pain is unavoidable, it should be relieved so as to prevent an increase in morbidity (Eland 1990). In addition, the severity of perceived pain may be increased by influences such as anxiety or lack of sleep. These issues will also be discussed in this section.

Increased morbidity

Unrelieved pain causes physiological and psychological problems (Eland 1990). The former include respiratory and cardiovascular problems and fluid and electrolyte loss. The Royal College of Surgeons and the College of Anaesthetists (RCS & CA 1990) argue that one of the benefits of treating pain is to reduce morbidity.

Psychological problems

Williams (1987b) reports that anxiety and pain are linked, each being able to increase the other; it is also known that inadequate information increases anxiety in children (Glasper & Stradling 1989). Therefore it is important to pre-empt and minimize anxiety by providing information. However, information given to children must be at a level which they can understand to prevent any misinterpretation and to clarify misbeliefs (Rodin 1983; Bielby 1984; Eiser & Patterson 1984). For example, Eiser (1987) suggests that children under 7

years perceive illness as punishment, Jago (1985) argues that hospitalization may be seen as a punishment by children aged five to ten years, and Eiser & Patterson (1984) state that children aged five to ten years associate hospital with pain. Consequently, the importance of preparing children for hospitalization and all that it involves cannot be stressed highly enough. It is possible that unrelieved pain experienced in hospital may contribute to the association between hospitalization and pain and should therefore be prevented.

Unavoidable pain

Relieving a child's pain caused by an invasive procedure is likely to make the experience less traumatic. If the pain is not prevented or relieved the child is likely to be more anxious, particularly if the procedure has to be repeated, e.g. bone marrow puncture. Analgesic administration by nurses to children is reported as being poor (Eland 1990; Elander *et al.* 1991). It is also known that children receive fewer analgesics than adults (Schechter *et al.* 1986; Eland 1990); for example, Schechter *et al.* examined 90 children and 90 adults with similar conditions and found that the adults were given twice as many narcotics as the children. In addition, they found that younger children were less likely to have opiates prescribed than older children. In the author's experience, even if younger children are prescribed opiates they are rarely, if ever, given (Gillies 1991, 1992). These situations should not occur when it is known that opiate administration is safe for children (Davis 1992; Burrows & Berde 1993).

Lack of sleep

Unrelieved pain is known to interrupt sleep in adults and it is suggested that this also occurs in children (Schechter 1989; Pfeil 1993). Conversely, lack of sleep may increase perceived pain. Healing occurs during non-rapid eye movement sleep (Kalat 1988). As rapid eye movement sleep starts about 90 minutes after falling asleep, Pfeil (1993) suggests that interruptions from pain, noise or vital sign recordings will not only disturb rapid eye movement sleep but also non-rapid eye movement sleep, thereby increasing perceived pain.

The answer to the question 'Why treat pain?' is simple: there is no reason not to (Burrows & Berde

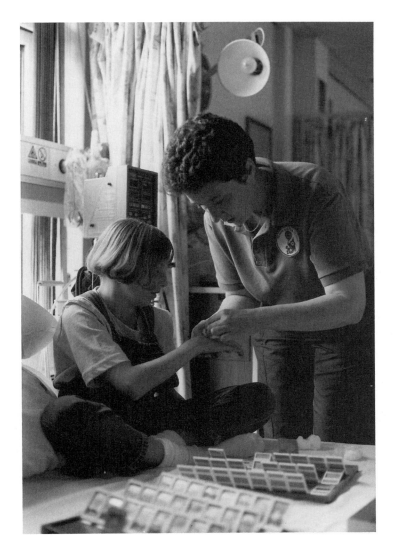

Fig. 12.1 The use of EMLA (eutetic mixture of local anaesthetics) cream can minimize the pain associated with siting intravenous cannulae or taking blood. *(Reproduced by permission of Jon Sparks.)*

1993) when that pain is caused by illness, disease, accident or invasive procedures. This is particularly important when it is known that either not treating or poorly managing pain will reduce the child's quality of life by causing lack of sleep, increased anxiety and increased morbidity. It should also be remembered that in the 1990s when finance is a consideration, it is likely that preventing or relieving pain will result in earlier discharge and so reduce cost (RCS & CA 1990).

MISCONCEPTIONS ABOUT PAIN

Misconceptions, otherwise known as myths or mis-beliefs, held by healthcare staff undoubtedly influence the assessment and management of children's pain. Some of the long-held beliefs about pain in children and adolescents have been noted repeatedly (Eland & Anderson 1977; Burokas 1985; Grunau & Craig 1987;

Alder 1990; Eland 1990). Examples of long-held beliefs about pain in children and adolescents are given in Table 12.3.

Table 12.3 Examples of long-held beliefs about pain in children and adolescents.

- Infants and children do not feel pain, when it is known that they do (Grunau & Craig 1987).
- Children do not remember pain, when it is known that they do (Schechter 1989; Burrows & Berde 1993).
- Children easily become dependent on opiates (Alder 1990; Burrows & Berde, 1993), when no literature has been found supporting this.
- Nursing and medical staff are more able to recognize the existence and rate the severity of pain than the children themselves (Burokas 1985), when it is well recognized that pain is a subjective phenomenon even for children and adolescents (McGrath & Unrah 1987; Devine 1990).
- Withdrawn children are coping with their pain, when in reality they are not admitting to it (Mather & Mackie 1983).
- Intramuscular injections are avoided by nursing and medical staff because of the belief that the injection is worse than the pain itself (Eland 1990).

In recent studies examining children's experiences of postoperative pain (Gillies 1991, 1992), the author found the results given in Table 12.4.

Traditional beliefs influence clinical practice in a negative manner. Children do suffer and in addition it is

reasonable to assume that because of their limited communication skills, they suffer more than adults. It is therefore essential that although health care staff need to be aware of the existence of misbeliefs, their practice should be research-based.

GOAL OF NURSING PRACTICE

The goal or aim of intended nursing practice is the basis upon which practice centres. Where pain relief is concerned, the goal is of paramount importance and is twofold:

(1) To completely eliminate the child's pain at best, or at least to reduce the amount of pain which the child is suffering.
(2) To achieve the standards of care set in relation to pain assessment and management and consequently to enable audit of that care.

Elimination or reduction of pain

The elimination of all pain is not always an achievable objective, particularly when the pain is chronic or caused by terminal disease. In such situations all efforts should be made to relieve the child's discomfort as much as possible. However, in other situations it may be possible to completely relieve the child's pain and this should be the ultimate goal.

In order to achieve these aims it is essential that nurses' perceptions of their role and practice do not differ, i.e. their practice is always what they think it is.

Table 12.4 Postoperative pain in children.

1:10 staff (doctors and children's nurses) and 1:3 mothers believed that postoperative pain cannot be prevented (Gillies 1991)	when	pain can be relieved or prevented safely using drugs (Burrows & Berde 1993).
24% of staff and 24% of mothers believed that children do not experience as much pain as adults (Gillies 1991)	when	children 'suffer pain in the same way as adults do' (Bray 1988).
Children experience more pain than staff and mothers realized (Gillies 1991, 1992)	when	children are given less strong analgesia less frequently than adults (Mather & Mackie 1983; Schechter *et al.* 1986; Eland 1990)

For example, if nurses offer analgesia regularly to children then the nursing documentation should show evidence of this, even if the treatment is refused. Otherwise it is difficult for other staff to know what has happened and to continue providing effective care. Similarly, different groups of healthcare staff should have the same aims. If aims differ this can result in compromised care for the child; for example, if doctors who prescribe believe that opiates should be given for as long as necessary after minor surgery, and nurses who administer believe that 24 hours is long enough, this is bound to influence practice, resulting in inadequate pain relief.

It is also important to discuss the aims of relieving pain with the parents because the staff's and parents' aims may differ (Eland 1990). If there is a difference, it is essential that both groups understand the other's feelings and aims. Of course, if possible the child should also be involved.

Standards of care and audit

Each hospital has standards of care against which its quality of care is measured. These standards must be achievable and measurable and are the tools which allow audit to take place. Setting standards relating to the assessment and management of pain is extremely difficult because no two situations are alike, in hospital or in the community, and also because it is impossible to say that one means of measuring pain will be of use for every child or in every different situation. A sample standard of care written on the assessment of pain is given in Fig. 12.2.

Yorkhill NHS Trust Hospitals

Central Ref. No. _____	Achieve Standard by *February 1994* _____
Local Ref. No. *Marjorie Gillies and a Pain Assessment Working Group*	Review Standard by *January 1995* _____
Topic *Individualised Care (01)* _____	Signature of Standard Setting Co-ordinator _____
Care Group *All In-Patients, RHSC* _____	Signature of Director of Nursing/Quality _____
Sub-topic *Assessment of Pain (2)* _____	

Date of unit validation _____

Standard statement   *Each patient will be assessed individually for their actual level and potential for pain.* _____

Structure	Process	Outcome
Patient *Parents* *Nurse – Registered or Learner (C2, C3, C4)* *– Competent in Pain Assessment or Educated in Pain Assessment* *Doctor* *Choice of assessment tools appropriate to developmental stage* *Nursing history* *Nursing care plan* *Pain assessment sheet*	*The Nurse will:* *– know family term for "pain"* *– explain the appropriate tool to each child on admission* *– listen to and reassure child* *– observe child's behaviour* *– ensure child understands assessment tool before using it (if self-report appropriate)* *– measure child's pain using an objective pain scale (where appropriate)* *– review recent pain-related management from nursing notes* *– involve and listen to parents* *– involve medical staff once specified criteria reached*	*Potential pain will be anticipated* *Presence of child's pain will be recognised* *Child will understand and be able to use appropriate self-report scale* *Child's pain level will be measured* *The need for pain relief will be effectively anticipated and organised.*

Fig. 12.2 Example of a nursing standard on the assessment of pain in children. (Published with permission from The Yorkhill NHS Trust, Glasgow)

PAIN ASSESSMENT

As in any nursing situation, a problem has to be appraised before any action can be taken. However, before going into details of how pain can be assessed, three questions need to be addressed:

(1) What is assessment?
(2) Why assess pain?
(3) Who should do this?

What is assessment?

A general definition of assessment, as given in Collins English Dictionary, is 'a judgement of worth or importance'. However, the assessment of pain is described by McCaffery & Beebe (1989) as 'a beginning step in understanding and working towards the patients' goal'. It could be argued that nurses judge situations all the time, but how does each nurse know that her or his assessment is accurate? When a child's pain is being considered the pain belongs to the child and not to the nurse. Pain is subjective and that means that no one else knows how severe another individual's pain is; the judgement has to be made by children themselves, providing communication is possible.

Why assess pain?

Assessment (of anything) is essential if effective and efficient management and evaluation are to follow. Effective pain relief cannot be given if the issues influencing the pain and the severity of the pain are not clarified. It follows that evaluation would be difficult, or even impossible, if the initial assessment and management are incomplete.

The provision of high quality health care is not only topical in the 1990s, professionally, but is demanded by the general public through the Patients' Charter. Less than the best is unacceptable practice. Professionally, standards of nursing care are being set and audit is taking place in medicine and nursing. In general, standards provide an expected level against which care can be measured, thus allowing audit. More specifically, in order to assess pain it has to be accurately measured.

Regardless of their profession, every health care worker is accountable to their patients for all aspects of their care, and that includes pain relief. Where children are concerned, they should be given the benefit of the doubt and if there is any question about their comfort or discomfort, pain relief should be evaluated. Nurses must remember that their role includes acting as children's advocates. If nurses do not assess and manage pain effectively they are failing the children who depend upon them. It is equally important to remember that nurses are also accountable to their profession (UKCC 1989, 1992), their peers and their employers for patient care. In addition, there is the question of ownership: all nurses want 'their' hospital to be known as the best, and part of that objective involves measuring to assess quality. Finally, it is unethical, immoral and inhuman not to treat a child's pain when the pain can be measured and effective management exists.

Who should assess pain?

Responsibility for the assessment of pain could be said to lie with professionals, parents or children. There are advantages and disadvantages for each group. Professionals know more about medical and nursing care but they do not know each child or family intimately. Nursing staff see more of patients than the medical staff who have other commitments away from the wards. Attitudes such as 'You shouldn't have pain' from both parents and staff, influence assessment (Gillies 1991). Neither parents nor staff have any right to make such statements to any child who may be in pain.

Parents obviously know their child better than anyone else but because of that relationship it may be difficult for them to be objective about their own child. Three other difficulties exist:

(1) Some mothers will state that their child is not in pain but will indicate that the child is in pain with an analogue scale (Gillies, 1991).
(2) Small numbers of parents do not tell staff if their child continues to have pain after being given analgesia (Gillies 1991).
(3) It is also possible that a small number of mothers may not recognize anxiety and pain in their child because of maternal anxiety.

So because the pain is theirs, should assessment be left to

the children themselves? A major problem with relying on verbal communication is that even if they have language skills, many children do not always admit to being sore (Fig. 12.3). However, a child may deny pain verbally but indicate the presence and severity of pain using a measurement tool (Gillies 1991). So, where age and maturity permit, pain should be assessed by children themselves. Where they are too young to use self-report, there is no alternative to objective measurement by others.

> Q: 'Are you sore anywhere now?'
> A: *'Yes.'*
>
> Q: 'Why are you sore?'
> A: *'Thingy's sore.'*
>
> Q: 'Where are you sore?'
> A: *(points to operation site)*
>
> Q: 'Is it sore there all the time?'
> A: *'Yes'*
>
> Q: 'Can you tell me what your sore bits feel like?'
> A: *'A wee bit (sore)'*
>
> Q: 'What helps you to get less sore?'
> A: *'Don't know – a bath.'*
>
> Q: 'Do you tell anyone if you're sore?'
> A: *'No.'*
>
> Q: 'Why not?'
> A: *'They'll laugh at me.'*

Fig. 12.3 Extract from an interview with a 6 year old boy who had had an orchidopexy the previous day (Gillies 1991).

The question of who should assess children's pain is clearly a complex issue, to which the only answer is a combination of the child, the parent and professionals, considering each child's situation individually. Children's, mothers' and staff's perceptions of what is sore may differ and this could negatively affect the assessment and management of the child's pain. For example, in one study children, particularly five to seven year olds, indicated that their pain was worse than either their mothers or the researcher had believed (Gillies 1991).

Issues for consideration when assessing pain

Children are thought to suffer pain the same way as adults (Bray 1988). However, in addition to influences such as culture or emotion, children's perception of and understanding of pain is influenced by maturational stage, specifically comprehension and language skills. Consequently, recognition of children's pain is not always straightforward.

Influences on children's pain

It is essential to think about issues which influence pain. Although those listed in Table 12.5 are discussed briefly, they may all be interconnected (Fig. 12.4). Physiological and emotional factors and type and cause of pain have already been discussed earlier in this chapter.

Emotional state, in particular anxiety or fear, is likely to increase a child's perception of pain. It is very easy to confuse pain and anxiety, and difficult to separate them. Therefore, if anxiety is lessened by explanation, by giving information or by having a parent present, then it follows that pain should be less.

Undoubtedly the most important influential factor in children's pain is their maturational or developmental stage because of the effect that this has on their abilities to communicate and understand. Younger children will be less able to communicate their needs or make themselves understood, because of their limited vocabulary (Beales 1986; Mills 1989; Swanwick 1990); for example, babies and toddlers may be misinterpreted by adults because they have not yet developed appropriate language skills; older children may not understand why they have pain because, at their stage of cognitive development, abstract thought develops and they may look for alternative reasons for their pain, e.g. mis-

Table 12.5 Influences on pain.

> ■ developmental stage
> ■ communication
> ■ type and cause of pain
> ■ emotional state
> ■ behaviour
> ■ culture
> ■ gender

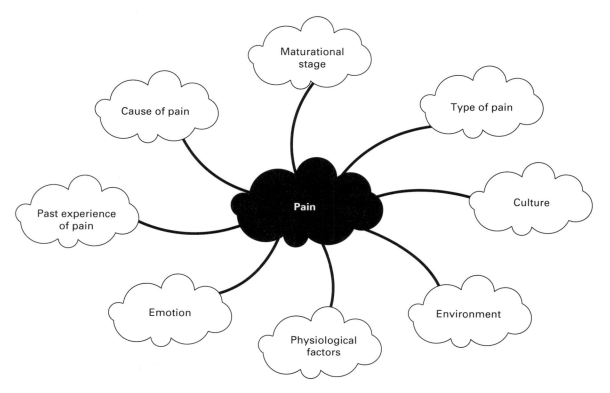

Fig. 12.4   The relationship of influences on children's pain.

behaviour; adolescents on the other hand are able to make themselves understood but may not do so, e.g. to promote a macho image.

Children's experiences and descriptions of pain are related to their developmental stage (Gaffney & Dunne 1987; Swanwick 1990; McCready *et al.* 1991). In general, older children are able to understand more than younger ones, and the more a child understands and can communicate, the more effective he or she will be in coping with pain. Difficulties in comprehension arise when children are given inappropriate or inadequate information. This occurs when age-related comprehension is not considered by staff; for example, one study reports that older children, aged eight to 11 years, rather than younger children, aged five to seven years, were prepared for what was to happen in hospital (Gillies 1991). It is just as important if not more so to prepare young children for what is to happen.

Young children may have previous experience of pain and do remember painful experiences (Tesler *et al.* 1983; Schechter 1989). Although these memories are often

negative, children also develop learned responses to pain, some of which are positive; for example, Chinese children learn to associate acupuncture needles with pleasant experiences (Adams 1989). Nevertheless, it must be remembered that children have numerous experiences as they mature and consequently it is likely to be difficult attributing an older child's pain behaviour to a painful experience when the child was younger.

Other influences on a child's experience of pain include gender and culture, which are not easily separated. Males and females and different cultures perceive and react to pain differently. In western cultures males are expected to feel less pain than females (Hosking & Welchew 1985; Lyall 1991), whereas Jews or Italians freely complain, even though their concepts of how to relieve their pain differ (Adams 1989).

In the author's experience, female nurses and doctors and mothers expect boys to hide their pain more than girls, and male nurses and doctors expect girls to hide their pain more than boys (Gillies 1991). Eskimos laugh at pain, while Americans do not (Adams 1989), and

American children seem to have a bigger vocabulary of words describing pain than Scottish children.

The environment in which a child is cared for is important. Noise interrupts sleep and high levels of noise are thought to delay healing (Bentley *et al.* 1977). Anxious people are said to be more sensitive to noise than relaxed individuals (Dias 1992). Children aged five to ten years find night-time in hospital 'too noisy" and it is also the most worrying time of day for them (Jago 1985). Unless proved otherwise, the possibility that children's perception of pain may increase at night, when in an unfamiliar, noisy environment, should not be forgotten.

It should now be easier to understand why pain is a subjective experience and why it is complex to assess. Although none of these influences are new, their importance is now more widely recognized. When all the possible influences are considered it can only be assumed that the level of pain experienced by any individual, whether a baby, toddler, child or adolescent, is unique to that person. Pain is therefore what the child says it is – a totally subjective experience (McGrath & Unrah 1987; Devine 1990). No other individual, whether a healthcare professional with expert knowledge or a parent who knows the child intimately, should

ever suggest that the child's pain is less severe than the child says it is.

Problems with current methods of pain assessment

Nurses have traditionally assessed pain, and still do, by relying on verbal and non-verbal communication with the children or by observing their behaviour, and by vital sign recordings. Difficulties are known to exist with the reliability of these methods for pain assessment, and these include the problem of how to measure communication and behaviour.

Verbal communication is determined by a child's maturity – what he understands and wants to tell you. Adults do not always understand when children try to talk about their pain; however, children are more likely to tell their parents than the staff if they are sore. In addition, children of all ages will deny pain, particularly if they think that their complaint will result in an injection. Culture also plays a part in determining language; for example, many Scottish children use the word 'jag' for an injection (Table 12.7). Examples of children of different ages talking about pain and related behaviour are given in Tables 12.6 to 12.10, which are based

Table 12.6 'Can you tell me what your sore (body part) is like just now?'

Age	Sex	Operation	Answer
3yr	M	excision of haemangioma	'strawberry'
3yr 6 mth	M	orchidopexy	'a wee bit sore'
4yr 2mth	M	orchidopexy	'fine; it was a wee bit sore'
4yr 11mth	M	inguinal hernia repair	'sore'
5yr	F	inguinal hernia repair	'fallen'*
5yr 8mth	M	hydrocele repair	'leg's lost'*
6yr 8 mth	M	orchidopexy	'hitting with a rock and bouncing off'
7yr 1mth	M	orchidopexy	'very bad'
8yr 5mth	F	bat ear repair	'bleeding a bit with salt going into it'
9yr	M	orchidopexy	'nippy'
9yr 2mth	M	bat ear repair	'very sore'

* These two children had not had local anaesthesia.

Table 12.7 'What frightens you most about hospital?'

Age	Sex	Operation	Answer
6yr 1mth	M	hypospadias	'jags'
8yr	M	orchidopexy	'jags and operations'
9yr 10mth	M	hypospadias	'pain after operations'
11yr	M	circumcision	'jags'
12yr	M	orchidopexy	'jags'

Table 12.8 'If you feel like crying when you are sore, why do you not cry?'

Age	Sex	Operation	Answer
8yr 2mth	M	bat ear repair	'embarrassed'
11yr 2mth	F	bat ear repair	'stop myself; get embarassed'

Table 12.9 'Why do you not tell anyone if you are sore?'

Age	Sex	Operation	Answer
5yr 3mth	M	inguinal hernia repair	'some people are bad and just laugh'
6yr	M	orchidopexy	'laugh at me'
7yr 1mth	M	orchidopexy	'mum said not to'
7yr 6mth	M	orchidopexy	'don't want them to know'
13yr	M	ligation of varicocele	'don't want them to know – get me into trouble'
15yr	M	urethral fistula repair	'no point in wasting their [nurses'] time'

Table 12.10 'Do you do anything to make your hurt go away?'

Age	Sex	Operation	Answer
5yr	M	hydrocele repair	'TV or colour in – doesn't work'
6yr 9mth	M	orchidopexy	'play games or watch TV'
8yr	M	orchidopexy	'play games or watch TV'
11yr 2mth	F	bat ear repair	'TV – to forget'
11yr 7mth	M	orchidopexy	'try to ignore pain'

on interviews with children following minor surgery (Gillies 1991, 1992).

Although talking to children about pain is essential, asking general questions such as 'How are you feeling?' will usually not elicit information about pain, only responses such as 'fine or 'Okay'. However, when asked specific questions such as 'Are you sore?' many children will say 'yes' if they are. It is more likely that a child who complains of pain actually is suffering than that a child who denies pain is pain-free. It is equally important to listen to an admission of pain and not readily accept a denial of pain. Time spent building a relationship with a child will be beneficial because it is more likely to result in information about the child's pain than a brief 'How do you feel?' in passing. It is easy to accept a child's answer of 'fine' when the nurse is busy.

Many children are able to describe their pain (Gillies 1991) but descriptions may be complex and not easily understood by adults. They may be associated with pain e.g. very sore, with other sensations, e.g. burning, or with blood e.g. bleeding (Table 12.6).

Non-verbal communication is equally unreliable; for example, a crying child may be homesick or not allowed their sweets, while a crying baby may be hungry or bored. It is also important to be aware of receiving (unspoken) information from children about their pain. The recognition of either an increase in the severity of pain or a change to acute pain in a child with chronic illness is essential, so that the pain is treated before it gets out of control.

Although it is recommended that children are given as much information as possible, there is an ethical argument that informing a child of impending pain may increase their anxiety and pain (Zeltzer & LeBaron 1986). In addition, children will readily misinterpret information which is misheard or not given in full. Eiser (1987) cites an example of a newly diagnosed diabetic child who thought he was going to 'die of betes'. It is absolutely essential that the explanation is given in language which each child will understand but is also given sensitively so as not to frighten the child.

Observing a child's behaviour is a commonly used method of assessing pain for many healthcare professionals. However, it is not systematic; there are many variables and observer bias exists (Alder 1990; Eland 1990; Lloyd-Thomas 1990). The behaviour of a child in pain is not predictable. Children may be active when in pain; in fact, increased activity can be a sign of pain

(Burokas 1985; Eland 1985b). Children, especially eight to 11 year olds, will make an effort to distract themselves from pain, e.g. by watching television or by getting up to play (Gillies 1991). It cannot be assumed that active children are not in pain – they may be.

Similarly, being asleep is not necessarily an indicator of being pain-free; it may be exhaustion partly caused by pain. It is also worth noting that most children having surgery think that they have to be brave afterwards (Gillies 1991) and it follows that this will influence their behaviour. A quiet youngster or baby does not necessarily mean that the child is comfortable – it may mean extreme pain.

Crying has been examined from the research rather than practical viewpoint. Many reports describe different cries caused by hunger or pain in babies but with varied conclusions as to their validity and reliability (Owens & Todt 1984; Johnston & Strada 1986; Gauntlet 1987). Grunau & Craig (1987) stated that crying behaviour is affected by gender and conscious level; for example, boys cry sooner than girls with a heel stab and alert babies cry quicker than sleeping babies. To date, no conclusive evidence has been reached about its value as a measure of pain in children under five years (Barr 1989).

Irritability, depression or being withdrawn are also signs of pain, but other causes for these must also be considered. A child admitted to hospital is likely to be frightened anyway, but whether the admission is elective for treatment or emergency because of pain will influence the child's behaviour.

Many nurses and doctors have traditionally been taught that children cannot localize their pain. The author has not found this to be true; the majority of children aged five years or more will point to the site of their pain when asked to do so (Gillies 1991). In addition, it is believed that although children may not be able to name the site of their pain, they are able to locate it on a body outline (Eland 1985a; Alder 1990). Behaviour is therefore difficult to assess and is clearly an unreliable indicator of pain when used alone.

Physiological measures such as blood pressure are easy to take but one cannot categorically state that a child is in pain because its blood pressure is elevated; there may be another reason, such as crying caused by hunger or a medical reason such as renal problems. Measurement of neurochemical secretion in children who have pain has been carried out, but raises ethical problems in accessing blood samples from children. Changes have been found in neurochemical secretion but the reason for this is unknown. Nevertheless, it is suggested that physiological responses may be of direct use in pain measurement (McIntosh *et al.* 1993).

Communication, behaviour and physiological measures are unreliable when used on their own but they may be useful in conjunction with other assessment such as facial expression. In order to improve the measurement of pain various formal methods of assessing pain in children of different ages and adolescents have been developed but not widely implemented. They include verbal communication, objective observation, and scales (some self-reporting, i.e. controlled by the child). They are described briefly below but it is important to note that many are being tested to check if they really do what they are supposed to do.

How to recognize pain by developmental stage

It is crucial that all healthcare professionals working with children understand that a range of behaviours may be displayed by children of different ages when they are in pain. Jean Piaget's stages of development have been associated with the perception of and reaction to pain (Mills 1989; Swanwick 1990; McCready *et al.* 1991). It is impossible to say exactly how any individual will react to pain but the guidelines in Table 12.11, based on Piaget's stages of development, will give an idea of what may be expected from children and adolescents at their different stages of maturation.

Assessment: preschool children

Preschool children are difficult to assess and there are few different methods of assessing their pain. Where babies, toddlers and preschool children are concerned, their ability to vocalize their feelings is obviously even more hampered by their developmental stage.

The behaviour of infants who may be experiencing pain has been examined repeatedly (Owens & Todt 1984; Johnston & Strada 1986; Grunau & Craig 1987; Mills 1989; McIntosh *et al.* 1993). Johnston and Strada (1986) concluded that facial expression could be the

Table 12.11 Recognition of pain, by Piaget's stages of development. Developed from Beales (1986), Gaffney & Dunne (1986), Mills (1989), Swanwick (1990) and McGeady *et al.* (1991).

Infants	0–2 years	Babies of one month perceive localized pain (by withdrawal of the limb); pain is not understood; from 6 months can recall painful experiences; verbal reports of pain and location may occur about 18 months; security develops with consistency.
Preoperational stage	2–7 years	Pain is physical and is present on the surface of the body, i.e. everything is taken at face value; pain may be interpreted as punishment; pain cannot be related to positive future outcomes; cannot reason beyond the present; do not understand how treatment, e.g. analgesics, help pain; a concrete object is needed for reassurance.
Concrete operations	7–12 years	Cause and effect begin to be understood, e.g. reason for immunisation; treatment which appears unrelated to illness is accepted; begin to perceive psychological pain; begin to question, but do not necessarily understand what is happening, rather than taking everything at face value.
Formed logical operations	12–18 years	Begin to think abstractly, understanding cause and effect; logical reasoning develops; will accept that organs can malfunction; may hide or deny pain to avoid appearing 'weak'; psychological factors may be understood as contributing to disease; understand that short-term discomfort may lead to long-term cure; may worry constantly if knowledge is incomplete.

most consistent indicator of pain when they observed 14 infants having immunization. They described typical findings in facial expression as a lowered brow, broadening of the nostrils, a square mouth and tightly closed eyes. Mills (1989) observed 32 children aged from birth to 36 months and described their behaviour according to age-bands within the group. More recently, McIntosh *et al.* (1993) studied the variability of physiological response to heel prick in 35 preterm infants. It was concluded that the infants' behaviour does vary but that the cause could not definitely be attributed to pain.

The inability of infants to communicate verbally the presence or severity of pain means that the findings of any study cannot be said to represent actual pain behaviour. Other causes for the change in behaviour may also exist. It follows that if assessment is difficult, effective management will also be difficult to measure. Nevertheless this does not mean that infants' pain should be ignored; they have as much right to effective pain management as any other age-group.

Objective pain scales are based on the assessment of several different factors, each of which may be influenced by pain. These assessments are made by someone other than the patient. They may be geared either to specific age-groups (Toddler Preschooler Postoperative Pain Scale) or are designed with particular patient groups in mind; for example, a French scale (Gustave-Roussy) exists for measuring pain in oncology children. A series of examples follows:

(1) The Children's Hospital of Eastern Ontario Pain Scale (CHEOPS) was developed in Canada and has been used to measure postoperative pain in children aged one to five years, following minor surgery. It consists of six behaviours: crying, facial expression, vocal expression, body position, touch and leg movement, which are rated by a healthcare professional. It has been compared with other types of measure, e.g. visual analogue scales (McGrath *et al.* 1985) and another objective scale (Norden *et al.* 1991a) and compared favourably with both. However, there is currently doubt about the usefulness of it (Professor McGrath, pers. comm. 1991; Watt-Watson & Donovan 1992).

(2) An American measure, the Objective Pain Scale, is a five point scale in which blood pressure, crying agitation, movement and either verbal expression or body language are measured, using a 0, 1, 2 scoring

system with definitions. A total score of 6/10 or more provides the criterion for intervention with strong analgesics, e.g. opiates. It has been used in children aged eight months to 13 years and, providing it is used by trained observers, it measures postoperative pain in preschool children in the clinical situation (Norden et al., 1991b) (Fig. 12.5).

(3) The author adapted Norden's Objective Pain Scale to a six point scale which assessed pulse rate, facial expression, crying, movement, agitation, and either verbal expression or body language (Table 12.12). Initial impressions are that it may be useful, but further validation is required (Gillies 1992).

(4) The Toddler Preschooler Postoperative Pain Scale is another American behavioural scale, which has been used to assess postoperative pain in children aged one to five years. The measure consists of nine behaviours categorized into vocal, facial or bodily pain expression. Evidence suggests developmental trends – e.g. one to two year olds used more bodily and less vocal expression than three–four year olds – and also that the tool is reliable in young children postoperatively (Tarbell & Cohen 1990; Tarbell *et al.* 1991; Tarbell *et al.* 1992).

(5) The Gustave-Roussy Child Pain Scale (Fig. 12.6) is French in origin and was developed for use four hourly in children aged two to six years with prolonged cancer pain. This scale consists of ten items, with a choice of five responses to each item (Gauvain-Piquard *et al.* 1991). Although it is complex, it may also be of use for children with chronic pain, but not for frequent, quick assessments of acute pain.

Reported difficulties with objective measurement included potential observer bias when staff assess pain, either because of their own emotional response or from their own experiences (Alder 1990).

Assessment: school age children and adolescents

The methods of assessing pain in school-age children and adolescents are more varied and complex.

(1) Verbal assessment is a potentially useful tool for adolescents, but not for younger patients because of the potential limitations in their language skills.

Objective pain scale
Operational definitions

Behaviour	Score	Definition
Blood Pressure (systolic)		
</ = 10% preop	0	
> 10–20% preop	1	
> 20% preop	2	
Crying		
Not crying	0	Awake and not crying or asleep.
Crying but responds to TLC	1	Crying is controlled by being touched, reassured or held by nurse/parent.
Crying, does not respond to TLC	2	Crying uncontrollably. Measures to comfort child are unsuccessful.
Movement		
None	0	Asleep or if patient is awake, lying or playing quietly.
Restless	1	Child unable to sit or lie still. Frequent position changes. No threat of self harm.
Thrashing	2	Child kicking and/or squirming. Potential for self harm. Has to be protected or restrained for safety.
Agitation		
Asleep or calm	0	Asleep or awake and calm.
Mild	1	Tense, voice quivering. Responds rationally to questions and/or responds to attempts to console.
Hysterical	2	Does not appear rational, eyes wide. May be clinging to nurse/parent. Does not respond to attempts to console.
Verbal Evaluation or Body Language		
Asleep or states no pain (Preverbal child – no special posture)	0	
Mild pain or cannot localize	1	Complains of general feeling of discomfort, but unable to describe location of pain or states pain is mild in nature.
(Preverbal child – **flexing extremities**)		
Moderate pain and can localize	2	Legs drawn up. Arms may be folded across body. Complains of pain that is bothersome and is able to point to or describe location of pain. Holding, guarding, or touching location of pain.
(Preverbal child – holding location of pain)		Infants with legs drawn up, fists clenched.

For a score > or = 6, patient receives a narcotic analgesic.

Fig. 12.5 The Objective Pain Scale (Norden, J., Hannellah, R. *et al.*, (1991a) *Anesthesia Analgesia.* **72**, 5199). (Published with permission from J. Norden, Nursing Research Associate, Children's Research Institute, Children's National Medical Center, Washington DC)

Table 12.12 The Objective Pain Scale (modified).

Behaviour			
Apex/pulse			
</= 10% preop	0		
> 10–20% preop	1		
> 20% preop	2	(	)
Facial expression			
Smiling	0		
Blank expression, frowning	1		
Crying	2	(	)
Crying			
Not crying	0	(	)
Crying, but responds to TLC	1		
Crying, does not respond to TLC	2	(	)
Movement			
None	0		
Restless	1		
Thrashing	2	(	)
Agitation			
Asleep or calm	0		
Mild	1		
Hysterical	2	(	)
Verbal evaluation or body language			
Asleep or states no pain	0		
Mild pain or cannot localize	1		
Moderate pain and can localize	2	(	)
or			
Asleep or no special posture	0		
Flexing extremities	1		
Holding location of pain	2	(	)
	Total	(	)

Objective pain scale definitions (modified).
Apex
</= 10% preoperative value
> 10–20% preoperative value
> 20% preoperative value

Facial expression	
Smiling	obviously relaxed and happy
Blank expression, frowning	not relaxed or happy, in some distress, pouting lip/asleep
Crying	crying and in obvious distress/unhappy

NB If the child is asleep, facial expression is categorised as '1', otherwise there could be a presumption that the child is pain-free and asleep, or asleep with pain. With the middle choice, either is possible in a mild form.

Table 12.12   (cont.).

Crying	
Not crying	awake and not crying/asleep
Crying, but responds to TLC	crying is controlled by being touched, reassured or held by nurse/parent
Crying, does not respond to TLC	crying uncontrollably
	measures to comfort child are unsuccessful
Movement	
None	asleep/if awake lying or playing quietly/fully mobile
Restless	child unable to sit or lie still,
	frequent position changes,
	no threat of self-harm,
	mobility self-restricted
Thrashing	child kicking and/or squirming, potential for self-harm, has to be protected or restrained for safety, cannot mobilise
Agitation	
Asleep or calm	asleep or awake and calm
Mild	tense, voice quivering
	responds rationally to questions and/or responds to attempts to console
Hysterical	does not appear rational, eyes wide, may be clinging to nurse/patient, does not respond to attempts to console
Verbal evaluation or body language	
Verbal child	
Asleep or states no pain	
Mild pain or cannot localize	complains of general feeling of discomfort but unable to describe location of pain or states pain is mild in nature
Moderate pain and can localize	complains of pain that is bothersome and is able to describe location of pain
Preverbal child	
No special posture	
Flexing extremities	legs drawn up, arms may be folded across body
Holding location of pain	holding, guarding or touching location of pain, infants with legs drawn up, fists clenched

Many children are able to describe their pain (Abu-Saad *et al.* 1990; Gillies 1991), but McGrath & Unrah (1987) note that descriptions are difficult to quantify in terms of measurement. For example, how severe is 'very sore' in comparison with 'sore' when considering how to relieve pain? In addition, when asked the same question about pain by their mother and staff, children may respond differently, i.e. they admit pain to their mothers but not to staff

(Savedra *et al.* 1989). Developmental differences in descriptions were reported by Savedra *et al.* (1982). For example, Alder (1990) describes the use of the word 'lemon' as a description for pain by a child.

It is essential for the nurses caring for each child to know which word each individual child and family uses for pain and also to know how each child behaves when it is or is not in pain. The author found that children use three principal words for 'pain' – sore, painful and hurt (Gillies 1991), so in theory each child could use a different term for 'pain' from the child in the next bed. It is therefore just as important to know the family word for pain as it is to know how the child refers to, for example, 'needing the toilet'. This information can be collected as part of the admission process in hospital or at the first visit in the community.

(2) Colour is reported as being an effective measure for the children who use it to illustrate their pain (Eland & Anderson 1977; Latham 1987; Maunuksela *et al.* 1987; Varni & Walco 1988; Savedra *et al.* 1989; Devine 1990). However, children who are most aware of this link are aged four to six years; because analytical thinking develops with age, the colour association diminishes as age increases.

The concept of the Eland Colour Tool (Fig. 12.7) involves each child choosing colours representing, for example, severe, moderate, mild and no pain. A body outline is then coloured with the chosen colours, indicating the location and severity of the child's pain. Although children from different cultures tend to choose red as representative of severe pain, e.g. American children (Eland & Anderson 1977; Savedra *et al.* 1982) and Scottish children (Gillies 1991), this is not exclusive. Other colours may be chosen, therefore it is important to offer the child a choice of colours (Varni & Walco 1988).

(3) The author used an adapted version of the Eland Colour Tool in children aged five to seven years (Gillies 1991). The adaptation was simple: the choice of colours was reduced from four to three (severe, little and no pain) and the body image was altered to two images, one female and one male, each with back and front views (Fig. 12.8).

For those children who understood it the tool seemed to be a sensitive measure, i.e. it did what it was supposed to do. However, there were two problems: first, a quarter of the children did not understand the concept of colour and pain; and second, it was very time-consuming for every day use. There are recent suggestions that age, gender and ethnicity make no difference to choice of colour (Savedra *et al.* 1989); however, the validity and reliability of using colour to assess pain are now in question (Watt-Watson & Donovan 1992).

(4) Hester's Poker Chip Tool involves the child choosing between one and four chips, i.e. pieces of 'hurt'.

Hester (1979) used this with children aged four to seven years who were having immunizations, and reported that it correlated highly with verbal and motor behaviour. Wong & Baker (1988) compared analogue scales, the Poker Chip Tool and a faces scale and concluded that the poker chip was the most reliable for older children, but suggested that different age groups preferred different methods of assessment. One further paper confirms the Poker Chip tool's validity and reliability (Hester *et al.* 1990), but there has been little other literature describing the use of this measure. In addition, it is not known how culturally sensitive this tool would be when used in the UK.

(5) The Oucher Scale (Beyer & Aradine 1986, 1987) is a vertical thermometer which represents no pain to severe pain and is aimed at different age groups. It is a poster which takes the form of a vertical scale. It looks like a thermometer and on one side has a series of faces depicting severe pain to no pain for young children, and on the other side has a 1–100 scale aimed at older children and adolescents. However, it is argued that children have difficulty differentiating between the two scales (Bieri *et al.* 1990).

(6) Visual analogue scales may be simple 1–10 cm lines which may be numerical, e.g. 1,2,3 ... 9,10 (0 being no pain and 10 being the worst pain ever), or simply 'no pain' at one end and 'the sorest it could be' at the other end (Fig. 12.9). They are described as being reliable and valid (Beasley & Tibbals 1987; Devine 1990) and are said to be a very effective means of assessing pain in children of different ages from five years up to adolescent (Savedra *et al.* 1987; Thomson *et al.* 1987; Varni *et al.* 1987; Broadman *et al.* 1988; Broome & Lillas 1989; Jennings 1990; Savedra *et al.* 1990).

The author has developed a 1–10 cm analogue scale (Fig. 12.10) on a red triangle, in the shape of a 6 in ruler, and has used it successfully with youngsters aged eight to 11 years (Gillies 1991). Its use with children aged five to seven years and with adolescents is currently being assessed.

Although well-liked, visual analogue scales have their problems. Maunuksela *et al.* (1987) and Bieri *et al.* (1990) state that because of their small size, visual analogue scales are unsuitable for children, and Savedra & Tesler (1989) report that while being a sensitive measure of pain, visual analogue scales

THE GUSTAV-ROUSSY CHILD PAIN SCALE
(DOULEUR ENFANT GUSTAVE-ROUSSY – DEGR®)

1989

LABEL

Date: .... Observer's name: ....

ITEM 1: ANTALGIC REST POSITION

The child avoids certain painful positions or adopts a particular position in order to relieve a painful area. This item should be studied when the child is sitting or lying down with no physical activity. It should not be confused with the antalgic position during movement.
SCORING:
0: no antalgic position: the child is at ease.
1: The child seems to avoid certain positions.
2: The child avoids certain positions but this does not seem to bother him.
3: The child chooses a certain antalgic position and seems to be fairly comfortable.
4: The child continually tries to find an antalgic position, without really being comfortable.

ITEM 2: LACK OF EXPRESSIVENESS

Concerns the ability of the child to register and express feelings by his tone of voice, eyes and facial expression. Should be scored when the child is active e.g. during games, meals, and chatter.
SCORING:
0: The child is lively, active and expressive.
1: The child seems a little apathetic.
2: One or more of the following: lifeless features; dejected expression; monotonous voice and mumbled words; slow speech.
3: Several of the above signs are clearly visible.
4: Rigid features, wide-eyed look, vacant stare, laborious speech.

ITEM 3: SPONTANEOUS PROTECTION OF PAINFUL AREAS

The child seems continuously to avoid all contact with painful areas.
SCORING:
0: The child shows no desire for self-protection.
1: The child avoids knocking one or more areas of his body.
2: The child protects his body by avoiding or pushing away anything that might touch him.
3: The child takes a great deal of trouble to avoid contact with a particular part of his body.
4: The child is totally preoccupied with protecting the area in question.

ITEM 4: SOMATIC COMPLAINTS

This item concerns the way in which the child says he is in pain, either spontaneously or when asked, during the period of observation.
SCORING:
0: The child never complains.
1: Neutral complaints:
   – no emotional emphasis, just mentions pain incidentally;
   – expresses pain without insistence or particular effort.
2: One or more of the following:
   – the child's manner leads the observer to ask "what's the matter, does it hurt?";
   – the child whines when complaining of pain;
   – the child grimaces when complaining of pain.
3: In addition to score 2, the child
   – attracts someone's attention to say he is in pain.
   – asks for medicine.
4: The child groans, sobs or pleads when complaining of pain.

ITEM 5: ANTALGIC BEHAVIOUR DURING MOVEMENT

The child spontaneously avoids all movements or tries not to move part of his body. To be scored during sequences of movements (e.g.: walking) possibly induced. Motor slowing should not be noted here.
SCORING:
0: The child moves without any difficulty. His movements are supple and easy.
1: The child moves with some difficulty, and sometimes a little unnaturally.
2: The child is careful when making certain movements.
3: The child clearly avoids certain movements, and moves, in general, with great care.
4: The child must be helped to avoid unduly painful movements.

ITEM 6: LACK OF INTEREST IN SURROUNDINGS

Concerns the child's available energy for interaction with his environment.
SCORING:
0: The child is full of energy, takes an interest in his surroundings, and is able to concentrate and amuse himself.
1: The child is interested in his surroundings but is unenthusiastic.
2: The child is easily bored, but can be stimulated.
3: The child drags himself about, is unable to play and looks on passively.
4: The child is apathetic and totally indifferent.

ITEM 7: CONTROL EXERTED BY THE CHILD WHEN MOVED
(passive mobilisation)

When the child is moved for a meal, bath, etc. he is wary, says how he wants to be moved, resists or holds onto the adult's hand.
SCORING:
0: The child lets himself be moved with no trouble.
1: The child is attentive when being moved.
2: In addition to score 1, the child shows he must be moved with care.
3: In addition to score 2, the child resists certain gestures or guides the person moving him.
4: The child resists all movements or prevents any movement from being made without his consent.

ITEM 8: THE CHILD POINTS OUT PAINFUL AREAS

Either spontaneously or when asked, the child locates his pain.
SCORING:
0: The child never mentions any part of his body as being painful.
1: The child only speaks about a painful sensation in a vaguely defined area, without giving further details.
2: In addition to score 1, the child vaguely indicates the area concerned.
3: The child points exactly to a painful area with his hand.
4: In addition to score 3, the child describes precisely, the part that hurts.

ITEM 9: REACTIONS WHEN PAINFUL AREAS EXAMINED

When a painful area is examined, the child resists, pulls away or reacts emotionally. Only the child's reactions to the examination should be noted, and not any previous reactions.
SCORING:
o: No reaction on examination.
1: The child seems a little apprehensive when the examination actually begins.
2: During the examination, one or more of the following: stiffness of the area examined, face twitch, sudden crying, or blocking of breathing.
3: In addition to score 2, the child changes codlour, sweats, whines or tries to stop the examination.
4: Examination of painful areas is virtually impossible because of the child's reaction.

ITEM 10: SLOWNESS AND INFREQUENCY OF MOVEMENTS

The child's movements are slow, restricted and rather stiff, even some distance away from painful areas. The trunk and large joints are particularly motionless. Should be scored in relation to a normal child's movements.
SCORING:
0: The child's movements are ample, lively, quick and varied, and give him pleasure.
1: The child is a little slow, and lacks momentum.
2: One or more of the following: hesitation before making a movement, restricted movements, slow gestures, infrequent motor initiatives
3: Several of the above signs are clearly visible.
4: The child remains in a fixed position, although there is nothing to stop him moving.

Pain: 1 + 3 + 5 + 7 + 9 = | | |

Voluntary Expression of Pain: 4 + 8 = | | |

Psycho Motor Atonia: 2 + 6 + 10 = | | |

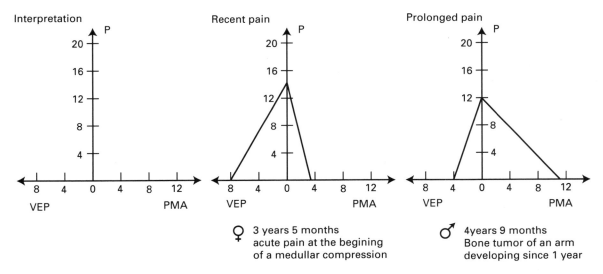

D.E.G.R.® SCALE (2–6 year old children)

For EACH ITEM circle the score which corresponds most closely to the child's condition during the last four hours using the following example:
  0: No sign
  1: You are unsure if the sign is present or not
  2: The sign is present but slight
  3: The sign is clearly present
  4: The sign is severe

Base your scores on the maximum intensity seen in the last four hours.

Before using this scale, write to:
  Dr. A. GAUVAIN-PIQUARD
  Psychiatry and Psycho-Oncology Unit
  Gustave-Roussy Institute – Rue Camille Desmoulins – 94805 VILLEJUIF FRANCE

Interpretation   Recent pain   Prolonged pain

♀ 3 years 5 months
acute pain at the begining
of a medullar compression

♂ 4years 9 months
Bone tumor of an arm
developing since 1 year

Fig. 12.6 The Gustave-Roussy Child Pain Scale. (Published with permission from Dr Annie Gauvain-Piquard, Unite de Psychiatrie et d'oncopsychologie, Institut Gustave-Roussy, Cedex, France)

are disliked by children. The ability of preschool children to use vertical scales in preference to horizontal scales is reported inconsistently (Aradine *et al.* 1988; Varni & Walco 1988; Gillies 1992).

(7) A faces scale is a different type of analogue scale which involves the child choosing one of a series of faces showing different emotions depicting 'no pain' to 'severe pain' (Fig. 12.11). There are variations of the faces scale, which have been regularly reported (Baker & Wong 1987; Snell 1988; Wong & Baker 1988; Savedra *et al.* 1989). Children as young as three years are described as using faces scales effectively (Beyer & Aradine 1986; Douthit 1990) and they are useful in both acute and chronic pain (Bieri *et al.* 1990). However, Broadman *et al.* (1988) argue that visual analogue scales, including faces scales, are of no value in young children.

One disadvantage of faces scales is that they are potentially unreliable because the faces may represent emotion rather than pain. In the author's experience children aged five to seven years chose the smiling face (representing no pain) when there were other indicators that they were in pain (Gillies 1991). This has also been noted by pain specialists in Australia (Juniper, 1992). It is accepted that pain and emotion are linked; however, it is suggested that if the series of faces excludes a smiling one and tears (Juniper, 1992) then emotion will not be confused with pain (Bierei *et al.* 1990).

(8) The McGill Pain Questionnaire (Melzack 1975; Melzack & Katz 1992) is a complex pain measure which makes many different measures and also takes a medical history. It has been extensively used in adults and less so in adolescents. Its uses include

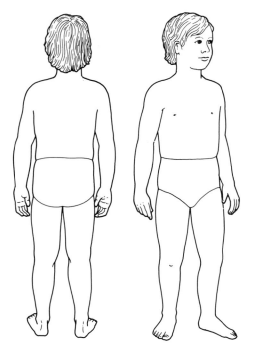

Fig. 12.7 The Eland Colour Tool – body outline. (Published with permission from Dr Joann Eland, Associate Professor, University of Iowa, USA)

postoperative pain but its primary use is for chronic pain. It also exists in a shortened form (Melzack 1987).

(9) The Adolescent Paediatric Pain Tool (Savedra *et al.* 1990; Tesler *et al.* 1991) is specifically geared to adolescents for postoperative pain assessment. It involves colouring the location of pain, marking a word graphic rating scale (no pain to the worst possible pain) and choosing words from a series describing pain. It has been used extensively in the USA.

The recognition of pain and deciding which measure(s) to use is not simple. Self-report is of most value because it allows subjective reporting; however, self-report tools must be understood by the child and also by the staff administering them, before they are used (Maunuksela *et al.* 1987). Where possible, more than one method of assessment should be used to allow for variations in situations, pain, etc. (Savedra *et al.* 1989). Cultural differences must be remembered: Salim (1993) from India reported difficulties using assessment tools developed in

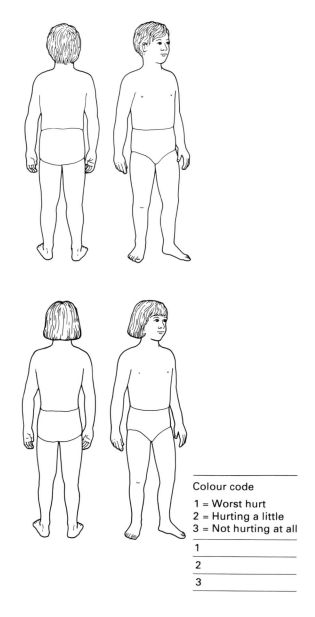

Colour code

1 = Worst hurt
2 = Hurting a little
3 = Not hurting at all

1
2
3

Fig. 12.8 Body outline – adapted from the Eland Colour Tool.

the western world. Finally, where objective measurement is the method of choice it is of paramount importance that children's maturation and their consequential language skills and behaviour are understood by those carrying out the assessment. A guide to recognizing pain is given in Table 12.13.

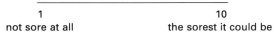

1   10
not sore at all   the sorest it could be

Fig. 12.9   A 1–10 cm visual analogue scale.

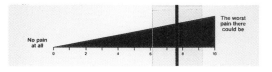

Fig. 12.10   Coloured visual analogue scale.

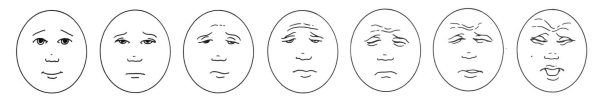

Fig. 12.11   A faces scale. (Published with permission from Dr G.D. Champion, Division of Paediatrics, The Prince of Wales Children's Hospital, Randwick, Australia)

Table 12.13   Guidelines on how to recognise pain in children.

- Physiological signs of pain: dilated pupils, pallor, increased respiratory rate, increased pulse rate, or change in blood pressure.
- Assess developmental stage.
- Observe behaviour and emotional state.
- Consider culture and gender.
- What is causing the pain?
- Assess the environment.
- Know about the child's past experience of pain, the family word for pain etc.
- Use appropriate methods of formal assessment.

MANAGEMENT OF PAIN

The effective management of pain is dependent upon accurate assessment in addition to meeting the objective or goal. Although management is usually attempted using drugs there is a slow move to using alternative therapies. In general, nurses administer drugs which doctors prescribe; nevertheless, healthcare staff should work together in achieving the relief of pain. This practice should be research-based. However, erratic prescribing by doctors, misinterpretation of prescriptions by nurses, and underestimation of strength or quantity of required analgesics all contribute to under-

treatment (Mather & Mackie 1983; Eland 1990; Kuhn *et al.* 1990).

Interesting differences in perceptions exist between different groups of staff; for example, in one study about a third of doctors expected children to have moderate to severe pain on the first postoperative day after minor surgery, and yet four in five nurses expected this. In fact, just over half the children had such pain (Gillies 1991). It is obviously important to be aware of potential problems arising from differing perceptions about pain. Children's perceptions of what relieves their pain differ: younger children aged five to seven years believe that topical remedies (e.g. sticking plaster) help, whereas older children (eight to 11) believe that medicine helps (Gillies 1991).

Pharmacological management

The type and frequency of analgesic administration is crucial; however, concern about overdosage and dependency often prevents strong analgesics from being administered to children. Literature describing the numbers of children who have become dependent on opiates given to relieve pain is either non-existent or rare and the case for withholding strong analgesics from young children no longer exists (Burrows & Berde 1993).

The method of administration varies. Analgesics may be administered orally, rectally or by injection (subcutaneous, intramuscular, intravenous). In general terms, milder analgesics such as paracetamol are given orally and strong analgesics are given by injection. Both mild and strong analgesics may be given rectally.

Traditionally, injections given to relieve pain were intramuscular and this is often still the method of choice in a one-off situation. This method brings its own problems, i.e. children are afraid of injections from a young age and many adults are afraid of giving injections to children and consequently may not do so. The intramuscular method should be kept to a minimum (McCready *et al.* 1991). In some instances, it has been superseded by the intravenous method, either if there is an IV line in place or where several doses will be required, thus preventing repeated injections. The drug may be given as a bolus via the IV line or as a continuous infusion.

The intravenous method is faster-acting but it creates a fear of overdosage and dependency for the nurses and doctors involved, resulting in inadequate pain relief for the child. In some instances, e.g. terminal care where long term pain relief is required but so is maintaining as good a quality of life as possible, subcutaneous opiates may be given. However, these also have to be resited. In some instances, such as terminal care, a central venous line may be used.

A recent development is the concept of patient-controlled analgesia (PCA), which has been used in adults for some time but is relatively new in children's nursing. PCA involves intravenous administration of small frequent doses of titrated opiates using an electronic pump which is controlled by the child. Safety mechanisms are present to prevent overdosage and regular checks are made by nursing staff. This method maintains a constant level of opiate in the blood circulation compared with the peak and trough situation which arises with bolus administration.

Gillespie & Morton (1992) report the successful use of PCA postoperatively in children as young as five years, but more recently it has been reported as useful in children aged three years or more (Llewellyn 1993). It is essential that the child understands the procedure *before* it is required. In addition, where the child is unable to control the administration of the drug, parent-controlled and nurse-controlled analgesia have been used. However, they are not without difficulties. With both methods people other than the child are making decisions about when pain relief is required. A second problem with parent-controlled analgesia is that giving parents ultimate control of their child's pain relief can create disagreements between family members, and so it is argued by some that parent-controlled analgesia should not be an option.

One problem with using drugs to relieve pain is the potential for misinterpreting prescriptions: for example, if analgesia is prescribed 'prn' it is unlikely to be given on a regular basis, even if the drug prescribed is mild; 'prn' is often misinterpreted as meaning 'only if absolutely necessary' when it actually means 'as necessary'. In addition, when opiates are prescribed for children they tend to be given occasionally or not at all. One of the principal reasons for this is staff concern about side-effects, dosage and addictive properties. Undertreatment of children's pain is often due to practice based on popular misconceptions.

Non-pharmacological management of pain

There are several different methods of relieving pain which do not involve the use of drugs. They include distraction, transcutaneous electrical nerve stimulation (TENS) in which pain is inhibited by stimulating large receptor fibres in the skin, and hypnosis which works by reducing attention to pain (Nie *et al.* 1989). Acupuncture and aromatherapy may also be of use. Although there are few reports of non-pharmacological methods of pain relief in children, Kuttner (1993) reports the successful use of hypnosis in children with chronic pain, and Eland (1991) describes using transcutaneous electrical nerve stimulation with children for phantom pain following amputation, and also for repeated venepuncture in haematology children.

The relief of anxiety and related pain using explanation, structured play (eg puppetry), relaxation or distraction are more widely recognized (Beyer & Levin 1987; McCaffery & Beebe 1989; Save the Children 1989). Although little is known about the extent to which children actively use distraction, in the author's experience about one half of children aged 5–11 years admit to using distraction, e.g. television, when they have pain (Gillies 1991). Means of distracting children of different ages include a cuddle or a soother for infants, or for older children talking, counting or watching television or videos (McCready *et al.* 1991).

It is important to consider mothers' perceptions of

their children's condition: a mother who believes that her child is in pain will become more anxious herself. Unless the child's pain is relieved, maternal anxiety will increase. The cycle of transferred anxiety and the possibility of a related increase in the child's pain may result. If the child is not in pain, attempts should be made to relieve the mother's anxiety. Mothers' expectations may be unrealistic but should be discussed with them; many mothers expect analgesia to completely relieve their child's pain, but this is not always possible. A mother who asks for analgesia for her child will expect it to be given quickly, but it is not always possible for registered nurses to stop what they are doing immediately to organize analgesia. Nevertheless, nurses must be aware that every mother is concerned only for the welfare of her child and that nothing and no one else matters.

Difficulties with pain management in school age children also exist. Management can be influenced by staff's personal experience of pain (Holm *et al.* 1989) or by the gender of the patient (Gillies 1991; Lyall 1991); for example, Lyall argues that nurses report pain in men less than in women. In addition, healthcare workers' knowledge about pain management is limited but could be improved by including specific training about the management of pain in training curricula (Watt-Watson 1987; RCS & CA 1990; Fields 1991). Guidelines for the management of pain are given in Table 12.14.

Table 12.14 Guidelines for managing pain.

- Remember to treat each child individually.
- Has the pain been effectively assessed?
- Give the prescribed analgesic.
- Reassess the pain severity, giving time for the drug to take effect.
- Listen to the child's verbal and non-verbal communication.
- If the child is still distressed, is the cause still pain?
- If the child is still in pain, ask for medical advice about using other drugs.
- Consider using available, appropriate nonpharmacological methods of pain relief.
- If communication is unclear give the child the benefit of the doubt and treat his distress as pain.

EVALUATION

Evaluation is the time to reflect on when care could or should be altered. It is the final stage of the assessment–management cycle. It depends upon accurate assessment and consequent management of pain in addition to good communication skills on the part of the staff involved.

Documenting each stage of the cycle – assessment, management and evaluation – provides the written information required by future staff to reappraise each child's individual care. If any one of the following are incomplete or absent then evaluation cannot take place:

- Appropriate assessment using relevant measures.
- Agreement in the aim of care for each child.
- Attempts at eliminating or reducing any discomfort.
- Accurate written documentation and oral communication.

Many healthcare staff believe that they evaluate care effectively but in practice this is not the case; for example, observation of the child's behaviour to check the effectiveness of analgesia is not recommended because observation alone is known to be unreliable. Talking to the child is more appropriate; however that does not mean wakening a sleeping child just to ask if their pain is better! Effective evaluation is just as important as any other part of the assessment–management cycle.

CONCLUSION

Pain is clearly a complex symptom of great importance for the caring professions. It is essential to assess and manage pain as effectively as possible in order to relieve or minimize unnecessary suffering. Practice based upon research findings will allow the current belief in misconceptions to diminish.

Assessment of pain involves examining all the issues which influence pain and, consequently, being able to measure or make a judgement about its existence and severity. In order to manage pain effectively and efficiently it must be assessed first. Pain may be assessed by:

- Using the admission process to establish the family word for pain.
- Documenting all aspects of pain assessment and management routinely.
- Listening to the child and being honest; trusting relationships are paramount.
- Asking specific questions about pain rather than general questions.
- Observing but not entirely relying upon behaviour.
- Considering the child's developmental stage and using appropriate measures.
- Involving the parents but not relying purely on their judgement.
- Involving the child, parent and staff in the assessment, and giving the benefit of any doubt to the child: it is the child's pain and he or she has to live with it.

The management of pain should be an ongoing process rather than a dose of analgesia given once. If this is carried out hand-in-hand with assessment and evaluation, if documentation is faultless and standards of care are maintained, then children's pain should become much less traumatic in both physical and emotional terms. Staff will also benefit by having increased job satisfaction.

REFERENCES AND FURTHER READING

Abu-Saad, H., Kroonen, E. & Halfens, R. (1990) On the development of a multidimensional Dutch pain assessment tool for children. *Pain*, 43, 249–56.

Abu-Saad, H., Pool, H. & Tulkens, D.B. (1994) Further validity testing of the Abu-Saad Paediatric assessment tool. *Journal of Advanced Nursing*, 13, 1063–71.

Adams, J. (1989) Pain Assessment: Part II. The Special Challenges of Assessing Pain in Children. *Dimensions in Oncology Nursing*, 3(3), 25–31.

Alder, S. (1990) Taking children at their word. *Professional Nurse*, 5(8), 398–402.

Alderson, P. (1992) *Children and Pain*. Action for Sick Children, London.

Aradine, C.R., Beyer, J.E. & Tompkins, J.M.(1988) Children's pain perception before and after analgesia: A study of instrument construct validity and related tissues. *Journal of Pediatric Nursing*, 3, 1, 11–23.

Baker, C. & Wong, D. (1987) QUEST: a process of pain assessment in children. *Orthopaedic Nursing*, 6(1), 11–21.

Barr, R. (1989) Pain In Children. In *Textbook on Pain* (eds P.D. Wall & R. Melzack), p.574. Churchill Livingstone, Edinburgh.

Beales, J. (1986) Cognitive Development and the Experience of Pain. *Nursing*, 3(11), 408–10.

Beasley, S.W. & Tibbals, J. (1987) Efficacy and safety of continuous morphine infusion for post-operative analgesia in the paediatric surgical ward. *Australia and New Zealand Journal of Surgery*, 57, 233–7.

Bentley, S., Murphy, F. & Dudley, H. (1977) Perceived noise in surgical wards and an intensive care area: an objective analysis. *British Medical Journal*, 10 December, 1503–5.

Beyer, J.E. & Aradine, C.R. (1986) Content validity of an instrument to measure young children's perceptions of their pain. *Journal of Pediatric Nursing*, 1, 386–95.

Beyer, J.E. & Aradine, C.R. (1987) Patterns of pediatric pain intensity: a methodological investigation of a self-report scale. *Clinical Journal of Pain*, 3, 130–41.

Beyer, J.E. & Levin, C. (1987) Issues and advances in pain control in children. *Nursing Clinics of North America*, 22(3), 661–76.

Bielby, E. (1984) A childish concept. *Nursing Mirror*, 159(18), 26–8.

Bieri, D., Reeve, R.A., Champion, G.D., Addicoat, L. & Ziegler, J.B. (1990) The faces pain scale for the self-assessment of the severity of pain experienced by children: development, initial validation, and preliminary investigation for ratio scale properties. *Pain*, 41, 139–50.

Bray, R.J. (1988) Management of Perioperative Pain in Children. *Hospital Update*, pp. 1565–76.

Broadman, L., Rice, L. & Hannallah, R. (1988). Comparison of a physiological and visual analogue scale in children. *Canadian Journal of Anaesthesia*, 35, 137–8.

Broome, M.E. & Lillis, P.P. (1989) A descriptive analysis of the paediatric pain management research. *Applied Nursing Research*, 2(2), 74–81.

Burke, S.O. & Jerrett, M. (1989) Pain management across age groups. *Western Journal of Nursing Research*, 11(2), 164–80.

Burokas, L. (1985) Factors affecting nurses' decisions to medicate paediatric patients after surgery. *Heart and Lung*, 14, 373–9.

Burrows, F.A. & Berde, C.B. (1993) Optimal pain relief in infants and children. *British Medical Journal*, 307, 815–16.

Carter, B. (1990) A Universal Experience. *Paediatric Nursing*, 2(7), 8–10.

Carter, B. (1994) *Child and Infant Pain: Principles of Nursing Care and Management*. Chapman and Hall, London.

Davis, H. (1992) Conference report: talking points in pain research. *Hospital Update*, 165–7.

Devine, T. (1990) Pain management in paediatric oncology.

Paediatric Nursing, 2(7), 10–13.

Dias, B. (1992) Things that go bump. *Nursing Times*, 88(38), 36–8.

Dilworth, N.M. & MacKellar, A. (1987) Pain relief for the paediatric surgical patient. *Journal of Paediatric Surgery*, 22, 264–6.

Douthit, J.L. (1990) Patient care guidelines: psychosocial assessment and management of pediatric pain. *Journal of Emergency Nursing*, 16(3), 168–70.

Eiser, C. (1987) What children think about hospitals and illness. *The Professional Nurse*, Nov., 53–4.

Eiser, C. & Patterson, D. (1984) Children's perceptions of hospital. *International Journal of Nursing Studies*, 21(1), 45–50.

Eland, J. (1985) The role of the nurse in children's pain. In *Recent Advances in Nursing: Perspectives of Pain* (ed. L. Copp), pp. 29–45. Churchill Livingstone, Edinburgh.

Eland, J. (1985b) The child who is hurting. *Seminars in Oncology Nursing*, 1(2), 116–22. In Pain Management in Paediatric Oncology (1990, T. Devine). *Paediatric Nursing*, 2(7), 10–13.

Eland, J. (1990) Pain In Children. *Nursing Clinics of North America*, 25(4), 871–84.

Eland, J. (1991) The use of TENS with children who have cancer pain. *Journal of Pain and Symptom Management*, 6(3), 145, abstract 12.

Eland, J. & Anderson, J. (1977) The Experience of Pain in Children. In *Pain. A Source Book for Nurses and Other Health Professionals* (ed. A. Jacox), pp. 453–76. Little, Brown, Boston.

Elander, G., Lindberg, T. & Quarnstrom, B. (1991) Pain relief in infants after major surgery: a descriptive study. *Journal of Pediatric Surgery*, 26(2), 128–31.

Fields, H.L. (ed.) (1991) *Core Curriculum for Professional Education in Pain*. International Association for the Study of Pain, Seattle.

Fordham, M. (1986) Neurophysiological Pain Theories. *Nursing*, 10, 365–72.

Gaffney, A. & Dunne, E. (1986) Developmental aspects of children's definition of pain. *Pain*, 26, 105–17.

Gaffney, A. & Dunne, E.A. (1987) Children's understanding of the causality of pain. *Pain*, 29, 91–104.

Gauntlet, I.S. (1987) Analgesia in the Neonate. *British Journal of Hospital Medicine*, 37(6), 518–19.

Gauvain-Piquard, A., Rodary, C., Rezvani, A. & Lemerle, J. (1987) Pain in children aged 2–6 years: a new observational rating scale elaborated in a pediatric oncology unit – preliminary report. *Pain*, 31, 177–88.

Gauvain-Piquard, A., Rodary, C., Francois, P., Rezvani, A., Kalifa, C., Lecuyer, N., Cosse, M. & Lesbros, F. (1991) Validity assessment of DEGR^R scale for observational rating of 2–6 year-old child pain. *Journal of Pain and Symptom Management*, 6(3), 171.

Gillespie, J.A. & Morton, N.S. (1992) Patient-controlled analgesia for children: a review. *Paediatric Anaesthesia*, 2, 51–9.

Gillies, M.L. (1991) A Study of Postoperative Pain in Children and Adolescents. *Health Bulletin*, 52(3), 193–6.

Gillies, M.L. (1992) Postoperative Pain in Children under Five Years. Unpublished.

Glasper, A. (1990) Accompanying children. Astra/NAWCH Nursing Standard Special Supplement. *Paediatric Nursing*, 2, 2.

Glasper, A. & Stradling, P. (1989) Preparing children for admission. *Paediatric Nursing*, 1(5), 18–20.

Grunau, R.V.E. & Craig, K.D. (1987) Pain expression in neonates: facial action and cry. *Pain*, 28, 395–410.

Gureno, M.A. & Reisinger, C.L. (1991) Patient controlled analgesia for the young pediatric patient. *Pediatric Nursing*, 17(3), 251–4.

Hayward, J. (1987) *Information – a prescription against pain*. Research Project 120, reprinted 1987, Series 2 No. 5. Royal College of Nursing, London.

Hester, N.K. (1979) The pre-operational child's reaction to immunisation. *Nursing Research*, 28, 250–4.

Hester, N.K., Foster, R.L. & Kristensen, K. (1990) Measurement of pain in children: generalizability and validity of the pain ladder and the poker chip tool. In *Advances in Pain Research and Therapy: Pediatric Pain* (eds D. Tyler & E. Krane), pp. 79–84. Raven Press, New York.

Holm, K., Cohen, F., Dudas, S., Medema, P. & Allen, B. (1989) Effect of personal pain experience on pain assessment. *IMAGE: Journal of Nursing Scholarship*, 21(2), 72–5.

Hosking, J. & Welchew, E. (1985) *Postoperative pain: Understanding its nature and how to treat it*. Faber and Faber, London.

Jago, D. (1985) Communicating with children in hospital. *Maternal and Child Health*, 12(6), 186–8.

Jennings, P. (1990) Thalassaemia. Levels of knowledge. *Paediatric Nursing*, 2(7), 22–3.

Johnston, C.C. & Strada, M.E. (1986) Acute pain response in infants: a multidimensional description. *Pain*, 24, 373–82.

Juniper, K. (1992) Personal Communication.

Kalat, J. (1988) Biological Psychology (3rd edn) Wadsworth Publishing, Belmont, California. In Sleep disturbance at home and in hospital (M. Pfeil 1993). *Paediatric Nursing*, 5(7), 14–16.

Kuhn, S., Cooke, K., Jones, J. & Mucklow, J. (1990) Perceptions of pain relief after surgery. *British Medical Journal*, 300, 1687–90.

Kuttner, L. (1993) Hypnotic interventions for children in pain. In *Pain in Infants, Children and Adolescents* (eds N. Schechter, C. Berde & M. Yaster), pp. 229–36. Williams and Wilkins, London.

Latham, J. (1987) *Pain Control* (2nd edn). Austen Cornish Publishers Ltd in association with The Lisa Sainsbury Foundation, Reading.

Llewellyn, N. (1993) The use of patient controlled analgesic for paediatric postoperative pain management. *Paediatric Nursing*, 5(5), 12–15.

Lloyd-Thomas, A.R. (1990) Pain Management in Paediatric Patients. *British Journal of Anaesthesia*, 64, 85–104.

Lyall, J. (1991) Real men don't cry? *Nursing Times*, 87(18), 21.

Mather, L. & Mackie, L. (1983) The incidence of postoperative pain in children. *Pain*, 15, 271–82.

Maunuksela, E. Olkkola, K. & Korpela, R. (1987) Measurement of pain in children with self-reporting and behavioural assessment. *Clinical Pharmacology and Therapeutics*, 42, 137–41.

McCaffery, M. & Beebe, A. (1989) *PAIN. Clinical Manual for Nursing Practice*. Mosby, St. Louis.

McCready, M., MacDavitt, K. & O'Sullivan, K.K. (1991) Children and pain: easing the hurt. *Orthopaedic Nursing*, 10(6), 33–42.

McGrath, P.A. (1989) Evaluating a child's pain. *Journal of Pain and Symptom Management*, 4(4), 198–214.

McGrath, P. & Unrah, A. (1987) *Pain in Children and Adolescents*. Elsevier Science Publishers, Amsterdam.

McGrath, P.J., Johnson, G., Goodman, J.T., Schillinger, J., Dunn, J. & Chapman, J-A. (1985) CHEOPS: A behavioural scale for rating postoperative pain in children. *Advances in Pain Research and Therapy*, 9, 395–402.

McIntosh, N., Van Veen, L. & Brameyer, H. (1993) The pain of heel prick and its measurement in preterm infants. *Pain*, 52(1), 71–4.

Melzack, R. (1975) The McGill Pain Questionnaire – major properties and scoring methods. *Pain*, 1, 277–99.

Melzack, R. (1987) The short-form McGill pain questionnaire. *Pain*, 30, 191–7.

Melzack, R. & Wall, P.D. (1965) Pain mechanisms: a new theory. *Science*, 150, 971–9.

Melzack, R. & Katz, J. (1992) The McGill pain questionnaire: appraisal and current status. In *Handbook of Pain Assessment* (eds D. Turk & R. Melzack), pp. 152–68. The Guildford Press, London.

Merksey, H. (1979) Pain terms: a list with definitions and notes on usage. Recommended by the IASP subcommittee on taxonomy. *Pain*, 6, 249–52. In *Textbook of Pain* (2nd edn) (P.D. Wall & R. Melzack, 1989). Churchill Livingstone, Edinburgh.

Mills, N.M. (1989) Pain behaviour in infants and toddlers. *Journal of Pain and Symptom Management*, 4(4), 184–90.

Nie, V.M., Hunter, M. & Allan, D. (1989) The Central Nervous System. In *Physiology for Nursing Practice* (eds S. Hinchliff & S. Montague), pp. 88–139. Balliere Tindall, London.

Norden, J., Hannallah, R., Getson, P., O'Donnell, R., Kelliher, G. & Walker, N. (1991a) Concurrent validation of an objective pain scale for infants and children. *Anesthesiology*, 72, 199.

Norden, J., Hannallah, R., Getson, P., O'Donnell, R., Kelliher, G. & Walker, N. (1991b) Reliability of an objective pain scale in children. *Journal of Pain and Symptom Management*, 6(3), 196.

Owens, M.E. & Todt E.H. (1984) Pain in infancy: neonatal reaction to a heel-lance. *Pain*, 20, 77–86.

Page, G.G. (1991) Chronic pain and the child with juvenile rheumatoid arthritis. *Journal of Pediatric Health Care*, 5(1), 18–23.

Page, G. & Halvorsen, M. (1991) Pediatric nurses: the assessment and control of pain in preverbal infants. *Journal of Pediatric Nursing*, 6(2), 99–106.

Pakoulas, C., Ring, H. & Tew, D. (1984) Only when it hurts: an 8-year-old's view of medicine. *Midwife Health Visitor & Community Nurse*, 20, 160–61.

Pfeil, M. (1993) Sleep disturbance at home and in hospital. *Paediatric Nursing*, 5(7), 14–16.

Pilowsky, I. (1988) An outline curriculum on pain for medical schools. *Pain*, 33, 1–2.

Price, S. (1992) Student nurses' assessment of children in pain. *Journal of Advanced Nursing*, 17, 441–7.

RCS & CA (1990) *Commission on the Provision of Surgical Services. Report of the Working Party on Pain After Surgery*. Royal College of Surgeons of England and the College of Anaesthetists. Royal College of Surgeons, London.

Rodin, J. (1983) *Will This Hurt?* Royal College of Nursing, London.

Salim, B.M. (1993) Pakistan coin pain scale. *Pain*, 52, 373–4.

Savedra, M. & Tesler, M. (1989) Assessing children's and adolescents' pain. *Pediatrician*, 16, 24–9.

Savedra, M., Gibbons, P., Tesler, M., Ward, J.A. & Wegner, C. (1982) How do children describe pain? A tentative assessment. *Pain*, 14, 95–104.

Savedra, M., Tesler, M., Ward, J., Holzemer, W. & Wilkie, D. (1987) Children's preference for pain intensity scales. *Pain*, Supplement 4, 234.

Savedra, M.L., Tesler, M.D., Holzemer, W.L., Wilkie, D.J. & Ward, J.A. (1989) Pain location: validity and reliability of body outline markings by hospitalised children and adolescents. *Research in Nursing and Health*, 12, 307–14.

Savedra, M., Tesler, M., Holzemer, W., Wilkie, D. & Ward, J.A. (1990) Testing a tool to assess postoperative paediatric and adolescent pain. *Advances in Pain Research Therapy*, 15, 85–93.

Save the Children (1989) *Hospital: A Deprived Environment for Children? A Case for Hospital Playschemes*, pp. 10–14. Save the Children, London.

Schechter, N.L. (1989) The undertreatment of pain in children. *Pediatric Clinics of North America*, **36**(4), 781–92.

Schechter, N.L., Allen, D.A. & Hanson, K. (1986) Status of pediatric pain control: a comparison of hospital analgesic usage in children and adults. *Pediatrics*, 77, 11–15.

Snell, J. (1988) Face Values. *Nursing Times*, **84**(17), 22–3.

Swanwick, M. (1990) Knowledge and control. *Paediatric Nursing*, **2**(5), 18–20.

Tarbell, S. & Cohen, I. (1990) The assessment of postoperative pain in young children. *Pain*, Abstract S302.

Tarbell, S.E., Marsh, J.L. & Cohen, I.T. (1991) Reliability and validity of the pain assessment scale for measuring postoperative pain in young children. *Journal of Pain and Symptom Management*, **6**(3), 196.

Tarbell, S., Cohen, I. & Marsh, J. (1992) The Toddler-Preschooler Postoperative Pain Scale: an observational scale for measuring postoperative pain in children aged 1–5. Preliminary report. *Pain*, 50, 273–80.

Tesler, M., Ward, J., Savedra, M., Wegner, C.B. & Gibbons, P. (1983) Developing an instrument for eliciting children's description of pain. *Perceptual Motor Skills*, 56, 315–21.

Tesler, M., Savedra, M., Holzemer, W., Wilkie, D.J., Ward, J.A. & Paul, S.M. (1991) The word-graphic rating scale as a measure of children's and adolescents' pain intensity. *Research in Nursing and Health*, 14, 361–71.

Thomson, K.L., Varni, J.W. & Hanson, V. (1987) Comprehensive assessment of pain in juvenile rheumatoid arthritis: an empirical model. *Journal of Paediatric Psychology*, **12**(2), 241–55.

UKCC (1989) *Exercising Accountability*. United Kingdom Central Council for Nursing, Midwifery and Health Visiting, London.

UKCC (1992) *Code of Professional Conduct* (2nd edition). United Kingdom Central Council for Nursing, Midwifery and Health Visiting, London.

Varni, J.W. & Walco, G.A. (1988) Chronic and recurrent pain associated with paediatric chronic diseases. *Issues in Comprehensive Pediatric Nursing*, 11, 145–58.

Varni, J.W., Thompson, K.L. & Hanson, V. (1987) The Varni/Thompson Paediatric Pain Questionnaire: I. Chronic musculoskeletal pain in juvenile rheumatoid arthritis. *Pain*, 28, 27–38.

Wall, P.D. (1978) The gate control theory of pain mechanisms. A re-examination and re-statement. *Brain*, 101, 1–18.

Wall, P.D. & Melzack, R. (eds) (1989) *Textbook of Pain* (2nd edn). Churchill Livingstone, Edinburgh.

Watt-Watson, J.H. (1987) Nurses' knowledge of pain issues: a survey. *Journal of Pain and Symptom Management*, **2**(4), 207–11.

Watt-Watson, J. & Donovan, M.I. (1992) *Pain Management. Nursing Perspective.* Mosby Year Book, Sydney.

Williams, J. (1987a) Managing Paediatric Pain. *Nursing Times*, **83**(36), 36–39.

Williams, M. (1987b) Pain and the person. In *Pain Control* (J. Latham 1987) (2nd edition). Austen Cornish Publishers Ltd in association with The Lisa Sainsbury Foundation, Reading.

Wilson, J.F., Brockopp, G.W., Kryst, S., Steger, H. & Witt, W.O. (1992) Medical students' attitudes toward pain before and after a brief course on pain. *Pain*, 50, 251–6.

Wong, D.L. & Baker, C.M. (1988). Pain in children: comparison of assessment scales. *Pediatric Nursing*, 14, 9–17, 34–5.

Zeltzer, L. & LeBaron, S. (1986) Assessment of acute pain and anxiety and chemotherapy-related nausea and vomiting in children and adolescents. *Hospital Journal*, **2**(3), 75–98.

Chapter 13

Pharmacological Management

Annette K. Dearmun and Rhoda Welsh

INTRODUCTION

It could be argued that both improvements in the prevention, identification and treatment of common diseases and pharmacological advances have contributed to alterations in the progress and overall management of many childhood ailments. For example, the availability of antibiotic therapy has to a great extent limited the effects of infection and subsequently reduced mortality, and the range of analgesics has enabled more effective pharmacological pain management.

Fradd (1990) argues that the most complex and hazardous role of the children's nurse lies within the administration of medicines. Misreading the prescription chart, administration by the incorrect route or an incorrect drug or dose may have potentially lethal consequences. There are several principles which should underpin practice in relation to drug administration:

- The individual nurse is responsible and accountable for their own decisions and actions.
- They must be able to defend those decisions and actions as being in the best interest of the patient (child and family).
- They must only undertake work for which they are trained and are competent to perform (UKCC 1992).

The main purpose of this chapter is to introduce a range of pharmacological issues which should be considered by the children's nurse in order that they might operate within the principles previously identified.

Section one addresses some of the problems associated with licensing of drugs to be used in children. Section two provides an overview of the ways in which drugs act, and with particular reference to the neonate discusses some of the factors affecting the child's physiological response to drugs. The third section identifies the routes by which drugs are given and explores particular considerations when administering drugs by these routes. Section four discusses wider issues including nurse prescribing and self/parent medication schemes.

LICENSING DRUGS FOR USE IN CHILDREN

All drugs are issued under licence and when discussing the licensing of drugs for use in children there are several relevant issues to consider. Although most marketed drugs are used in children, only a very few have specific indications for use within this population. This in effect means that many drugs are used outside the terms of their product licences. One example of this is the controversy surrounding the oral use of vitamin K (Thompson (1992).

If a drug, prescribed for an identified group of patients, is not included on the data sheet the use of this drug is considered to be 'unlicensed'. The licence for several commonly used hospital drugs specifically excludes their use in children under twelve years; this has led to children being referred to as 'therapeutic orphans'.

The Department of Health (DoH 1985) maintains that the practitioner takes full responsibility when prescribing such drugs and in the event of an adverse reaction they may be called upon to justify their actions. It appears that the practitioner who prescribes the drug, at the present time a doctor, takes on the full responsibility for the consequences of their actions (Leonard 1994). However, the nurse is often the person who actually gives the drug and thus there are implications for children's nurses. They need to be aware of the potential risks and side effects of all drugs they are giving and should ensure that there is early recognition and reporting of any adverse reactions. Unfortunately there seems to be no central data bank through which to share information and therefore knowledge regarding the safety and efficacy of drugs in children is scarce. This may change as the European Community law recognizes that simplified procedures are needed to ensure that useful compounds can still be marketed.

It may be interesting to consider some of the reasons for the reluctance to market or issue licences for use of drugs in children under twelve. It may be a question of commercial viability; for example, babies only represent a small market and there may be insufficient financial incentive for a pharmaceutical company to establish a safe neonatal dose. The need for additional pharmacological or therapeutic research creates ethical issues and there may be risks of toxic side effects associated with the research. Obtaining reliable data on these effects on children may require repeated estimation of serum levels and this may be unethical, difficult and expensive. Many drugs are already in use and thus pharmaceutical companies may lack the incentive to perform clinical trials. Overall it seems that there are very few occasions when companies simultaneously apply for licences for children and adults.

referred to as the 'first pass effect'. As the liver is not fully matured and some of the complex enzymes are not refined, many drugs are 'poorly handled' by babies.

All the above may affect children differently because of their immature body systems, thus exacerbating the iatrogenic effects of drug therapy.

THE WAYS IN WHICH DRUGS ACT

As mentioned previously it is important for the children's nurse to understand the ways in which drugs work as this may enhance understanding of the potential risks associated with drug administration. The following outlines some of the basic principles of drug action:

- Drugs do not, on their own, create functions but modify existing functions within the body; in other words they interrupt or potentiate physiologic processes.
- Drug actions are produced by any of the following:

  (1) altering the chemical properties of a body fluid;
  (2) interacting with a cell membrane;
  (3) binding to specific receptors;
  (4) creating changes in protein synthesis.

  Drug action is determined by how the drug interacts with the body.

- All drugs have multiple actions and may affect more than one physiological process; thus it may be seen that the risk of side effects is increased if more than one drug is administered simultaneously.
- Once in the body the drug is converted into a soluble form so that it can be excreted in the urine. This means that many drugs pass through the kidneys and it is a reason for exercising caution when giving drugs to babies, because of the unsophisticated kidney function, and to children who have renal impairment.
- The process of conversion or metabolism takes place mainly within the microsomes of the liver. This organ receives a blood supply from the hepatic portal vein and is thus well placed for absorption from the gastrointestinal tract. Therefore all drugs given orally are taken up by the liver fairly rapidly; this is

FACTORS THAT AFFECT DOSE AND RESPONSE

Due to the rapid changes in growth of the infants over the first few months doses need to be regularly reviewed. Dosage regimes which are extrapolated from adult data will probably be inaccurate because other differences such as age, maturity of body systems and specific effects of the disease processes need to be taken into account as these additional factors increase the risks of toxicity.

The fact, mentioned previously, that most drugs protocols are not established for use with children is crucial and should be remembered when exploring other factors which may influence the pharmacokinetic phase of drug administration, namely absorption, distribution, metabolism and excretion.

The first of these is related to the degree and rate of absorption. This may be particularly pertinent when considering administration of drugs via the oral, rectal, percutaneous and intramuscular routes.

The stomach and the small intestine are major sites for absorption. When giving oral drugs the bioavailability or fraction of drug that reaches the systemic circulation will depend upon the pharmaceutical properties of the drug as well as the pH of gastric contents and gut motility. Some drugs are chemically unstable at a low pH and are thus inactive when given orally, for example benzylpenicillin. Most drugs are absorbed from the gut by diffusion and the rate of absorption may be influenced by food (McPherson 1993).

Newborn, particularly premature, babies have a greatly reduced gastric acid secretion, having a lower, more alkaline gastric pH of about 6–8 compared with the adult values of about 2. Additionally, in the neonate gastric emptying time is prolonged and intestinal peristalsis is slower. Diarrhoea and malabsorption may affect absorption of drugs in terms of both rate and volume, leading to increased toxicity or reduced efficiency. Because of the unpredictability of absorption there may be higher serum concentrations of some drugs and lower concentrations of others.

All the factors affecting absorption when giving drugs orally are relevant to the nurse when planning care to administer drugs at the optimum time. A major reason for recommending drug ingestion with food is to avoid gastric irritation but food can interact with drugs to alter their absorption (McPherson 1993).

An alternative to oral administration may be giving drugs into the rectum. This may be very useful if the child is vomiting or experiencing a convulsion. Analgesia is often given via this route, for example, suppositories. These can be given in theatre whilst the child is anaesthetized, thus avoiding the potential distress associated with rectal administration. However, absorption by this route may be erratic leading to unreliable serum levels. The acceptability of this method of administration may also be determined by cultural acceptance, for example it seems to be more acceptable in the rest of Europe than in Britain.

The skin is a useful route of administering drugs to babies. Percutaneous absorption may be substantially increased in new-born infants because of both the under developed epidermal barrier and increased skin hydration. This is further increased where skin is burnt or excoriated. This has particular implications for the application of topical agents, for example steroids to children with eczema, or if substances are applied to excoriated skin where disposable nappies create an occlusive dressing.

If a drug cannot be given orally or rectally, for example if the child is unable to absorb drugs due to vomiting or diarrhoea or if the child is physiologically unstable, parenteral administration may be necessary, including subcutaneous, intramuscular and intravenous routes.

The aim of the subcutaneous method is to inject the drug into the subcutaneous layer rather than into the active muscles. The most common drugs given by this route are heparin and insulin. Absorption of the drug may be delayed when the perfusion to the skin is impaired, for example in situations when a child is in physiological shock.

Absorption of drugs given intramuscularly tends to be erratic for several reasons. First, the rate and extent of intramuscular absorption may change rapidly in relation to actual muscle mass, and to changes in relative blood flow to various muscles. Second, the variability and unreliability of absorption is particularly problematic in babies because they usually have limited muscle mass. Generally, wherever possible, this method should be avoided in children because it is painful.

Increasingly drugs are being given intravenously. However, there are several problems associated with this route (Livesley 1993, 1994), including:

- Obtaining a drug in a suitable form for administration.
- Difficult access in neonates due to small veins.
- The hazards associated with the irritant and hypertonic characteristics of some intravenous drugs leading to necrosis if the injections infiltrate the tissues.
- Limited access, which often means that more than one drug is injected into the same site. This also introduces the potential problems of incompatibility of drugs and subsequent interactions.

Many of the intravenous drugs widely prescribed for infants and children are produced only in adult strengths, therefore small doses need to be reconstituted or diluted and this raises questions about stability. It is necessary to use displacement values for dry powder injectables, and children's nurses need to be able to calculate drug doses with accuracy. Volumes used to flush lines before and after intravenous medications should be kept to a minimum and included on the fluid balance sheet. Some hospitals are producing 'standard infusion strengths' for commonly infused drugs by providing worksheets to identify the correct methods to prepare drugs, and lists of compatible diluents. Many children's units set standards for intravenous drug administration which include guidelines about who is eligible to take on this role and the training required (Fig. 13.1).

Inhalation is a useful route of administration for young children with asthma or cystic fibrosis. Drugs are usually given by nebulisers or inhalers. A 'spacer' can be used in those children under three years and the baby inhales the drug by normal tidal breathing.

One of the most important components of pharmacological management is that treatment is delivered effectively. However, even with good techniques much of the medication is deposited in the upper airways and

1. *Preparation and education of nurses to give intravenous drugs*

Standard: All nurses who administer intravenous drugs will be competent to do so and the risks associated with intravenous therapy will be minimized
Each nurse who undertakes this role:

1.1 Meets the criteria set out in the policy   Yes   No

Comments:

1.2 Is conversant with the health authority (trust) policies related to this area   Yes   No

Comments:

1.3 Has completed the distance learning pack, (including additional information related   Yes   No
to paediatrics)

Comments:

1.4 Has been assessed by a competent peer, or assessed themselves as competent to   Yes   No
give IV drugs via bolus, bag and burette

Comments:

1.5 Has completed a competence certificate, a copy of which is kept in the ward file and   Yes   No
own profile

Comments:

1.6 Has attended an update within the last year to keep abreast of current practice and   Yes   No
innovations

Comments:

2. *Care of the intravenous infusion and cannula site*

Standard: All children requiring an intravenous infusion will be managed safely and appropriately

2.1 All children and families were verbally prepared by a nurse for the IV therapy   Yes   No

(a) EMLA cream was used appropriately   Yes   No

(b) Play preparation was used   Yes   No

Comments:

2.2 The preparation was documented in the nursing care plan   Yes   No

Comments:

2.3 A copy of the policy for care of IV sites is kept:

(a) in the area where the IV drugs are prepared   Yes   No

(b) in the staff orientation folder or equivalent   Yes   No

Comments:

2.4 A qualified nurse accepts accountability for supervising unqualified (including bank/   Yes   No
agency) nurses who may be caring for children with an IV infusion

Comments:

2.5 Each ward has a representative who liaises with other paediatric wards six monthly and updates literature kept on the ward	Yes	No
Comments:		
The site selected was recorded in the care plan (nursing notes)	Yes	No
A sterile dressing, e.g. Vecaflex, Opsite, Bioclusive, was applied	Yes	No
There was minimal bandaging and the site could be easily observed	Yes	No
Moulded splints were used	Yes	No
1 in pink elastoplast (backed) was used to secure the splint in place	Yes	No
The condition of the site was documented in the nursing evaluation at shift handover	Yes	No
The pump being used was appropriate for the product which is being infused	Yes	No
The clamp between the bag and burette was clamped	Yes	No
There is evidence that the intravenous site is checked regularly	Yes	No
The criteria for the use of intravenous pumps are applied	Yes	No
The fluid balance is recorded hourly	Yes	No
Comments:		

Fig. 13.1   Standards for intravenous care (Children's Unit, Oxford Radcliffe Hospital 1994).

subsequently swallowed (Gregson *et al.* 1993). The nurse, in recognizing that the inhaler device requires differing levels of skill and co-ordination, can avoid poor technique by planning appropriate education programmes.

Some drugs are given intrathecally directly into the cerebral spinal fluid. It is important to be aware that the formulations and dosages often differ significantly from intravenous or intramuscular preparations.

DISTRIBUTION OF DRUGS

Many factors are involved in drug distribution, including distribution of body fluids, the levels of plasma protein in the blood, and the permeability of the blood brain barrier.

The total body fluid as a percentage of body weight has been estimated at 85% in premature infants compared with 60% in adults, and the distribution between intracellular and extracellular fluid differs. Newborn babies have a much higher extracellular volume (Table 13.1). The usual therapeutic dose of drug given to a child who is in shock or dehydrated, may lead to

increased levels and increased side effects. In contrast, if the child has oedema the serum levels will be decreased and the effectiveness of the drug reduced.

The binding or affinity of drugs to albumin plasma proteins will be decreased in newborn infants for several reasons: there is decreased plasma protein concentration, providing fewer binding sites for some drugs, and altered binding capacity together with endogenous substances which inhibit binding. All these factors lead to increased concentrations of free unbound drug in the serum and the tissues. This is highly relevant as it explains the increase in toxic effects.

The pH of body fluid, for example in acidosis seen in

Table 13.1   Percentage of extracellular fluid and percentage body fat.

Age	Extracellular fluid % of body weight	% Body fat
Premature	50%	3%
Full term	45%	12%
1 year	25%	
Adult	20%	20%

dehydration, enhances or inhibits the effects of some drugs. The amount of body fat is substantially lower in the neonate compared to the adult and this also affects the distribution of drug therapy (Table 13.1).

Development of the blood brain barrier is incomplete in the newborn, therefore there is increased permeability to certain drugs into the cerebral spinal fluid and hence the brain. Lipid soluble drugs, for example some general anaesthetic agents, sedatives and narcotic analgesics, readily enter the brain and result in higher sensitivity sometimes leading to respiratory depression.

METABOLISM

Many drugs are metabolized in the liver, involving synthetic and non-synthetic pathways. The former includes such processes as oxidation, reduction and hydrolysis, and in the latter there is conjugation. Drug metabolism is substantially slower in infants than in older children and adults because there are differences in the maturation of the liver in these metabolic pathways.

ELIMINATION

Drugs and their metabolites are often eliminated by the kidney. Neonates, in particular, have reduced glomerular filtration rate and poor tubular function, leading to increased toxicity. Renal function of the neonate is 30%–40% (per unit of body surface area) less than an adult's. Many drugs in the neonate are eliminated unchanged by the kidneys.

THE DIFFERING REQUIREMENTS OF THE NEONATE

When considering any pharmacological issue it should be remembered that the physiology of the infant and child is not only immature but also a dynamic process changing rapidly from week to week (Smith 1985). This is one of the reasons for regular measurement of serum levels, especially when administering potentially toxic drugs. The clinical relevance of immaturity has been summarized by Rylance *et al.* (1991) and may be useful to consider the main factors in order to understand the rationale behind the different doses prescribed for neonates:

- Neonates have less plasma than adults and hence fewer binding sites for drugs. Therefore pharmacological activity may be achieved with lower doses of lightly protein bound drugs.
- Highly water soluble drugs produce lower plasma concentrations because newborn babies have a greater proportion of total body fluid. Therefore larger doses in mg/kg may be required compared to adults.
- Drug elimination is slower in neonates due to the immature liver (less drug metabolism) and kidneys (less drug excretion). To avoid accumulation and subsequent toxic effects the intervals between doses may be longer, and weight related total daily doses may be required.
- Liver enzyme processes and renal clearance may rapidly improve over several weeks, associated with growth, and thus it is necessary to adjust the dose as the drug is eliminated more rapidly.
- The longer half life of drugs (time taken for the plasma concentration to fall to half its previous level) in neonates means loading doses are required to achieve a more rapid pharmacological response.
- The marked inter and intra patient variation of the newborn increases the requirement to closely monitor effects, and thus blood level monitoring is essential for potentially toxic drugs.

All these factors may affect the response to drugs in the infant and child. The nurse needs to have a sound knowledge of both pharmacological and physiological principles of drug action. By applying these it may be possible to predict the likely toxic effects of drugs on the child and plan care accordingly.

DRUG CALCULATIONS

'There are few fortunate nurses who can honestly say they have never made a drug error – many live with the fact that they have.' (Glasper & Oliver 1984)

The dose prescribed is usually calculated on the child's actual weight rather than age because weight at a certain age can be variable. An alternative approach, often used to calculate cytotoxic drugs where precision is very important, is to estimate surface area. This is determined using a weight and height nomogram. These can be found in *The Paediatric Prescriber* (Catzell 1981).

$$\frac{\text{amount required} \times \text{dilution}}{\text{amount in stock}} = \frac{250\,\text{mg} \times 2\,\text{ml}}{500\,\text{mg}} = 1\,\text{ml}$$

- The amount required is the prescribed dose.
- The amount in stock is the amount of drug contained in all or part of the volume in the bottle or vial.
- The dilution is the amount of liquid in which the given quantity of the drug is dissolved

Fig. 13.2 Drug calculation formula (Glasper & Oliver 1984).

However, if a nurse is uncertain about the dose of drug prescribed there are several useful reference sources. The British National Formulary (1994), issued annually, usually contains sufficient information regarding the appropriate doses for those over twelve years old. The Data Sheet Compendium (ABPI 1993–4), which sets out the patient group for which the drug is intended together with information about indications for use, side effects and contraindications, provides a more detailed source. Many units have developed their own in-house list of drug dosage regimes, or have adopted one of the formularies that are currently available in the UK, for example the *Paediatric Vade Meacum* (Insley) or the *Alder Hey Book of Children's Doses* (1990).

The nurse should take particular care when checking prescription charts, should ensure that correct age and weight are recorded, and should be alert to prescription errors. All dosages need to be calculated carefully. The chance of error can be reduced if all nurses use the same method of calculation, for example the drug calculation formula (Fig. 13.1).

Mason (1993) recognized the fact that the administration of drugs to children is more complex because of the variables in body weight and surface area, and she suggested that drug administration mistakes are commonly associated with the calculation and administration phases. In response to the need to ensure that nurses were appropriately educated on these aspects, she designed a simulation game for use with students.

DRUG ADMINISTRATION

Problems in the administration of drugs in children are common for a number of reasons:

- A suitable dosage form may not be available and volumes may be large.
- The child may refuse to take the medicine.
- In the case of oral medications, the child may vomit due to the medication.
- There may be limited intravenous access.

There are persuasive arguments for giving drugs orally whenever possible, for example via tablets, capsules, liquids, drops and powders (Taylor & Helliwell 1992). However, in order to manufacture a drug in oral form the medicinal compound needs to be water soluble and therefore by this criterion some drugs may be excluded.

Assumptions are made that medicine in liquid form is more suitable for children because it is thought to be easier to swallow, allows minute adjustments in dosage and is faster acting (Taylor & Helliwell 1992). However, Manley *et al.* (1994) undertook a small survey to investigate the administration of long term medication to children and found that liquids had disadvantages and in general tablets were more popular with the parents and children. The reasons offered for this were that the dose was more accurate and easier to swallow, and there was less spillage and mess. The disadvantages of liquids appeared to be that they were less portable, were unpalatable because of taste or texture, and had a short shelf life and poor stability and because of this often needed to be refrigerated and replaced frequently.

Where possible sugar free preparations should be used as this will reduce the risk of dental decay. This is a particular consideration when giving oral medications over a long period as there are iatrogenic effects of sweetened medicines on children's oral health (Manley *et al.* 1994).

Advice to parents regarding safety and effectiveness in relation to giving medicines to children at home, should include information regarding:

- The special care that may be needed in relation to storage instructions and expiry dates, as inactive or toxic products may be produced if these are exceeded

(Taylor & Helliwell 1992). This is particularly relevant when the pharmacy produces their own liquid formulations of drugs.

■ The actual dose prescribed – this is important because sometimes concentrations are altered to keep volumes to a minimum in order that the child has to take less volume of an unpleasant tasting medicine.

■ The timing and frequency of administration – for instance, the timing between each dose and whether it should be given before or after meals, with fluids or milk. It has been suggested that giving the baby medicine before a feed may be more successful because the baby is hungry, may be less likely to vomit and if they do vomit they will not vomit the whole feed only the drug.

■ Techniques that may make administration easier – for example, it is sometimes easier to use a specially designed oral syringe in preference to a spoon, because there may be less chance of spillage. These syringes include special adapters which allow easier access to the medicine in the bottle and generally

Table 13.2 Using a nursing model as a framework within which to consider drug administration (© Dearmun, 1995).

Activities of daily living	Questions in relation to drug administration
Maintaining safety	Has an appropriate drug and dose been prescribed? Is it the correct dose, route, time and date? Has the prescribed dose been measured correctly? Is it going to be given to the right child? Who is the most appropriate person to administer this drug?
Communication	How can adherence to treatment be encouraged? Are medicines already being given regularly at home? Has the prescription chart been signed? Has adequate information been provided for the child and family? Have the family agreed to take part in a self medication scheme?
Eating and drinking	Should the medication be given before/after or with food? Is the drug likely to induce vomiting? Is there a drink/sweet available to counteract any unpleasant taste?
Elimination	Is this drug likely to induce diarrhoea, for example antibiotics.
Playing	What strategies can be used to gain co-operation, for example preparation and play.
Sleep & rest	Can timing of drugs be planned to minimize disruption to sleep patterns?
Breathing, maintaining temperature	What are the potential side effects associated with this drug and will these effects be exacerbated due to the immaturity of the child's physiological systems or illness? What are the known side effects? What actions should be taken in the event of an adverse reaction?
Hygiene	Does the administration of this drug have implications for mouth care, for example is a sugar free preparation being given to avoid dental caries? Is a cytotoxic agent being given? Is this drug likely to create excoriation of the skin, for example enzyme preparations?
Mobilising	Where is the best place to give this drug? Can the child select a position most comfortable for them, for example sitting on a parent's knee?

they are much safer to use; indeed the use of ordinary syringes should be discouraged and even oral syringes should be used with care since rapid administration may result in the child aspirating the liquid. Another method is to place the teat in the baby's mouth and slowly syringe the medicine into the teat whilst the baby is sucking at it.

■ Foods or other drugs that should be avoided as they may be incompatible due to known side effects.

Both nurses and parents recognize that oral drug administration may be a challenge. If, due to the child's age, co-operation is not a realistic expectation, the only alternative may be to wrap the baby up securely in order to administer the medication. Parents may find this distressing and may need to be given support and the opportunity to discuss their feelings; it may also be useful to reiterate the rationale for treatment. If this distress continues unresolved the treatment may not be continued or completed once the child is at home.

When the child is older appropriate age related strategies to gain a child's co-operation can be employed. Fradd (1990) suggests that the key to successful drug administration lies to a great extent in the preparation; for example, 'giving it' to a favourite toy or allowing time to play. Other strategies include using distraction, providing simple honest explanations about what the medicine will do or how it will help, and offering a degree of choice and responsibility. Overall a positive attitude which rewards and praises positive and ignores negative behaviour is likely to be most effective.

Various techniques may be employed to make the drugs more palatable but it is especially important that the characteristic of the drug is known in order to undertake this safely. This is illustrated in Table 13.3. If there is any doubt the pharmacist should be consulted.

Adherence to treatment regimes may depend on several factors including the disease that is being treated and its duration; for example, many endocrine disorders require a lifetime of treatment, in contrast to an infection when a course of antibiotics of five to seven days' duration will suffice. A study found that at best only 69% of patients took their medication (Evans & Spelman 1983). One might speculate that the adherence to treatment may be improved in children if carefully supervised by their parents; nevertheless it may still be necessary to consider methods to increase co-operation.

The nurse should assess and support the capabilities of the family and co-operation may be further enhanced by the quality of information given to the parents (Fig. 13.3). This should include the reasons for the medication, when it should be given and why, and how to recognize potential side effects (Williams 1991). The dosage measurement should be made as simple as possible.

Table 13.3 Measures to make the drugs more palatable.

Techniques to make drugs more palatable	Contra indications
Capsules may be emptied out and mixed with yoghurt or a small amount of jam and some tablets may be crushed prior to administration.	Some tablets should not be crushed, for example sustained release preparations and drugs that have an enteric coating, as these are designed to avoid irritation to the stomach lining.
Some medicines taste better when they are cold and can be mixed with ice cream.	Some drugs bind to milk protein, particularly iron preparations. This is one of the main reasons for not adding them to the baby's milk bottle.
It is usually possible to flavour preparations with a little orange juice or blackcurrent juice just prior to administration without affecting the stability.	Adding flavourings may be a problem as these sometimes alter the pH of the preparation and thus their absorption.

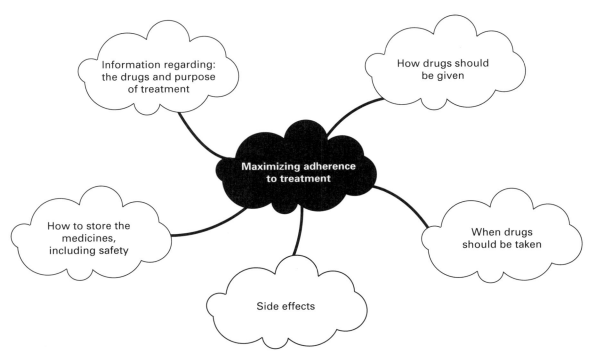

Fig. 13.3   Information to be given to parents.

Self/parent medication schemes

'Doing the drugs' may be incompatible with the named nurse or primary nursing systems and one could question the necessity to undertake drugs rounds. Abolishing this task may pave the way for parents to work with their individual nurse to become more involved in administering drugs.

Several hospitals have introduced self/parent medication schemes, where either the parents or the older child administer their own drugs. These schemes are usually most appropriate when the child is likely to be on long term medication. The co-operation of the pharmacist is essential as he or she will be required to supply all children's drugs on a 'named basis'. The drugs are then kept in lockable boxes by the bedside. Parents have a key and, after undertaking an appropriate

teaching programme, sign to accept responsibility for the storage and checking of their child's drugs.

Woodhouse (1990) undertook a survey in order to evaluate the introduction of such a scheme into the oncology unit in Birmingham. It was found that all parents who returned the questionnaire were 'happy to take on the responsibility' although nurses, when questioned, were concerned about accountability. Fradd (1990) described a system where the nurse had an educational and supervisory role and accountability was shared. It seems logical when parents have a vested interest in their child receiving the correct dose at the correct time, that, where negotiated and agreed, handing over this responsibility is completely congruent to a partnership approach to the nursing of children.

However, there need to be guidelines regarding:

■ The selection of and negotiation with the parents/ young adults.
■ Clear designation and acceptance of responsibility.
■ Precise documentation using record cards.

- Ways of auditing that the drugs have been given according to the treatment protocols.
- The storage and security of drugs.
- The production of comprehensive information leaflets.

Nurse prescribing

The Royal College of Nursing (RCN 1992) states that 'the right to prescribe drugs will only be extended to community nurses with the appropriate training'. It is likely therefore that this role will extend to community children's nurses and will enable them to prescribe a limited number of medicines and dressings. Gown (1989) identified three levels of nurse prescribing as:

- 'Initial prescribing' where the community nurse could prescribe independently from a 'nurses formulary'.
- A 'secondary level' where they could prescribe within a 'group protocol'.
- A simple level where they could alter the timing and dosage of medicines within specified guidelines.

Glenhill (1994) maintains that having nurses prescribing is not without risk and suggests that nurses will be required to attain a certain level of education and competence. To fulfil this standard it is recognized that the nurse needs to have a sound knowledge of pharmacology in order to fully appreciate the implications of their prescribing, in particular, any long term effects (Ashurst 1993).

CONCLUSION

It could be argued that developmental and pharmacological aspects are interrelated and have physiological, psychological and social dimensions. Each stage in a child's development brings with it different considerations.

Sometimes drugs taken by the mother during pregnancy can have an effect on the fetus, causing congenital abnormalities. These are known as teratogens. Probably the most well publicized of these was thalidimide. During labour narcotics given to the mother may depress the baby's respiratory system. After birth,

drugs taken by the mother whilst breast feeding may pass into the mother's milk and have an effect on the baby.

During the neonatal period there may be difficulties in the administration of drugs due to physiological imma-turity and constant change in growth, weight and general maturity of body systems. The nurse who is aware of the ways in which drugs act will be in a position to anticipate possible problems and side effects and take appropriate action. During the first year drug handling becomes less of a problem because there is improved pharmacokinetic handling, absorption, metabolism and excretion.

In the toddler/pre-school age group the emphasis becomes one of encouraging acceptance of the medication and a focus upon safety to avoid self poisoning. These challenges are most common in the 18 months to three years age group and may be interrelated with a child's quest for autonomy and their need to explore their environment. Unfortunately the incidence of infections and the risk of febrile convulsions is higher in this age group and therefore there is an increased need to administer antipyretic agents, for example paracetamol or antibiotics. The nurse who understands this stage of development will be able to discuss with the parents techniques to encourage the toddler to accept medicines, and can offer advice regarding avoidance of accidental ingestion.

When the child reaches school age, if they are involved in decisions about their care and are provided with information about the medications they are taking, they are often more co-operative.

Adolescence is often associated with challenges regarding the adherence to therapeutic regimes. In this age group the medications are usually required long term to reduce the physiological effects of an underlying disease, for example insulin therapy in the case of diabetes (Smith 1991). Drugs taken to improve a prognosis, for example steroid therapy in renal failure, may have side effects which the young adult finds unacceptable. A further aspect in relation to this age group is possible experimentation with tobacco (Stewart & Orme 1991), alcohol, solvents, and illegal drugs or missuse of prescribed drugs (Harding-Price 1993).

This chapter has addressed several of these aspects that are pertinent to children's nurses. It is necessary to explore all these areas in order to acquire a working knowledge of the drugs commonly administered and the likely physiological responses to drug therapy, and also necessary to maintain a questioning approach to ensure safe and effective practice.

REFERENCES AND FURTHER READING

ABPI (Association of British Pharmaceutical Industry) (1994–95). *Data Sheet Compendium* Datapharm Publications, London.

Alder Hey Book of Children's Doses (1990) (5th edn). Alder Hey, Liverpool.

Ashurst, S. (1993) Nurses must improve their knowledge of pharmacology. *British Journal of Nursing*, 2(12), 608.

British National Formulary (1994) No. 26. British Medical Association and Royal Pharmaceutical Society, London.

Buchanan, N. (1987) In *Avery's Drug Treatment* (ed. T.M. Speight) (3rd edn), p. 118–59. Adis Press, Auckland.

Callaghan, S. (1990) Doing the round alone. *Nursing Times*, 86(44), 36–8.

Catzell, P. (1981) *The Paediatric Prescriber*, 5th edn. Blackwell Science, Oxford.

Crown, J. (1989) *Report of the Advisory Group in Nurse Prescribing*. DoH, London.

Di-Piro, Talbert, Hayes, Yee, Mateke & Posey (eds) (1992) *Pharmacotherapy: Pathophysiologic Approach*, 2nd edn, pp. 56–63. Elsevier Science Publishing, New York.

DoH (1985) *A Guide to the Provisions Affecting Doctors and Dentists, Medicines Act leaflet*, MAL30. HMSO, London.

DoH (1992) *Prophylaxis Against Vitamin K Deficiency. Bleeding in Infants.* HMSO, London.

Evans, L. & Spelman, M. (1983) The problem of non compliance with drug therapy. *Drugs*, 25, 63–73.

Federal Drug Agency vs Unapproved Drug Use (1993) *Paediatrics*, March, A26.

Fradd, E. (1990) Sharing Accountability. *Paediatric Nursing*, 2(3), 6–8.

Gadomski, A. & Horton, L. (1992) The need for rational therapeutics in use of cough and cold medicine in infants. *Paediatrics*, 89, 774–6.

Gaukroger, P.B. (1991) Paediatric Analgesia: Which Drug? Which Dose? *Drugs*, 41, 52–9.

Glasper, A. & Oliver, R.W. (1984) A simple guide to infant calculations. *Nursing*, 2(22), 649–50.

Glenhill, E. (1994) Implications of nurse prescribing. *British Journal of Nursing*, 3(9), 439–40.

Gregson, R., Kelly, P. & Warner, J. (1993) Education for control: management principles and inhaler techniques for childhood asthma. *Child Health*, 1(1), 16.

Harding-Price, D. (1993) A sensitive response without discrimination: drug misuse in children and adolescents. *Professional Nurse*, 8(7), 419–22.

Insley, J. (ed.) *Paediatric Vade Mecum* (annual). Edward Arnold, London.

Johnson, L. & Giles, R. (1993) Prescription for change. *Nursing Times*, 89(16), 42–5.

Livesley, J. (1993) Reducing the risks: the management of paediatric intravenous therapy. *Child Health*, 1(1), 68–71.

Livesley, J. (1994) Peripheral IV therapy in children. *Paediatric Nursing*, 6(4), 24–30.

Lloyd, G. (1990) Opioids: routes of administration. *Professional Nurse*, 5(12), 634–6.

Manley, M.C.G. (1994) A spoonful of sugar helps the medicine go down: perspectives on the use of sugar in children's medicine. *Social Science & Medicine*, 39(6), 833–40.

Manley, G., Sheiham, A. & Eadsforth, W. (1994) Sugar-coated care? *Nursing Times*, 90(7), 34–5.

Mason, G. (1993) Medicine round: a simulation game. *Paediatric Nursing*, 5(3), 16–19.

McPherson, G. (1993) Absorbing effects. *Nursing Times*, 89(32), 30–32.

Moon, A. (1988) Juggs and Herrings. *Nursing Times*, 84, 27 July, 58–60.

Mulholland, P. (1991) *The Pharmaceutical Journal*, 5 January, p. 24.

Prescribing unlicensed drugs or using drugs for unlicensed indications (1992) *Drugs and Therapeutics Bulletin*, 30, 97–9.

RCN (1992) Factsheet: *Nurse Prescribing*. Royal College of Nursing, London.

Rylance, G., Harvey, D. & Aranda, J.U. (1991) *Neonatal Clinical Pharmacology and Therapeutics*, Chapter 1. Butterworth-Heinemann, London.

Smith, S. (1985) Drugs at different ages. *Nursing Times*, 9 January, 37–9.

Smith, J. (1991) An extra source of conflict, diabetes in adolescence. In *Child Care: Some Nursing Perspectives* (ed. A. Glasper), pp. 171–7. Wolfe Publishing, London.

Stewart, A. & Orme, J. (1991) Why do adolescents smoke? In *Child Care: Some Nursing Perspectives* (ed. A. Glasper), Chapter 23, 153–8. Wolfe Publishing, London.

Taylor, D. & Helliwell, M. (1992) Liquid preparations for oral administration. *Professional Nurse*, 8(3), 163–7.

Thompson, J. (1992) Vitamin controversy. *Nursing Times*, 88(24), 19.

UKCC (1986) *Administration of medicines.* UKCC, London.

UKCC (1992) *Code of Professional Conduct for the Nurse Midwife and Health Visitor.* UKCC, London.

UKCC (1992) *The Scope of Professional Practice.* United Kingdom Central Council for Nursing, Midwifery and Health Visiting, London.

Valman, H.B. (1993) Febrile convulsions. *British Medical Journal*, 306, 1743–5.

Williams, B. (1991) Medication education. *Nursing Times*, 87(29), 50–52.

Woodhouse, S. (1990) Why have medicine rounds? *Paediatric Nursing*, 2(10), 9–12.

INTRODUCTION

Complementary therapy is a broad term which encompasses many different therapies, some of which are considered in terms of their possible applications to child health care. Complementary therapies differ from traditional medical treatment in that they make assumptions about health and illness. Practitioners consider their work to be holistic in that it treats the whole person and not purely the physical symptoms of illness. Thus the psychological and physiological are seen as inseparable; a treatment that affects the body will also affect the mind. Complementary therapies can be broadly divided into two categories: touch and energy therapies (Fig. 14.1). Alternative concepts about health and illness are particularly apparent in some of the energy therapies, such as reflexology and shiatsu.

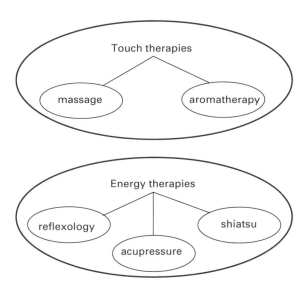

Fig. 14.1 Touch and energy therapies.

The common factor in the therapies discussed is the use of touch as the medium through which treatment is delivered. Human touch is believed to play an important role in child development, and can be particularly useful in working with children who may have not developed language skills. In this chapter the importance of touch is discussed before reviewing two of the most commonly used touch therapies – massage and aromatherapy.

Other complementary therapies are then reviewed under the term energy therapies. These include therapies such as reflexology, shiatsu and acupressure, which use touch to balance the energy forces present in the body. Each of these therapies may individually, or in combinations with other treatments, contribute to the effective holistic management of the sick child.

Many nurses see the potential benefits in using complementary therapies and are eager to utilize them to promote an improved quality of patient care. Ersser (1990) highlights a number of issues related to the use of complementary therapies by nurses. Nurses should, however, remember that competence in such therapies requires dedication, the right training and the appropriate support (Rankin-Box 1992). Nurses must consider both the UKCC's Code of Professional Conduct (UKCC 1992a) and the UKCC's Scope of Professional Practice (UKCC 1992b) when considering using any such therapies.

TOUCH THERAPIES

Touch is a primitive form of communication and it is seen to be the earliest means of communicating (LeMay 1986). The extent to which people touch each other varies enormously across different cultures (Feltham 1991; Carruthers 1992). The Eskimo baby is placed in the back of the mother's parka from birth and never leaves her until walking; the Indian baby is massaged daily from one month old. Western societies, particularly the British, are renowned for their reticence about touching their children and each other, and the British have been described as a 'non-touch' culture (Jourard 1968; Berry 1986). Montagu (1986) argues that children who lack loving touch may become withdrawn, insecure, and in extreme cases fail to mature into happy, healthy and socially confident adults. It is therefore suggested that touch plays an important role in child development as it fulfils a fundamental human need and is an important component of nonverbal communication (Tilton 1992).

The quality of touch is of supreme importance; the softest stroking movement is enough to convey sympathy, understanding and reassurance, whereas smacking conveys displeasure and punishment. Mitchell *et al.*

(1985) identify different types of touching between nurse and child and categorizes them:

- Spontaneous touch – incidental touching by the nurse or parent.
- Procedural touch – touching to perform nursing procedures.
- Nonprocedural touch – parental touching such as stroking or kissing.

Mitchell *et al.* (1985) monitored the child's intracranial pressure response to different types of touch and found that quite profound decreases in intracranial pressure, with subsequent stabilization, followed parental stroking. Surprisingly, nurses were found to minimize tactile contact when caring for children and this was especially so with the very ill child. Touch is a relatively well understood component in nursing babies and very young children but less so in respect to nursing older children. As children grow older and their repertoire of communication skills develops, being touched begins to need permission or consent. However, touch can still play an important role in communication particularly when the older child/young adult, who may be experiencing illness for the first time, finds it difficult to verbally express feelings about their illness.

Massage

The oldest of the touch therapies is massage, a simple and easy treatment for nurses, parents and carers to perform although guidelines need to be considered and followed (Beck 1988). In the west techniques called Swedish massage use effective and appropriate strokes belonging to the classifications of stroking, effleurage, and petrissage/pressure manipulations. Massage strokes are not only psychologically comforting but they also have a wide range of physiological benefits:

- Increase circulation and blood flow to the tissues.
- Encourage healing by oxygenating and providing essential nutrients to the tissues.
- Remove metabolites of ill health through the increased flow of lymph.

Dunn (1992) showed that massage resulted in a decrease in heart rate and blood pressure, and reduced muscle tension. Studies into the psychological benefits of massage have mostly used qualitative methodologies and a range of benefits have been identified. Massage can help in the way that children:

- Perceive their pain.
- Cope with illness.
- Perceive their illness.

In nursing, massage has been applied in several areas. Baby massage has achieved great popularity in recent years and is thought to enhance care by promoting bonding. Adamson (1993) asserts that massage may be used therapeutically when a baby has colic or constipation or psychologically to promote a sense of security and wellbeing. Goleman (1988) demonstrated that the importance of massage to child development is critical. Premature babies massaged for fifteen minutes three times a day gained weight 47% faster, developed a more mature nervous system and were discharged from hospital six days earlier than babies who were not massaged. Massage strokes are noninvasive, promote a feeling of security and are generally well accepted by parents and professionals. Massage is gaining recognition and acceptance within the current context of health care delivery.

Potential applications in nursing children

A range of applications can be considered for massage within nursing practice, and it is as appropriate in the hospital setting as in the community setting. Parents can be taught relatively quickly by the experienced, trained nurse to use massage strokes to provide support and intervention for the child.

Pain – Massage can provide not only psychological support by means of the physical human contact but can also, through stimulating large C fibres, have an effect on the 'gate' located in the dorsal horn of the spinal column, thus mediating the pain response (McCaffery & Beebe 1989; Melzack & Wall 1965, 1988). When treating a child who is in pain or distress the hand movements should be lengthened into long, slow strokes as these are particularly effective in soothing sensory nerve endings and blocking pain impulses.

Constipation – Constipation massage consists of effleurage strokes following the line of the large intestine, followed by circular kneading movements using the fingertips or the palm of the hand (depending on the age of the child) and then repeating the effleurage strokes (Fig. 14.2). Diaphragmatic breathing can also be included to increase the internal pressure within the abdomen (Emly 1993). However, the nurse should always assess the child's other health problems and it may be that increasing abdominal pressure is contra-indicated.

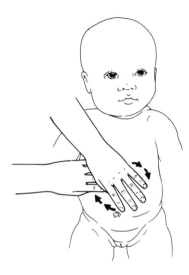

Fig. 14.2   Effleurage strokes to abdomen.

Baby massage – There is no fixed sequence for massaging a baby but the movements should be gentle and flowing. The limbs may be grasped and stroked from top to bottom with slight traction. The baby's back may be stroked from top to bottom encompassing the sides of the body. Firmer kneading strokes should be stroked down the chest area and from behind the waist to the pubis. These stroking movements should be firm and steady as if one were smoothing the creases from a piece of silk. The whole surface area of the baby's body should feel cosseted and protected. The nurse must ensure that the baby is warm and safe throughout – babies massaged with oil become somewhat slippery.

Aromatherapy

Aromatherapy uses natural, aromatic oils which aromatherapists believe influence physical health through the absorption of essential oils into the blood stream,

and psychological health by the effect of odour on the limbic system (Davis 1988; Ryman 1991). Combined with specific massage techniques, aromatherapy treatments offer a powerful intervention in both the promotion of health and in managing problems. An essential oil is a volatile liquid present in tiny sacs in plants. The oil is made up of numerous different organic molecules which when combined give the essential oil its own distinctive aroma and a range of therapeutic values. The individual components have been found to be less effective than the whole oil – a synergistic effect is said to exist.

Engen (1988) asserts that a newborn baby responds to odour, discriminating between its breastfeeding mother and another mother. Research suggests that smell memories can last longer than visual memories and can last throughout life. Whilst it is only recently that research findings concerning the differential effects of essential oils are starting to be generated and published, the initial findings look promising. Torii *et al.* (1988), for example, found an 80% agreement in discrimination between oils that are said to relax and those that are believed to act as stimulants.

The aromatherapist uses essential oils in conjunction with a specialized massage technique to promote both psychological and physiological effects. The extent and diversity of physiological effects of essential oils is vast and beyond the remit of this chapter. However, some recent papers demonstrate some of the range of effects that essential oils can have psychologically. Warm *et al.* (1990) argues that mentha piperita (peppermint) will help to increase accurate vigilance performance. Melaleuca alternifolia (tea tree) is effective on candida albicans (Belaiche 1985). Origanum marjorana (marjoram) is shown to be effective against 25 bacteria including aspergillus and salmonella (Deans & Svoboda (1990). Betts (1994) suggests that cananga odorata (ylang-ylang) may reduce seizures in epilepsy.

Lavender oil, currently widely used in hospitals, has been shown to have a soporific effect and is therefore considered beneficial in reducing anxiety and encouraging sleep. However not all lavenders have the same effect; some are extremely stimulating to the respiratory system and some have an excellent healing effect. Buckle (1992) argues that care must be taken to use the correct lavender for the required effect. In studies carried out on an adult cardiac intensive care unit, lavandula burnatti (a hybrid between lavandula angustifolia and lavandula latifolia) was shown to be helpful in reducing anxiety and increasing coping levels. Traditionally, lavandula angustifolia is said to have this effect, and lavandula latifolia is used for its expectorant effect.

The use of aromatherapy can be very beneficial when caring for sick children, perhaps particularly in relation to calming and soothing a distressed child and helping them cope with the anxiety associated with so many aspects of being in hospital. However, the essential oils used to provide these aromas and treatments have many diverse effects and should be well understood before attempting this therapy. Nurses, carers and mothers wishing to use aromas should understand the essential oils, their effects and the many contra-indications to their use, and should seek advice from a qualified therapist.

It is strongly recommended that a qualified aromatherapist or nurse-aromatherapist, who is able to prescribe the appropriate essential oils, is employed in the hospital situation. Essential oils should be referred to by their Latin names to ensure that the appropriate oil giving the correct effect is chosen. There are, for example, some ten eucalyptus, five thyme, and six lavender oils currently on the market. Differentiating between these oils and choosing the right oil takes knowledge, experience and skill, which need to be developed through appropriate training courses.

Potential applications in nursing children

Hardy (1991) suggests that essential oils can complement orthodox treatments and that sometimes they reduce the need for sedating or tranquillising drugs. Again the range of possible interventions and uses of essential oils is vast and has both physical and therapeutic effects:

Sedation/Relaxation – Adding one drop of lavandula angustifolia to a tablespoon of full fat milk and introducing this to a bath of warm water before bathing the child can help to calm and relax the anxious child, and could be used with good effect preoperatively.

Skin irritation/pyrexia – One drop of mentha piperita (peppermint) essential oil added to a bottle containing two pints of water can be used to reduce the skin irritation experienced in association with chickenpox, for example. The bottle should be shaken well before every application. Davis (1988) suggests that this mixture can be used to cool a child with a pyrexia as peppermint is

acknowledged as reducing temperature. Peppermint should be used with great care on children and the dose mentioned above should not be exceeded.

Coughs/colds/respiratory tract infections – One drop of eucalyptus globulus (eucalyptus) added to a bowl of cold water by the child's bed allows slow release of the vapour into the room and gently affects the nasal passages, sinuses and lungs throughout the night. This is particularly helpful in relieving symptoms associated with coughs, colds and lung infections.

Nappy rash/candida infection – One drop of melaleuca alternifolia (tea tree) added to a tablespoon of milk and then added to a half pint of water can be used as a mouthwash. Tea tree added to a bland cream can be used as an excellent treatment for nappy rash and candida.

All essential oils must be diluted before use on the skin and this is particularly important in respect of young children and babies. Normally a 0.5–2% dilution is appropriate, although the therapist would again need to assess the child individually to determine the most appropriate dilution. However, guidelines do exist that indicate appropriate, safe dilutions for use with children (Table 14.1).

Table 14.1 Recommended dilutions for essential oils.

	Age of child (years)	Dilution %
Babies	0–1	0.5
Children	1–5	1
Children	6–12	1.5
Adolescent	13–18	2

Aromatherapists use a blend of essential oil and carrier oil for treating the child. Carrier oils are used as a medium for dilution of the essential oils, and for the massage (Table 14.2).

Aromatherapy can be used effectively as a means of treating 'normal' childhood problems, as can be seen in this case study.

Sophie, a five year old girl, was reported to have an abundance of energy and had difficulty in getting to

Table 14.2 Drops of essential oil required to make appropriate dilutions.

% solution being made	Number of drops used in 100 ml of carrier oil
0.5	10
1	20
1.5	30
2	40

sleep at night. She was referred for aromatherapy treatment. She was also described as being disobedient. After a comprehensive assessment the aims of treatment were decided to be to reduce her hyperactivity and to encourage her to settle to sleep at night.

It was important to involve Sophie in all aspects of the treatment so the final selection of oils was done by encouraging her to smell and then choose three oils from six suitable oils chosen by the therapist for their relaxing or calming effects. Sophie enjoyed choosing the oils and quickly found her favourites; the blend was then made up by the therapist (Table 14.3).

The massage was begun on Sophie's back as this is an area that is suited well to getting her used to the type of strokes (touch) that will be employed throughout the treatment. Sophie was talkative and restless at the beginning of the treatment but became more relaxed as the treatment progressed, allowing the whole body to be massaged. A considerable time was spent on long strokes of effleurage performed sufficiently deeply to prevent tickling, progressing to

the legs, then effleurage to the hair and kneading to the scalp. By the end of the treatment Sophie was quiet and tranquil – a deep state of relaxation. Sophie was encouraged to rub a small amount of the prepared blend on her arms at night to help her recall the relaxation and thus prolong the effects of the treatment.

Sophie's mother reported a peacefulness which lasted over a week, a greater ease in bedtime rituals and a general improvement in Sophie's behaviour. The combination of the soporific effects of the chosen oils and the slow stroking massage movements produced the desired effect of calming hyperactivity. Restfulness was apparent in her general demeanour and an overall feeling of well-being seemed to be a positive side effect.

ENERGY THERAPIES

Eastern philosophy believes in a system of energies running through the body in channels or zones, a concept not widely accepted within present western thinking. In health a balanced condition prevails, and this energy or vital force flows smoothly along the connected channels supplying and maintaining all parts of the body. Where the energies are out of balance or blocked, the body develops patterns of ill health. The treatments in this group are various pressures to rebalance these energies.

Table 14.3 Therapeutic blend and rationale for choice of oils for Sophie.

Lavender (*Lavandula angustifolia*)	2 drops (0.1 ml)	A natural, safe sedative chosen for sleeplessness and to calm during waking hours (Hardy 1991).
Mandarin (*Citrus reticulata*)	2 drops (0.1 ml)	A sedative particularly helpful for restlessness in children (Lawless 1992).
Benzoin (*Styrax benzoin*)	1 drop (0.05 ml)	A sedative with a warming effect which gives a positive, calming but euphoric effect (Dye 1992).
Sweet almond (*Prunus amygdalas*)	25 ml	A general carrier oil for diluting essential oils to a safe percentage.

Reflexology

Energy is believed to flow through the body in ten equal vertical zones ending in the fingers and toes (Norman 1988; Hall 1991). By applying pressure in one of these zones an effect is caused elsewhere in the body. Today, reflexology is almost always applied to the feet as the most effective area to influence these energies. The reflexes map out specific areas and organs in the body, which when pressed release a flush of energy through the zone to the appropriate region which is considered to be blocked due to ill health.

Reflexology is best used as a method of elimination. These eliminating effects are documented by an increase in urine flow, micturition and an increase in faecal output. This is an excellent treatment for children with constipation and digestive upsets of all kinds. Also effective is pressure to the lung areas for congestive lung conditions; this improves the elimination of mucus and, when combined with positioning, drains the lungs. As asserted by Norman (1988) reflexology should be practised very gently in children and babies (about half the normal pressure used for adults and very light pressure for babies). As a beginner treating children it is hard to believe that gentle pressure of this nature can have any effect, but used wrongly it can produce such a surge of energy through the zones as to be detrimental to the child.

Potential applications in nursing children

Relaxation – Stroking the feet has been found to be particularly relaxing to the child. However, whether this can be considered to be true reflexology or simple stroking movements is difficult to say.

Shiatsu

Chinese philosophy approaches health in a concept of duality. This means that things function in relation to each other and is expressed as yin and yang (Fig. 14.3). The belief is that one state is always affected by its opposite; for example, rest is affected by movement; heat is affected by cold. Neither extreme is seen in Eastern terms as being the optimum state and it is believed that a balance should exist between the two states of yin and yang. Therefore illness, as opposed to

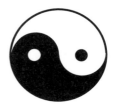

Fig. 14.3   The symbol of yin and yang.

wellness and good health, is merely a balance between these. The two states are continually in a state of flux. Shiatsu treatment is based on an attempt to balance yin and yang energies (Gulliver 1988). Oriental medicine considers that energy (chi) circulates round the body in channels called meridians and that this flow of energy has a direction which can be altered to produce an effect.

Nonspecific shiatsu gives children a feeling of lightness, relaxation, renewed energy and wellbeing. Occasionally temporary discomforts may occur, such as tiredness, headaches, aching muscles and possibly emotional sensitivity. These discomforts would be very temporary. Shiatsu techniques on babies should be introduced in a very relaxed way by stroking all the meridian lines along with other massage strokes. More specific shiatsu techniques may be performed on older children, increasing the pressure slightly on the meridian lines and changing energy levels.

Potential applications in nursing children

Anxiety, lack of energy, sleeplessness and pain – The sick child who has too little energy, is depleted of sleep and experiencing anxiety and pain, may be stroked very gently along the meridian lines in the direction of the flow of energy. This increases the child's natural energies and improves general wellbeing. Running the meridians with the whole hand can give a quick energizing massage.

Hyperactivity – The hyperactive child can be calmed by reducing the energies and this can be achieved by stroking the meridian lines against the flow of energy with more depth and 'flicking off' the body at the end of the stroke.

Acupressure

This treatment is acupuncture without needles. Points are pressed quite strongly with thumbs or fingers, almost to the point of pain. This has two effects. First, manual pressure causes the body to release two kinds of opiate peptides within the central nervous system, particularly beta-endorphins, which modulate pain, and dynorphins, which act on the gating mechanism in the spinal cord (Saks 1992). Second, the depth of the pressure stimulates touch receptors in the skin, sending faster impulses than pain impulses. By the time the pain stimuli reach the spinal cord, the gate (as described in the gate-control theory) is already closed (Macnish 1991).

Potential applications in nursing children

Nausea and vomiting – Nausea and vomiting can be helped by a 15 second thumb pressure on pericardium 6 (an acupressure point); this is seen to be useful in Stannard's (1989) study using acupressure bands on this point on patients undergoing chemotherapy. This point is found on the inside of the forearm, two of the child's finger widths above the wrist fold between the radius and ulna (Fig. 14.4). Pressure is applied to this point in a downward direction for 15 seconds.

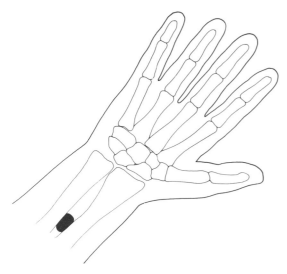

Fig. 14.4   Pericardium 6 – point for nausea and vomiting.

TRAINING, EDUCATION AND PRACTICE ISSUES IN COMPLEMENTARY THERAPIES

As the use of complementary therapies within society grows, there is increased pressure from both within and outside the profession for nurses to incorporate them into their own practice. Indeed many nurses see the use of complementary therapies as an attractive addition to their range of skills. However, rather than rushing headlong into the use of such therapies nurses must consider whether or not they are qualified to use them. Gradually, ratified training courses are being developed for nurses to encourage the development of safe and effective practitioners/therapists. Issues related to standardizing courses and accreditation of prior learning are under review by the RCN Complementary Therapies forum. This level of scrutiny can only be of benefit as this will help to safeguard both the client and the therapist.

Nurses must ensure that they practice appropriately and are governed by the Code of Professional Conduct (UKCC 1992a). Nurses should also consider ongoing study within their own chosen field once they have completed their training. This provides the therapist with opportunities for discussion with fellow therapists and regular updating. It also reduces the potential isolation that the therapist may feel if working on their own.

The *Nursing Times* (1994) offers five prerequisites that a nurse should consider before practising in a clinical setting (Table 14.4). All these issues must be considered, as must the need for regulating individual therapies if safe, high quality practice is to be delivered to clients, and the use of therapies within mainstream nursing care is to be justified (Rankin-Box 1993).

CONCLUSIONS AND RECOMMENDATIONS

Complementary therapies can play an important role in looking after the healthcare needs of children. The therapies discussed are easy to administer in both the hospital and community and they require very little equipment. They are cost effective and some of the

Table 14.4 Prerequisites that a nurse should consider before practising in a clinical setting. (From *Nursing Times*, 1994 - modified format).

Have I undergone a recognized training and been awarded proof of having completed the course?	The UKCC Scope of Professional Practice leaves it to the individual nurse to decide his or her competency in a particular technique or area of care. However, as the field of complementary medicine is still largely unregulated, it is important that nurses are seen to have gained best possible qualifications in the therapies they intend to use.
Is there research based evidence that the therapy I wish to practice is of benefit to the patients to whom I intend to offer it?	A nurse who cannot justify the care given to a patient leaves him or herself open to litigation and investigation by the UKCC if, as a result of the use of a complementary therapy, a patient suffers.
Do I have permission to use the therapy from my employer, line manager, the doctor, the patient and his or her relatives?	Gaining informed consent for a particular intervention should always be a priority. It is also important that when a nurse intends to introduce a new form of care into his or her practice, it is done with the full support of managers and colleagues.
Are there any contraindications for the use of the therapy with the patients to whom I intend to offer it?	There is a danger that a complementary therapy may be seen as being safe because it is considered 'natural' or 'holistic'. This is not necessarily so, and nurses must be aware of the circumstances under which a complementary therapy should not be used.
Would a professional therapist be better able to treat the patient?	Employing a therapist or using volunteer practitioners may free a nurse's time for other essential nursing care. This may benefit patients more than trying to incorporate the use of complementary therapies into a nurse's already busy schedule.

simpler techniques can be self administered by the parents or the children themselves. Most importantly, the complementary treatments discussed are non-invasive and they do not hurt. Whilst complementary therapies have been held to be effective for a wide range of problems (Table 14.5), it is only within the last ten years that systematic evaluations have started to appear. Whilst more research is undoubtedly needed, initial results appear promising. There is reason to believe that complementary therapies have a role to play in modern child healthcare.

In some parts of the world therapies may be used as an alternative to conventional treatment rather than as complementary to other forms of treatment. In China, for example, acupuncture is used to provide anaesthesia; in France essential oils are administered internally to kill bacterial and fungal infections and are used by some medical practitioners in preference over conventional pharmacological therapy. However in the UK complementary therapies are generally used in addition to conventional medicine rather than in opposition to it

or as a sole means of treatment (Murray & Shepherd 1988).

The two disciplines (conventional and complementary) work together very successfully to bring about healing of the whole person, which is one of the major aims of the complementary therapist. Currently there is a swing back to the natural therapies as drug therapy often fails to live up to expectations. Current health initiatives encourage individuals to take responsibility for their own and their children's health, and allowing parents to have access to an extended range of treatments will facilitate them exercising their rights and responsibilities. Nursing as a profession is increasingly concerned with delivering high quality care that aims to be child and family centred and based on an individualistic and holistic philosophy. The opportunity to develop holistic and complementary therapy skills offers a development of the nursing role and is well suited to the caring and artistic component of nursing practice.

Table 14.5 Appropriate therapies for individual problems.

	Aromatherapy	Massage	Reflexology	Shiatsu
Anxiety	✓	✓		✓
Arthritis (rheumatoid)	✓			
Asthma	✓	✓	✓	✓
Bronchitis	✓		✓	✓
Colds	✓		✓	
Colic	✓	✓	✓	✓
Constipation	✓	✓	✓	✓
Diarrhoea	✓		✓	
Eczema	✓	✓		
Eneuresis	✓			✓
Hyperactivity	✓	✓	✓	✓
Infectious disease	✓			
Insomnia	✓	✓	✓	✓
Learning difficulties	✓	✓	✓	✓
Low energy	✓	✓		✓
Low grade infection	✓		✓	
Nausea and vomiting	✓			✓
Pain	✓	✓	✓	✓
Physical handicap	✓	✓	✓	✓
Stress/fear	✓	✓	✓	✓
Fungal infection	✓			

REFERENCES AND FURTHER READING

Adamson, S. (1993) Hands on Therapy. *Health Visitor*, 66(2).

Arnould-Taylor, W. (1977) *The Principles and Practice of Physical Therapy*. Stanley Thornes, Cheltenham.

Auckett, A. (1982) *Baby Massage*. Thorsons, London.

Beck, M. (1988) *The Theory and Practice of Therapeutic Massage*. Milady Publishing, London.

Belaiche, P. (1985) Treatment of vaginal infections of *candida albicans* with essential oil of *Melaleuca alternifolia*. *Phytotherapie*, 15, 13–15.

Berry, A. (1986) Knowledge at one's fingertips. *Nursing Times*, 3 December, 56–7.

Betts, T. (1994) Sniffing the breeze. *Aromatherapy Quarterly*, Spring, 19–22.

Booth, C., Johnson-Crowley, N. & Barnard, K. (1985) Infant massage and exercise – worth the effort? *Maternal and Child Nursing*, 10(3), 184–9.

Buckle, J. (1992) Which Lavender Oils? *Nursing Times*, 88(32).

Buckle, J. (1993) Aromatherapy. *Nursing Times*, 89(20).

Carruthers, A-M. (1992) A force to promote bonding and wellbeing. Therapeutic touch and massage. *Professional Nurse*, Feb, 297–300.

Chaitow, L. (1980) *Neuromuscular Technique*, p. 39. Thorsons, London.

Davis, P. (1988) *Aromatherapy, an A–Z*, p. 261. C.W. Daniel, Essex.

Dawes, J. & Harrold, F. (1990) *Massage Cures*. Thorsons, London.

Deans, S. & Svoboda, K. (1990) The antimicrobial properties of marjoram (*Origanum Marjorana L.*) volatile oil. *Flavour and Fragrance Journal*, 5(3), 187–90.

Dunn, C. (1992) *Staying in Touch – a report on a randomised controlled trial*. Battle Hospital, Reading.

Dye, J. (1992) *Aromatherapy for Women and Children*, p. 47. C.W. Daniel, Saffron Walden.

Emly, M. (1993) Abdominal Massage. *Nursing Times*, 89(3).

Engen, T. (1988) The acquisition of odour hedonics. *Perfumery* (eds S. Van Toller & G. Dodd), pp. 80–83. Chapman & Hall, London.

Ersser, S. (1990) Touch and Go. *Nursing Standard*, 4(28), 39.

Feltham, E. (1991) Therapeutic touch and massage. *Nursing Standard*, 5(45), 26–8.

Field, T. & Scafidi, F.S. (1987) Massage of preterm newborns to improve growth and development. *Pediatric Nursing*, 13(6), 385–7.

Goleman, D. (1988) The experience of touch: research points to a critical role. *The New York Times*, 2 February, p. C1.

Gulliver, N. (1988) Shiatsu. In *Complementary Therapies: a guide for nurses and the caring professions* (ed. D.F. Rankin-Box). Croom Helm, London.

Hall, N.M. (1991) *Reflexology A Way to Better Health*. Gateway Books, Bath.

Hardy, M. (1991) Sweet Scented Dreams. *International Journal of Aromatherapy*, 3(2).

Heinl, H. (1982) *The Baby Massage Book*. Coventure, London.

Jourard, S.M. (1968) *Disclosing Man to Himself*. Van Nostrand, Princeton.

Kramer, N. (1990) Comparison of therapeutic touch and causal touch in stress reduction of hospitalised children. *Pediatric Nursing*, 16(5), 483–5.

Krieger, D., Peper, E. & Ancoli, S. (1979) Therapeutic touch: searching for evidence of physiological change. *American Journal of Nursing*, 79, 660–62.

Larsen, J. (1990) Infants' colic and belly massage. *Practitioner*, 234, 22 April, 396–7.

Lawless, J. (1992) *The Encyclopaedia of Essential Oils*, p. 125. Element Books, Shaftesbury.

Leboyer, F. (1977) *Loving Hands*. Jarrold & Sons, Norwich.

LeMay, A. (1986) The Human Connection. *Nursing Times*, 19 Nov, 29–30.

Macnish, S. (1991) The Soothing Touch. *International Journal of Aromatherapy*, 3(1).

Maxwell-Hudson, C. (1991) *The Complete Book of Massage*. Dorling Kindersley, London.

McCaffery, M. & Beebe, A. (1989) *Pain: Clinical Manual for Nursing Practice*. Mosby, St. Louis.

Melzack, R. & Wall, P.D. (1965) Pain mechanisms: a new theory. *Science*, 150, 971–9.

Melzack, R. & Wall, P.D. (1988) *The Challenge of Pain*, 2nd edn. Penguin Books, Harmondsworth.

Mitchell, P., Habermann-Little, B., Johnson, F., VanInwegen-Scott, D. & Tyler, D. (1985) Critically ill children: the importance of touch in a high-technology environment. *Nursing Administration Quarterly*, 9(4).

Montague, A. (1978) *Touching*. Harper & Row, New York.

Montagu, A. (1986) *Touching, The Human Significance of Skin*, p. 262. Harper & Row, New York.

Murray, J. & Shepherd, S. (1988) Alternative or additional medicine? – a new dilemma for doctors. *Journal of the Royal College of Physicians*, 38, pp. 511–14.

Nelson, D., Heitman, R. & Jennings, C. (1986) Effects of tactile stimulation on premature infants' weight gain. *Journal of Obstetric, Gyneocologic and Neonatal Nursing*, May/June, 262–267.

Norman, L. (1988) *The Reflexology Handbook*, pp. 194–217. Piatkus, London.

Nursing Times (1994) *Nursing Times Guide to Using Complementary Therapies in Nursing*. Nursing Times, London.

Patterson, L. (1990) Baby massage in the neonatal unit. *Nursing: Journal of Practice Education and Management*, 4(23), 19–22.

Peneol, D. & Franchomme, P. (1990) *L'Aromatherapie Exactement*. Roger Jollois Publishers, Paris.

Polden, S. & Beadslee, C. (1990) Contacts experienced by neonates in intensive care environments. *Maternal-Child Nursing Journal*, 16(3), 207–26.

Rankin-Box, D. (1992) Complementary Therapies in 1992. *Nursing*, 4(47), 27–8.

Rankin-Box, D. (1993) Innovation in Practice. *Complementary Therapies in Nursing*, 1, 30–33.

Ryman, D. (1991) *Aromatherapy. The Encyclopedia of Plants and Oils and How they Help You*. Piatkus, London.

Saks, M. (1992) *Alternative Medicine in Britain*, p. 223. Clarendon Press, Oxford.

Stannard, D. (1989) Pressure prevents nausea . . . acupressure band. *Nursing Times*, 85(4), 33–4.

Tilton, J. (1992) Massage in Medicine. *Journal of Community Nursing*, Oct, 4–6.

Torii, S., Fukuda, H., Kanemoto, H., Miyanchi, R., Hamauzu, Y. & Kawasaki, M. (1988) Contingent negative variation (CNV) and the psychological effects of odour. *Perfumery, the Psychology and Biology of Fragrance* (eds S. Toller & G.H. Dodd), pp. 107–18. Chapman & Hall, London.

Tutton, E. (1991) An exploration of touch and its use in nursing. In *Therapy* (eds R. McMahon & A. Pearson). Chapman & Hall, London.

UKCC (1992a) *Code of Professional Conduct for the Nurse, Midwife and Health Visitor*. United Kingdom Central Council for Nursing, Midwifery and Health Visiting, London.

UKCC (1992b) *The Scope of Professional Practice*. United Kingdom Central Council for Nursing, Midwifery and Health Visiting, London.

Warm, J.S., Dember, W.N. & Parasuraman, R. (1990) Effects of fragrances on vigilance performance and stress. *Perfumer and Flavorist*, 15, 15–18.

Watson, W. (1975) The meanings of touch: geriatric nursing. *Journal of Communication*, 25, 104–10.

White-Traut, R. & Carrier Goldman, M. (1988) Premature baby massage: is it safe? *Pediatric Nursing*, 14(4), 285–9.

INTRODUCTION

It is now recognized that children and their families in receipt of health care should be attended to by practitioners who have been specifically educated for that purpose. A series of reforms initiated by the Platt Report (MoH 1959) helped to promote a child/family-centred philosophy of healthcare for all interested professional groups, by promoting a psychosocial approach to healthcare provision. In addition to these reforms children's nurses are increasingly influenced by the growing number of conceptual frameworks which have been developed to describe and guide nursing practice (While 1991).

This chapter will initially assess the relevance of nursing models as frameworks for child health nursing practice, and will then examine the utility of three conceptual frameworks using a case study approach. The chapter concludes with a brief consideration of how to choose an appropriate framework to guide practice, and with some suggestions for a way forward for child health nursing.

NURSING MODELS ADAPTED AND/OR DEVELOPED FOR USE BY CHILDREN'S NURSES

A nursing model is, essentially, a representation of how nursing is, should, or could be practised. It offers a philosophy, aims and objectives for providing care. These elements are usually defined and organized within four main concepts which could be considered to be central to nursing practice: person, nursing, health and environment (Fawcett 1989). The components of nursing models have been described in depth elsewhere (Aggleton & Chalmers 1986; Pearson & Vaughan 1986; Salvage & Kershaw 1990) and readers are advised to consult these or other similar texts for a more detailed overview.

There is an abundance of nursing models which have been developed and promoted as conceptual frameworks to provide guidelines for nurses, and that can be adapted for any client group. Nevertheless, Miles (1985) complained that no model had emerged that was designed specifically to guide children's nursing and suggested

that this was because a medical focus of care still predominated in child health practices. There have since been several attempts to devise or adapt conceptual frameworks for this purpose (Casey 1988; Cheetham 1988; Clarke 1988; MacDonald 1988; While 1991; Mason 1993; Welch 1993).

Yet in spite of this it seems that no studies have been conducted in the UK to assess the extent to which nursing models have actually been used in the child healthcare setting, or of their actual/potential value in this field. A review of recent literature suggests tht the models put forward by Roper *et al.* (1990), Roy (1976) and Orem (1991) have been applied in a limited number of places. There is also growing interest in Casey's (1988) partnership model which was designed specifically for the child healthcare setting. Other models, for example King (1971) and Henderson (1966), are also used but are less frequently cited.

This situation is not unique to children's nursing (Johnson 1986; Draper 1992) and many authors challenge the value of nursing models as realistic guides for practice. Johnson (1986), for example, states that models are merely speculative ideologies, whilst Webb (1984) suggests that they amount to no more than a collection of unverified assumptions which reflect the authors' value systems. Hardy (1986) also complains that the perspectives of the consumer (i.e. the patient/client) are not usually considered and that models promote jargon and specialized concepts which require lengthy orientation. However, there are many writers who support the concept of model-based nursing practice (Salvage & Kershaw 1990; Millar 1990; Walsh 1991), pointing out that these frameworks represent an important milestone in the development of British nursing practice. Problems associated with their application to clinical practice can often be related more to the wholesale acceptance of assumptions put forward in a given model, or of their interpretation for nursing practice, than to the basic concepts of the models themselves.

Whether the currently available models are of any real use for children's nurses will depend largely on the philosophies and commitment of individual and collective users. However, before any children's nurse is tempted to reject them out-of-hand, perhaps they should consider once again the research conducted by Pamela Hawthorne (1974). Hawthorne showed that nurses provided task orientated rather than client or family centred care, partly as a result of inadequate education relating to all aspects of child development. Since there was no mention of care planning in the study, it could be assumed that care was recorded in the standard nursing record systems in which the necessary nursing actions related to medical diagnoses were usually described. Thus planned physical care would be carried out, but it is evident from Hawthorne's conclusions that nurses neglected to identify properly the nursing needs of children which did not arise directly from the medical diagnoses.

It could be argued that Hawthorne's (1974) research highlighted the consequences of providing nursing care that lacked any meaningful philosophy and/or any meaningful framework to guide experienced and inexperienced nurses alike. This study has been influential in the advancement of children's nursing, in particular for improving standards of care by urging nurses to recognize that their practice should focus on the psychosocial needs of the children and not just their medical diagnoses. The use of nursing models as one means to achieve this may help nurses reflect on their professional values and beliefs. However, it is disappointing that there is still relatively little which has been written regarding the practical application of nursing models in the child health setting. The following case studies will therefore offer an interpretation of ways in which certain models can be used to provide family-centred care. Although suggestions for further reading are provided it is not the intention of this chapter to supply in-depth details related to any medical diagnoses or treatments cited in the case studies. Readers are advised to refer to relevant chapters in this text for more detailed information.

APPLYING OREM'S SELF-CARE DEFICIT MODEL FOR THE PROVISION OF HOME-BASED NURSING CARE

Dorothea Orem devised this nursing model in the late 1950s and since that time the concepts for nursing practice have been continuously reviewed and updated, most recently in the 1991 edition of the text (Orem 1991). It is based upon the systems and developmental theories (Fawcett 1989; Orem 1991). The model has

been devised from Orem's theory of self-care which is defined as: '... the personal care that human beings require each day and that may be modified by health state, environmental conditions, the effects of medical care and other factors' (Orem 1991). It is argued that self-care is a learned, goal oriented activity of individuals and recognized that in relation to children, self-care acts may be undertaken by responsible adults acting on their behalf. This sub-concept of self-care is described as dependent care and it incorporates all the therapeutic activities performed by responsible others, for any socially dependent individuals.

Included in Orem's model are two other theories related to self-care: the self-care deficit theory of nursing, and the theory of nursing systems. The self-care deficit theory of nursing has its origins in what Orem describes as the proper object of nursing; that is, that nursing is a response to an individual's/group's recurring incapacity to care for themselves or their dependents when action is limited because of health care needs. The theory of nursing systems is the organizing component of the model because it establishes the form nursing will take, that is whether to provide total, partial or supportive care, and the relationship between child, family and nurse.

The need for self-care or dependent care arises from care which is required momentarily, or for a duration, for a particular purpose. Orem (1991) defines such purposes as therapeutic self-care demands and there are three types:

(1) Universal – which includes eight components related to life function, common to all individuals.
(2) Developmental – which describe major developmental milestones.
(3) Health deviation – which arise because of ill-health (Elliott 1991; Orem 1991).

When the therapeutic self-care demands of a person or their dependent(s) exceed their ability to meet such demands, a deficit exists.

If the deficit is related to the health of the person or their dependent(s), nursing and/or other types of professional healthcare may be required (Fig. 15.1).

Orem (1991) utilizes the nursing process framework and identifies four main stages:

(1) Diagnosis (assessment).
(2) Prescription (planning).

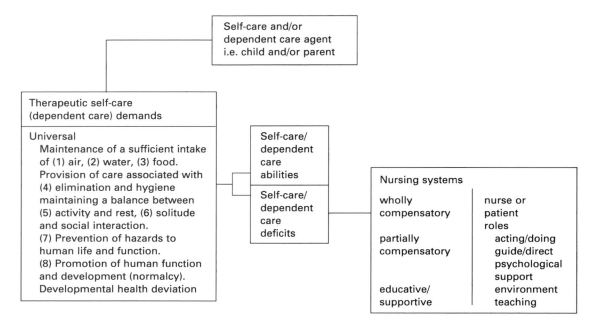

Fig. 15.1   Overview of Orem's self-care deficit nursing model.

(3) Treatment/regulation (intervention).

(4) Case management (evaluation).

It can be seen that these stages equate to those which are more commonly referred to in the UK and Cavanagh (1991) offers a very useful comparison of both approaches. Orem proposes that the purpose of assessment is to diagnose a person's needs for nursing care. Planning involves deciding upon the level and extent of nursing care which may be required, that is, whether the nurse needs to provide wholly compensatory, partially compensatory or educative/supportive care. The decision is based on the child's abilities and/or the presence of others to provide dependent care. It also specifies the actions which will be necessary to achieve therapeutic care. The final two steps incorporate the provision and continuing evaluation of nursing care.

This model offers an important way forward in the development of a philosophy for the nursing care of children and their families. It promotes partnership by encouraging nurses to assess the self-care abilities of a child in relation to development, and to assess the role to be played by families of children with health problems and needs. Orem (1991) suggests that parents providing dependent care may contribute to ongoing nursing care

with supervision. It is also possible to combine the nursing actions with those of the child/family to meet the child's therapeutic self-care demands and to regulate or promote their abilities for self/dependent care.

However, there are several identified limitations to the self-care approach. For example, the model comprises jargon which may be difficult to interpret; it assumes that potential clients favour a self-care approach to health care delivery and it may be seen to reduce people into a series of systems and subsystems. In spite of this, there is increasing evidence that children's nurses in the UK are overcoming such limitations and in doing so are recognizing the potential of Orem's model to guide their practice (Stephenson 1987; Cheetham 1988; Elliott 1991; Welch 1993a).

Case study 1 shows how Orem's model has been adapted to promote self-care for a family whose child has experienced lengthy hospitalization, and enables them to meet his needs at home.

Case Study 1

Jason Williams is a boy of four months who has had malabsorption caused by nonspecific enterocolitis (intractable diarrhoea) since he was five weeks old. In spite of exhaustive investigations, the cause for the diarrhoea has yet to be identified and attempts to re-introduce oral feeding have not been successful. Jason is currently receiving total parenteral nutrition (TPN) (Table 15.1) whilst efforts to determine and treat the cause of his diarrhoea continue. Jason faces the prospect of long-term supportive therapy to maintain his nutritional needs, and therefore it is considered desirable by both his parents and the healthcare team that he should be cared for in his home environment as this would promote optimal development (Sinclair & Whyte 1987).

Jason is the only child of Evelyn and Mike Williams, both in their late thirties, and they live on the outskirts of a large city 15 miles from the hospital where Jason is being treated. Mrs Williams stopped working as a primary school teacher when her son was born; her husband is a manager for a cement company. The family live in a semi-detached house and

although there are no relatives living close by, they have many friends in their neighbourhood. Jason's most recent admission to hospital has been for five weeks, and for most of the time he has been receiving TPN. His weight has been gradually increasing during the past two weeks, and apart from his weight and height he has reached the developmental mile-stones consistent for a child of his age.

Jason's mother provides most of his daytime care, apart from management of his TPN. Both parents have been taught the principles of intravenous feed-ing via a central venous line, and of administration of medications, and have been told about the benefits and potential complications of TPN therapy (James & Mott 1988; Stapleford 1990). Nursing care, which has promoted family participation from the outset, is now focusing on Mr and Mrs Williams' dependent care abilities (on behalf of their son) in preparation for Jason's aftercare and subsequent support in the community (see care plan 1).

Table 15.1 Total parenteral nutrition (TPN) – the provision of all nutritional requirements by the intravenous route.

> - It provides complete intravenous caloric support and access to a positive nitrogen balance and homeostatic control of fluid, electrolyte and metabolic function.
> - TPN was first used in 1968 (Hazinski 1984) and is now widely established as a means to supply nutrition to nutritionally compromized patients. Developments in TPN have increased its potential for successful usage. For example:
>   - Increased understanding of nutritional needs during illness.
>   - Development of safer, more efficient equipment (e.g. silicone catheters).
>   - Formulation and preparation of daily feeding programmes.
>   - Utilization of a multidisciplinary approach to care (Atkins 1989).
>
> TPN is used more as a supportive than a curative therapy for infants and children and it may be used over long periods of time. It is required when there is evidence of protein calorie malnutrition (PCM) and when it is not possible to provide nutritional support directly to the gastro-intestinal tract (enteral nutrition) (Silk 1989).

Assessment

It can be seen from Jason's care plan that assessment, using Orem's (1991) therapeutic self-care demands as a framework, has focused upon his current self-care abil-ities and the dependent care he is receiving from his parents. This is followed by the identification of self or dependent care deficits, allowing for nursing or family diagnoses to be made. Such an approach has immediate advantages for children's nurses who seek to promote family-centred care, by highlighting what a child can do for him/herself in relation to his/her development and health state, and what care parents (or other primary carers) are able to do on their chid's behalf. In Jason's case he is too young to contribute to most of his needs and so the emphasis is placed on his parents' dependent care abilities/deficits.

When using a self/dependent care approach it is essential that any nursing diagnoses are agreed on with the family, especially if the diagnosis is based on a dependent care deficit. Nursing and family perceptions of self or dependent care abilities and/or deficits may differ markedly. It is therefore important for nursing staff to negotiate with relevant family members when differences of opinion exist, if successful self/dependent

Care plan 1 – Assessment of Jason Williams

Therapeutic self-care demands	Self-care abilities	Dependent care given	Self or dependent care deficits
Universal self-care requisites			
(1) Maintaining a sufficient intake of air	Maintains own airway. Breaths normally, colour pink. Respiratory rate 22/min.	Able to provide additional support when necessary, e.g. assisting with optimal sleeping position.	None
(2) (3) Maintaining a sufficient intake of water and food	Cannot tolerate oral feeds – tolerating TPN therapy via a central line and is gaining weight (weight 5.5 kg).	Mrs Williams provides 4 hourly mouth care and feeds Jason with clear fluids when this is allowed (see diet sheet). Both parents help to monitor TPN and care for IV central line and assist with administration of Jason's medications. Parents have knowledge of principles of TPN therapy.	Jason is underweight for his age (birth weight 3.72 kg). Parents unable to manage TPN independently. Jason is too young to be self-caring.
(4) Provision of care associated with elimination and hygiene	Able to urinate without difficulty; faeces very soft and usually foul smelling, loose and dark green in appearance. Skin on buttocks slightly excoriated. Is able to cry when nappy is wet or dirty.	Mrs Williams maintains Jason's hygiene needs, frequent nappy changes and application of barrier cream to buttocks. She monitors and reports on the amount and consistency of Jason's faecal output.	Parents may be unsure how to cope with changes in Jason's elimination patterns when he is discharged. Jason is too young to be self-caring.
(5) Maintaining a balance between activity and rest	Plays with soft toys in cot and mobiles; enjoys the attention of parents and hospital staff and being taken for walks in his pram. Cries quickly if left alone. Rest: usually settles by 9pm and sleeps continuously until 5am unless he soils his nappy or there are problems with his TPN therapy; sleeps for 1–2 hrs in the am and again in the pm.	Mrs Williams is with Jason until he settles for the night; both parents provide most stimulation for him and are knowledgeable about play appropriate for his stage of development. Mrs Williams feels she will cope well with Jason at home if he continues these activity/rest routines.	None at present; for re-assessment three days after discharge.
(6) Maintaining a balance between solitude and social interaction	Enjoys the company of others and being talked to – attempts to respond verbally and laughs easily. Cries if left alone, particularly if his mum leaves the room; is used to being in a room on his own at night and does not cry as soon as he wakes, unless he is cold or dirty.	Both parents interact with Jason very well and are very attentive towards him. Mrs Williams says she gets frustrated at times because she feels isolated because of Jason's special needs. She is worried about how this will affect her life in the longer term, and both her and her husband's contact with others.	Parents (especially mother) may need relief from providing dependant care at intervals, to facilitate long-term coping patterns.
(7) Maintaining safety	Unable to maintain own safety due to young age.	Parents able to maintain Jason's safety needs; they are aware of potential hazards in the home and hospital environments and have already taken many measures to promote Jason's safety after discharge.	None
(8) Being normal	Unable to express awareness of self due to young age.	Parents feel Jason is developing well in spite of his illness and do not think he is different from others.	None

Care plan 1 – Assessment of Jason Williams (contd.)

Therapeutic self-care demands	Self-care abilities	Dependent care given	Self or dependent care deficits
Developmental self-care requisites (1) Initiating and maintaining conditions which promote all aspects of child development.	Gross motor: able to raise head and trunk from cot and roll from side to side; head balance is good. Fine motor: able to grasp objects and plays with hands; vocalizes well making sounds; sight and hearing appear normal; enjoys attention and interaction	Both parents able to maintain and promote Jason's growth and development: have good knowledge of normal development milestones and show great interest in Jason's abilities.	None
(2) Provisions of care to prevent conditions which may adversely affect child development.	Unable to prevent problems occurring due to his young age.	Parents feel able to promote an optimal developmental environment; however, they are worried about the effects of long-term use of TPN.	Parents need to be advised re. preventing developmental problems whilst Jason is on TPN at home.
Health deviation self-care requisites (1) Attending to the effects of pathological conditions	Unable to do so due to young age.	Parents aware of how to seek support to care for Jason at home. The primary healthcare team is aware of Jason's pending discharge and a community paediatric nurse has already been in contact with the family and conducted a home assessment. Parents have a good relationship with their GP and feel confident in their relationship with her and her ability to support them.	Parents may not be aware of all the community resources available to support them.
(2) Learning to live with the effects of pathological conditions and medical care in a way which promotes personal development	Unaware of illness state due to young age.	Parents have not been given a definite medical diagnosis for their son's health problems. They are frustrated by this and are hopeful he will make a complete recovery.	Parents may not have accepted that their son requires long-term medical/nursing care.

Care plan 1 – Planning, implementation/evaluation for Jason Williams

Nursing/family diagnosis	Goal	Nursing care	Family care	Eval. date	Evaluation
(1) Parents have a knowledge deficit related to home management of TPN	For parents to demonstrate their ability to manage Jason's TPN.	With Jason's parents: (1) Review principles of TPN therapy. (2) Provide detailed instructions in writing. (3) Demonstrate care procedures. (4) Observe parents carrying out procedures until they reach competence. (5) Inform parents how fluids and equipment will be delivered and stored. (6) Review potential problems of TPN and how parents should deal with them.	With Jason's nurse: (1) Describe the principles of TPN therapy. (2) Practice care procedures until both feel competent to work independently. (3) State how they will receive and store fluids/equipment. (4) Describe potential problems and how they will deal with them. (5) Ensure written instructions and advice have been provided.	(1) In 24 hr (2–5) in 4 days	
(2) Jason may have altered elimination patterns at home (exacerbation of acute diarrhoea)	For Jason's parents to be prepared to manage this potential problem.	(1) Ensure Jason's parents are aware of who to contact if this occurs. (2) Review how parents will manage his elimination and hygiene routines at home and offer advice if appropriate.	(1) State how they will seek help if a problem arises. (2) Describe how they will continue to manage Jason's elimination and hygiene routines at home.	In 24 hrs	
(3) Parents (especially mum) may feel isolated when meeting Jason's special needs at home	For Jason's parents to feel they will receive adequate support at home	(1) Ascertain what social support may be already available. (2) Discuss with both parents their potential for taking breaks from dependent care. (3) Discuss parents' plans for organizing Jason's routines to maximize free time (e.g. TPN will be administered at night).	(1) Review own social support systems and possible deficits. (2) Discuss possible assistance that might be needed in order to take breaks. (3) Start to plan for desired routines re. Jason's care once they are discharged.	In 4 days	
(4) Parents are anxious re. the effects of long-term use of TPN on Jason's development	For parents to be made aware of factors related to TPN therapy which may adversely affect Jason's development.	(1) Review with parents potential factors which may adversely affect Jason's development, how to manage them or how to seek support. (2) Review community (or other) resources parents may utilize.	(1) Discuss any potential problems one or both may feel unable to cope with and how they might cope or seek assistance.	In 4 days	
(5) Parents are frustrated because no medical diagnosis has been made	For parents to be kept up-to-date with results of investigations and future plans for Jason's medical care.	(1) Review with parents their understanding of Jason's current health stage. (2) Check with them what arrangements have been made for ongoing medical care and whether they feel satisfied with this. (3) Arrange for parents to see Jason's consultant if necessary.	(1) Outline perceptions of Jason's health state. (2) Review arrangements for medical follow-up and if this is satisfactory for the whole family. (3) Discuss situation with Jason's consultant, if desired.	In 4 days	

care is to be a reality. In such cases nurses should draw on their specialist knowledge of a given problem and then help child/family members to apply it to their unique situation. Jason's parents will have to cope with his special needs related to his treatment as well as his dependence on them as an infant, and so nursing (family) diagnoses highlight their knowledge, psychomotor deficits and psychosocial needs.

Planning, implementation and evaluation

Planning care for Jason involves setting goals to address each diagnosis which has been made, and outlining what care will be provided by nursing staff and what care will be carried out by his parents. A date is also set to make a summative evaluation, although care will also be continuously evaluated on a formative basis. The care plan could also be used to document the nursing system that will be utilized, that is, wholly or partially compensatory, or educative/supportive, and to record formative evaluations in the forms of progress notes. These particular features have not been illustrated on Jason's plan.

By organizing care in this way, children's nurses can facilitate the achievement of goals for independent self/dependent care and negotiate nurse and family roles. In fact, Orem's self-care deficit theory of nursing has already helped children's nurses to negotiate with children and/or their families, rather than to make assumptions regarding children's or their families' abilities for self/dependent care (Wesolowski 1988; Elliott 1991; Biehler 1992). Jason's care plan demonstrates that nursing actions are aimed at increasing the family's independence in preparation for his discharge, but only where deficits have been agreed upon by both the nurse and his parents.

In addition to the nursing systems designed for implementing care, Orem (1991) also identifies five helping methods which may be chosen by the nurse:

- Acting or doing for another.
- Guiding another.
- Supporting another.
- Teaching another.
- Providing an environment that supports development.

These helping methods can also be utilized for dependent care purposes; however, it is important to consider who is accountable for care given by a child/parent (Charles Edwards & Casey 1992). Mrs Williams is already providing for the majority of Jason's self-care needs and so nursing care is based mainly on an educative/supportive system using any of the helping methods outlined above, as appropriate.

Evaluation of care for the Williams family will focus on whether the set goals have been achieved and, consequently, whether the family are ready to go home and provide for Jason's self-care needs with community care support. The success of this phase of care depends upon input from self/dependent carers or parents who should be encouraged to offer their own evaluation of the situation. In this way nursing staff using the self-care framework will continue to place children and their families at the centre of the nursing process. It will also increase the validity of any judgements made, and will reinforce the importance of negotiation for promoting self/dependent care.

Discussion

Case study 1 illustrates the potential benefits of Orem's self-care deficit model for nursing if applied to child/family centred care. The identification of family routines and family roles related to dependent care, and the self-care abilities of children as they develop, all contribute to optimizing development for a child who is beset by health problems. In this situation the self-care approach facilitates parental involvement which is so crucial at his time of life. Other users of Orem's model have illustrated ways in which it can facilitate the child's involvement either in conjunction with, or independently from, other family members (Eichelberger *et al.* 1980; Wesolowski 1988). The recognition of developmental and health deviation self-care requisites means that assessment is thorough, highlighting the child's social situation and emotional/psychological qualities, his or her ability to adapt during illness, and their knowledge of the circumstances they find themselves in.

In spite of these positive attributes, Orem's nursing model may not be an appropriate framework for all children and their families. Elliott (1991), for example, points out that some parents are not always in a position to provide dependent care away from the family home due to other commitments or social restrictions. In addition, children capable of providing their own self-care may feel that they are being 'left to get on with things' at a time when they might benefit from increased dependent or nursing care. There is also the potential for overlap between developmental/health deviation and universal self-care requisites; for example, children's universal self-care requisites are continuously undergoing change as they develop.

Finally, it must be remembered that like many other models, Orem's framework was not devised exclusively for children and their families, although recently the author has made many alterations to enhance a more user-friendly approach in a family context (Orem 1991). If children's nurses and families are attracted by the underlying philosophy and dependent-care concept, they may need to adapt it further to suit particular situations, to alter some of the terminology to ease communication, and to promote its use amongst other health care professionals.

APPLYING ROPER, LOGAN AND TIERNEY'S ACTIVITIES OF LIVING MODEL TO CARE FOR A YOUNG BOY IN HOSPITAL

Nancy Roper commenced work on a nursing model in the mid 1970s as part of a Master of Science degree at Edinburgh University (Roper 1976). She was later joined by Winifred Logan and Alison Tierney and together they developed Roper's ideas into a conceptual framework which was first published in 1980 (Roper *et al.* 1986). The model is based upon human needs theory and is influenced by behavioural and developmental theories. It is also described as having the foundations of systems theory (Newton 1991). Roper *et al.* (1990) were inspired by the work of Virginia Henderson (1966) when creating their model which is widely accepted as the first British attempt at a major conceptual framework for nursing practice. Roper *et al.* continued to develop the work throughout the 1980s and the latest edition was published in 1990.

The activities of living (A/L) model is based upon a model for living and focuses on a person's individuality

and independence in 12 activities of living. Nursing is defined as:

'Helping patients to prevent, alleviate or solve, or cope with actual or potential problems related to the activities of living' (Roper *et al.* 1990)

Five components can be identified within this framework, all of which are closely interrelated (Fig. 15.2). In both the model for living and the model for nursing the first four components are identical. The fifth component changes from individuality in living (Fig. 15.2) to individuality in nursing (Fig. 15.3). The Roper *et al.* model also uses a four stage nursing process to individualize patient care:

(1) Assessing.
(2) Planning.
(3) Implementing .
(4) Evaluating.

Roper *et al.* stress that using terms such as assessing helps to underpin the active and dynamic nature of the nursing process (Fig. 15.4). The authors do not identify nursing diagnosis as a stage of care within their framework, but recognize that the identification of patients' problems corresponds to this phase of care. The development and use of child health nursing diagnoses within the UK has recently been initiated in some settings (Hamilton 1990; Mason & Webb 1993); however, the concept has not been widely applied in clinical practice.

Roper *et al.* (1990) advocate that patients should, as far as possible, be active participants in their care in order to encourage personal responsibility for health and to protect personal autonomy in illness. In the case of children, the authors suggest that family members may participate on their behalf as they would usually do at home.

This option of family participation is not expanded upon in the model and consequently offers no real guidance for children's nurses, who view children and their families as partners in care. Where the model has been applied to the care of children (for example, Jones & While 1991; Newton 1991), there is little indication of active participation by the child or family in the care planning process. A study by Webb & Mason (1993) also shows that nurses who were using Roper *et al.*'s framework in one children's hospital, failed to acknowledge most of the care provided by children and their families in their care plans. Case Study 2 will

Model of living

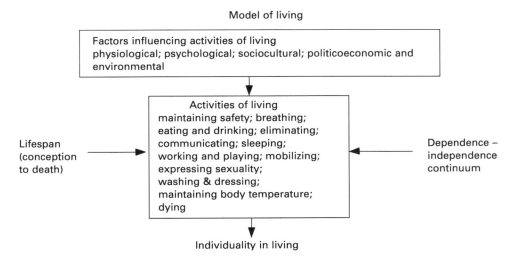

Fig. 15.2 Overview of Roper *et al.*'s (1990) activities of living model (1).

Model of nursing

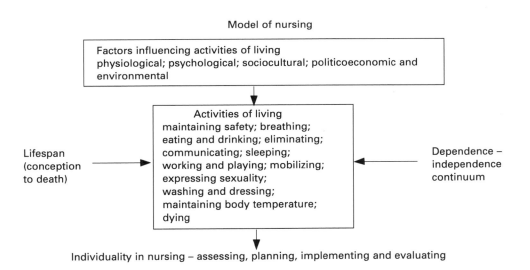

Fig. 15.3 Overview of Roper *et al.*'s (1990) activities of living model (2).

therefore offer an alternative adaptation of the Roper *et al.* model for the care of a hospitalized child and its family, which illustrates the participative process.

Case study 2

Ian Denton is a ten year old boy who was knocked down by a car. He sustained multiple superficial grazes to his arms, legs and face and a full thickness friction burn to his right thigh. This latter injury necessitated the application of a thin-split skin graft (taken from Ian's left thigh) under general anaesthetic (Table 15.2).

Ian is the youngest in a family of five children ranging in age from ten to seventeen years. He is the third son for Andy and Sarah Denton and they form

Assessing ────────▶ Planning

- Collecting information from or about the patient.
- Reviewing the information.
- Identifying patients' problems.
- Identifying priorities among problems.

- To prevent potential problems from becoming actual ones.
- To solve actual problems.
- To alleviate problems which cannot be solved.
- To help patients cope with problems.
- Setting goals and preparing a plan.

Evaluating

- Determining if goals have been achieved.
- Re-assessing, continuing or re-planning care.
- Terminating care.

Implementing ↓

- Putting the care plan into action to achieve the aims of the planning process.
- Helping patients to prevent, alleviate, solve or cope with problems.

Fig. 15.4   Overview of Roper _et al._'s (1990) nursing process. (Adapted from written text in Chapter 5 of Roper _et al._ 1990.)

Table 15.2   Thin-split skin graft (Macallan & Jackson 1971; Norris & House 1991).

- Skin is detached from the donor site.
- Skin is detached as a thin split or a thick split depending upon the requirements of the situation.
- Since the skin is also detached from its blood supply, its survival will depend upon receiving enough nourishment and oxygen until new capillaries grow into it.

part of a large extended family who live in a town on the Scottish/English border. Mrs Denton works part-time as a secretary for an accountancy firm and her husband is an unemployed engineer. All five children are still attending school and consequently the family are receiving financial support from the State. The family interact well together and although no one is resident in hospital with Ian, there are usually visitors with him all day, particularly his father, who is with him from 10AM until 7PM daily.

Ian has now been in hospital for three days and it is 14 hours since he underwent surgery to replace skin on his right thigh. He is anxious to resume his usual activities and so nursing care will focus upon helping Ian to achieve maximum independence in his A/L (see care plan 2). The standard pre and post-operative care which is essential for all children requiring surgery is

contained in a standardized care plan for Ian and is not included in this case study.

Assessment

In using the Roper _et al._ (1990) model for Ian's assessment, the focus has been on a comparison of his normal abilities/level of independence and any present changes which have occurred since his accident and surgery, in each A/L. Jones & White (1991) point out that such an approach allows nursing staff to make a full developmental assessment of a child, as well as identifying any actual or potential problems they may have as a result of illness or other health problem. It also enables nurses to assess a child's normal routines and the part their family has to play in this. In Ian's case he is already independent in most of his A/L, with guidance, supervision and support from his parents and other family members.

In order to promote Ian's and his father's participative roles in the care planning process, the assessment records their interpretation of Ian's needs, rather than the nurse's perception of the situation, as much as possible. The identification of potential problems also highlights those of the father so that his usual parenting role is not undermined and his need for support in order to cope with Ian's problems is not undermined. The activity of dying is replaced with Ian's perception of his personal health state. This will still encourage him to assess his level of health, but without focusing on death and dying

Care plan 2 – Assessment of Ian Denton

Activities of living	Usual routines and family care	Present situation (if different from usual)	Actual (a) potential (p) problems of child/family
Mobilising	Usually very active; likes to swim and play football.	On bedrest although not immobile; unable to mobilize freely due to pain in both thighs since surgery; father assisting Ian with some movement but is worried he may increase Ian's pain.	Ian has reduced mobility due to pain in both thighs and the effects of surgery. (a) Mr Denton has knowledge deficit related to correct lifting/handling techniques for Ian. (a)
Maintaining safety	Able to maintain own safety at home and at school; receives some guidance from parents and teachers.	Is weak and less orientated than usual due to the effects of the anaesthetic; father is able to maintain Ian's safety needs and is aware of potential dangers on the ward and the effects of anaesthetic.	Mr Denton will need support from nursing/medical staff if Ian experiences any latent effects from anaesthetic (p) (see post-op. care plan).
Communicating	Interacts well with family and friends and is confident and outgoing.	Interacts well with other children on the ward; father is helping Ian to communicate his needs and feelings to the appropriate people; Ian states that he is no longer anxious about hospital care but is missing his pet dog; he has plenty of visitors: mother comes each evening at bedtime.	
Working/playing	Attends a local primary school, is a member of the junior football team and states he has many friends. He joins in a lot of family social activities and has a pet dog, Toby.	Ian has been showing signs of boredom since admission and demands a lot of his father's attention. Father states that Ian is not used to relying on TV and board games etc. for pleasure, preferring to be 'out and about'.	Ian may become increasingly bored due to the effects of reduced mobility and the constraints of hospitalization. (p) Mr Denton may become tired trying to entertain Ian all the time. (p)
Expressing sexuality	Ian is pre-pubescent; most of his friends are boys at this time and he likes to wear what he considers to be fashionable.	No change	
Sleeping	Ian sleeps approximately 10hrs/night.	Ian's sleep patterns have altered slightly since admission, but he sleeps approximately 8 hrs/night.	Ian may have difficulty sleeping due to pain in both thighs. (p)
Eating and drinking	Prefers meat dishes, coke and puddings; weight 30kg.	Has been fasting since surgery but is now drinking fluids freely; intravenous infusion discontinued 3 hrs ago.	Ian may have altered eating patterns (anorexia) due to the effects of pain and surgery.
Eliminating	Bowels open daily; expressed no problems with eliminating.	Has passed urine since surgery; father is helping Ian to use a urinary bottle and will carry him/wheel him to the bathroom if he needs more privacy.	

Care plan 2 – Assessment of Ian Denton (cont.)

Activities of living	Usual routines and family care	Present situation (if different from usual)	Actual (a) potential (p) problems of child/family
Breathing	Respirations 16/bpm; no history of respiratory problems.	No change	
Washing and dressing	Attends to all own hygiene needs at home and at school.	Manages most of his own hygiene needs but requires some assistance whilst mobility is restricted; father is able to provide supportive care. Ian has two wounds, one on each thigh, as a result of surgery. Both have dressings on (see wound care plan). Ian and his father are not aware of what care the wound sites will require.	Ian and his father have a knowledge deficit related to management of his new skin graft and wound site. (a) Ian may experience discomfort and distress when his dressings are changed. (p)
Maintaining body temperature	Usually maintains own temperature with some guidance from parents. Temp. 36.8°C	Ian's temperature is being monitored more closely (4 hrly) since surgery, to detect early signs of wound infection; temperature remains within normal limits.	
Perception of personal health state	Ian feels he is fit and well for his age. He states that he is never usually sick and that he is more active than a lot of his friends.	Ian feels that his injuries are not as serious as they might have been; he expects to recover quickly (he has not seen his skin graft or donor site) and is aware he may have a scar. He is anxious about the effects of the accident on his ability to play football etc. Father is also anxious about this.	Ian and his father are anxious about the effects of Ian's injuries on his sporting activities. (a) Ian may develop a negative body image when he sees his new skin graft and donor site. (p)

Care plan 2 – Planning, implementation/evaluation for Ian Denton

Goals	s/t short term l/t long term	Nursing care	Family care	Eval. date	Evaluation
(1) To recommence limited mobility. (2) To keep levels of pain to a minimum. (3) To resume usual mobility patterns. (4) To be free from pain.	s/t s/t l/t l/t	(1) Administer post-op. analgesia to Ian as prescribed if he complains of pain. (2) Check dressings to ensure they are not too tight or soiled: show father how to do this. (3) Help Ian and his father to decide upon optimum positions of comfort in bed/in a chair. (4) Help Ian to gradually mobilize, starting with sitting in a chair, weight bearing, walking as directed by his doctor; show father how to assist at each stage. s/t	(1) Father will assist with administration of analgesia to Ian. (2) Father and Ian will check dressing sites and observe for any changes or soiling: support from nursing staff will be offered. (3) Ian, assisted by his father, will commence mobility programme; father will describe appropriate lifting/handling techniques for Ian to Ian's nurse and will gradually take over his care with minimum assistance.	s/t end of each shift l/t start eval. in 3 days then daily	

Care plan 2 – Planning, implementation/evaluation for Ian Denton (cont.)

Goals	s/t short term l/t long term	Nursing care	Family care	Eval. date	Evaluation
		(5) Re-assess (with Ian and father) mobility patterns and level of pain in 3 days' time. l/t	(4) Ian, assisted by his father, will assess and adopt the most comfortable positions for him in a bed/chair. (5) Father and Ian will re-assess Ian's mobility and pain levels with Ian's nurse, in 3 days' time.		
(1) For Ian to use his time constructively in hospital. s/t (2) For Ian & his father to liaise with healthcare team re. longer term rehabilitation for him. l/t		(1) Explain alternative activities that Ian and his father may engage in; playleader will also advise. (2) Encourage family and friends to continue to visit regularly. (3) Encourage Mr Denton to take breaks from Ian's care when other family members are present. (4) With other healthcare staff, help Ian and his father to address long term rehabilitation and resumption of usually activity levels (outdoor).	(1) Ian and his father will select desirable activities for Ian on a day to day basis. (2) Ian will have the company of family and friends to help to pass the time. (3) Mr Denton will negotiate with Ian when he will go for meals and other breaks, when the family are present. (4) Ian and his father will, with hospital staff, plan appropriate exercises and build-up of activity to enable Ian to resume his usual activity levels.	s/t daily l/t start in 3 days then daily	
For Ian to sleep 8–10 hrs each night, undisturbed. s/t		(1) Assess pain/anxiety levels at Ian's bedtime. (2) Administer analgesia as required. (3) If Ian wakes, stay with him and help him adopt position of comfort.	(1) Ian and his father will monitor pain patterns. (2) Father/mother will remain with Ian until he is settled for the night.	every pm and night shift	
For Ian to resume his usual eating habits. s/t		(1) Offer Ian meals at times he is used to eating. (2) Offer Ian food he likes. (3) Inform Ian and his father of the benefits of a nutritious diet for wound healing.	(1) Father will encourage Ian to resume his normal eating patterns. (2) Father and Ian will monitor what Ian eats to ensure diet promotes wound healing.	daily	
(1) For Ian and his father to assist with dressing changes. s/t (2) For Ian and his father to be able to care for Ian's new skin graft and donor site independently. l/t		(1) Explain wound care regime to Ian and his father (use wound care plan). (2) Ensure Ian is fully aware of what to expect when dressings are changed; offer analgesia before dressing changes. (3) Teach Ian and his father how to care for a new skin graft and donor sites (use wound care plan).	(1) Ian and his father will participate with Ian's dressing changes. (2) Ian will describe what he expects at dressing time; father and nurse will offer support and feedback. (3) Father and Ian will demonstrate how to care for Ian's skin graft and donor site, supervized by Ian's nurse, until they reach competence.	s/t before and after dressing change l/t start when wounds exposed then daily	

Care plan 2 – Planning, implementation/evaluation for Ian Denton (cont.)

Goals	s/t short term l/t long term	Nursing care	Family care	Eval. date	Evaluation
		(4) Offer written instructions for home use. (5) Observe Ian and father caring for new skin graft and donor site until they are competent.	(4) Father will ensure that they have written instructions to take home for long term use.		
For Ian to develop a positive body image and outlook for his future (especially in relation to sporting interests) l/t		(1) Assess Ian's reaction when he sees his skin graft and donor site. (2) Show Ian pictures of healed donor sites and skin grafts. (3) Re-inforce the positive effects of the wound care regime to promote future resumption of activity levels.	(1) Ian to assess his own wound sites and describe how they should heal; father to support Ian with this. (2) Ian and his father will describe the benefits of promoting optimal wound healing for Ian. (3) Ian and his father will be aware of Ian's full recovery potential.	start at first dressing change then daily	

when it is clearly not appropriate to his situation. This adaptation of the Roper *et al.* (1990) framework for assessment has been influenced by Orem's (1991) dependent care concept and, consequently, success is dependent upon negotiation between family members and nursing staff.

Planning, implementation and evaluation

Planning care for Ian and his father involves setting short and long term goals for all the problems identified in the assessment process, and outlining the nursing care that will be needed to achieve the set goals. Roper *et al.* (1990) argue that the identification of potential problems helps nurses to highlight their health education/health promotion roles. In Ian's case this approach enables nursing staff to consider the long term needs he and his family may have in relation to his health care and once again the process has been adapted to incorporate family care. This adds a positive dimension to the Roper *et al.* problem orientated model because it may encourage nurses to apply the concept of participation and at the same time to record activities the family can accomplish without nursing support.

Roper *et al.* (1990) state that implementing care should help patients to prevent, alleviate, solve or cope

with their identified problems. Many nurses formatively evaluate the care they (or the family) are giving in the form of progress notes. Such notes are only of value if they are offering feedback which is not already written into the plan, or if they record a child/family's feelings regarding progress in care. In Ian's case progress notes may be used for the above purposes although they are not presented in the study. Evaluation of Ian's and his father's care will focus upon whether their short term goals have been met and whether their long term needs are being satisfactorily addressed according to the original plan of care. The evaluation process should be a joint venture between child, family and nurse and as with previous stages of care, this necessitates some alterations in the Roper *et al.*'s original framework. One means of achieving this may be to record the result of family and nursing actions in different columns, or alternatively to record care from the family's perspective and then from the nurse's perspective. The latter approach will be used to record the Denton family's care.

Discussion

Case Study 2 demonstrates ways in which the Roper *et al.* framework can be adapted to promote a family centred approach to nursing care. It has also been used in at least two different settings as the basis for the development of children's nursing models (Clark & Bishop 1988; Clarke 1988; Macdonald 1988). Notwithstanding its potential in the child care setting, the model's focus on individuality and the physiological basis of the twelve A/L make this an unlikely tool to effectively guide children's nurses who assist families with long term, complex and/or specifically psychosocial needs. Although Roper *et al.* draw attention to five factors which influence each A/L, these factors cannot always be readily identified within the constraints of the twelve A/L in the framework. Walsh (1991) also questions the model's value for other client groups for similar reasons, arguing that it is too physically orientated, reductionist and fragmented.

In spite of such criticisms the model is widely established in the UK in both clinical practice and education (Newton 1991; McCaugherty 1992). The British origin and user friendly terminology have facilitated its rapid integration into many health care settings, including the child health areas. The twelve A/L offer a simple and popular framework for assessment and subsequent care planning, and perhaps because of this it is likely to be successfully applied if used for children with short term physically based needs, for example day surgery. This is, of course, assuming that appropriate adaptations are made to promote family participation and the age related psychological needs are highlighted.

APPLYING CASEY'S PARTNERSHIP IN CARE MODEL FOR A YOUNG ADULT IN HOSPITAL USING ROY'S ASSESSMENT FRAMEWORK

As mentioned in the introduction, the publication of the Platt Report (MoH 1959) heralded a new beginning for children with health problems/needs. It provoked a series of reforms, research studies and clinical education initiatives, designed to improve the standards of psychosocial care for children, especially if separated from their families. Although recommendations were not immediately adopted by children's nurses, particularly in relation to the involvement of families in hospital based care (Hawthorne 1974), significant improvements in nursing care have since been established (Cleary *et al.*

1986; Ball *et al.* 1988; Casey & Mobbs 1988; Marriott 1990; Evans 1992; Audit Commission 1993; Campbell & Summersgill 1993). However, it could be argued that there has been a lack, until recently, of a nursing model to promote family centred care.

It is now several years since Casey (1988) first published her conceptual framework for child health nursing. Unable to find a model which adequately reflected her philosophy, Casey decided to develop her own. It has since been adopted as both an education and a practice model in the health authority where she works (Casey 1988; Farrell 1992). It is also becoming increasingly popular in other child health settings because of the focus on the specialist needs of this client group (Purcell 1993). The philosophy states that:

'The care of children, well or sick, is best carried out by their families, with varying degrees of assistance from members of a suitably qualified health care team whenever necessary.' (Casey 1988).

The model is derived from an adaptation of nursing's central concepts: the child; the family (person); health; environment; and children's nursing (nursing) (Fig. 15.5).

In her model Casey does not describe how nurses should function within a nursing process context, although key nursing roles are identified as: carer; providing support; teaching and referral to other health professionals (Farrell 1992). There are also some guidelines for assessment which focus upon an analysis of family care routines, the child's present physiological/psychological condition, the nursing care that is required in relation to the child's medical diagnosis and the abilities the child/family already have to enable them to participate in care. Within these criteria Casey (1988) advises that nurses should consider the child's developmental stage, and his/her understanding of and likely reactions to, the situation.

Unlike other models there is very little structure in the partnership in care framework. Instead Casey (1988) aims to encourage nurses to be flexible and adaptable in the planning and delivery of care. She defends the decision not to include a specific assessment structure within the model by arguing that the many specialities within children's nursing will have different priorities for care. Thus a more open framework allows nurses to apply a variety of assessment tools to suit their clients'

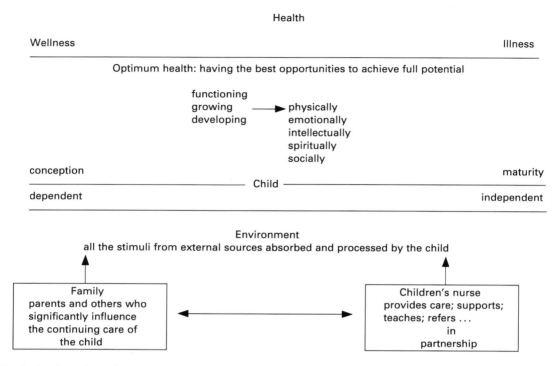

Fig. 15.5 Overview of Casey's partnership in care model (Source: Casey, 1988)

needs. Casey sees this as an advantage because the model offers a general philosophy and description of children's nursing which can then be interpreted accordingly by others. This concept has been successfully applied by Purcell (1993) who uses a biomedical framework to assess and plan care for critically ill children within the central targets of the partnership model.

The Casey model focuses throughout on the child and family, therefore any assessment tool may be utilized within the philosophy of partnership. In the case of children with projected long term healthcare needs, frameworks should be adapted or developed in a way which encourages an in-depth analysis of the situation. Roy's (1976) adaptation model offers an ideal framework for such situations because of the two stage assessment process (Table 15.3). Roy developed this model from theories of stress and adaptation. It is suggested that nursing aims to promote a person's physical and psychological adaptation to health related stressors. Roy was inspired, in part, by personal experience of the great resilience shown by children when responding to major health changes (Mason 1993). In case study 3

Roy's assessment framework will be used as a structure to promote Casey's concept of partnership in care.

Case study 3 centres upon the care of a fifteen year old girl who presented to her GP with a history of intermittent abdominal pain, anorexia, weight loss and diarrhoea. By utilizing Roy's (1976) assessment framework, four adaptive modes are used to guide a two-level assessment:

(1) First level – assessment of a person's behaviours in each of the modes.
(2) Second level – assessment of factors influencing those behaviours.

This is followed by problem identification (nursing diagnosis), goal setting, intervention and evaluation (Roy 1976; Rambo 1984) (Table 15.3). In this study the aim is to demonstrate how partnership and negotiation can be used to help a client to adapt to an altered health state.

Table 15.3   Roy's assessment framework adapted for use with Casey's model.

First level assessment: Behaviours (Roy)		Second level assessment: Influencing factors (Roy) (Casey)

Physiological mode
  exercise and rest
  nutrition
  elimination
  fluid and electrolytes
  oxygen
  circulation
  regulation
	focal
	contextual
	residual
	stimuli
		Routine family care
		
		Child's present health status

		Provision of nursing/family care

Interdependence
  dependence v. independence
Role function
  primary (e.g. age)
  secondary (e.g. parent)
  tertiary (e.g. writer)
Self-concept
  physical self
  personal self
	problem
	identification
	goal setting
	
	intervention
	
	evaluation
		Nursing care required
		
		Child and/or family participation

Case study 3

Kathleen O'Hara is fifteen years old and is the only child of Tom and Margaret O'Hara. Kathleen's parents are divorced although they share the responsibility for her upbringing and welfare. She lives with her mother and stays with her father and his girlfriend on alternate weekends and occasional nights during the week. This arrangement has been consistent for the two years since her parents separated. Kathleen attends a local secondary school and has a good academic record, although she has a history of truancy with two of her school friends.

Kathleen and her mother live in a flat with two cats near the centre of a large city. Mrs O'Hara did not work prior to her divorce but has since taken on two part-time cleaning posts for five afternoons and evenings each week. Kathleen first started to complain of abdominal pain eight weeks ago. She visited her GP at that time but no diagnosis was made and no follow-up ordered. Kathleen continued to experience the symptoms but did not tell either parent. When her mother noticed that Kathleen was losing weight she took her back to her GP and, following referral, a tentative diagnosis of Crohn's disease was made (Elias & Hawkins 1985; Jones & Irving 1993).

Kathleen has now been admitted to hospital for investigations. Nursing care will focus on a detailed assessment which aims to promote partnership between the O'Hara family and healthcare staff (see care plan 3).

Assessment

Assessment of Kathleen has revealed that she is experiencing many physiological and psychological problems associated with disordered gastrointestinal function. This is exacerbated by the fact that she is at an age when the need to feel 'normal' and fit in with her peers is of paramount importance (Shelley 1993). By utilizing Roy's (1976) framework, nursing staff are able to conduct an indepth physical and psychological assessment of Kathleen's situation and health problems. In order to promote Kathleen's and her mother's involvement in the care planning process, however, Roy's criteria for assessment have been subsumed into Casey's (1988) family centred model. Consequently the assessment data reveal relevant family roles, Kathleen's current health status and her relationships with family and significant others.

Care plan 3 – Assessment of Kathleen O'Hara

Adaptive modes	First level assessment Behaviours	Second level assessment Influencing factors			Nursing diagnosis
		Routine family care and present health status			
		Focal	Contextual	Residual	
Nutrition, fluid and electrolytes	Usually eats a lot of fast foods (e.g. chips, burgers) and soda drinks; eats at irregular times and avoids vegetables. Likes to drink tea. Kathleen is now anorexic because she states that eating and drinking are usually followed by abdominal pain, cramps and diarrhoea (for the past twelve weeks). Her skin is dry.	Oral intake is usually followed by cramps and abdominal pain.	Associates eating as the possible cause of her discomfort.		Kathleen is anorexic due to intermittent abdominal pain and abdominal cramps. Weight 43 kg.
Elimination and hygiene	Has had altered elimination patterns for several months – has experienced acute diarrhoea (intermittently) for approximately three months. Kathleen states this is made worse by the foul smell of her stools, causing anxiety, and says she has tried to hide this from family and friends.	Embarrassed by foul smell of stools, causing feelings of anxiety.	Worried about reactions of others to the odour, especially in public settings.	Elimination is usually a private and personal activity.	Kathleen is experiencing acute diarrhoea, usually following consumption of food and drinks. Kathleen is embarrassed and anxious about the smell associated with her faecal output.
Oxygen, circulation, regulation	Kathleen's baseline observations are within normal limits (see TPR chart). She states that during episodes of pain, her respiratory rate increases and sometimes she feels clammy.				
Exercise and rest	Kathleen usually enjoys ice skating and disco dancing. She also likes reading crime books and thrillers and being with her friends. Has been getting increasingly lethargic due to above symptoms and often feels weak, even with mild exercise. She is now reluctant to go out due to elimination patterns.	Pain and embarrassment are reducing activity levels. Lack of appropriate nutrition is causing increased weakness.			Kathleen is becoming increasingly weak and lethargic due to the effects of abdominal pain, abdominal cramps and diarrhoea.

Care plan 3 – Assessment of Kathleen O'Hara (cont.)

Adaptive modes	First level assessment Behaviours	Second level assessment Influencing factors			Nursing diagnosis
		Routine family care and present health status			
		Focal	Contextual	Residual	
Interdependence	Kathleen is in mid-puberty. She attends most of her needs independently, with guidance and support from her parents. She feels she has had to become more independent since her parents divorced, and experiences loneliness in the evening when her mother is at work. This has, she says, encouraged her to play truant and stay out with friends. She feels uncomfortable discussing this with her mother because she says that the latter is trying so hard for her. Kathleen now thinks hospital will be too restricting.	Impact of empty house when she returns from school. Feels sense of belonging with friends. Dependent upon mother for emotional support.	Her parents' divorce. Friends provide company and support. Used to having mother there all the time, and her father.	Her family life differs from friends. Need to belong to a peer group very important for Kathleen; has had previous experience of a more secure family unit.	Kathleen is experiencing feelings of loneliness and isolation at home, especially when her mother is out at work. Kathleen is experiencing feelings of insecurity in her relationships with others, since her parents divorce.
Role function	Kathleen is the only daughter of Tom/Margaret O'Hara. She has good relationships with both but says she is closer to her mother. She is a pupil at secondary school and has many friends. She is studying for GCSE exams and spends half a day a week at the ice rink with friends.				
Self concept	Kathleen states she does not like her physical appearance. She feels she is too tall (5 ft 5 in) and is worried that she has lost so much weight (6 kg over past two months). She feels she has lost confidence in going out with her friends because of her weight loss and diarrhoea.	Altered body appearance and altered body image.		Potential reactions of friends/family to her perceived altered body image.	Kathleen has developed a negative self-concept due to effects of diarrhoea and weight loss.

Care plan 3 – Planning, implementing, evaluating care

Goals	Nursing care	Family care	Eval. date	Evaluation
With Kathleen, her mother and medical staff, to find and treat cause of diarrhoea.	(1) Offer nutritious diet: high protein, high calorie, low fat, low residue. (2) Offer antispasmodics as prescribed. (3) Administer nutritional supplements as prescribed. (4) Encourage adequate oral intake by explaining benefits of above diet and effects of the medication. (5) Encourage Kathleen to monitor her own oral intake and for her mother to support her in this. (6) Assist with medical diagnosis. (7) Prepare Kathleen for specific investigations as appropriate.	(1) Kathleen will select foods, with assistance, to promote optimal nutrition. (2) Kathleen will tell staff if she experiences discomfort and ask for medication if appropriate. (3) Kathleen and her mother will monitor her oral intake and make assessments of the nutritional value of the food she is eating. (4) Kathleen and her mother will be told of any investigations necessary for diagnosis and will be supported in preparation for this by health care staff.	When oral intake is resumed daily: for re-assessment after completion of tests for diagnosis	
For Kathleen to be able to tolerate adequate food and fluid intake with minimal abdominal pain and cramping.	(1) As indicated, to withhold oral intake. (2) To administer and monitor intravenous fluids as prescribed (refer to IVI prescription sheet: IVIs ordered initially for first 48 hours). (3) To teach Kathleen and her mother about the principles and management of IV therapy to encourage their participation in this process. (4) To assist Kathleen and her mother with perianal care as appropriate. (5) To nurse Kathleen in a cubicle of her own to promote privacy. (6) To provide bed pans, commode and air freshener in room to facilitate hygiene needs. (7) To assist Kathleen with her hygiene needs as appropriate. (8) Assist with medical diagnosis.	(1) Kathleen will refrain from oral intake to facilitate medical diagnosis and rest her bowel. (2) Kathleen and her mother assist with the management and observation of Kathleen's IVI as appropriate. Kathleen's mother will provide most support in this, to facilitate Kathleen's rest. (3) Kathleen's mother will assist her with all her hygiene needs until she feels able to resume her own care independently.	Daily and as indicated during each day	

Care plan 3 – Planning, implementing, evaluating care (cont.)

Goals	Nursing care	Family care	Eval. date	Evaluation
For Kathleen to be able to balance activity and rest patterns without experiencing undue tiredness/weakness.	(1) Provide a quiet environment and promote rest. (2) Ensure Kathleen is not subjected to frequent medical/nursing assessment and care without suitable rest periods. (3) Negotiate with Kathleen and her mother who will visit and the length of visiting periods. (4) Ensure Kathleen is provided with suitable activities to promote rest, relaxation and distraction.	(1) Kathleen and her mother will negotiate suitable rest periods during the day, in conjunction with medical staff. (2) Kathleen to plan visiting arrangements of family and friends, in negotiation with her mother and nurse. (3) Kathleen's mother will bring Kathleen's books etc. into hospital as requested by Kathleen. (4) Kathleen will seek assistance from nurse/ medical staff if she is unable to promote rest.	Daily	
For Kathleen and her mother to be able to explore Kathleen's feelings of loneliness and insecurity together, and with other family and friends as appropriate	(1) Ensure Kathleen and her mother have enough privacy together. (2) Offer support if Kathleen and her mother become too distressed together. (3) Spend time with Kathleen and her mother, together and on an individual basis as appropriate. (4) Facilitate involvement of other family members and friends as appropriate. (5) Offer family counselling services to Kathleen and her mother.	(1) Kathleen and her mother to spend time together to explore their feelings and Kathleen's loneliness. (2) Kathleen and her mother to consider possible solution to Kathleen's feelings of loneliness and insecurity. (3) Kathleen and her mother to determine if others should be involved (e.g. father). (4) Kathleen and her mother to seek guidance from nurse or family counsellor as appropriate.	For continuous monitor and evaluation with Kathleen and her mother daily or as indicated.	
For Kathleen to increase her self-esteem in response to health care and family intervention.	As for above goal.	As for above goal.	in 7 days	

This is important for the O'Hara family because although Kathleen is still a minor and dependent upon her parents' support for her continued development and welfare, she is also approaching maturity and is in need of space and independence. In this case Casey's (1988) concept of partnership in care can be balanced between negotiating family care with Kathleen as the central focus and/or negotiating Kathleen's independent participative role. Roy's (1976) criteria for assessment highlight Kathleen's current health needs whilst Casey's (1988) framework helps nursing staff/family to determine the scope for participation.

Planning, implementation and evaluation

Planning, implementing and evaluating care now centres wholly upon the negotiated roles identified during assessment. Goals are set for Kathleen's care and at this point nursing staff should use their specialist knowledge of the situation to guide the development of a realistic care plan. Nursing and family care can then be set out in a format similar to that presented in case study 2.

When adopting a negotiated care approach nursing staff must work within, or develop, policy guidelines which set out criteria for children and families' self-recording of the care they are giving and for the accountability of the nursing team in the overall process. Another important consideration at this stage is the maintenance of confidentiality. Where appropriate any child who is able to understand should be informed about those who will have access to their nursing care plan and where it will usually be kept.

Evaluating care determines whether or not set goals have been achieved and whether or not the negotiation process has been effective. In Kathleen's case this will involve an analysis of her level of adaptation to her altered health state, hence the choice of Roy's assessment process, and whether or not family care and nursing care was delivered according to the plan.

Discussion

Case study 3 illustrates the potential of Casey's (1988) partnership in care philosophy for children and their families with health care needs. Unlike the models used in the previous two case studies, the child and family are the primary focus in Casey's model and nurses can select an assessment tool of their choice for the organization and delivery of care. In this example the client, Kathleen, has an altered health state which may have long term (complex) physical, psychological and social implications for herself and her family. An assessment tool which facilitates an in-depth analysis of her situation, for long term use or referral, is therefore considered to be the most appropriate. In other situations, for example in short term care, a less sophisticated tool could be used. Experienced children's nurses can also devise their own criteria to suit the needs of their particular client group.

Whilst much has been written about the benefits of family centred care and partnership, surprisingly little attention has been paid to this first attempt to develop a children's nursing model which is not based on, or adapted from, other more established models. Casey's model offers children's nurses a starting point for isolating and describing the phenomena unique to their nursing role. There is clearly a need, therefore, for more widespread applications of Casey's (1988) framework, in order to assess its potential as a leading model for child health nursing and to validate its concepts of partnership and negotiation among children, families, nurses and other health care professionals.

CONCLUSION

This chapter has examined the utility of three conceptual frameworks for child health nursing practice. Like many other nursing models, each has its potential benefits and limitations for use with this client group. Orem's (1991) model is perhaps the most well developed and has been subject to widespread analysis, applications, research and further development. It also offers clear guidelines for involving families and significant others in the care process, not seen in many other models. However it is highly structured, complex and contains jargon which may be difficult to understand and apply to different situations. The Roper *et al.* (1990) model is both familiar and well established in the UK and it too promotes the concept of participation in care. However, it does not explore child/family centred care, and its main focus of twelve activities of living is said to be rather physiologically based and self-limiting for facilitating a thorough psychosocial assessment.

In contrast, Casey's (1988) model has as its major strength a primary focus on children and their families. It is flexible and adaptable and allows nurses to choose their own structure for assessment. It is also one of the first frameworks devised specifically for children's nurses and its philosophy for care is one which is supported by other interested healthcare professionals. Thus it has the potential to provide a basis for collaborative care planning. However, the model still requires further application and testing to determine its utility and validity for child healthcare.

There are several other frameworks which may be chosen and since a major objective of children's nursing is to offer a caring service for its clients, the following suggestions are presented as a guide for selecting or developing the most appropriate framework to deliver such a service. This list is not exhaustive and should be seen only as a starting point in a selection process:

- The framework should offer a philosophy which is sympathetic to child/family care.
- The nursing process component of the model should offer an appropriate structure to highlight the needs of a particular client group.
- It should be sufficiently flexible to assist nurses in focusing upon the needs of an individual child and family.
- It should be sufficiently flexible to support children and families who, for whatever reason, cannot or do not wish to participate in the care process.
- The framework should offer appropriate definitions of and guidelines for child healthcare.
- The entire healthcare team should subscribe to the principles underpinning the framework, if the families are to benefit from these approaches.
- There should be policies to support the implementation of the framework, particularly in relation to the legal and ethical implications associated with the family's participation in care.

To conclude it could be argued that historically the organization and delivery of nursing care for children and their families has been influenced by models of care, formal or informal, which are not generally sympathetic to all the needs, rights or wishes of their clients. Whilst it is evident that this situation is changing, children's nurses need to be more proactive in establishing their role within the healthcare team. Collectively they can initiate, implement and validate family centred care and the development or adaptation of frameworks to guide practice, based upon an appropriate philosophy, is one means of achieving this.

REFERENCES AND FURTHER READING

Aggleton, P. & Chalmers, H. (1986) *Nursing Models and the Nursing Process*. Macmillan Education Ltd, Hampshire.

Atkins, S. (1989) Parenteral nutrition – the nurse's role. *Surgical Nurse*, 4, 13–17.

Audit Commission (1993) *Children First – A Study Of Hospital Services*. NHS report No 7. HMSO, London.

Ball, M., Glasper, A. & Yerrell, P. (1988) How well do we perform? Parents' perceptions of paediatric care. *Professional Nurse*, 4(3), 115–18.

Biehler, B.A. (1992) Impact of role-sets on implementing self-care theory with children. *Paediatric Nursing*, 18(1), 30–34.

Bruce, E. (1989) Thermal injuries. *Paediatric Nursing*, 1(9), 8–9.

Campbell, S. & Summersgill, P. (1993) Keeping it in the family. *Child Health*, 1(1), 17–20.

Casey, A. (1988) A partnership with child and family. *Senior Nurse*, 8(4), 8–9.

Casey, A. (1993) Development and use of the partnership model of nursing care. In *Recent Advances in Child Health Care* (eds A. Glasper & A. Tucker), Chapter 14, pp. 183–93. Scutari Press, London.

Casey, A. & Mobbs, S. (1988) Partnership in practice. *Nursing Times*, 84(44), 67–8.

Cavanagh, S. (1991) Orem and the nursing process: new directions for the 1990s. *Nursing Practice*, 4(4), 26–8 (in association with *Nursing Standard*).

Charles-Edwards, I. & Casey, A. (1992) Parental involvement and voluntary consent. *Paediatric Nursing*, 4(1), 16–18.

Cheetham, T. (1988) Model care in the surgical ward. *Senior Nurse*, 8(4), 10–12.

Clark, J. & Bishop, J. (1988) Model-making. *Nursing Times*, 84(27), 37–40.

Clarke, D. (1988) Framework for care. *Nursing Times*, 84(35), 33–5.

Cleary, J., Gray, O.P., Hall, D.J., Rowlandson, P.H., Sainsbury, C.P.O. & Davies, M.M. (1986) Parental involvement in the lives of children in hospital. *Archives of Disease in Childhood*, 61(8), 779–87.

Colliss, V. (1990) Pre-and post-operative management. *Paediatric Nursing*, 2(5), 16–17.

Dearmun, A.K. (1992) Perceptions of parental participation. *Paediatric Nursing*, 4(7), 6–9.

Department of Health (1991) *Welfare of Children and Young People in Hospital*. HMSO, London.

Dragone, M.A. (1990) Perspectives of chronically-ill adolescents and parents on health care needs. *Pediatric Nursing*, 16(1), 45–50.

Draper, J. (1992) The impact of nursing models. *Senior Nurse*, 12(3), 38–9.

Eichelberger, K.M., Kaufman, D.H., Rundahl, M.E. & Schwartz, N.E. (1980) Self-care nursing plan: helping children to help themselves. *Paediatric Nursing*, 6, 9–13.

Elias, E. & Hawkins, C. (1985) *Lecture Notes On Gastroenterology*. Blackwell Science, Oxford.

Elliott, B. (1991) Caring for a child with atopic eczema using Orem's self-care model. In *Caring for Children* (ed. A. While), pp. 70–87. Edward Arnold, London.

Evans, M. (1992) Extending the parental role – involving parents in paediatric care. *Professional Nurse*, 7(12), 774–6.

Farrell, M. (1992) Partnership in care – paediatric nursing model. *British Journal of Nursing*, 1(4), 175–6.

Fawcett, J. (1989) *Analysis and Evaluation of Conceptual Models of Nursing*, 2nd edn. F A Davis Company, Philadelphia.

Galligan, A.C. (1979) Using Roy's concept of adaptation to care for young children. *American Journal of Maternal/Child Nursing*, 4(1), 24–8.

Glasper, A. (1987) Help or hazard? (parents in the anaesthetic room). *Nursing Times*, 83(52), 85.

Hamilton, W. (1990) *The Hamilton Classification Scheme and Glossary for Nursing Diagnoses in Child and Adolescent Mental Health Care*. Teach-In Publications, Clydebank, Scotland.

Happs, S. (1994) Nursing: concepts, theories and models. In *The Child and Family. Contemporary Nursing Issues in Child Health and Care* (ed. B. Lindsay). Bailliere Tindall, London.

Hardy, L. (1986) Identifying the place of theoretical frameworks in an evolving discipline. *Journal of Advanced Nursing*, 11(1), 103–7.

Hawthorn, P. (1974) *Nurse, I Want My Mummy*. Study of Nursing Care. Project Reports Series 1, No. 3. Royal College of Nursing, London.

Hazinski, M.F. (1984) *Nursing Care Of The Critically Ill Child*. The C V Mosby Company, St Louis.

Henderson, V. (1966) *The Nature Of Nursing*. Macmillan, New York.

Jacques, S. (1985) A route to home. *Nursing Mirror*, 161(4), 24–8.

James, S.R. & Mott, S.C. (1988) *Child Health Nursing: Essential Care Of Children and Families*. Addison-Wesley Publishing Co Inc, Menlo Park, California.

Johnson, M. (1986) Model of Perfection. *Nursing Times*, 82(5), 42–3.

Jones, D.J. & Irving, M.H. (eds) (1993) *ABC Of Colorectal Diseases*. B.M.J. Publishing Group, London.

Jones, K. & While, A. (1991) Caring for a child undergoing circumcision using Roper's Model. In *Caring for Children* (ed. A. While), pp. 39–47. Edward Arnold, London.

King, I. (1971) *Toward A Theory Of Nursing: General Concepts Of Human Behaviour*. John Wiley, New York.

Macallan, E.S. & Jackson, I.T. (1971) *Plastic Surgery And Burns Treatment*. Heinemann Medical Books, London.

MacDonald, A. (1988) A model for children's nursing. *Nursing Times*, 84(34), 52–5.

MacKenzie, H. (1991) Caring for a neonate in hospital using Roy's adaptation model. In *Caring For Children* (ed. A. While), pp. 15–27. Edward Arnold, London.

Marcoux, C. (1990) Central venous access devices in children. *Pediatric Nursing*, 16(2), 123–33.

Marriott, S. (1990) Parent Power. *Nursing Times*, 86(34), 68.

Mason, G. (1993) Partners in care: Roy's adaptation model in child care. *Child Health*, 1(1), 38–42.

Mason, G. & Webb, C. (1993) Nursing diagnosis – a review of the literature. *British Journal of Clinical Nursing Studies*, 2(2), 67–74.

Mason, G. & Webb, C. (1994) Time to paint a clearer picture: child health nursing diagnosis. *Child Health*, 2(91), 1010–15.

McCaugherty, D. (1992) The Roper nursing model as an educational and research tool. *British Journal of Nursing*, 1(9), 455–9.

Michie, B. (1988) Making sense of total parenteral nutrition. *Nursing Times*, 84(20), 46–7.

Miles, I. (1985) A suitable case for treatment. *Nursing Times*, 81(18), 48–50.

Millar, B. (1990) The benefits of nursing models. *Surgical Nurse*, 5, 5–14.

MoH (1959) *Report Of The Committee On The Welfare Of Children In Hospital* (Platt Report). HMSO, London.

Morgan, J. (1985) Paediatric lifeline. *Nursing Mirror*, 161(4), 29–31.

Mount, M. (1993) Self-care to home care: the way forward. *Paediatric Nursing*, 5(5), 20–23.

Mueller, M. (1990) What's the use of models. *Paediatric Nursing*, 2(6), 8–10.

Mughal, M. & Irving, M. (1986) Home parenteral nutrition in the United Kingdom and Ireland: a report of 200 cases. The *Lancet*, 2, 383–7.

Newton, C. (1991) *The Roper–Logan–Tierney Model In Action*. The Macmillan Press, Hampshire.

Norris, M.K. & House, M.A. (1991) *Organ and Tissue Transplantation – Nursing Care From Procurement Through Rehabilitation*. F A Davis Company, Philadelphia.

Orem, D.E. (1991) *Nursing – Concepts Of Practice*, 4th edn, p. 61. Mosby-Year-Book Inc., St Louis.

Pearson, A. & Vaughan, B. (1986) *Nursing Models for Practice*. Heinemann Nursing, London.

Purcell, C. (1993) Holistic care of a critically ill child. *Intensive and Critical Care Nursing*, 9, 108–15.

Rambo, B.J. (1984) *Adaptation Nursing – Assessment & Intervention*. W B Saunders Co, London.

Rodgers, B.L. (1984) Home parenteral nutrition: principles of management. *Nursing Practitioner*, March, 42–52.

Roper, N. (1976) A model for nursing and nursology. *Journal of Advanced Nursing*, 1(3), 219–27.

Roper, N., Logan, W. & Tierney, A. (1986) Nursing models: a process of construction and refinement. In *Models for Nursing* (eds B. Kershaw & J. Salvage), pp. 25–38. John Wiley & Sons, Chichester.

Roper, N., Logan, W. & Tierney, A. (1990) *The Elements of Nursing*, 3rd edn., p. 37. Churchill Livingstone, London.

Roy, C. (1976) *Introduction To Nursing: An Adaptation Model*. Prentice-Hall Inc., New Jersey.

Salvage, J. & Kershaw, B. (eds) (1990) *Models for Nursing 2*. Scutari Press, London.

Senior, J. (1990) Post-operative pain relief. *Paediatric Nursing*, 2(9), 10.

Shelley, H. (1993) Adolescent needs in hospital. *Paediatric Nursing*, 5(9), 16–18.

Silk, D.B.A. (1989) Enteral and parenteral nutrition. *Gastroenterology In Practice*, Feb/Mar, 21–30.

Sinclair, H. & Whyte, D. (1987) Perspectives on community care for children. In *Nursing Care Of Children In Health And Illness* (Recent Advances In Nursing), 16, 1–15. Longman Group UK, London.

Stapleford, P. (1990) Parenteral nutrition in children. *Paediatric Nursing*, 2(6), 18–21.

Stephenson, P. (1987) Models for Action. *Nursing Times*, 83(29), 62–3.

Thomas, L. (supplement ed.) (1990) Children in surgery. *Nursing Standard Special Supplement*, Astra/NAWCH, 4(24), 1–14.

Wallace, E. (1993) Nursing a teenager with burns (using Roper *et al*'s model). *British Journal of Nursing*, 2(5), 278–81.

Walsh, M. (1991) *Models in Clinical Nursing: The Way Forward*. Bailliere Tindall, London.

Webb, C. (1984) On the eighth day God created the nursing process and nobody rested. *Senior Nurse*, 1(33), 22–5.

Webb, C. & Mason, G. (1993) Nursing diagnosis in sick children's nursing. *British Journal of Clinical Nursing Studies*, 2(5), 279–86.

Welch, L. (1993a) Applying Orem's Model. *Paediatric Nursing*, 5(6), 14–16.

Welch, L. (1993b) Orem and Roy: two concepts of nursing. *Paediatric Nursing*, 5(5), 24–6.

Wesolowski, C.A. (1988) Self-contracts for chronically ill children. *Journal of Maternal Child Nursing*, 13(1), 20–23.

West, R. & Harris, B. (1988) Adolescents: how healthy are they? *The Practitioner*, 232(1459), 1314–16.

While, A. (ed.) (1991) *Caring for Children*. Edward Arnold, London.

Wright, S.G. (1990) *Building and Using a Model of Nursing*, 2nd edn. Edward Arnold, London.

INTRODUCTION

This chapter focuses on the special problems that the child and their family will experience as a result of changes from normal respiratory function. The impact of respiratory illness will be examined and the role of the nurse in helping the child and family meet these needs will be explored. The underlying principles of effective, therapeutic nursing care of the child in relation to play, pain management, reassurance, and preparation apply equally to the child with respiratory problems but this chapter will focus more specifically on those related to disordered respiratory function. In caring for and supporting a child experiencing respiratory problems the nurse must be aware of the many facets of the nursing role including:

- Assessment.
- Planning, and implementing care.
- Evaluating care.
- Acting as advocate for the child and family.
- Providing emotional/psychological support.
- Offering health education and promotion.
- Liaison with other members of the multi-disciplinary team.
- Standard setting.

Respiratory disorders are relatively common in childhood and the consequences for the child are potentially serious (Wooler 1993) due to overall immaturity of the respiratory tract, both structurally and functionally. It should be remembered that the most common cause of cardiac arrest in infants and children is hypoxia (Tunstall & McCarthy 1993) and this emphasizes the need for any respiratory problem in children to be viewed seriously. Respiratory problems can arise as primary disorders from disease, trauma or malformation/structural anomaly, and as secondary disorders from disease elsewhere in the body. However, three broad categories of respiratory problems can be identified:

(1) Respiratory infections.
(2) Allergic responses.
(3) Mechanical disturbances.

There is, however, overlap between these categories and when caring for the child with respiratory needs it is often the child's age and stage of development that will be the crucial factor in both their response to the respiratory challenge and in the need for and type of intervention and care required. Respiratory problems can present as acute, chronic and acute on chronic – each type of presentation requires the nurse to utilize good assessment and planning skills and provide a high quality of nursing care and support.

This chapter aims to investigate how this nursing care can be best delivered. Section one will deal with the principles underlying respiratory assessment, since effective assessment is a crucial part of the nurse's role in meeting the child's immediate and long term needs.

Section two of the chapter will examine the child experiencing the effects of respiratory infection and the role of the nurse in meeting their needs. Bronchiolitis will be looked at to highlight the respiratory management issues related to the infant, and croup and epiglottitis will allow the needs of the young child to be considered. The child with tonsillitis will also be considered due to the potential need for surgical intervention.

Section three will explore issues related to the care and management of children experiencing the chronic disorders of asthma and cystic fibrosis. Although the interventions and the underlying pathologies are different, there are similarities both in their need to adhere to drug regimes and the impact that a chronic illness can have on the family. The nurse's role as health educator/promoter will be considered.

In section four the care of a child with a foreign body in situ will be considered, as will the care of the family who have experienced a baby dying from sudden infant death syndrome/cot death.

Overall this chapter aims to highlight the importance of the nurse's role in supporting and caring for the child with respiratory difficulties and in promoting an optimum level of health and wellbeing.

PRINCIPLES UNDERLYING RESPIRATORY ASSESSMENT

Effective, thorough and ongoing assessment is a crucial part of the nurse's role and care should be taken to ensure that the child is not unduly inconvenienced by it. Often a child presenting with respiratory problems is anxious and perhaps distressed and the nurse must always consider the need to prepare the child for the assessment. Aspects that may seem to be routine to the nurse, for example the use of a stethoscope, may be perceived as being threatening by the child. The nurse requires a sound knowledge base of normal physiological and anatomical functioning in order to ensure that effective and appropriate use is made of the data/information collected.

The child's level of development and the maturity of the respiratory system will have an effect on both the nature and severity of their symptoms and type of problem. Children are vulnerable to respiratory challenges for several reasons:

- 'Their relatively high need for oxygen.
- The high metabolic rate needed for growth.
- The immaturity of their lungs.
- Infants and young children have relatively fewer alveoli and therefore a reduced alveolar surface area (Engel 1989).

Ramsay (1989) states that respiratory assessment involves four components:

- History taking from child and parents.
- Observation of the child.
- Physical examination.
- Laboratory investigation.

Factors which may influence the child's respiratory status

The nurse must be aware of the factors which may influence the child's breathing and these should be taken into consideration when assessing and analysing the results of that assessment. Factors which influence the child's normal respiratory rate or pattern include age, medications, position, pyrexia, level of activity, emotional status, pollution, and pathological states (Engel 1989; Ramsay 1989). The age of the child influences both the rate and rhythm of respiratory rate; the infant and younger child have a faster respiratory rate than that of the older child/adult and the rate is prone to dramatic increases in the presence of pyrexia, disease, anxiety and distress (Engel 1989). If the child or infant becomes pyrexial the additional metabolic demand results in an increase of both rate and depth; equally hypothermia

will result in a decrease in respiratory rate. Distress, crying and fear will also increase the rate and depth of respiration, although Ramsay (1989) proposes that sad or depressed children will have a slower respiratory rate. Changes in the child's activity pattern will influence respiratory effort and rate and this should be borne in mind when assessing the child.

Other pathological disorders such as raised intracranial pressure, systematic infection and respiratory disorders themselves, will all impact on the child's normal respiratory rate. All these factors must be considered when assessing the child, but the overall aims of respiratory assessment are first to determine the severity of the child's respiratory distress (Brunner & Suddarth 1991) and to ensure that prompt and appropriate action is taken as a result of the assessment.

Observing the child's respiratory status/needs

Whenever possible the child's respiratory rate and pattern should be assessed while the child is calm and prior to commencing any other procedures; the child's respirations should be observed over a full minute since their rate may be irregular. More accurate readings will be achieved if the child is unaware that their respirations are being counted, as knowledge of being observed may result in the rate being modified. Young children and infants may present challenges/difficulties in terms of accurately observing their respirations; in this situation it is appropriate either to use a stethoscope to listen to the child's breath sounds or to place a hand on the child's chest to determine inspiratory rises of the chest.

The nurse should remember that respiratory movements in the infant are primarily driven by the diaphragm and therefore respiration in this age group is performed by observing abdominal movements (Whaley & Wong 1991). In fact abdominal/diaphragmatic movement is common in the child under the age of about six years. Note must be taken of the depth and rhythm of the child's breathing as these can give significant clues to the nature of the problem that the child is experiencing. Shallow breathing, for example, may indicate metabolic acidosis; a prolonged period of expiration is indicative of asthma; 'rattling' respiration may result from a respiratory tract infection; and periodic Cheyne-Stokes breathing may indicate raised intracranial pressure; bradypnoea may be indicative of over-sedation.

Not only should the rhythm and rate of respirations be assessed but note should also be taken of the child's chest movements which again can indicate a significant underlying anomaly. The movement of the chest should be symmetrical and should be co-ordinated with the child's breathing. For children under the age of about seven years the normal breathing pattern will involve the use of abdominal muscles, so that use of the costal muscles may indicate that the child has abdominal pain and is favouring the costal muscles. In contrast children who normally use their costal muscles for breathing, that is those over seven years old, who revert to abdominal breathing may be experiencing costal muscle pain. An urgent sign to take note of is the use of accessory muscles (including nasal flaring) and any retractions (intercostal, subcostal, suprasternal, substernal and clavicular). These indicate air hunger and, unless intervention occurs, possible respiratory failure; they indicate a severe effort on the child's behalf to oxygenate themselves adequately and they act as a severe drain on the child's physical and emotional resources.

Physical examination of the child's respiratory status/needs

Additionally the nurse should palpate, percuss and ausculate the child's chest as part of a comprehensive assessment. The nurse can assess the adequacy and equality of air conductance by assessing the absence or presence of fremitus. Fremitus refers to the vibration felt through the chest wall; this vibration can be triggered by feeling for the transmission of the child's voice through the palmar surfaces of the hand held on the chest wall. Fremitus should be equal on both sides of the chest, although the intensity is modified by factors including the child's age and the tone of their voice. Decreased fremitus is indicative of asthma or a pneumothorax whereas increased fremitus can reflect pneumonia.

Percussion is used to assess the 'amounts of gaseous, liquid or solid material in the underlying lung tissue and to determine diaphragmatic movement and resting levels' (Smith Millet 1992). Unusual dullness in the percussive note may reflect fluid or tissue mass in the lungs. Auscultation aims to assess airflow into and through the lungs, the absence or presence of mucous, any obstruction to the airflow, and the overall condition of the lung tissue itself. The nurse should assess for normal breath sounds (vesicular sounds) and should be able to determine both the characteristics and location of these sounds.

Assessment for vesicular sounds allows the nurse to become aware of abnormal or adventitious sounds. Adventitious sounds can generally be classified as rales/crackles, rhonchi, wheezes, stridor, and pleural friction rubs. Rales tend to occur on inspiration and are generally heard on inspiration; they indicate pneumonia, pulmonary oedema, congestive cardiac failure and bronchitis and are indicative of fluid in the alveoli, bronchioles and/or bronchi (Engel 1989). Rhonchi are continuous sounds usually occurring during expiration and are described as sonorous, as heard in bronchitis, indicative of tracheal and large bronchi involvement, or as sibilant, as heard in asthma, indicative of obstruction and oedema in the smaller airways. Wheezes tend to be described as sonorous, musical and whistling; they are usually heard on expiration and can reflect foreign body aspiration, asthma and bronchiolitis. Inflamed pleural surfaces result in the characteristic pleural friction rub; it is usually heard on inspiration and may be described as grating or rubbing and may be either low or high pitched.

A major indicator of the adequacy of the child's overall perfusion relates to the child's colour, and assessment for any level of cyanosis should be made. Peripheral cyanosis (cyanosed nail beds) may indicate vasoconstriction as a result of peripheral shut down, whereas central cyanosis (cyanosed lips and trunk) is indicative of a more significant drop in the oxygen carrying capacity of the blood. However, cyanosis must be considered along with other factors as it is not a reliable indicator of the extent of the hypoxemia that the child is experiencing if it is taken in isolation (Clancy & Jones 1993).

Another factor that needs to be assessed is whether or not clubbing of the nails is present. Clubbing usually indicates the chronic hypoxaemia that is seen in cystic fibrosis. Additionally the child should be observed for any signs of restlessness and apprehension as well as decreases in conscious level as this can indicate air hunger/hypoxia. The nurse should also assess the child for the presence of a cough (infants under the age of six months cannot cough) and whether it is dry or productive, as this may indicate the presence of infection. Sputum should also be noted by the nurse during the assessment process, sputum being indicative of infection, disease processes such as cystic fibrosis, pulmonary oedema and irritation/inflammation. As such the nurse should note the absence or presence of sputum and provide a description of it; for example, purulent frothy, tenacious, mucopurulent or bloodstained. The nurse should also note whether the child has experienced any unusual weight gain or loss as these may indicate fluid retention (weight gain) or a chronic pulmonary disease (weight loss).

All these factors need to be assessed and documented and the implications of them noted. Single symptoms may be indicative of an underlying problem but often it is the integration of symptoms and linkage with other signs and symptoms that allow the nurse to draw appropriate conclusions and plan relevant therapeutic care.

Physical examination of the chest is important as it can indicate both normal development and abnormal development which may indicate an underlying disease process. Vitamin D deficiency may result in swellings on either side of the sternum (rachitic rosary). Chronic chest disease such as asthma may result in the development of a barrel shaped chest which is the result of hyperinflation. Pigeon chest (pectus carinatum) where the sternum protrudes, and pectus excavatum where the sternum is depressed, should also be noted as both may compromise adequate lung expansion. Pectus excavatum may be seen in children with chronic active allergies.

As can be seen, assessment of the child's respiratory competence is an important responsibility that requires the nurse to utilize a wide range of skills and consider a variety of factors, based on a broad knowledge base (Fig. 16.1). Effective assessment is vital in both ensuring early detection of problems and in monitoring and assessing the progress of treatment and care (Engel 1989).

Assessing the child's respiratory status/needs through a nursing history

A vital part of the assessment of a child with respiratory problems lies with the nursing history; this is important because it allows the nurse to assess and understand the child's normal pattern and to determine what inter-

ventions are appropriate and indicated. The previously mentioned aspects of assessment will also need consideration, thus the restrictions that the present problem has imposed can be seen. The nurse needs to consider the nursing history from a holistic perspective since respiratory problems inevitably have some degree of impact on all the child's activities. The nurse should assess the impact that the respiratory defect has on the child's sleeping pattern, whether it results in modification of the child's eating and drinking, whether it disrupts or alters their pattern of playing and mobility, whether it affects the child's ability to communicate, whether the child is experiencing any pain in relation to the respiratory problem and, importantly, if it affects the child's emotional security.

The impact of the child's illness on their family should not be underestimated and should be seen as an important component of the overall assessment process. Obviously in the situation of a respiratory emergency some of this history taking will be condensed, but a comprehensive overall picture is still of vital importance. The nursing history should include the duration of the present problem and specific information relevant to the child's present symptoms, such as recent contact with infectious illness. It should also include information about the child's neonatal history as this can have a major impact on subsequent respiratory episodes (Smith Millet 1992).

Throughout the whole assessment process the need of the child to feel secure and safe is paramount and therefore appropriate explanation must be given. The child can be given the stethoscope to play with and warm before it is used for auscultation of their chest; this may reduce the child's fear of a seemingly threatening piece of hospital hardware/technology – the child may have perceived this innocuous piece of equipment as hard, cold and invasive. The child, whenever possible, should feel an important part of the assessment process. Moss (1981) emphasizes the need to involve the child throughout the assessment as this increases their feelings of control.

Investigations as a means of assessing the child's respiratory status/needs

As with all investigations that the child has to undergo, the nurse's prime role lies in effective communication

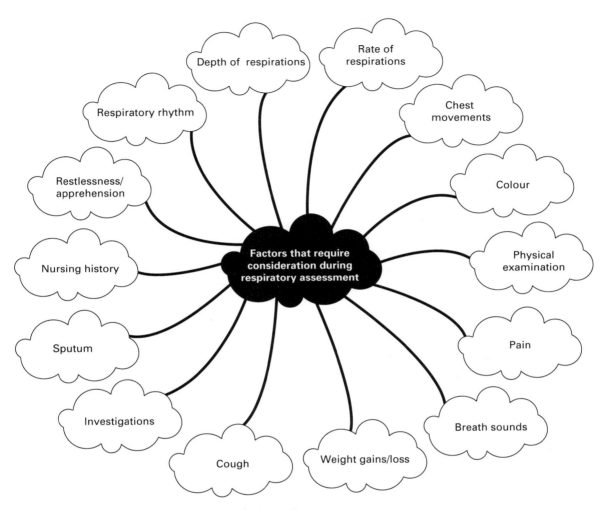

Fig. 16.1   Factors that the nurse must consider in respiratory assessment.

and preparation. This is especially important for the child with compromised respiratory effort where the distress associated with procedures such as X-rays, blood sampling, lung function tests, and 'routine' culture and sensitivity swabs can be mediated by appropriate preparation. Good preparation leading to a calm and co-operative approach by the child can result in a decrease in the stress placed on their compromised respiratory system.

As always, the nurse needs to consider the child's age, knowledge of the situation, coping style and developmental level in determining the best approach to preparing the child (Douglas 1993). A teaching role may also be important in the preparation of the child for

lung function tests, for example, where the nurse and the child's parents can be encouraged to learn how to use the equipment appropriately by practising using the mouthpiece and encouraging their child to breathe appropriately.

It is likely that the child requiring respiratory intervention will need to have arterial oxyhaemoglobin saturation assessed. It is infinitely preferable for the child, for this assessment to be undertaken using pulse oximetry or transcutaneous oxygen monitoring. Both these methods are noninvasive although the transcutaneous method, which uses a heated electrode, can result in blistering of the child's skin. Of the two noninvasive methods pulse oximetry is preferable as nontraumic, and data generated is readily updated. Arterial blood gas sampling is an important part of the assessment process as it can help determine the adequacy of lung function in oxygenating the blood.

Chest X-rays may be ordered to determine the presence of disease, changes in the pathological status of the lungs, the presence of lung deformities and the presence of foreign bodies, and to determine the correct or incorrect placement of monitoring lines, endotracheal tubes and chest drains.

The child may also be involved in lung function tests to determine their peak flow, vital capacity and lung spirometry. Chest aspiration may be performed either to examine the withdrawn fluid for the presence of malignant cells or for culture and sensitivity to determine specific bacterial growth or to reduce the fluid collection. Children who are undergoing investigation for diagnosis of cystic fibrosis will have a sweat test performed. The more specific/specialized tests and investigations should not overshadow the more routine tests such as nasal and throat swabs and sputum analysis, which can be equally upsetting for both the child and their family. The nurse should also remember that the child with a chronic illness who experiences repeated investigations will not get used to them, although they may cope with them, and will continue to need appropriate preparation and support.

NURSING CARE OF THE INFANT WITH BRONCHIOLITIS

The progression of symptoms from those of a seemingly simple upper respiratory tract infection and 'runny nose' to the distressed, irritable, tired baby with marked tachypnoea and dyspnoea is frightening for both the baby and the parents. A baby with bronchiolitis can need hospital admission and respiratory support as a matter of urgency, although increasingly infants and children with bronchiolitis who would previously have required admission to hospital for assessment and observation are being cared for in their own homes with the family being supported by the paediatric community nurse (Jones, pers. comm.). Strategies and protocols are developing to ensure that appropriate action is taken and support is given.

Those who require admission have a severe response

to the infection or are at high risk. The high risk group includes infants born preterm and who have an underlying/chronic pulmonary condition such as bronchopulmonary dysplasia. The nurse's role in meeting the needs of the infant and family focus on assessment, respiratory support and good communication to relieve their obvious and reasonable anxiety about the distress their baby is experiencing.

Bronchiolitis is an acute viral infection that has maximum impact on the bronchioles. It is characterized by both inflammatory and mechanical changes in the bronchioles (Ramsay 1989). The most common pathogen involved in bronchiolitis is the respiratory syncitial virus (RSV) which is responsible for being the most frequent cause of pneumonia in infancy (Dinwiddie 1991; Guerra *et al.* 1990). Most infants are able to deal effectively with RSV infection although the disease can become serious for a number of them.

Other pathogens implicated in bronchiolitis include adenovirus, parainfluenza virus, influenza virus and mycoplasma pneumonia (Brunner & Suddarth 1991). The virus enters the lower respiratory tract and invades the bronchiole epithelial cells. This leads to the cells sloughing away, increased secretion of mucus and oedema (Clancy & Jones 1993). The exudate produced accumulates in the narrowed airways, which become obstructed, and air trapping occurs with a resultant hyperinflation of the lung tissue. The trapped exudate causes atelectasis and collapse of the affected alveoli; a ventilation-perfusion mismatch may result with hypercapnea and hypoxaemia (Smith Millet 1992; Whaley & Wong 1991).

It takes between one and two weeks for the damaged epithelial cells to be restored to health (Guerra *et al.* 1990). In some rare situations the infant may require intensive respiratory support as a result of respiratory failure and exhaustion. Schweich (1990) reports that bronchiolitis increases predisposition to asthma. Bronchiolitis occurs in infants between two and 12 months of age with a peak incidence at six months old; it lasts seven to ten days and the prognosis is generally good. The nurse must be prepared to support the family through this crisis, reassuring them that the baby's needs are being met, and should involve them, whenever appropriate, in caring for their baby.

Nursing assessment

Assessment focuses on consideration of the level of respiratory distress and the effects that this is having on the infant's ability to function. Since bronchiolitis is characterized by progressive respiratory dysfunction before recovery, comprehensive assessment and consideration of trends must be made (Fig. 16.2).

accessory muscles and other signs of respiratory distress must be taken seriously as the risk of hypoxaemia and hypercapnea is very real in this age group. The nurse should also observe for hyperinflation of the chest, which manifests itself in a barrel shaped chest wall. The baby should be monitored, either by close observation or by the use of an apnoea device. Any apnoea attacks should again be carefully recorded (Table 16.1).

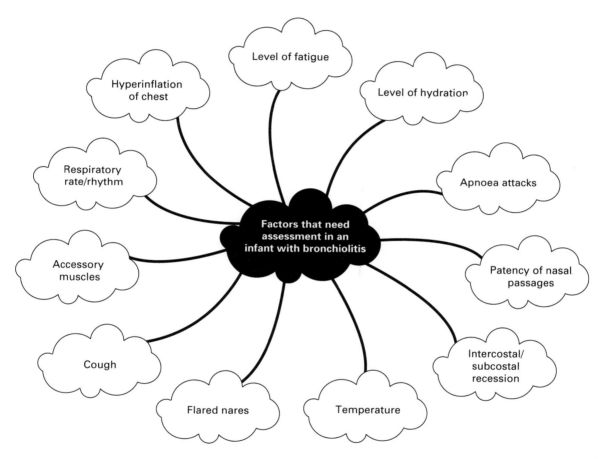

Fig. 16.2 Factors that require assessment in a baby with bronchiolitis.

Dyspnoea and dehydration are the two prime nursing problems to be considered. The infant's respiratory rate and rhythm, the degree of dyspnoea, tachypnoea, use of accessory muscles, the level of subcostal and intercostal retractions and flaring of the nares should be assessed and documented comprehensively; simply recording the respiratory rate is insufficient. Any increase in the use of

The nurse should also assess the baby's cough and record the type, frequency and other characteristics. Since young babies are obligatory nose breathers the nurse must assess the baby for patency of this part of their airway. The infant's temperature must be taken regularly as the infectious agent and the increased workload imposed by the respiratory distress can cause

Table 16.1 Characteristics that should be recorded about apnoea attacks.

- time
- duration
- colour change
- awake/asleep prior to attack
- respiratory pattern prior to attack
- position of baby
- associated trigger
- bradycardia
- action required (self limiting, gentle stimulus, resuscitation)
- additional comments

the infant to become pyrexial and therefore at risk from febrile convulsions.

Another major area of nursing assessment lies in determining the child's level of hydration. The infectious illness, pyrexia and respiratory distress can result in the infant losing more fluid than usual through insensible losses. Additionally, a poor intake of fluids often results from the infant being either too tired to suck or being unable to effectively co-ordinate sucking with breathing. The infant may also vomit as a consequence of the bouts of coughing. The infant's skin turgor, mucous membranes and anterior fontanelle as well as urinary output can help in the assessment of dehydration. The infant may also experience diarrhoea as a result of the viral infection, and gastro-intestinal status should be considered.

Another and perhaps less well considered aspect of nursing care at this stage relates to consideration of the infant's level of fatigue and exhaustion. The infant's ability to continue to cope with the respiratory distress must be considered and documented; the increasingly tired and exhausted infant is at risk from collapse. Intervention prior to collapse is always appropriate.

Nursing intervention: meeting the baby's needs

Respiratory support is essential for these infants and is the mainstay of all care. Correct and appropriate positioning of the infant reduces one stressor on the child's respiratory efforts. Sitting the baby in a suitable chair or nursing them on a 10–30° angle head-up tilted mattress may provide effective and almost immediate help. This position reduces pressures in the infant's diaphragm and facilitates abdominal breathing. The patency of the infant's airway needs to be maintained and gentle suction to the nasopharynx can greatly assist the infant's respiratory efforts. The aim with suctioning is to be as atraumatic (both physically and psychologically) as possible.

Infants should have their need to be 'sucked out' carefully assessed. This is achieved by considering the amount and type of secretions being produced, the effects that the secretions are having, and the general condition of the infant. In response to arterial blood gas results and/or pulse oximetry measurements, supplementary oxygen may be required and this must be monitored. The nurse needs to ensure that the environment is safe for this to occur and that the baby can be easily observed and is comfortable. Small infants generally manage well with oxygen supplied via a head box; older infants may require an oxygen tent. Humidity should be supplied to reduce the drying effects of the oxygen as well as to facilitate liquefaction of secretions. Any humidity supplied to small infants should be warmed as cold moist air may cause reflex bronchoconstriction.

For the baby experiencing moderate problems with bronchiolitis the use of an apnoea monitor is advisable, although the nurse should discuss the reasons for and benefits of the device with the parents, and should discuss its limitations; for example, the alarm may be triggered even when the baby is fine. Parents are often bewildered by the amount of technology and intervention their small baby requires and careful explanation of what is being used, why and how they can help is a vital part of the nurse's duties and responsibilities. The same applies to the use of pulse oximetry as a means of monitoring the baby's oxygenation. To the parents it can seem like a frightening set of figures and moving lights and lines, and the nurse should encourage them to focus on their baby rather than the machinery.

Managing the infant's level of hydration is important and when the baby is no longer able to maintain their fluid intake orally the usual short term option is the intravenous route. Intravenous fluids provide a route that places no stress on the infant as enteral routes can place an unnecessary strain on the infant. Nasogastric tubes are best avoided as they obscure part of the infant's air passage and bolus feeds can fill the stomach and may splint or partially splint the diaphragm, which again restricts the baby's respiratory efforts. Fluid and electrolyte balance need monitoring regularly.

Generally the care of the baby with bronchiolitis is supportive and drug therapy, apart from oxygen, is not indicated. However, in severe cases or in those infants classified as at high risk, ribovarin may be prescribed to combat RSV (Clancy & Jones 1993). Ribovarin is delivered by a small particle aerosol generator (SPAG) and the fine mist produced is inhaled into the lungs. Care needs to be taken when using ribovarin; precautions are advised especially for pregnant or lactating women (Clancy & Jones 1993). Bronchodilators are not generally indicated (Whaley & Wong 1991) and antibiotics are only of value if secondary infection occurs.

The nurse must also ensure that infection control is a priority due to the highly contagious nature of RSV. Ideally the infant with RSV should be nursed isolated and if this is not possible then the nurse should review the options and resources available to ensure that the risk is reduced to a minimum. McFarlane (1992) high-lights a number of ways of preventing the spread of RSV (Fig. 16.3). These can be part of the nurse's role as teacher and leader of care to both colleagues/other members of the multi-disciplinary team and the parents. Ensuring that the risk of cross infection is minimized is important and emphasizing this aspect of care to the parents is vital.

Evaluating the effectiveness of nursing support and the infant's recovery or progress is important and as the infant's respiratory status stabilizes and improves, the supportive therapy can gradually be withdrawn whilst close assessment continues. As the need for supplementary oxygen reduces, and the respiratory rate returns to normal, and dyspnoea decreases, the infant's usual feeding routine can be re-established. Parents need to be encouraged to take over all the infant's care so that they can recover any lost confidence. They need support and reassurance about managing at home, and the help from the paediatric community nurse can be essential at this time as she or he is an expert who is close at hand.

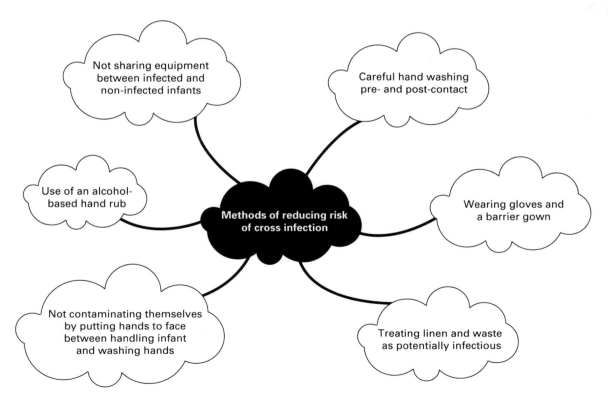

Fig. 16.3 Methods of reducing cross infection (developed from McFarlane 1992).

Parents may feel insecure in dealing with future coughs and colds as they may worry that their baby will develop bronchiolitis again. Reassurance should be given that as the infant develops, its resistance to infection will increase, and it should be suggested that they can enhance this by avoiding smoking near the baby and avoiding crowded places that have a higher likelihood of transmitting infections. The parents should also be taught about the signs of respiratory distress and when they should seek help.

NURSING THE CHILD WITH CROUP

Often the child with croup can be nursed at home and while the symptoms may appear worrying, parents can provide appropriate and adequate support and care although they may require education, support and advice from the paediatric community nurse. Children who are nused in their own homes need to be assessed regularly and the parents need to be advised about the signs and symptoms of needing urgent review or urgent help. The paediatric community nurse is in the ideal position to provide this educational role and also provide a level of emotional and 'professional' help. The parents can be advised that sitting with the child in a steamy bathroom can provide a good level of humidity to help ease their symptoms; a gentle reminder not to leave the child unsupervised in the bathroom should be given. However some children will require admission to hospital as the complications of croup, which include pneumonia and laryngeal obstruction, may prove fatal.

Croup is correctly considered a clinical syndrome characterized by a barking cough, inspiratory stridor and a hoarse voice (Wald 1990). Laryngotracheobronchitis (LTB) is most commonly seen in young children and infants, boys and girls being equally affected. The mild symptoms generally cause a level of anxiety in both the child and their parents, some sleepless nights caused by the barking cough and the need to keep the child's airway humidified. The severe symptoms which often occur in association with the initial infection are not generally seen in subsequent infections (Ramsay 1989). The infecting agent is normally viral, most commonly parainfluenza virus 1-2-3, but can also be respiratory syncitial virus, influenza virus and rhinovirus (Brunner & Suddarth 1991).

Secondary bacterial infection also occurs and coagulase positive staphylococci are most often implicated, although group A streptococcus, streptococcus viridans, hameophilus influenzae and gram negative enterics are cited by Wald (1990) as likely to be implicated as pathogens. Unlike epiglottitis, the onset and progression of the disease is gradual following a couple of days of mild illness with an upper respiratory tract infection. Careful assessment, managing the child's airway and constant psychological care and support provide an appropriate background to meeting the needs of the child with croup.

Nursing assessment

Assessment focuses on the effects that the infection is having on the child's respiratory system and overall status. Laryngeal oedema, along with tenacious secretions in the lower respiratory tract, and generalized oedema of the respiratory tract make breathing difficult for the child. Inspiratory stridor is caused by the laryngeal oedema, and the hoarse voice by oedematous vocal cords. An overall assessment of the child with croup usually gives a picture of a child who is:

- Mouth breathing due to blockage of the nose and nasopharynx with secretions.
- Coughing in an attempt to expel secretions from their lungs.
- Breathing with a characteristic inspiratory stridor in an attempt to draw air through the oedematous larynx.
- Showing signs of increasing respiratory effort and exhaustion.

Hypoxia may result and in severe cases retention of carbon dioxide in the lungs leads to respiratory failure and eventually cessation of breathing (Whaley & Wong 1991). Pneumonia is reported to occur in 50% of children with laryngotracheobronchitis (Wald 1991).

Assessment includes observing the child for signs of increasing respiratory distress, including use of accessory muscles and nasal flaring. The child's colour, perfusion, signs of pallor and cyanosis should be noted. Due to the infection the child's temperature should be recorded regularly as hyperpyrexia may be problematic. Tachycardia should be noted and reported. The nurse assessing the child should be concerned about the potential for rapid respiratory deterioration if the following symptoms occur:

- Tachycardia.
- Tachypnoea.
- Flaring nares.
- Intercostal, suprasternal and substernal recession.
- An increased/increasing level of distress and agitation.

The child's ability to take and tolerate oral fluids, and the overall fluid balance, should be established. The respiratory distress experienced by the child may make taking oral fluids problematic and their level of agitation and tiredness may result in the child being fractious with fluids. The child's risk of aspiration when coughing must also be assessed and the need for intravenous fluids considered. The child's respiratory status is not allowed to deteriorate without appropriate action taking place and the nurse should consider the family's coping strategies and their ability to deal with their child's illness.

Nursing intervention: meeting the child's needs

Physical management focuses on maintaining the child's airway. However, the child is likely to feel anxious and frightened by their admission to hospital and the nurse can ease some of both their physical and emotional distress by providing a friendly and reassuring presence for both the parents and the child.

If the croup is mild–moderate, an appropriate level of humidity may be all that is required to ease the child's respiratory distress. Humidified oxygen may be indicated if pulse oximetry or arterial blood gases show that the child is hypoxaemic. The anxious, distressed, infected child will also benefit by being nursed in a cool environment as this will help to reduce their pyrexia and may make them feel more comfortable. Antipyretics may be prescribed and administered according to hospital protocol. Due to the viral nature of most infections antibiotics are not normally indicated.

If the child's condition requires managing with placement of an endotracheal tube or tracheostomy tube, the most appropriate place is in theatre and, due to the oedema, the child will usually be intubated with a

tube of narrower diameter than the one that would usually be selected for their age. Careful management of the tube is vital (Table 16.2).

Table 16.2 Factors in effective management of endotracheal tube.

- Tube should be well secured, not dragging.
- Tube should have good connections, which fit rebreathing circuit.
- Tapes should be clean and dry.
- Skin care should be provided to prevent excoriation.
- Spare ET, cut to size, and laryngoscope available.
- Appropriate suction technique.

The nurse needs to ensure that chest movement is equal and that the child is positioned comfortably. Warmed, humidified oxygen should be delivered to the ET tube and suction applied appropriately to the tube to maintain its patency. The child requiring an endotracheal tube in situ needs a high level of psychological support; they need a great deal of reassurance and comforting. The parents can be encouraged to help the child in this way although it should be acknowledged that they may find it difficult to comfort their child when they are distressed themselves. The nurse can encourage the child to play quietly, listen to stories or watch the television as appropriate. Initially the child will often be too tired to play. Encouraging the parents to talk and touch the child makes the parents feel they are valued and have something positive to offer their child. As the laryngeal oedema subsides, a leak around the ET tube becomes evident and this strongly indicates that extubation is possible.

Careful preparation of the child and family for extubation is important and close assessment of the child, pre, intra and post extubation is vital (Clancy & Jones 1993). Supplemental humidified oxygen needs to be continued by head box or face mask as appropriate for a period after extubation until the child can be weaned off this and can breathe room air again. Throughout the period that the child is experiencing respiratory distress, intravenous fluids are indicated to ensure that their level of hydration is maintained appropriately. Rest is also important and should be seen as a nursing priority. Grouping care, minimizing disturbances, and creating a restful atmosphere can promote the child's opportunities to rest and sleep, thus conserving their energy (Whaley & Wong 1991).

As the child recovers, the need to prepare the parents and child for discharge becomes apparent and parents need to be aware that the child may sound 'croupy' for some time afterwards. Warm, moist air such as in the bathroom can still be used to quieten noisy respirations. Parents also need to be advised of the importance of ensuring that the child continues to drink appropriate volumes of fluid. Encouraging the child to sleep and rest and to generally recover from their experience of being in hospital or being ill at home is an important component of aftercare.

Conclusion

In conclusion therefore, the nurse's role is vital. An ongoing and high level of critical assessment is the basis for clinical decision making in respect of children with croup. The need to preempt respiratory collapse is at the forefront of the nurse's aims, and elective intervention at the appropriate time (not too early, not too late) is a crucial part of intervention. These children experience a gradually deteriorating condition that infrequently requires a high level of technological intervention and as such the impact of the illness on them must be considered.

NURSING THE CHILD WITH EPIGLOTTITIS

As with many childhood infections, in epiglottitis the child can suddenly deteriorate creating an extreme level of anxiety for both the child and their family. Epiglottitis requires urgent and expert attention and calls upon a considerable level of interpersonal and intrapersonal skills on the part of the nurse. Creating a calm and reassuring environment as well as assisting with management of the condition is vital. The speed at which the child deteriorates and the symptoms they present with are frightening; they may go to bed asymptomatic, apart from what may be seen to be the beginnings of a cold, and awake several hours later distressed and acutely symptomatic.

Epiglottitis should always be considered a potential respiratory emergency (Clancy & Jones 1993). The nurse should be aware that resources, including suitably experienced staff, for potential intubation or for formation of tracheostomy should be available. Epiglottitis generally affects children between the ages of three and seven years (Whaley & Wong 1991), although Smith Millett (1991) suggests that most cases are seen in children aged one to five years.

Epiglottitis results from bacterial infection, most commonly haemophilus influenza type-B although pneumococcus, staphylococcus aureus and β. haemolytic streptococcus are causative agents. In epiglottitis, the epiglottis becomes markedly oedematous and the false cords and the aryepiglottic folds obstruct the laryngeal outlet during inspiration. Epiglottitis can be fulminant with total occlusion of the child's airway; this can occur suddenly and is most often precipitated by either an attempt to examine the child's throat or by lying the child down to examine them. Neither of these procedures should be attempted in the child with suspected epiglottitis unless full support for intubation is available.

Nursing assessment

Assessment must be comprehensive, careful and undertaken in as calm a way as possible (Table 16.3).

Table 16.3 Features of epiglottitis.

Three classic symptoms ■ drooling ■ agitation ■ absence of spontaneous cough Additional features ■ position ■ inspiratory stridor (croaking) ■ expiratory snore ■ sore throat ■ thick muffled voice ■ tachycardia ■ pyrexia High risk features (indicating near total obstruction) ■ lethargy ■ decrease in both inspiratory and expiratory breath sounds ■ cyanosis

The nurse should explain carefully to the child what they are going to do and generally assessment should be performed whilst the child is being reassured, held and cuddled by the parents. Separating the child from its parents is both unnecessary and dangerous if the child becomes stressed and anxious. An overall quick assessment will usually demonstrate that the child has three classic symptoms: drooling, agitation and absence of a spontaneous cough. In the presence of these three symptoms a diagnosis of epiglottitis should be assumed until proven otherwise.

Assessment of the child's respiratory status involves assessing the way in which the child is actually managing to breathe. They automatically adopt an upright sitting position, leaning forward, chin thrust forward, mouth open and their tongues protruding. This position facilitates chest movements and on no account should this be discouraged. The child has a severe inspiratory stridor (Brunner & Suddarth 1991) and this tends to make a characteristic croaking sound, the child's expirations sounding like snoring. The child's colour should be assessed regularly. The difficulty associated with breathing, the very sore throat, the unusual noise of their breathing and their thick, muffled voice, all add to the child's emotional distress and thus to their respiratory distress. The respiratory distress can result in hypoxia and the child will display a level of restlessness and agitation. The nurse must assess and record all of these symptoms, including the presence of drooling and mouth breathing.

Any tachycardia and pyrexia should be noted. Assessment of the child's hydrational status should also be performed, although oral fluids are not usually indicated as the child experiences difficulty in swallowing even their own secretions. As the child's condition deteriorates the nurse should be aware that lethargy, a decrease in the sounds of both inspiration and expiration, and cyanosis indicate that the child is at extreme risk from total obstruction. Much of the nurse's role constitutes a high level of assessment and observation so that pre-emptive intubation is performed at the appropriate moment. The nurse requires and must insist on having the close support of an experienced, skilled anaesthetist (for intubation) and in some hospitals the presence of an equally experienced ENT surgeon can be of value in case a tracheostomy is required (Lord 1988 pers. comm.). Assessment of the child's throat can only be considered if emergency support is available. Diagnosis is made from the presenting symptoms and from a lateral neck X-ray which indicates supra-epiglottic oedema. Normally this is done using a portable X-ray machine with the child continuing to be nursed on the parent's lap. Further assessment involves epiglottal swabs once the child has been intubated.

Nursing intervention: meeting the child's needs

The nurse's prime role in caring for the child with epiglottitis is that of maintaining a patent airway. Endotracheal intubation is indicated to maintain patency of the airway; however, if intubation is not required, an extremely vigilant level of observation and assessment by the nurse and regular review by the medical team is indicated until the oedema starts to diminish and the child's symptoms disappear in response to antibiotic therapy (Whaley & Wong 1991). Prior to endotracheal intubation, the nurse is responsible for ensuring that as calm an atmosphere as possible prevails, that the parents and the child are reassured and informed of the need to intubate, and are told what this entails. Protecting the child from unnecessary examination or intervention and liaising with appropriate members of the multidisciplinary team is also important.

In respect to intubation a smaller diameter endotracheal tube than usually expected for the child must be available and cut to size, and an appropriate tracheostomy tube should be available. Intubation is often carried out in the operating theatre providing that the transfer of the child is carried out gently and is not seen to be an additional stressor. Oral intubation with the child still sitting up is generally performed and once this airway has been established a more secure nasotracheal tube can usually be placed in situ. Humidified oxygen to the tube is usually sufficient to stabilize the child. In practice smaller lumen tubes tend to be short in overall length and this can result in a situation where the endotracheal tube is only just long enough. In these situations it is essential that nothing disturbs the position of the tube as the need to reintubate the child (if the tube becomes displaced/malpositioned) increases the level of risk (and difficulty in replacing the tube). Some children may require further respiratory support from either continuous positive airways pressure or intermittent positive pressure ventilation (Ramsay 1989).

The child is usually prescribed a course of broad

spectrum intravenous antibiotics prior to identifying the specific nature of the infecting pathogen. The child may also receive corticosteroid therapy for the first 24–48 hours (Clancy & Jones 1993), although this is not always the treatment of choice. During the period of intubation the child continues to drool as they find it painful to swallow, and the nurse needs to ensure that their pillows and clothes are kept clean and dry.

A high level of psychological support is needed for both the child and their family. Often it appears that the parents' initial relief that the endotracheal tube or tracheostomy has brought about such a radical response and relief of the child's respiratory distress, is replaced by anxiety about the tube itself and the consequences of it being in place. Some children may require a light level of sedation to help them tolerate the tube, but it is preferable that the child complies with the tube through a high level of skilled nursing care and family support. The child usually sleeps after intubation due to the level of exhaustion that they experience.

Intravenous fluids are used to maintain fluid and electrolyte balance until the child is able to be extubated and able to swallow an appropriate amount; at this point the antibiotics are prescribed for the oral route of administration. Normally 24 to 48 hours after the commencement of antibiotic therapy, the epiglottal oedema has diminished and the child is able to swallow. The nurse must always help to manage the child's pyrexia, and appropriate antipyretics are indicated if the child's temperature is above 38°C. The pyrexia also responds to the antibiotic therapy. As the child recovers, swallowing becomes easier and the child may be able to make some speech noises around the endotracheal tube.

Extubation is usually possible within 24 to 36 hours. Again the nurse must closely assess the child post-extubation to ensure that they are able to maintain their respiratory status with no distress. Once extubated the child's usual routine in respect to eating, drinking and playing can be re-introduced and the intravenous fluids discontinued. Throughout the whole admission parents are likely to feel anxious and distressed and will often be exhausted both emotionally and physically. The nurse should see that they are kept informed of their child's progress and encouraged to rest. As the child improves the importance of the antibiotics must be stressed so that once the child is discharged home they continue to have the antibiotics at the regular prescribed intervals, and they complete the course of treatment.

Conclusion

For both the child and the parents epiglottitis comes as a sudden, unpredicted and potentially catastrophic emergency and the parents may often feel guilty that their child became so ill without them realizing it. The nurse needs to reassure them that it is an illness trajectory that is impossible to predict in the early stages and they are in no way to blame for the child needing hospital admission and such 'aggressive' intervention. They should also be assured that as the child grows and develops they are less at risk from recurrence. The child also needs plenty of psychological support as this may have been their first contact with hospital. Playing with the child, reassuring them and helping the family support the child are all important aspects of nursing care. Investing special care and support can obviate some of the child's fear and anxiety if for whatever reason, the child needs to come into hospital again.

CARE OF THE CHILD WITH TONSILLITIS AND TONSILLECTOMY

Tonsillectomy is an elective operation without undue complications, which tends not to need an excessive amount of physical preparation. However, this does not mean that the child views it as a simple, easily understood and atraumatic experience (Sharman 1985). One of the most important psychological needs that the nurse needs to meet is that of providing a high level of support and reassurance to the child who is admitted to hospital well and healthy and goes home post-operatively feeling worse than when they arrived. Good preparation, using appropriate techniques that are adequately audited and evaluated, can help to ensure that the child's exposure to the hospital environment is as atraumatic as possible. Hammerschlag (1990) reports that sore throat is the most common reason for children and young adults going to the doctor.

Nursing assessment

The nurse's role in assessment relates mainly to the effects that the specific infection is having on the individual child. The tonsils are masses of lymphoid tissue that provide a first line of defence against respiratory infections and as such are important. Inflamed tonsils create special problems for children because their tonsillar growth exceeds somatic growth in the first ten years of life, so the tonsils appear large in the child (Brunner & Suddarth 1991). Mostly tonsillitis is viral although some tonsillitis episodes are caused by β-haemolytic steptococcus. The inflamed tonsils can obstruct airflow and make eating difficult.

The nurse needs to assess the child with tonsillitis for sore throat, mild pyrexia, headache (mild), and loss of appetite. The nurse can assess for redness and exudate in the pharyngeal area. The child's hoarse voice and productive cough can also be indicative of tonsillitis. Although the presenting symptoms may appear mild the nurse should always assess for signs of respiratory distress which could be associated with the enlarged tonsils/obstructed airway.

The child's level of hydration and nutrition must also be assessed since the sore throat will often make them reluctant to take oral fluids or diet or they may experience difficulty in swallowing. Children with tonsillitis often mouth breath which, along with poor fluid intake, makes the mucous membranes of the orophraynx dry and irritated, and halitosis is not uncommon. An important part of the assessment process lies with the nurse establishing the frequency of episodes and the onset of symptoms (Smith Millet 1992).

Nursing intervention: meeting the child's needs

The child with tonsillitis basically requires supportive care since the illness itself is self limiting. Cold drinks, mild analgesics, a soft diet, salt water gargles and throat sprays can all be used to minimize the child's discomfort. Antibiotic therapy is only indicated if the tonsillitis is identified as being of bacterial origin. The nurse needs to ensure that parents understand the importance of any medication that has been prescribed and that they are aware of the symptoms associated with respiratory distress, that indicate the need to seek further help.

However, some children may be referred after repeated episodes of tonsillectomy. The debate surrounding the value of tonsillectomy continues and tonsillectomy remains the most frequently performed surgical proce-

dure on children beyond the neonatal period (Whaley & Wong 1991). As with any surgical procedure there are risks involved and children should not be exposed to these risks unnecessarily. Contraindications to tonsillectomy include cleft palate, acute infection at the proposed time of surgery, and uncontrolled systemic diseases and blood dyscrasias (Whaley & Wong 1991).

For the child requiring tonsillectomy the usual careful planning and preparation by the nurse for admission to hospital, the surgery itself, and the recovery afterwards are all vital. What may be considered by some nurses as a routine operation is a potentially very frightening and painful episode for the child – a situation of going into hospital feeling well and leaving with a sore throat and some perhaps frightening memories. Keeping the child safe involves ensuring that their psychological as well as physical needs are met.

Post operatively the prime aims of nursing care are to ensure that the child is safe (primarily not at risk from bleeding and/or airway obstruction) and comfortable. The child needs to be nursed on their side or abdomen to facilitate drainage of secretions. Parents and the child should be told that the child will probably have some old blood in their mouth, nose and on their teeth when they return from theatre; preparation for the sight of their child is often sufficient to allay their fears. The nurse needs to assess for the presence of fresh blood which would indicate continued bleeding from the tonsillar bed, and should try to prevent bleeding from occurring. This can be achieved by encouraging cool fluids (once the child has recovered from the anaesthetic), and the use of a good suction technique if the child's secretions are building up (trauma to the orpharynx must be avoided). The nurse should also discourage the child from coughing too frequently or trying to clear their throat too vigorously.

The child's overwhelming concern during the postoperative recovery will be the pain they experience; their throat will be very sore and the judicious use of mild analgesia, other pain management strategies and cool/cold drinks can be of real help in easing the pain. The nurse caring for the child postoperatively needs to regularly assess the child for signs of haemorrhage. Signs include tachycardia, tachypnoea, pallor, vomiting bright red blood, increased swallowing, and restlessness. If suspicious of continued bleeding the nurse must inform the surgeon immediately as the child may need to return to theatre for intervention. Children are at risk from haemorrhage post-tonsillectomy due to the very vascular nature of the tonsillar tissue and the fact that they can covertly lose a large amount of blood and be at considerable risk from hypovolaemic shock.

As the child's recovery continues soft diet can be introduced and the child is usually discharged within twelve hours. Care continues at home by the parents, and the nurse needs to ensure that they are fully prepared to continue their child's care, by providing them with information and advice including the encouragement of an appropriate diet (one which is not irritating), use of cool drinks and mild analgesics to combat the pain, and avoidance of the use of gargles and very vigorous tooth brushing (Whaley & Wong 1991).

For children recovering from tonsillitis much of the care is supportive in terms of helping them to deal with some of the trauma they have experienced. Hopefully with therapeutic nursing interventions and good preparation for the operation and stay in hospital, children will have good memories of the nurses who cared for them and of their hospital stay.

NURSING THE CHILD WITH ASTHMA

The nurse caring for and meeting the needs of the child with asthma requires a sound knowledge base from which to work. This will include an understanding of the causes of asthma, the physical and emotional impact that it has on the child, and the preventative, prophylactic and 'emergency' care that may be considered. The need to work in partnership with the child, their family and other health care professionals is seen as vital, and partnership is seen by Gregson *et al.* (1993) as the key to successful management of childhood asthma.

An understanding of asthma is crucial as it is one of the most common causes of childhood ill health (Rees & Price 1989; Gregson *et al.* 1993; Wooler 1994). The prevalence of asthma in children is increasing (Warner *et al.* 1989) and this has been particularly noticeable over the past twenty years. Burr *et al.* (1989) and Burney *et al.* (1990) both report changes in the prevalence of asthma. A variety of factors have been implicated in this increase, notably environmental factors such as air pollution (nitrous dioxide NO_2, pavement level ozone, sulphur dioxide SO_2, acid air and particulates), and tobacco

smoke (active and passive) (NAC 1993b). *Asthmanews* (1993) reports a study undertaken in Atlanta, Georgia, during 1991 in which a strong link was established between the levels of ozone in the atmosphere and the number of emergency visits to the hospital made by children with asthma.

Estimates about the number of children with asthma vary: 12–15% (Wooler 1994); at least 11% (Rees & Price 1989); 1:10 (NAC 4 1993) and 10–15% (Asthma Training Centre 1991). The size of the problem is clearly seen but the size of the problem for the children themselves may be less obvious. Carter (1993) highlights the impact that asthma can have on the child's schooling, with 1:8 of nine year olds who wheeze losing more than 30 days schooling annually, and Rees & Price (1989) suggest that 30% of children who are asthmatic miss in excess of three weeks' schooling every year. Additionally asthma is shown to have an impact on the child's sleep pattern. Action Asthma (1993) in a survey of 20 000 asthmatic children aged 4–17 years, found that 5% of the children lost sleep to asthma every night; 60% reported feeling sleepy in class the following day and 1:3 were woken by asthma symptoms once a week.

Asthma is more common in boys than girls (2:1) before adolescence, but affects boys and girls equally after adolescence (Smith Millet, 1992). Most (80%) of children are symptomatic before their fifth birthday, with about 30% of them being symptomatic before the age of two years. A number of children have associated allergies and/or a family history. Gregson *et al.* (1993) report that 80% of children have a family history of allergic disease, with 30% of them having eczema. Ramsay (1989) reports that asthmatic children can be broadly categorized, with 75% of asthmatic children experiencing infrequent attacks mostly associated with upper respiratory tract infections (URTIs), while 22% experience severe and more frequent attacks resulting from a number of triggers/factors. The remaining 3% of children have chest deformities and a permanent underlying lung function problem as a result of their severe bronchoconstriction.

Despite the fact that asthma is acknowledged as such a common condition there remain problems with diagnosis and mismanagement (Wooler 1993).

Asthma is difficult to define due to the variety of symptoms, but it has recently been defined as:

'a condition in which episodic wheeze and/or cough

occur in a clinical setting where asthma is likely and other, rarer conditions have been excluded.' (International Paediatric Asthma Consensus Group, 1992).

In essence it is an obstructive airways disease which is usually reversible and is characterized by three major mechanisms which result in reduction of airway lumen size and give rise to the characteristic cough, wheeze and shortness of breath. The mechanisms involved are: an increased bronchoconstrictor response, oedema, and hypersecretion of mucous (Wooler 1993).

Nursing assessment

Assessment will include observing the child's respiratory rate and their pattern of breathing; use of accessory muscles, recession and the child's colour should be noted. The child's pulse should be taken and the presence of pulsus paradox noted. Pulsus paradox increases with the increasing severity of the attack until the point where respiratory failure is imminent; at this point it decreases. The overall level of respiratory distress should be assessed and the child's level of tiredness and anxiety should be noted. The position that the child adopts, usually sitting up, can also be helpful in assessing the difficulty that the child is experiencing.

The type and frequency of the child's cough should be noted, as should the nature and amount of any expectorated sputum as this may indicate an underlying respiratory tract infection. Care needs to be taken in determining any factors which may have precipitated the attack, and the duration and characteristics of it. The nurse should observe the child for sweating and signs of dehydration. The child's ability, or more significantly inability, to communicate and the infant's ability or inability to cry should be noted as this can reflect the severity of the attack. The nurse needs to assess the affects that the asthma attack is having/is likely to have on the child's normal activities, including sleeping and eating and drinking.

Nursing intervention: meeting the needs of child with acute, severe asthma

The child experiencing an acute severe asthma attack that requires hospital care will need experienced nursing care and medical support. Overwhelmingly the child with asthma needs to be nursed in a supportive environment; this means that they should not be separated from their parents unnecessarily and the nurse should offer support, information and reassurance to both the child and their family. Humidified oxygen therapy is required to save the child's life; oxygen is the most important drug that can be administered to the child since children with acute asthma die from hypoxaemia. Additionally the humidity can facilitate expectoration of sputum and thus ease this part of the child's dyspnoea.

Humidified oxygen needs to be delivered by an appropriate method which is dependent on the age of the child and the child's tolerance of means of delivery. Older children will often tolerate oxygen via a face mask and care should be taken to ensure that the mask is comfortable. For smaller children the option of using an oxygen tent may be considered, although some young children may become distressed by being nursed in a tent which can be perceived as being noisy, damp and isolating (oxygen tents tend to make observing the child difficult since visibility is compromised). In this situation the child is more appropriately nursed on a parent's or the nurse's lap. Regardless of the means of delivery the nurse must ensure that the child's colour, respiratory effort and level of fatigue can be easily observed and should maintain vigilant assessment of their response to treatment.

Nebulized salbutomol (nebulized with oxygen) is often prescribed two to four hourly and the effect of this intervention requires monitoring. If the child is able to use a peak flow meter, pre and postnebulizer recordings can be made to see the efficacy of this treatment. However, the child with a very severe attack will often be incapable, due to the respiratory distress and their fatigue, of complying with a request to generate a peak expiratory flow rate (PEFR) reading. Intravenous aminophylline is indicated when the child does not respond to nebulized treatment, and the nurse should be aware of the risk of tachycardia and cardiac arrhythmias associated with the administration of this drug (Efthimiou 1992).

Oral corticosteroids may be used short term and intravenous corticosteroid therapy may be indicated in severe status asthmaticus. An intravenous infusion to maintain the child's hydration may be indicated if the child is too breathless to take oral fluids, and the nurse should ensure that this infusion is given safely and effectively. Oral fluids can usually be given once the child is breathing more easily.

The overall aim of nursing care is to reassure and comfort the child whilst reducing the child's respiratory distress. The nurse should also ensure that all cares and interventions, wherever appropriate, are organized to facilitate periods of rest and sleep. In rare cases the child in status asthmaticus requires transfer to the intensive care unit for ventilation. Throughout a severe attack treatment effectiveness needs monitoring through the measurement of arterial blood gases and by pulse oximetry; this ensures that treatment is responsive to the child's changing condition.

As the child's condition improves, the intravenous treatment, if used, is withdrawn and then the frequency of the nebulized bronchodilator is reduced. Ongoing assessment of the child's tolerance of this reduction in treatment is vital and PEFR (in older/school age children) is an important indicator of this tolerance. The move towards a return to the child's usual drug regime is

made and the nurse needs to ensure that both the child, where appropriate, and the family fully understand the protocols and are competent in using the various pieces of equipment such as inhalers and spacers (Gregson *et al.* 1993). Technique can be checked whilst the child is awaiting discharge and any deficits in knowledge can be met by the nurse using suitable teaching programme. Difficulties related to complying with the treatment may also be discussed and hopefully overcome. The final aim of treatment must be prevention of further occurrence or, if this is not possible, reduction of the severity of subsequent attacks.

Nursing intervention: meeting the needs of the child with nonacute asthma

The child with asthma will often be managed within the community and should be able to take part in most activities. Prophylactic treatment, whilst not curing

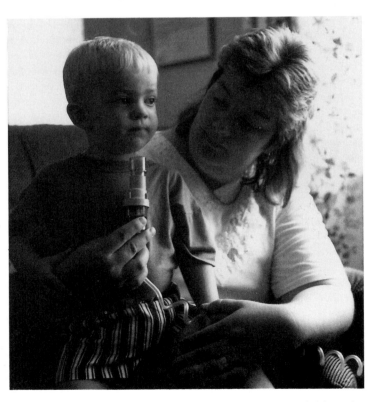

Fig. 16.4 The family is paramount in providing ongoing management of their child's asthma. *(Reproduced by permission of Jon Sparks.)*

asthma, results in reduction of asthma symptoms, and optimum asthma management, from a pharmacological perspective, means using the right drugs at the right level and at the right times to meet the individual child's needs. One crucial factor within pharmacological management is that the drugs are delivered effectively and this can be a major component of the nurse's role. Ensuring good inhaler technique and compliance with the treatment regime is part of the teaching, supporting and health promoting aspect of nursing care.

Warner *et al.* (1989) proposes that treatment regimes

example, can be difficult for young children with small fingers to manipulate. Nebulisers provide a suitable route for administration although they should not be relied on as the sole means of treatment delivery. Oral medication, to ensure bronchodilation, is a useful route for the very young child but the drawbacks to this approach arise from the fact that larger doses are needed and the effects are delayed as a result of the drug not being directed straight to the lungs (Gregson *et al.* 1993). The appropriateness of a delivery system is closely related to the child's age (Table 16.4).

Table 16.4   Delivery systems appropriate for different age children (developed from Hurrell 1993, Gregson *et al.* 1993).

Age	Delivery system	Comments
0–3 yrs	■ Metered dose inhaler with spacer and inverted face mask. Medication is inhaled during normal tidal breathing. ■ Oral agents such as Ventolin syrup if the above system is inappropriate. ■ Steroids can be delivered via the spacer.	■ Inverting the mask angles the spacer and allows the one way valve to fall open
3–5 yrs	■ Metered dose inhaler (MDI) and spacer as the child can usually use the spacer mouth piece directly. One puff medication: four deep breaths in and out.	■ Nurses can encourage deep slow breaths, getting the child to pretend they are blowing up a balloon.
5–12 yrs	■ Dry powder device, or breath activated inhaler. ■ Bronchodilator steroid therapies can be delivered by dry powder.	■ Dry powder devices should also be supplied with a spacer so that the child can still manage an effective dose if they become quite wheezy and short of breath as they may not have sufficient breath strength to activate the device.
12 yrs +	■ Dry powder devices, breath activated device, MDI.	■ Compliance with treatment or bad technique habits may decrease effectiveness of the therapy.

should reflect the severity and frequency of the child's symptoms and that there is usually a progression from bronchodilator, as required, to non steroidal and to steroidal prophylaxis. Asthma management aims to control any underlying inflammatory response – this is the role of prophylactic therapy – and then treat breakthrough symptoms, if any, with bronchodilators.

Asthma medication falls into three main forms of administration: inhalers, nebulisers and the oral route. Each has its advantages and disadvantages. Inhalers, for

Ensuring that treatment is fun rather than a chore can increase the effectiveness and adherence. Decorating the child's spacer can cheer up a fairly boring piece of equipment and *Asthmanews* (1993) reports the development of a ninja turtle backpack nebulizer which has been designed to be child friendly.

Regardless of the treatment regime decided on or the means of delivery of the treatment, the nurse must bear in mind that nonadherence to treatment has been reported as one of the commonest reasons for poor asthma control. Furthermore, Hurrell (1993) suggests that nonadherence may be implicated in a number of preventable asthma deaths. It may result from an inability to use a treatment device correctly, or resistance/dislike of using the device, or a result of embarrassment. This is supported by Eiser (1991) who reports that some children may feel shame and embarrassment about their diagnosis. This is something that the nurse should be attuned to so that it can be discussed with the child and their family.

Prior to starting any education programme about managing a child's asthma, the nurse should remember that the child needs to be closely involved and feel some level of ownership of both their asthma and the means of managing it. Richards (1991) reports that it is increasingly important to educate the child as well as the parents so that the child can play an active part in monitoring and managing themselves. The introduction of peak flow meters on prescription in 1990 has allowed much closer home monitoring of asthma status. In terms of choosing the right device for the child, consideration of a number of factors must be made. These include:

- Assessment of the child's cognitive and motor ability to determine their ability to use particular devices, both prophylactically and in an acute situation.
- Exploration of the child's attitude to both their diagnosis and the treatment so that any fears can be reduced and eliminated and a suitable knowledge base laid down (Hurrell 1993; Richards 1991).
- Consideration of any changes in the child's life, such as starting school, as devices that were acceptable at home, such as the large spacer devices, may be inappropriate for use at school.

Close monitoring by the nurse is recommended by Richards (1991) so that the child adjusts to such changes as atraumatically as possible. Hurrell (1991) emphasizes the need for careful consultation between the child and the nurse to ensure that the most appropriate device/medication is prescribed and that relevant, consistent information is given when educating the child.

The child and family need to be closely involved in evaluating the efficacy of the treatment and this can partly be done by maintaining an asthma diary. Diary cards, provided by the National Asthma Campaign for example, allow the child or family to document daily symptoms and where possible/appropriate the PEFR.

Close monitoring of the child's asthma status ensures that treatment effectively manages the condition so that the minimum effective dose of drugs can be given.

Ensuring that the child has sufficient information is vital. Richards (1991) emphasizes the central role of the child in the information giving–receiving process, and by closely involving the child in any assessment or consultation a clearer picture of the effects and limitations that asthma may impose on the child emerges. Richards (1991) goes on to propose that even very young children need to be involved so that they can appreciate the effects upon their asthma and what happens during an exacerbation. One area that needs to be explored with any child relates to factors which trigger an attack. Health education and promotion can be achieved by encouraging the family to minimize contact where possible with these risk factors (Fig. 16.5).

The nurse may, in consultation with the family, suggest ways that they can help to reduce the trigger factors by maintaining a relatively allergen/trigger free environment (Fig. 16.6). Problems resulting from dust and the dust mite can be minimized by daily damp dusting and vacuuming when the child is not present. Parents should be encouraged not to smoke in the child's presence as the smoke can trigger an attack. Keeping the house warm and free of damp, restricting the child's diet by avoiding allergens as appropriate, and encouraging the parents to give the child toys that are easy to keep dust free and clean, are all ways in which the parent, with the support of the nurse, can minimize risk factors.

Teaching the child relaxation strategies may also be beneficial. It should not be presumed that failing to follow advice is reflective of an uncaring attitude; it may simply be unrealistic to follow the advice. Over-protection of the child should be avoided.

Conclusion

Asthma care requires the full support and co-operation of the multidisciplinary team. Experts both within the community and the hospital setting, who have effective communication channels and use them, provide a support network that will ensure high quality asthma management. Of paramount importance, however, is the support offered to the child and their family. Nevin & Nevin (1992) discuss some ways in which they feel

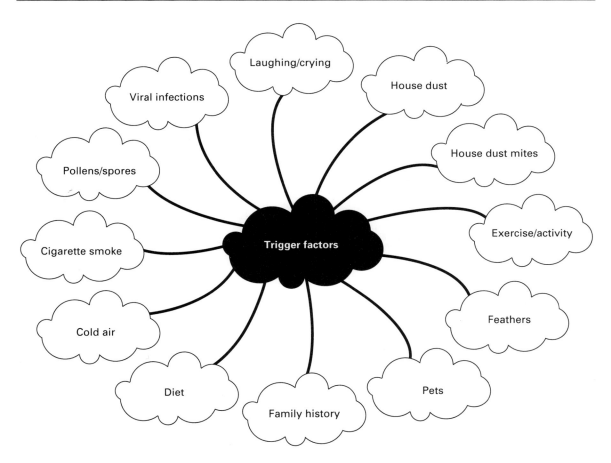

Fig. 16.5 Trigger factors associated with asthma.

that the nurse can offer support. Whilst they identify the nurse's role in caring for the child during an acute attack, they also state 'Help us and you automatically help the child' (Nevin & Nevin 1992). They potently describe the impact that asthma has had on the functioning of their family and this should always be considered as an important issue by the nurse. Parents often feel vulnerable, distressed and anxious when faced with making decisions about their children, and benefit can be derived from a voluntary group. Swallow & Thompson (1992) describe how one small support group was initiated and the successes that it has achieved. The National Asthma Society also provides an excellent service.

NURSING THE CHILD WITH CYSTIC FIBROSIS

Children with cystic fibrosis are members of a family who have to cope every day with the treatment involved in managing a generalized, multisystem disease which, at present, cannot be cured. Cystic fibrosis is a genetic, chronic, life threatening disorder. It is the most common cause of chronic suppurative pulmonary disease in Caucasian children and young adults (Byers 1989; Gill 1993). In the early 1990s cystic fibrosis affected approximately 8000 people in Great Britain (Jennings 1992a).

Historically many children with cystic fibrosis died from malnutrition and diarrhoea in early infancy (Taylor, 1993) and the prognosis was poor. When cystic

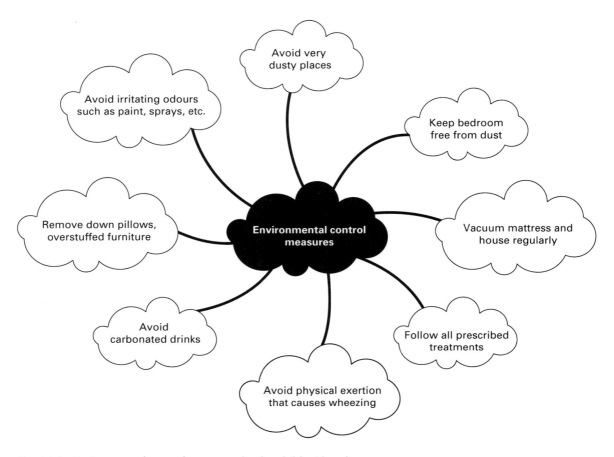

Fig. 16.6 Environmental control measures for the child with asthma.

fibrosis was first recognized in the 1930s, 90% of the affected children died before their first birthday (Ramsay 1989). Millar (1994) reports that as little as ten years ago children with cystic fibrosis were not expected to survive to adulthood, although there is now the probability that survival into their thirties and beyond is possible for babies being currently diagnosed. Caring for the child with cystic fibrosis needs to be set against changes in prognosis, management, and the increasing emphasis on care in the community. The context of cystic fibrosis care has demanded that health care professionals respond and provide treatment and care that is less disruptive of the child's lifestyle and the family's normal functioning.

Cystic fibrosis affects the child's exocrine glands and has its greatest impact on the lungs and the pancreas. It additionally affects the gastrointestinal tract, salivary glands, liver, reproductive tract, nose, paranasal sinuses and sweat glands (Smith Millet 1992; Ramsay 1989). The specific gene responsible for cystic fibrosis was identified in 1989. Every child is affected differently but the condition is progressive and the most common reason for morbidity is respiratory disease. The overriding aim of treatment for any child is to provide optimum treatment and promotion of a good quality of life (Byers 1989).

Basically children with cystic fibrosis overproduce very viscous mucous secretions which result in obstruction, particularly in the pulmonary and gastrointestinal system, resulting in chronic bronchial pulmonary disease and offensive, loose bowel motions. Pancreatic obstruction and malabsorption is evident very early in life, whereas lung involvement takes a little longer to present. Secondary infection is problematic throughout life and this is part of a vicious cycle of infection, increased mucus secretion, infection which results in brochiectasis, pulmonary fibrosis, cor pulmonale and eventually death.

Bronchiectasis is evident in nearly all children with cystic fibrosis after the age of 18 months (Rosenstein 1990). Regular, prophylactic courses of intravenous antibiotics are used to combat infection, along with chest physiotherapy to remove secretions, and nutritional support and management. Thus the impact that cystic fibrosis has on the whole family and what might be considered a 'normal' family schedule can begin to be imagined. The nurse must be aware of the implications and impact that cystic fibrosis has on an individual family whenever called upon to care for the child. Needs assessment must consider the whole family, and the fact that cystic fibrosis is a chronic, life threatening disorder should also be borne in mind.

Cystic fibrosis is diagnosed using the sweat test (after two sweat sodium levels over 70 mmols/l). If the sweat test is inconclusive fat estimation from a three day stool collection, and assessment of pancreatic enzymes, may be performed. These tests support the clinical findings which include failure to thrive and chest pathology.

Nursing assessment

The assessment of a child with cystic fibrosis is fundamental to good management, and assessment as always should be ongoing, dynamic and comprehensive. Assessment also allows early signs of deterioration/improvement to be detected so that modifications to treatment and care can be made. Assessment basically involves carefully monitoring and evaluating all systems that could be/are affected by the condition; thus assessment focuses on the child's respiratory and nutritional status, their fluid and electrolyte balance, infection status, elimination and psychosocial needs.

Children with cystic fibrosis present with different features at different points during their life. Ramsay (1989) identifies three stages: neonate, early infancy and later childhood. Meconium ileus is seen in about 10–15% of neonates who are later diagnosed as having cystic fibrosis (Goodchild & Dodge 1985). Later on the young child presents with recurrent chest infection, a harsh cough and noisy and wheezy breathing – some 40% of cystic children present with these symptoms. A

further 30% display symptoms of malabsorption, including poor weight gain, steatorrhoea and rectal prolapse. A smaller number of children (5%) sweat excessively, taste salty when kissed and are at risk from dehydration. Older children may develop cirrhosis, sinusitis, diabetes mellitus and recurrent abdominal pain, and may experience delayed puberty (Ramsay 1989).

Respiratory assessment focuses on the child's pulmonary function, involving lung function tests such as PEFR and vital capacity. The child's oxygenation status is assessed primarily through the use of a noninvasive method of pulse oximetry, although arterial blood gases may also be required. The nurse also needs to assess the child's colour, respiratory rate and rhythm, chest movements – especially signs of recession and retraction – and any dyspnoea, and sputum for signs of infection or haemoptysis. This information requires careful documentation. Nutritional status is assessed through anthropometric measurements and by looking for dysfunction of the pancreas and for nausea and vomiting. Electrolyte balance is also considered and the nurse should be aware of the potential for the child to develop diabetes mellitus and this should be screened for. The nurse needs to ask the child (or family where appropriate) about the colour, consistency, frequency and odour of the child's stools.

This level of information provides a sound base line from which to manage the child's care. Byers (1989) states that 'treatment is for life' and the implication of this must be that assessment is for life as well. The child's psychosocial status is a priority and time must be given to allow the child to articulate their feelings and worries and to support them through any difficulties they experience. The impact on the whole family is also an important area to consider.

Nursing intervention: meeting the child's needs

Management aims to reduce the morbidity associated with the condition and to ensure an optimum quality of life. Byers (1989) highlights a number of factors which influence overall successful management of the child (Fig. 16.7).

In respect to respiratory management, care focuses on the prevention of infection, the removal of thickened

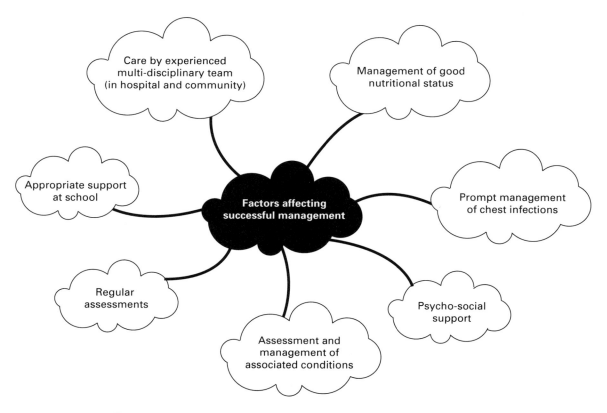

Fig. 16.7   Factors affecting successful management (developed from Byers 1989).

secretions from the lungs and prompt intervention if the child's respiratory status deteriorates. The most important aspect of respiratory care lies with chest physiotherapy and breathing exercises. The aim of respiratory care is to ensure that the child's respiratory rate is within normal limits, that they do not experience dyspnoea and that their breathing does not unduly restrict their usual activities. Breathing exercises are an important part of the child's routine as they can help the child overcome breathlessness, can reduce the tightness in their chest associated with coughing bouts, loosen secretions, and keep the chest wall mobile (Webber & Pryor 1991).

Forced expiration technique (FET) is a means of encouraging the expectoration of more sputum than is possible with a normal cough. Chest physiotherapy is usually performed for fifteen minutes three times a day, and through postural drainage (tipping) and clapping the child's chest the tenacious secretions from all areas of

the lungs can be expectorated. A systematic approach is taken to this and all areas of the chest are covered (Fig 16.8).

As the child matures they are able to take over some and then all aspects of postural drainage so that by the time they are adolescents they should be able to manage independently of their parents – an important part of growing up with or without cystic fibrosis. Postural drainage is a somewhat time-consuming but vital part of the child's care and should be made as much fun as possible; the child should be as relaxed as possible. Treatment is given more frequently when the child has an infection.

Ensuring the child's co-operation is an important part of this process; this may be problematic during adolescence when the regime may seem particularly restrictive and one which sets them apart from their peers. Adolescents with cystic fibrosis have to deal with all the usual problems of this transition as well as the condition

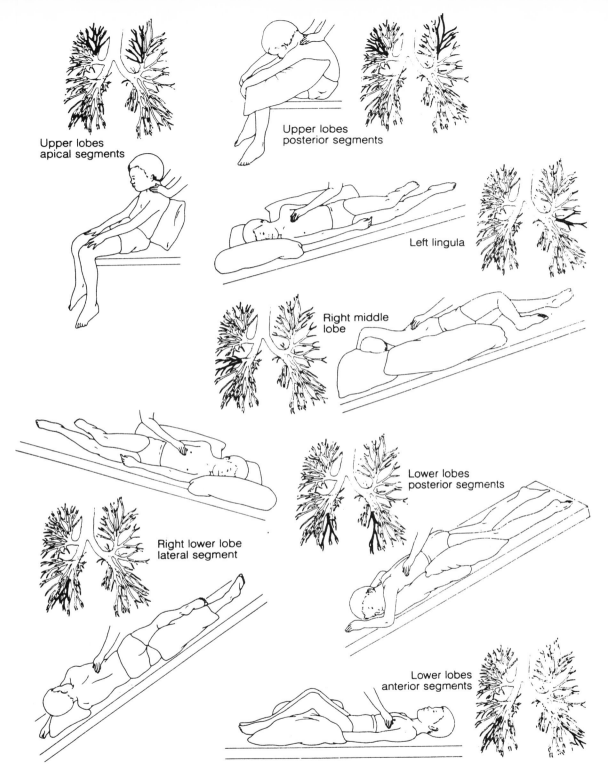

Upper lobes
apical segments

Upper lobes
posterior segments

Left lingula

Right middle
lobe

Lower lobes
posterior segments

Right lower lobe
lateral segment

Lower lobes
anterior segments

Fig. 16.8 Postural drainage. Position for draining upper lobes, anterior segments, is the same as the position for draining lower lobes, anterior segments. (Source: Brunner & Suddarth 1991; *reproduced courtesy of J.B. Lippincott Co, USA*)

itself and this imposes special strains on them (Bray 1989). Additionally the child should be encouraged to exercise as this helps to keep the child fit and healthy and is a good way of mobilizing secretions. Intermittent aerosol therapy may be used pre, post or both pre and post postural drainage to allow drugs to be delivered in droplet form directly to the surface of the lungs. Some antibiotics can be nebulized, as can bronchodilators.

Children with cystic fibrosis are susceptible to chest infections, the most common being staphylococcus aureus and pseudomonas aeruginosa. Staph. aureus is commonly found in the lungs of children with cystic fibrosis and long term (permanent) oral antibiotic therapy is indicated as a means of minimizing damage to the lung tissue (Ellis 1991). Colonisation with *pseudomonas aeruginosa* is also prevalent. Ellis (1991) reports that 74% of children in one clinic were colonized and required frequent intravenous treatment with antibiotics. Pseudomonas exacerbates the child's respiratory problems and must therefore be controlled.

The need for such regular intravenous treatment used to have major implications not only for ways in which drugs were given but also for where the treatment was carried out. Children are notoriously distressed by the thought of needles and therefore the prospect of needing many intravenous drugs, with all that that implies, would or could be overwhelmingly daunting for the child with a lifelong need for treatment. As a result Port-a-Caths ('implantable access systems') have become the route of choice, although intravenous cannulae may still be used in some circumstances.

The disruption that the traditional two week admission to hospital for the therapy imposed on both the child and the family has now been superseded in many instances by care in the community, with the parent or the child where appropriate administering the medication and managing their care (Ellis 1991; Sidey 1989; Kendrick 1993). The role of the nurse in this context is as educator, advisor and supporter. Gill (1993) describes the nurse's role as being part of the care team, informing parents of available options. The nurse acts as a resource in partnership with the child and parents. Additionally the move from hospital to community care is reinforced in the guidance documents *The Welfare of Children and Young People in Hospital* (DoH, 1991). This is also supported by the Royal College of Nursing who advocate family participation in care and the reduction of hospital admissions and in-patient stays (RCN 1992).

The nurse in most home care schemes appears to act as a teacher of both knowledge and skills and this is seen in the context of their scope of practice (Gill, 1993). Catchpole (1989) indicates that there are a number of advantages to the child receiving intravenous antibiotic therapy at home. These advantages appear to focus on the reduction in disruption to family life, schooling or work, and the reduction in hospital admissions as well as a decrease in the potential for cross infection. Overwhelmingly the evidence from the home care schemes seems to support home care as being a welcome option for some families; it promotes flexibility and allows the family to more appropriately manage their condition rather than the condition managing them (Kendrick 1993). The value of the paediatric community nurse in respect to supporting these families cannot be underestimated.

Unfortunately some children may acquire Burkholderia cepacia (formerly classified as pseudomonas cepacia) and special consideration needs to be made in respect to infection control. Individual units and teams are developing protocols for reducing the risk of spreading this infection (Leaver 1994), whilst not making the child with the infection feel stigmatized and isolated.

Nutritional management is also an area of nursing focus since malabsorption remains a problem despite the use of pancreatic supplements. Respiratory infections place an additional stressor on the child's nutritional status and as a result a diet high in protein, carbohydrates and with a normal fat content is recommended (Byers 1989; Smith Millet 1991). Taylor (1993) suggests that a diet of 120–150% recommended daily allowance (RDA) of calories and protein should be encouraged.

Malabsorption is a problem for children with cystic fibrosis since over 85% of them produce inadequate amounts of pancreatic enzymes which leads to malabsorption of fat and protein. In addition, insufficient bicarbonate is produced in the pancreatic fluid, creating problems with intestinal enzyme function (Taylor 1993). Enzyme preparations which are taken with the child's food attempt to correct enzyme deficiency and the new high lipase preparations appear to be successful. The child's dietary intake and dietary supplements should be planned according to the individual child's specific needs and should be reviewed regularly. Without careful monitoring energy malnutrition can result and the child's growth can be stunted. Pancreatic enzymes can cause excoriation of the skin and this should be considered when planning the child's care.

Vitamin and mineral supplements often complement the diet and during periods of hot weather the child may also require supplementary sodium chloride. However, despite careful planning of the child's dietary intake, he or she may fail to complete their recommended intake especially in respect to fat intake. Taylor (1993) reports that in a study the well nourished patients had a significantly higher fat and energy intake than the malnourished ones. For those children who are unable to maintain an adequate dietary intake, enteral or total parenteral nutrition must be considered to ensure that the child gains weight and is in an optimum nutritional status to stave off infection. Children with cystic fibrosis requiring such nutritional support should wherever possible continue to receive care in their home, providing this is acceptable to the child and to their family and the appropriate skilled nurses are available to support and help to manage the care.

Psychological support and care must be ongoing and the child's needs assessed on an ongoing basis. The fact that the child (and family) appear to be coping should not lead the nurses to assume that no help is required. As the child gets older the problems that cystic fibrosis may result in will change and the family will need the nurse to act as a resource, friend and perhaps counsellor. Some studies have examined the issue of self-esteem in cystic fibrosis sufferers, and Krulik (1980) reports children with cystic fibrosis see themselves as younger than their chronological age although these findings are not confirmed by a later study by Simmons *et al.* (1985). Byers (1989) identifies a number of psychological problems that the adolescent with cystic fibrosis may experience (Fig. 16.9). Any of these problems must be treated with respect by the nurse, and discussed and solutions offered where appropriate.

In conclusion then, the role of the nurse in meeting

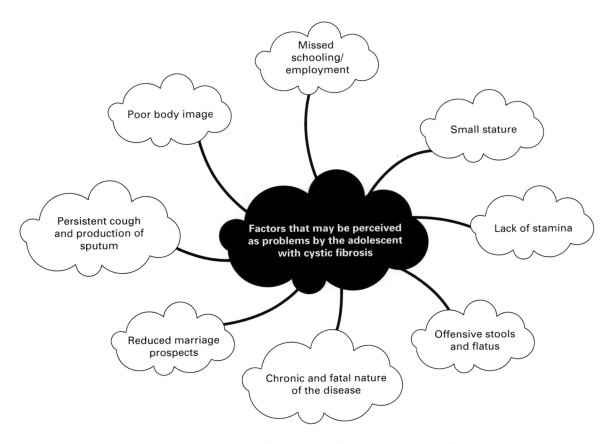

Fig. 16.9 Factors that may be perceived as problems by the adolescent with cystic fibrosis.

the needs of the child and the family can be seen to be more than instrumental (Ellis 1991), encompassing education, advocacy, advice, support, expert carer, and source of information, liaison and communication both within the hospital and increasingly within the community setting. The potential for community based strategies is clear and as Whyte (1990) emphasizes, the role of the nurse (paediatric community nurse) in ensuring family health by providing emotional and physical and practical day to day support is of profound importance. Supporting the family, particularly the mother, is also seen as vital in Jennings' (1992a) study. Parents are fairly independent and tend to cope because they adopt positive attitudes (Gibson 1988). The nurse has much to offer and to provide this must be confident in terms of knowledge and skills and must be prepared to work with the family.

NURSING THE CHILD WITH FOREIGN BODY ASPIRATION

Small children enjoy exploring the world, although this is not without risk and they are prone to place small objects into their mouths. Aspiration is a consequence of this, especially if the child is laughing, running or jumping. It occurs most commonly in children aged six months to three years and it remains a major cause of morbidity and mortality in children (Lorin 1990). Food is commonly the culprit, especially 'round' food, with peanuts being the most common food which is aspirated (Smith Millet 1992). However, children can be aspirate and obstruct on small toys, coins, buttons, paper clips and so on.

The response to aspiration will depend on a number of factors, including the nature of the object, the degree of obstruction which results and the site where it lodges. Dry food objects such as popcorn will swell when in contact with moist mucous membranes and this complicates matters. Most children who aspirate a foreign body may experience some mild symptoms which, although annoying, are not life threatening. Usually a localized inflammation results and the child may produce copious, purulent, foul smelling nasal secretions. Removal of the foreign body in these circumstances is usually uncomplicated and the child recovers from the experience quickly (Lorin 1990). Nurses can offer advice

and support to reduce the risk of the child aspirating again.

More complicated episodes of aspiration of foreign body result in asphyxia and inflammation of the lower respiratory tract. Lorin (1990) proposes that aspiration of foreign bodies into the larynx and trachea is the second commonest cause of accidental death in the home in children under the age of five years. After aspiration the child attempts to rid itself of the foreign body and will cough convulsively and become dyspnoeic. Signs of obstruction are dependent on the degree of obstruction, whether the foreign body is causing a total occlusion or partial occlusion, and the degree to which inhalation is impaired, exhalation is impaired, or whether air is unable to move either way past the obstruction.

Nursing assessment

Assessment is focused on the degree of respiratory dysfunction and includes assessing the child for signs of choking, wheezing, coughing and gagging, loss of colour, level of consciousness and signs of asphyxiation and cardiorespiratory arrest. Additionally signs and symptoms of respiratory tract infection should be looked for in children who have aspirated a foreign body in the days and/or weeks before presenting with a problem. The nurse will be involved in preparing the child for X-ray to determine the location of the foreign body, although a bronchoscopy or laryngoscopy is often required to locate non-radio-opaque objects.

Nursing intervention: meeting the child's needs

The child experiencing acute, complete obstruction is likely to be very distressed and will need both psychological and physical care from the nurse. The most immediate priority is to clear the airway and this may be done as an emergency in the community by using the Heimlich manoeuvre (abdominal thrust). This should only be performed if the child appears to be choking and deteriorating; otherwise, the child should be kept calm and taken to hospital facilities where direct sight of the obstruction can be made using laryngoscopy or bronchoscopy as appropriate. Whilst waiting for the child to have the bronchoscopy the nurse should ensure that the child is quiet and relaxed. After the procedure the child should not be given oral fluids until their gag reflex has returned, and they should be monitored for potential laryngeal oedema.

The nurse should ensure that the parents are aware of the dangers of foreign body aspiration and should teach them the Heimlich manoeuvre for future reference.

SUDDEN INFANT DEATH SYNDROME

Sudden infant death syndrome (SIDS), or cot death as it is sometimes called, is not a new problem. It remains the major cause of post-neonatal (six weeks to one year of age) mortality in industrialized countries (Stewart *et al.* 1993; Jones 1989). SIDS can be traced back to pre-Christian times even though many of those unexpected deaths were attributed to other causes such as overlaying (Golding *et al.* 1985). New and initially attractive theories have continued to be presented as proposed explanations, although no one theory or single explanation seems likely to answer the question of what causes sudden and unexpected infant death. The full picture of the number of sudden infant deaths went largely unrecorded until 1953 when the Ministry of Health investigated the problem and uncovered a much larger problem than had been anticipated (FSID 1994). Sudden infant death syndrome is said to be 'sudden infant's death, unexpected by history and unexplained by post-mortem.' (FSID 1994).

SIDS only became a registerable cause of death in 1971; prior to this many unexpected deaths had been attributed to other causes such as respiratory infection. Pathologists took some time to adopt the term and this has apparently skewed some of the statistics; in 1971 there were 0.61 such deaths per 1000 live births and in 1988 2.31 per 1000 live births. In perhaps more real terms, five babies per day were dying from SIDS in the late 1980s (Stewart *et al.* 1993). By 1992, after the introduction of the Back to Sleep campaign in 1991, the figures had dropped to 0.78 per 1000 live births, although regional variations do occur (FSID 1994).

For parents the sudden death of their baby is devastating and is complicated by the fact that there are no simple answers as to why their baby died (Limerick 1976). The apparent injustice of the situation is over-whelming (Golding *et al.* 1985). Parents often feel a desperate need to determine the cause of the death of their child and may experience guilt or even blame their spouse (Stewart *et al.* 1993; Raphael 1984). Guilt and blame are often heightened by relatives' and neighbours' response to the unexpected death of a baby. Police involvement often occurs in cases of sudden infant death and initially some responses may be hostile (Rajan 1994; Woodward *et al.* 1985). SIDS still remains difficult to explain and despite the wealth of theories no single cause has been identified. Current thinking proposes that babies who die suddenly, unexpectedly and without explanation at post mortem, did so as a result of a combination of factors/causes and at a time when they were vulnerable.

Nursing assessment of at-risk families

Many factors are seen to be associated with SIDS (Table 16.5) and these were used as the basis for the campaign launched in 1991, known as Reduce the Risk.

Potentially vulnerable babies can be identified by using risk assessment methods and then positively taking action to reduce the risks. Taylor (1992) talks of positively discriminating in favour of these babies receiving increased healthcare support, and Potrykus (1992) attributes 100 lives saved since 1975 in Sheffield to a strategy to positively discriminate towards at risk families. Other models of care involve first parent visiting, which aims to improve parents' confidence and self esteem and increase their knowledge. Profiles of the family are developed and provide a key to issues which could affect the babies' health and place them more at risk. Jones (1992) reports this as a useful strategy in reducing infant mortality whilst acknowledging that even active support from health visitors cannot combat poverty and deprivation.

Nursing intervention: meeting the needs of the family

Caring for the parents who have experienced the death of their baby in such a catastrophically sudden way involves many nursing skills and a knowledge/understanding of what impact/effect this will have on them, both short and long term. Bereavement care is vitally

Table 16.5   Factors associated with sudden infant death syndrome (developed from FSID 1994).

Infant factors	
Age of infant	78% cot deaths occur 1–6 months of age. Peak age 2–3 months of age.
Birth order	Higher birth order babies at increased risk.
Birth weight/gestation	Low birth weight and low gestation babies at increased risk.
Multiple births	Multiple birth babies at increased risk.
Sex of infant	Boys at increased risk (60:40%) compared with girls.
Maternal and parental factors	
Breast feeding	Various suggestions although breast feeding generally seen to be good practice.
Marriage	Babies born outside marriage at increased risk.
Maternal age	Babies born of young mothers at increased risk.
Short interpregnancy interval	Short interpregnancy interval increases risk for baby.
Smoking	During pregnancy increases the risk; some studies suggest that smoking after baby's birth increases risk.
Social and cultural factors	
Ethnic group	Decreased risk for babies of Asian origin who were born in the UK.
Sleeping location	Conflicting evidence as to whether to encourage bed sharing or not. FSID recommend not to share bed until baby is 6 months old.
Sleeping position	Sleeping prone increases the risk although there is some conflict about this.
Social class	Increased risk in social class IV and V compared with social class I, II, III.
Environmental factors	
Cities	Increased risk in cities compared with rural settings.
Housing	Increased risk in poor housing.
Infection	Increased risk if baby has infection/minor illness.
Season of year	Increased risk during the winter months.
Temperature	Increased risk if overheating occurs, such as in a hot room or if baby is overwrapped.

important if the families are to come to terms with their bereavement. Immediate and ongoing support is crucial for these families who will feel vulnerable about all of their children especially subsequent babies (Stewart *et al.* 1993). Skilled supportive care is often most appropriately offered by the family's health visitor, although there is a role for the paediatric community nurse. Professional help is required not only in the form of bereavement care but also in general preventative strategies and in specific strategies for families who have experienced sudden infant death. Bereavement support aims to 'help the family integrate the death into their lives and move forward with positive memories.' (Stewart *et al.* 1993).

This involves helping the parents cope with their own reactions/responses to the death. Families need support from health care professionals, through the bereavement process which involves support from the time of death, in the A & E department, in the initial week, and then ongoing support especially during subsequent pregnancies. Counselling skills are important and parents need the time and space to talk about their feelings and start the process of working through their grief. Home visiting and support is vital with subsequent children as this can help reduce both the actual risks of SIDS occurring again in the family and the family's vulnerability and anxiety. It also helps the parents feel that they are involved in reducing future risks.

REFERENCES AND FURTHER READING

Action Asthma (1993) *The Young Asthmatics Survey*. Allen & Hanburys, Middlesex.

Asthmanews (1993) *Ninja Turtle Nebulisers*, (new report), issue 36, p.3. National Asthma Campaign, London.

Asthma Training Centre (1991) *Asthma, who cares?* A manual to help parents who have asthma. The Asthma Training Centre, Stratford-upon-Avon.

Black, L., Hersher, L. & Steinschneider, A. (1987) Impact of the apnoea monitor on family life. *Pediatrics*, 62, 681–685.

Bray, P. (1989) *Cystic Fibrosis, A Guide For Parents and Sufferers*. Souvenir Press, London.

Brunner, L.S. & Suddarth, D.S. (1991) *The Lippincott Manual of Paediatric Nursing* (3rd edn). Harper Collins Nursing, London.

Burney, P.G.J., Chinn, S. & Roner, R.J. (1990) Has the pre-valence of asthma increased in childhood? Evidence from the national study of health and growth 1973–1986. *British Medical Journal*, 300, 1306–10.

Burr, M.L., Bulland, B.K., King, S. & Vaughan-Williams, E. (1989) Changes in asthma prevalence: world prevalence: worldwide surveys 15 years apart. *Archives of Disease in Childhood*, 64, 1452–6.

Byers, C. (1989) Managing cystic fibrosis. *Paediatric Nursing*, Sept., 14–16.

Carter, J. (1993) Charity profile: British Lung Foundation. *Child Health*, Oct/Nov., 110.

Castiglia, P.T. & Harbin, R.E. (1992) *Child Health Care Process and Practice*. J.B. Lippincott Company, Philadelphia.

Catchpole, A. (1989) Cystic fibrosis: intravenous treatment at home. *Nursing Times*, 85 (12) 40–2.

Clancy, M. & Jones, E. (1993) Care of the child with respiratory problems. In *Manual of Paediatric Intensive Care Nursing* (Ed. B. Carter), pp. 86–131. Chapman and Hall, London.

Deaves, D.M. (1993) An assessment of the value of health education in the prevention of childhood asthma. *Journal of Advanced Nursing*, 18, 354–65.

deFrain, J.D. & Ernst, L. (1978) The psychological effects of sudden infant death syndrome on surviving members. *Journal of Family Practice*, 6, 985–9.

Dinwiddie, R. (1991) *The Diagnosis and Management of Pediatric Respiratory Disease*. Churchill Livingstone, Edinburgh.

DoH (1991) *Welfare of Children and Young People in Hospital*. HMSO, London.

Douglas, J. (1993) *Psychology and Nursing Children*. The British Psychological Society, Macmillan BPS Books.

Efthimiou, J. (1992) The drug therapy of respiratory disorders. In *Textbook of Clinical Pharmacology and Drug Therapy* (eds D.G. Grahame-Smith & J.K. Aronson), pp 301–18. Oxford.

Eiser, C. (1991) It's OK having asthma . . . young children's beliefs about illness. *Child Care: Some Nursing Perspectives* (ed. A. Glasper) pp. 205–10. Wolfe Publishing Ltd, London.

Ellis, J. (1991) Let parents give the care: IV therapy at home in cystic fibrosis. In *Child Care: Some Nursing Perspectives* (ed. A. Glasper), pp 110–17. Wolfe Publishing Ltd, London.

Engel, J. (1989) *Pocket Guide to Pediatric Assessment*. The CV Mosby Company, St Louis.

Fleming, P.J., Gilbert, R., Azaz, Y., *et al* (1990) Interaction between bedding and sleeping position in the sudden infant death syndrome: a population based case-control study. *British Medical Journal*, 301, 85–9.

FSID (1991) *Reduce the Risk of Cot Death* (leaflet). Foundation for Study of Infant Death, London.

FSID (1992) Factfile 2: *Research background for advice to reduce the risk of cot death* (leaflet). Foundation for Study of Infant Death, London.

FSID (1994) Factfile 1: *Cot death – facts, figures and definitions*.

Foundation for Study of Infant Death, London.

Gantley, M., Davies, D.P., & Murcott, A. (1993) Sudden infant death syndrome: links with infant care practices. *British Medical Journal*, 306, 16–20.

Gibson, C. (1988) Perspectives in parental coping with a chronically ill child: the case of cystic fibrosis. *Issues in Comprehensive Children's Nursing*, 11, 33–41.

Gill, S. (1993) Home administration of intravenous antibiotics to children with cystic fibrosis. *British Journal of Nursing*, 2(15) 767–9.

Golding, J., Limerick, S. & Macfarlane, A. (1985) *Sudden Infant Death: Patterns, Puzzles, and Problems*. Open Books, Somerset.

Govan, J. (1994) What's in a name? *Cystic Fibrosis News*, 3, 14–15.

Goodchild, M., & Dodge, J. (1985) *Cystic Fibrosis Manual of Diagnosis and Management*, 2nd edn. W.B. Saunders, Philadelphia.

Gregson, R., Kelly, P. & Warner, J. (1993) Education for control management principles and inhaler techniques for childhood asthma. *Child Health*, 1(1) 10–16.

Guerra, I.C., Kemp, J.S. & Shearer, W.T. (1990) Bronchiolitis. In *Principles and Practice of Pediatrics* (eds. F.A. Oshi, C.D. Deangelis, R.D. Feigin & J.B. Warshaw) pp. 1332–4. J.B. Lippincott, Philadelphia.

Hammerschlag, M.R. (1990) Pharyngitis, In *Principles and Practice of Pediatrics* (eds F.A Oshi, C.D. Deangelis, R.D. Feigin & J.B. Warshaw) pp. 893–5. J.B. Lippincott, Philadelphia.

Hurrell, F. (1993) Choosing inhaler devices for children with asthma. *Paediatric Nursing*, 5(7) 22–4.

International Paediatric Asthma Consensus Group (1992) Follow-up statement. *Archives of Disease in Childhood*, 67, 240–48.

Jennings, P. (1992a) Coping mechanisms. *Paediatric Nursing*, 4(8) 13–15.

Jennings, P. (1992b) Coping strategies for mothers. *Paediatric Nursing*, 4(9) 24–6.

Jones, D.A. (1989) Sudden infant death syndrome. *British Medical Journal*, 298, 959.

Jones, J. (1992) Supporting mothers in their war of survival. *Health Visitor*, 65(11) 386.

Kendrick, R. (1993) Teaching children with cystic fibrosis and families to give IV therapy. *Paediatric Nursing*, 5(1) 22–3.

Krulik, T. (1980) Successful 'normalizing' tactics of parents of chronically ill children. *Journal of Advanced Nursing*, 5, 573–8.

Kubler-Ross, K.E. (1970) *On Death and Dying*. Macmillan, New York.

Leaver, J. (1994) Unpublished research dissertation, the Manchester Metropolitan University, Manchester.

Limerick, S. (1976) Counselling needs after a cot death.

Marriage Guidance, July/Aug, 118.

Limerick, S.R. (1992) Sudden infant death in historical perspective. *Journal of Clinical Pathology*, 45 (supplement), 3–6.

Lorin, M.I. (1990) Foreign bodies. In *Principles and Practice of Pediatrics* (eds F.A. Oshi, C.D Deangelis, R.D. Feigin & J.B. Warshaw), pp. 1348–50. J.B. Lippincott, Philadelphia.

McLaughlin, S. & Haase, L. (1994) Home is where the heart is. *Cystic Fibrosis News*, 4, 8–9.

Millar, B. (1994) Growing demand. *Nursing Times*, 90(8) 20.

Mitchell, E.H., Scragg, R., Stewart, A. *et al.* (1991) Results from the first year of the New Zealand cot death study. *New Zealand Journal of Medicine*, 104, 71–6.

Moss, J.R. (1981) Helping young children cope with physical examination. *Pediatric Nursing*, 7, 17–20.

NAC (1993a) Asthma at School 4. National Asthma Campaign, London.

NAC (1993b) Asthma and the Environment: Air Pollution 11. National Asthma Campaign, London.

Nevin, M. & Nevin, M. (1992) Help the parent and you help the child. *Paediatric Nursing*, Feb., 25–7.

Potrykus, C. (1992) What price prevention. *Health Visitor*, 65(11) 384.

Price, M., Carter, B. & Shelton Bendell, R. (1985) Maternal perceptions of sudden infant death syndrome. *Children's Health Care*, 14(1) 22–31.

Rajan, L. (1992) 'Not just dreaming': parents mourning pregnancy. *Health Visitor*, 65 (10) 354–7.

Ramsay, J. (1989) *Nursing the Child with Respiratory Problems*, p. 25. Chapman and Hall, London.

Raphael, B. (1984) *The Anatomy of Bereavement*. Hutchinson, London.

RCN (1992) Paediatric nursing, a philosophy of care. *Issues in Nursing and Health 10*. Royal College of Nursing, London.

Rees, J. & Price, J. (1989) *ABC of asthma*, 2nd edn. British Medical Journal, London.

Richards, S. (1991) Let them do it for themselves – teaching asthma self management to children. *Professional Nursing*, 7 (2) 130–33.

Rosenstein, B.J. (1990) Cystic fibrosis. In *Principles and Practice of Pediatrics* (eds F.A. Oshi, C.D. Deangelis, R.D. Feigin & J.B. Warshaw) pp. 1362–72. J.B. Lippincott, Philadelphia.

Schofield, P.M. (1987) Sudden infant death: parents' views of professional help. *Health Visitor*, 60, 109.

Schweich, P.J. (1990) Emergency medicine except poisoning. In *Principles and Practice of Paediatrics* (eds F.A. Oshi, C.D. Deangelis, R.D. Feigin & J.B. Warshaw) pp. 751–5. J.B. Lippincott, Philadelphia.

Sharman, W. (1985) Tonsillectomy through a child's eyes. Occasional paper. *Nursing Times*, **81** (8) 48–52.

Sidney, A. (1989) Intravenous home care. *Paediatric Nursing*, May, 14–15.

Simmons, R.J., Covey, M., Cowen, L., Keenan, N., Robertson, J. & Levinson, H. (1985) Emotional adjustments of early adolescents with cystic fibrosis. *Psychosomatic Medicine*, 47(2) 111–21.

Smith Millet, S.J. (1992) Alterations in respiratory function. In *Child Health Care Process and Practice* (eds P.T. Castiglia & R.E. Harbin) pp. 515–63. J.B. Lippincott Company, Philadelphia.

Stewart, A., Fleming, P. & Howell, T. (1993) Follow up support for families with subsequent children. *Health Visitor*, 66(7) 244–7.

Swallow, V. & Thompson, L. (1992) A parent's support group. *Paediatric Nursing*, Feb, 23–4.

Symes, J. (1991) What comfort this grief? *Professional Nurse*, 6(8) 437–41.

Taylor, C. (1992) Nutrition and the child with cystic fibrosis. *Paediatric Nursing*, 5(4) 26–8.

Tunstill, A. & Mccarthy, C. (1993) Care of the child with cardiovascular problems. In *Manual of Paediatric Intensive Care Nursing* (ed. B. Carter). Chapman and Hall, London.

Wald, E.R. (1990) Croup. In *Principles and Practice of Paediatrics* (eds F.A. Oshi, C.D. Deangelis, R.D. Feigin & J.B. Warshaw) pp. 905–8. J.B. Lippincott, Philadelphia.

Warner, J. et al (1989) Management of asthma, a consensus statement. *Archives of Disease in Childhood*, 64, 1065–79.

Watson, G. & Dimond, H. (1991) Supporting parents. *Health Visitor*, 64(4) 115.

Webber, B. & Pryor, J. (1991) *The Physical Treatment of Cystic Fibrosis*. Cystic Fibrosis Research Trust, Bromley.

Whaley, L.F. & Wong, D.L. (1991) *Nursing Care of Infants and Children*. Mosby Year Book, St Louis.

Whyte, D. (1990) The family with a chronically ill child. *Paediatric Nursing*, Nov, 21–3.

Williams, R. & Nikolaisen, S. (1992) Sudden infant death syndrome: parents' perceptions and responses to the loss of their infant. *Research in Nursing and Health*, 5(2) 55–61.

Woller, E. (1994) On course for knowledge. *Nursing Times*, 90(15) 42–4.

Woodward, S., Pope, A., Robson, W.J. & Hagan, O. (1985) Development counselling after sudden infant death. *British Medical Journal*, 290, 363–5.

Woolder, E. (1994) Asthma in children. *Paediatric Nursing*, 5(6) 22–7.

Woolsey, S.F. (1988) Support after sudden death. *American Journal of Nursing*, 1348–51.

Chapter 17

Nursing Support and Care: Meeting the Needs of the Child and Family with Altered Cardiovascular Function

Bernadette Carter and Ted Hewitt

INTRODUCTION

Within this chapter the special needs and problems of the child experiencing altered cardiac function will be examined. The effect of the child's experience will be explored in relation to the impact that it has on their family. Additionally, it will be examined in terms of delivering quality nursing care that aims to minimize the disruption to their lives.

The care of the child with cardiac health needs and deficits occurs both within the community and in hospital settings, although a higher level of activity is generally seen within the hospital environment where their child is admitted for investigations, acute management and surgery. During this period the child who may have been chronically ill becomes acutely and often critically ill. Discharge from hospital often signals a return to a quiescent period for the child's care needs or, in many cases, the child is convalescent moving towards a 'normal' cardiac state following corrective surgery.

Liaison between the community and hospital is vital and ensures that the child and their family are provided with support through all stages of the child's illness. The community nursing team can provide preparatory support and advice, ongoing education about medication and care, and support in relation to ensuring that the child's dietary intake is appropriate. The team is vital in encouraging both the child and their family to manage the health deficits, rather than let the heart deficits and needs manage the functioning of the family.

Children with identified cardiac needs can broadly be divided into two main categories. Children with congenital heart disease (CHD) comprise the largest category, whilst the children with acquired heart disease can be further subdivided into those experiencing infectious disease or coronary artery disease (Table 17.1).

In caring for the child with cardiac health needs the nurse must have a sound understanding of not only the haemodynamic consequences of the defect or condition, the treatment regime and medically based interventions, but just as importantly of the psychosocial effects that a life threatening disorder can have on the child's siblings and other members of the family. A holistic perspective should be taken when considering how to meet the child's needs from a nursing perspective.

Assessment remains a key component in planning the care of the child and their family and a partnership through the process of nursing the child is vitally important. The child must be seen to be central and should, whenever possible, be involved in making decisions concerning their care. Planning ways of over-

Table 17.1 Classification of cardiac health needs/deficits with examples of associated defects/conditions.

Congenital heart disease	Acquired heart disease
■ ventricular septal defect (VSD)* ■ patent ductus arteriosus (PDA)* ■ atrial septal defect (ASD)* ■ tetralogy of Fallot* ■ pulmonary stenosis* ■ coarctation of the aorta* ■ aortic stenosis* ■ transposition of the great arteries* ■ truncus arteriosus ■ pulmonary atresia ■ tricuspid atresia ■ hypoplastic left heart syndrome	Infectious disease ■ rheumatic fever ■ Kawasaki's arteritis ■ cardiomyopathies (although not always infectious in origin)
	Coronary artery disease

* The eight most common defects – regional differences may alter the order shown but are unlikely to exclude any of the defects listed (Jordan & Scott 1989)

coming the challenges presented by the child's deficits and of implementing and evaluating the effectiveness of nursing care strategies is fundamental to ensuring that quality care is delivered.

This chapter is divided into sections, for convenience of presentation, although it is acknowledged that they will overlap to a degree. First, the principles of assessing a child with a cardiac/cardiovascular deficit will be examined, and some of the factors that influence the child's cardiovascular status will be outlined. Second, the nursing care required to meet the needs of the child with congenital heart disease will be explored; the most common defects will be considered to provide a more comprehensive picture of the haemodynamic consequences of congenital heart disease. Additionally, defects in cardiac rhythm will be discussed as these frequently occur in conjunction with congenital problems. The section after that will provide information about acquired conditions, both those of infectious origin and those related to coronary artery disease. Additionally, issues related to cardiopulmonary resuscitation will be briefly addressed. The role of the nurse as health educator and health promoter will be highlighted, particularly in relation to coronary artery disease, as it is recognized that early prevention avoids problems in later life.

PRINCIPLES UNDERLYING CARDIOVASCULAR ASSESSMENT

Accurate, effective and ongoing assessment of the child's cardiovascular status provides a source of rich data which can be used to help determine the child's progress or possible deterioration. The nurse caring for the child needs to utilize a high level of skills in relation to communication (preparation, support and education), in addition to the observational and technical skills utilized in actually obtaining the recordings/measurements. The nurse must also be cognisant of the various developmental changes in relation to the circulation, from the embryonic circulation to post-natal circulation. An understanding of normal cardiac function allows the nurse to effectively assess and plan care for the child experiencing disordered cardiac function.

In a holistic assessment of the child's cardiovascular status, four key areas must be considered:

- History taking.
- Observation
- Physical examination.
- Investigations.

For a child who experiences regular and repeated assessment, the need to ensure adequate and appropriate preparation must be seen as a priority.

Assessing a child's cardiac health status/ needs through a nursing history

Gaining a comprehensive nursing history is a vital component of the assessment as it assists the nurse in building up a picture of all the child's/family's needs, coping and management strategies and concerns. It should include relevant factors relating to birth, previous children with cardiac problems, and health, especially in relation to infections, as well as specific questions pertaining to the child's weight gain, feeding habits, tendency to fatigue, exercise tolerance, weakness, respiratory status (dyspnoea, tachypnoea, shortness of breath, and frequent respiratory infection), cyanosis, dizziness, oedema, and developmental delay (Engel 1989; Talner 1990; Whaley & Wong 1991; Pitts-Wilhelm 1992). All of these provide an indication of how effectively or ineffectively the child is coping with the cardiac challenge (Fig. 17.1).

The nurse must be particularly sensitive to the parents' fears and concerns during the assessment process, as there may be anxieties about the assessment in relation to diagnosis, prognosis and potential treatment strategies (Pitts-Wilhelm 1992).

Observing the child's cardiac status/needs

The child should be observed for signs of respiratory and cardiovascular difficulty. Good observational technique by the nurse can support the nursing history gained from the parents and can allow further exploration and consideration of specific issues. The nurse should observe the child holistically before considering them systematically. Both their level and type of activity should be noted in addition to the duration and effect of activity on the child. The child's body posture is also indicative of particular dysfunction, for example children with Fal-

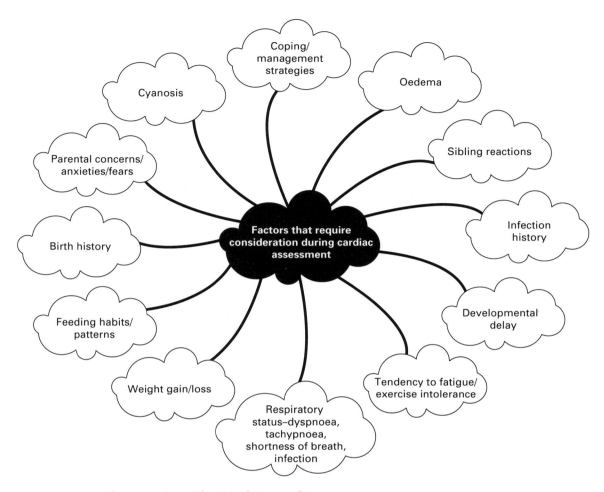

Fig. 17.1 Factors that require consideration during cardiac assessment.

lot's tetralogy tend to squat. However, Tunstill & McCarthy (1993) note that early surgical repair now means that squatting is rarely seen.

The nurse should observe for signs of respiratory difficulty as these may indicate either a respiratory infection or congestive cardiac failure. In these instances the child may display a cough, grunting respirations, flared nares, costal retractions and use of accessory muscles as well as a rattly chest. Equally important is the need to observe the child's colour for duskiness, cyanosis (central and peripheral), pallor, mottling and oedema. The site(s) and extent of any cyanosis should be carefully documented (Talner 1990). However, it is important to remember that the child's haemoglobin status will have a marked effect on the child's ability to demonstrate

cyanosis as a true reflection of the oxygen saturation of their blood. Very anaemic children and infants may have a very reduced haemoglobin level which does not produce a cyanotic response (Pitts-Wilhelm 1992). The nurse should not assume that the absence of cyanosis necessarily means that the child is adequately oxygenated.

The child's nail beds should be examined for possible clubbing, widening or lengthening. Although clubbing of the nail beds takes time to develop, the initial response to chronically deoxygenated blood is for the child's fingertips to become red and shiny. After this stage is reached, clubbing (usually initially of the thumb) itself develops. The child's chest should also be observed for equality of movement as asymmetrical chest movements are indicative of congestive cardiac failure. Additionally, any chest deformities should be noted as the shape of the chest wall can be distorted by an enlarged heart (Whaley & Wong 1989).

Physical examination of the child's cardiac status/needs

Palpation, percussion and auscultation help to reveal additional information on the child's cardiac status. Systematic examination of the child is necessary and the nurse must ensure that the child is well prepared as this may lead them to be more accepting of the examination.

Palpation of the chest enables the nurse to detect the apical pulse in young children and infants (Engel 1989), and if the nurse has knowledge of the appropriate location of the apical pulse it can enable them to determine if the heart is enlarged. However, a very dynamic apical pulse may indicate that the child is frightened, pyrexial or anaemic. Thrills and rubs (abnormal) can also be detected by palpation of the chest. Additionally, palpation of the peripheral pulses can demonstrate the strength, rate, equality and rhythm and this is useful information in precluding some diagnoses. In health, peripheral pulses are palpable, symmetrical and even in rhythm. Palpation of the abdomen allows the nurse to determine the presence/absence of hepatomegaly and/or splenomegaly. Percussion of the chest can be used in some circumstances to help determine cardiac size, although it is a less valuable method of doing this (Engel 1989).

Through auscultation heart sounds can be evaluated for quality, rate, intensity and rhythm. An effective technique takes time and skill to acquire (Pitts-Wilhelm 1992). The nurse should auscultate the aortic, pulmonary, mitral/apical and tricuspid areas and Erb's point. The nurse should be aware of the normal sounds so that any change/deviation from expected sounds can be documented. Additional sounds such as murmurs must also be noted, although it is important to be aware that some murmurs may be nonpathologic. Organic murmurs must be evaluated in relation to location, timing of occurrence in cardiac cycle, intensity (whether this varies when the child changes position), pitch, radiation to other areas, and quality (Engel 1989; Pitts-Wilhelm 1992).

The child's heart rate and rhythm should be noted

and considered in relation to the normal range for the child's age and in relation to the child's level of activity and temperature. Additionally, any discrepancies between the child's apical beat and peripheral pulses should be noted.

Blood pressure is an important component of the assessment and although it varies in response to the child's level of activity, the time of day, and the child's level of distress, it should not be missed out of a comprehensive assessment process. The nurse must ensure that an appropriately sized blood pressure cuff is used and that the technique for measuring blood pressure is accurate, otherwise inappropriate and misleading readings can result. It is advisable to take blood pressure readings on both upper and lower limbs as differences between the two can be indicative of disease.

Decreased urinary output and the presence of oedema are useful indicators of cardiac status/cardiac failure, and urinary output should be measured and tested.

CONGENITAL HEART DISEASE

Aetiology and epidemiology

Congenital heart disease (CHD) is the single most common congenital defect, accounting for some 30% of all congenital defects (Jordan & Scott 1989). Almost 100 types of abnormality have been described (Tunstill & McCarthy 1993). It is also commonly found associated with other congenital defects such as CHARGE and VARTA syndrome (Behrman & Kliegman 1990). CHD occurs in 8:1000 live births (Anderson *et al.* 1986). Early detection of CHD can be problematic due to the underlying haemodynamic changes that occur from fetal to extra uterine life (Lynch & Sweatt 1987). Symptoms may be masked by the increased pulmonary resistance of the neonate's circulation or they may not be present at birth. The cause of CHD has remained difficult to identify as the heart is formed in the first three to eight weeks of fetal life (Moore 1988). However, some factors are associated with CHD, such as inheritance, chromosomal aberrations, environmental factors (drugs, infections, maternal conditions) and familial recurrence (Jordan & Scott 1989; Lin 1990) (Table 17.2).

Table 17.2   Possible causes of congenital heart disease (developed from Jordan & Scott 1989; Lin 1990).

Inheritance	Either associated with a syndrome, e.g. Noonan syndrome, or as a single defect across both autosomal dominant and recessive transmission, with the associated risk of subsequent children having the problem.
Chromosomal aberrations	There is a significant association amongst the plethora of chromosomal defects with having a congenital heart defect, e.g. Down's Syndrome where there is a 40% incidence of a congenital heart defect.
Environmental factors	Drugs – a variety of agents have been associated with the occurrence of congenital heart defects: alcohol, amphetamines, phenytoin, lithium, sex hormones (oestrogens and progestogens).
	Infections – a number of viruses have been implicated in the development of a defect, if a mother is infected at the time of cardiac development: rubella, cytomegalovirus, herpes virus.
	Maternal conditions – may also be associated with defect development, particularly diabetes mellitus, systemic lupus erythromatosus.
Familial recurrence	Outside of association with already mentioned genetic factors the risk is considered to be between 1 and 3%, although this varies with each condition.

Probably the most commonly seen syndrome associated with CHD is Down's syndrome (Trisomy 21) where a 40% incidence of CHD is noted with most of these children presenting with an atrioventricular canal defect (Jordan & Scott 1989). CHD is thought to be multifactorial in nature (Lin 1990) and although this may be an appropriate understanding of the situation for the professionals, it is difficult for parents to deal with. Parents often feel the need to identify a reason for their child's problem as this may be a way of deflecting the blame they feel for their child/baby being ill.

Fetal circulation

At birth the cardiorespiratory system undergoes a number of changes that result in the baby being able to use its lungs to breathe. In utero oxygen is supplied to the fetus from the maternal blood via the inferior vena cava (IVC) and flows into the right atrium and then towards the foramen ovale (due to the shape of the right atrium). The foramen ovale allows flow of blood into the left atrium. Also present in the fetal circulation is the ductus arteriosus which allows the small volume of blood which does flow into the right ventricle to return to the systematic circulation (Fig. 17.2).

The sequence of events following birth is important since it is not until after these changes have occurred

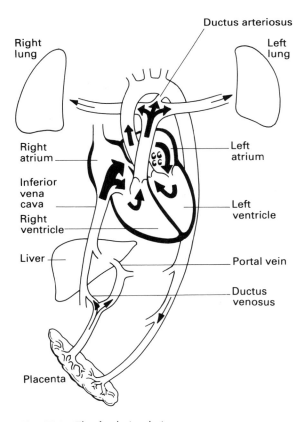

Fig. 17.2   The fetal circulation.

that the haemodynamic effects of the majority of heart defects begin to manifest themselves. The effects may appear quite rapidly as the ductus arteriosus closes, for example in pulmonary atresia. Alternatively the effects may only become apparent over a period of time; this can be seen in ventricular septal defect (VSD), which becomes evident in response to vascular resistance changes (Jordan & Scott 1989).

HAEMODYNAMICS OF CONGENITAL HEART DEFECTS

Traditionally CHDs have been classified as either cyanotic or acyanotic defects (Table 17.3), although this is not an entirely satisfactory classification system. An alternative approach is to categorize them in terms of their haemodynamic effects (Table 17.4), as it is these effects which have the most impact and significance on the actual care required by the child and their family.

as blood flow to the lungs is reduced there is little opportunity for gaseous exchange and the child becomes hypoxic. Second, at the same time desaturated venous blood may shunt from right to left across the foramen ovale and/or a ventricular septal defect (VSD). Initially at birth the baby may not appear either hypoxic or cyanosed, which may be due to blood flowing from the aorta through the ductus arteriosus (a left to right shunt) to the pulmonary arteries. As the ductus arteriosus closes, the baby becomes more hypoxic and cyanosed, although the extent of this depends on the degree of obstruction to flow. In pulmonary atresia the neonate is likely to become acutely ill as the ductus closes, and may require immediate emergency treatment. However, a baby with Fallot's tetralogy may not become so obviously ill until one to three months old (Jordan & Scott 1989).

Cyanosis is the result of hypoxia and the infant with acute hypoxia may experience problems with acidosis, metabolic disruption, possible major organ insult and potentially cardiac arrest. Chronic hypoxia/cyanosis may

Table 17.3 Congenital heart defects.

Acyanotic	Cyanotic
Raised pulmonary blood flow ■ Atrial septal defect ■ Ventricular septal defect ■ Endocardial cushion defect ■ Patent ductus arteriosus	Raised pulmonary blood flow ■ Transposition of the great arteries ■ Persistent truncus arteriosus ■ Total anomalous venous pulmonary venous return
Normal pulmonary blood flow ■ Coarctation of the aorta ■ Aortic stenosis ■ Pulmonary stenosis	
	Reduced pulmonary blood flow ■ Tetralogy of Fallot ■ Tricuspid atresia ■ Ebstein's anomaly

Haemodynamics of reduced pulmonary blood flow

These conditions occur when blood supply to the lungs is severely restricted at some point in the right side of the heart. The haemodynamic effect of this is two-fold. First,

result in a number of effects and complications (Table 17.5) including polycythaemia, clubbing, diminished stature, poor weight gain, lethargy, reduced exercise tolerance, increased risk of thrombus and embolism formation, infective endocarditis, cerebral abscess and metabolic acidosis (Kulik 1989).

Table 17.4 Defects grouped by associated haemodynamic categories.

Reduced pulmonary blood flow	Raised pulmonary blood flow (acyanotic)	Obstruction to ventricular blood flow
Tetralogy of Fallot Tricuspid atresia Pulmonary atresia with intact ventricular septum	Ventricular septal defect Patent ductus arteriosus Atrial septal defect	Coarctation of the aorta Aortic stenosis Hypoplastic left heart syndrome (HLHS) Pulmonary stenosis
	Raised pulmonary blood flow (cyanotic)	
	Truncus arteriosus Transposition of the great arteries with a VSD	

Table 17.5 Effects and complications of cyanosis in congenital heart disease.

Polycythaemia	Haematocrit is raised as the body responds to persistent hypoxia.
Finger 'clubbing'	Finger ends become thickened and flattened, thought to be due to polycythaemia and hypoxia.
Diminished stature, poor weight gain, lethargy, reduced exercise tolerance	
Increased risk of thrombus and embolism formation	Particularly if dehydration occurs. These may occur in any part of the body and have dire consequences, e.g. cerebrovascular obstruction or pulmonary embolism.
Infective endocarditis	May be a problem for these children and care needs to be taken to protect them from potential infection especially when undergoing dental treatment.
Cerebral abscess	Although rare in children under two years, may arise in older children with cyanotic defects.
Metabolic acidosis	Associated with potential hypoperfusion of the tissues.

Haemodynamics of raised pulmonary blood flow

Children with defects that result in raised pulmonary blood flow may present with differing symptomatic pictures which reflect the severity of the defect. In VSD for example there is usually a left to right shunt (left to right ventricle). This results in the normally lower pressure pulmonary circulation having to cope with a raised pressure and flow. The infant may not become symptomatic until three to six months of life (Jordan & Scott 1989). The severity of the signs and symptoms will vary with the underlying condition. Thus a child with an ASD may be asymptomatic, whereas a child with a large VSD can be very ill (Jordan & Scott 1989; Moynihan & King 1989). Regardless of age of presentation the clinical picture is generally typical, with failure to thrive and respiratory distress being the cardinal symptoms (Table 17.6).

Children with raised pulmonary blood flow may also present with cyanosis (Moynihan & King 1989). Whilst

Table 17.6   Raised pulmonary blood flow symptoms and clinical picture (developed from Gerraughty 1989; Jordan & Scott 1989).

Symptoms	Behavioural signs
Tachycardia ■ Rates persistently above normal. Tachypnoea and dyspnoea ■ More than 60/min in infants. ■ More than 40/min in older child. ■ May exhibit grunting respirations and/or signs of increased respiratory effort. Pulmonary oedema ■ Depending on the size of the L-R shunt, the more severe the greater the shunt. Sweating ■ Sometimes profound sweating as a result of the raised metabolic rate, and peripheral shutdown, as the child endeavours to regulate their body temperature.	Restlessness ■ Child is often restless and anxious looking. Feeding difficulties ■ Unwilling to feed due to respiratory state, often tiring and going to sleep without taking feed, even though hungry. ■ Apparent failure to thrive, does not gain weight easily, looks pale and thin. Tends to grow in length without increasing weight significantly. Chest infections ■ Frequent chest infections plague these children.

the cyanosis may not be as acute/marked as in those children who experience reduced pulmonary blood flow, it does effectively combine the symptomatic problems of both groups. Transposition of the great arteries (TGA) is the most common representative of this group. In TGA the aorta and the pulmonary artery are transposed so that the aorta arises from the right ventricle whilst the pulmonary artery arises from the left ventricle. The result is two separate circulations and when the ductus arteriosus closes severe cyanosis occurs (Tunstill & McCarthy 1993). Alternatively, as in truncus arteriosus, where the primitive truncus has not divided into the aorta and pulmonary artery, there is common mixing of systemic venous and pulmonary venous blood.

Obstruction to flow from the ventricles

If blood flow from the ventricles is obstructed, the ventricle is required to pump harder to push the blood past the obstruction; this pressure can be extremely high. In severe pulmonary stenosis for example pressures up to 200 mmHg have been reported (Jordan & Scott 1989). Children with an obstructive pathology of this

nature present with the symptoms of heart failure (the heart is unable to effectively supply the needs of the body). The child's actual symptoms depend on whether the left or right ventricle is obstructed (Table 17.7).

However, the child's symptoms (failure to thrive and tachypnoea) are similar to those seen in raised pulmonary blood flow conditions. But it should be noted that children with cardiomyopathy (failure of the myocardium) may also present with heart failure.

Conclusion

A clear understanding of the haemodynamic effects of the various defects allows the nurse to fully appreciate the physical effects on the child and their family and be able to anticipate their needs and to plan and provide appropriate and effective nursing care. However, despite the undoubted importance of cognisance of the physical defects and physiological effects, the nurse cannot see these problems in isolation from the child's psychosocial needs and still appreciate the potentially devastating effect that a cardiac defect can have on the functioning of the family. The nursing care of the child with a

Table 17.7 Heart failure due to right and left ventricular obstruction (developed from Gerraughty 1989; Jordan & Scott 1989).

Left ventricular obstruction	Right ventricular obstruction
In the symptomatic child there will be: ■ Tachycardia ■ Tachypnoea ■ Persistent dry cough ■ Sweating ■ Pulmonary oedema ■ Restlessness ■ Oedema – as a later developing sign	The child may be asymptomatic if not severe. The child may appear healthy looking, well nourished, moon faced and with a good colour (pink/red cheeks). The lips may also be pink. May tire on exertion due to inability to meet oxygen demand and raised cardiac output.
The severity of the obstruction will also affect the systemic blood pressure leading to possible acidosis and a low cardiac output state.	In severe or critical circumstances the child will appear cyanosed, breathless and fatigued even on minimal exertion. It is possible the child may experience myocardial ischaemic pain and syncope. In the newborn this condition may be fatal without urgent intervention.

congenital defect requires many skills and these are partly dependent on the nature of the defect itself and the age of the baby/child.

NURSING CARE OF THE INFANT WITH A CONGENITAL CARDIAC DEFECT

Whilst the cardiac anomalies themselves give rise to a range of symptoms, the differing levels of severity may be apparent in the child's cardiovascular status, requiring different types of management strategies. However, some common principles of care can be applied. Every child who has a cardiac defect is different and therefore requires individualized nursing care. The individuality of care may lie in the way that principles are applied, and care is planned and implemented. This section aims to address these principles and later considers specific aspects of assessment and care.

Two main aspects of care can be identified when nursing children with cardiac defects. First, the support, preparation and care of the child prior to, during and after diagnostic procedures. Second, the ongoing support and care needed to maintain and improve their cardiac status; this may involve caring for the child prior to and during transfer to a specialist regional unit, caring for the child

pre and post operatively, and facilitating medical support and management. Whilst these interventions meet the physiological needs, the child and their family will require a tremendous amount of psychological support to help them cope with the child's diagnosis, treatment and their associated fears and anxieties.

Nursing care of these families must start at the initial point of contact, continue throughout a potentially traumatic period of hospitalization, and continue into the community. Families of children with cardiac defects often require long term support to help them deal with the child's changing health needs. Initially the psychosocial support offered by the nurse may need to be most addressed to the parents of the newly diagnosed baby. However, as the child grows and develops they often need psychosocial support to deal with the effects that the defect has on them. It may curtail their activities of daily living and lead them to feel socially isolated.

The impact that chronic illness has on the child's psychological status has been studied (Stein & Jones Jessop 1984) as have the special needs of adolescents with CHD (Uzark *et al.* 1989; Gantt 1992; Uzark 1992). The nurse should be aware that congenital heart disease has both an immediate and long term impact on the infant/child and their family, and this awareness should be integral to planning care, even in the very early stages. Additionally the nurse should consider the needs of the siblings as research has recently recognized the stress that they experience as a result of a brother or sister in hospital. Simon (1993) highlights the need for the nurse to assess and support such siblings and suggests that contact with the hospital is desirable, as is the maintenance, as far as possible, of their usual pattern of activities.

When considering the complexity and multiplicity of needs, long and short term, nurses caring for a child with a cardiac defect must base their care planning, implementation and evaluating of care on a sound theoretical base. Holistic care is vital if all of the child's needs are to be met.

Nursing care during diagnostic procedures

Cardiac catheterization is one of the most valuable diagnostic procedures and although it is now a fairly common place procedure it is not without risk. Essentially it involves the introduction of a radio-opaque catheter through a peripheral vessel into the chambers of the heart. This allows assessment and monitoring of intra cardiac pressures, cardiac output, intra cardiac blood oxygen levels, ventricular and valvular function, and confirmation of diagnosis of congenital heart defects (Murphy Mayer 1986). In many centres echocardiogram has replaced cardiac catheterization in the diagnosis of defects (Coles 1994, pers. comm.).

Children and their families need adequate preparation from the whole of the multidisciplinary team. They need to be able to assimilate the information they have been given and to be provided with opportunities to ask for additional information and clarification of issues. As with any invasive procedure, psychological preparation is vital and play therapy is another important component of care. Petrillo & Sanger (1980) discuss the value of preparing children and their parents for surgery, invasive procedures and explaining about the illness. Play hospitals have been shown to be a good way of preparing children for hospital experiences (Eiser & Hanson 1991). Therapeutic play in hospital and in the community aims to allow the child control over their feelings and to release emotional distress (Thompson 1988; Douglas 1993; Eaton 1993). This type of emotional release is important for children with potentially long term health care needs and the prospect of repeated hospital admissions/contact.

Children who are to undergo cardiac catheterization

will need to be told about the procedure itself; what will happen to them, what they can do, what sort of equipment will be involved and who will be with them during the event. Age appropriate explanations are important and information needs to be repeated as necessary to ensure that the child grasps what is going to occur. Children are normally fasted for four to six hours before the procedure and sedation is given as prescribed. Additionally the nurse must ensure that the child's level of hydration and blood glucose level is maintained; this is particularly important if the child has a cyanotic heart lesion. The principles of preoperative care should be applied. Pre-emptive treatment is desirable.

After the procedure the nurse should be aware of the potential complications so that prompt treatment/action can be taken if required. Complications that may arise from cardiac catheterization include dysrhythmias, haemorrhage, reduced cardiac output, infection, adverse response to the contrast medium, cardiac perforation, arterial obstruction, phlebitis and hypoxia (Murphy Mayer 1986; Whaley & Wong 1991; Pitts-Wilhelm 1992). The range and potential severity of these complications results in the child needing close observation and monitoring of their vital signs, as well as specific issues related to the invasive nature of the procedure itself (Table 17.8).

Generally fluids are reintroduced once the child has recovered from the procedure and is able to tolerate them. Appropriate wound care (to the site of catheterization) must be given – local protocols will apply. Wound care management may be continued by the paediatric community nurse after the child has been discharged. As with any child discharged from hospital, good preparation for their return to the community is paramount. The child's parents must feel that they have been given adequate information and they should be given contact numbers and have the opportunity to discuss problems with a nurse. If as a result of the findings, it has been decided that the child will need surgery, the nurse should commence preparation of the child and their family for this eventuality.

Ongoing care and support of the child and family

Much of the care provided to children and their families with CHD is supportive: of the child's psychological

Table 17.8 Specific care and observations post cardiac catheterization (developed from Brunner & Suddarth, 1991).

Monitor vital signs; look especially for	■ Temperature: pyrexia can indicate infection; hypothermia may reflect the cardiac condition. ■ Pulse: changes in child's baseline rate and rhythm. ■ Respirations: changes to rate, rhythm, presence of dyspnoea. ■ Blood pressure: sudden drops.
Avoid potential dehydration	■ Introduce fluids as early as possible to prevent dehydration – a risk for children with cyanotic defects as polycythaemia increases the risk for thrombus formation.
Specific care required	■ Site of catheter insertion needs regular inspection for signs of haemorrhage, oozing, swelling, inflammation. ■ Area distal to the site of insertion of catheter needs to be checked for pallor, numbness, tingling, lowered temperature, decreased mobility, and change of colour. ■ Palpate the pulses distal to the insertion point and compare with contralateral ones. ■ Any of the above symptoms should warn the nurse that the child's circulation has altered and the vessel may be obstructing, and an appropriate response should be made.

needs, emotional needs and knowledge needs. Each aspect of support is important and requires a high level of input from the nurse. The type and intensity of interventions will reflect the child's actual needs at any time and the nurse must be able to assess the child/family on an ongoing basis so that appropriate interventions can be planned.

As stated earlier in this chapter, children with congenital cardiac defects present with broadly similar symptoms/health deficits and these will now be discussed in terms of the role of the nurse in meeting the child's needs. Children with a congenital cardiac defect experience problems due to the altered haemodynamics resulting in changes in oxygenation and blood flow. This gives rise to fatigue, dyspnoea, cyanosis, and recurrent respiratory infections due to the increased susceptibility of the lungs as a result of pulmonary vascular congestion. Due to the child's dyspnoea and associated difficulty in feeding, poor physical growth and weight gain results. Body image disturbances can arise from a multiplicity of causes including frequent hospitalization, scars (from surgical intervention), social isolation as a result of being different from their peers, and limitations in group activities. It may also result from family pressures not 'to do too much'.

Nursing care here aims to prevent maladaptive behaviour in the family and to ensure that the child has an appropriate level of self esteem and is not over protected by other members of the family. As previously mentioned, in order to achieve this the child and their family have an ongoing need for information, access to resources, advice and emotional support. The nurse should act as the child's/family's advocate and should employ strategies which will empower the family. This is a particularly important role once the child has been discharged from hospital as the child and their parents may feel particularly vulnerable and isolated.

The child's physical needs in relation to their cardiac defect can be discussed in terms of nutritional, respiratory and cardiac interventions. The child experiencing respiratory distress needs close monitoring of the level of distress and the response of the child to the therapy. If oxygen therapy is required the nurse must ensure that it is administered safely and that the effects are monitored. Mouth care is an important adjunct to oxygen therapy as this has a drying effect and there is risk from infection. Nursing the child sat at a 30° to 45° angle provides relief and reduces the pressure of the abdominal contents on the diaphragm, facilitating greater/improved lung expansion. Children can be nursed in comfortable chairs where appropriate or with the head of the bed elevated and pillows positioned to support them. Babies and infants can be nursed in a suitable infant reclining chair; measures should be taken to ensure that the baby is safely strapped into the chair.

If the child becomes hypoxic/increasingly cyanosed the nurse should intervene by calming and reassuring the child and either administering or increasing the delivery of oxygen. Another means of alleviating a cyanotic episode is to place the baby in the knee chest position (Higgins & Kashani 1986), where the child has pulmonary valve stenosis.

The nurse, and the parents, are key people in ensuring that the child receives an adequate nutritional and fluid input, and in evaluating their ability to tolerate it. One characteristic of CHD is inhibition of growth and Rønholt Hanson & Dørup (1993) propose a number of factors which may be associated with this (Fig. 17.3).

Infants with congenital cardiac defects are often thought of as difficult feeders; slow to take feeds, only able to tolerate small amounts and prone to vomiting. This means that a feeding plan needs to be developed based on small frequent feeds that do not tire the baby unnecessarily. The baby should be fed semi-erect as this facilitates lung expansion and special teats can be provided for bottle fed babies so that they do not have to expend energy. For the toddler or child a plan based on encouraging the child to eat a nutritious diet is important. Rønholt Hanson & Dørup (1993) advise that when children appear to be failing to thrive parents should be recommended to give their child vitamin/mineral supplements to facilitate normal and catch up growth. Monitoring the child's weight assists in determining the appropriateness of weight gain. However, genuine weight gain should not be confused with weight gain from fluid retention, which occurs in cardiac failure.

The nurse also needs to ensure that nursing care and the child's general activities are planned so that an appropriate balance between activity and rest is achieved. This should be done sympathetically so that the child does not feel restricted. Grouping care will ensure that the baby/child has periods which are not disturbed so that they can sleep, rest and relax.

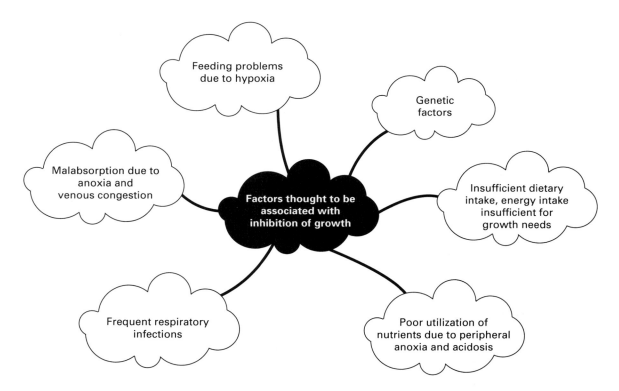

Fig. 17.3 Factors thought to be associated with inhibition of growth.

Parental needs in terms of needing psychosocial support have been discussed, but parents also need to learn how to care for their child at home and when to ask for help, as this is a valuable means of reducing their stress levels. Higgins & Kashani (1986) identify a number of parental learning needs (Fig. 17.4). This learning process is obviously ongoing and it needs to be commenced early during the child's stay in hospital.

CARE OF THE INFANT WITH PATENT DUCTUS ARTERIOSUS

Patent ductus arteriosus (PDA) occurs normally and essentially as part of the fetal circulation and only becomes problematic/abnormal if it persists after the birth of the baby (Mullins 1990). Patent ductus arteriosus is responsible for approximately 7% of CHD in full term infants. It is more commonly a problem seen in

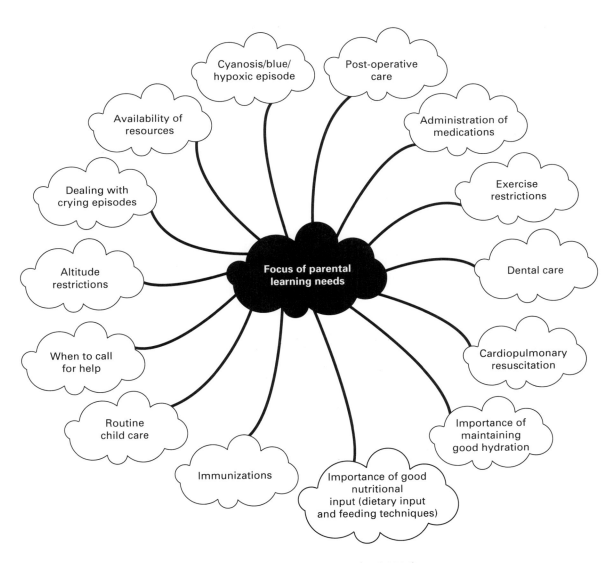

Fig. 17.4 Parental learning needs (developed from Higgins & Kashani 1986).

premature infants and is the result of lung immaturity and high pulmonary vascular pressures.

Functional closure of the duct usually occurs within 24 to 72 hours after birth and anatomical closure occurs within several weeks (Lynch & Sweatt 1987; Brunner & Suddarth 1991). If the ductus remains open the haemodynamic effects that result are dependent on both the size of the ductus and the pulmonary vascular resistance (PVR). Normally a small persistent ductus is asymptomatic but a large ductus can cause symptoms to develop early in infancy. A patent ductus results in a left to right shunt with blood from the aorta (higher pressure) being shunted across the duct to the pulmonary artery (lower pressure). This additional blood is recirculated through the lungs to the left side of the heart which results in an increased workload for the left heart and pulmonary vascular congestion, and potentially exerts an effect on right ventricle pressure. This can be detected by a characteristic murmur through the whole of systole. Diagnosis of PDA occurs through ECG and radiographic studies and echocardiography.

Often the PVR is high enough in the early stages of the infant's life to result in minimal shunting; however, as PVR decreases the defect becomes apparent as shunting increases. Infants with a large symptomatic ductus present with poor weight gain, difficulties feeding, lassitude, dyspnoea, and tachypnoea. They are prone to lower respiratory tract infections, atelectasis and endocarditis. Congestive heart failure can result from an unrelated PDA and this is an indication for closure in infancy.

Nursing assessment

Nursing assessment primarily focuses on the impact that the ductus is having upon the child and this will be related to their age and expected level of development and activity. If the infant is symptomatic then their ability to feed, gain weight and the amount of activity they can tolerate will need to be assessed. It is important to monitor their respiratory status and to note anything that contributes to/exacerbates their respiratory distress, level of dyspnoea, tachypnoea, colour change, and use of accessory muscles.

Nursing intervention: meeting the child's needs

Again the nursing interventions required will depend on the infant/child's age and the severity of the defect. Careful consideration of nutritional input (and the frequency and type of feeds) is vital in order to provide the child with maximum nutritional input with minimal expenditure of energy. Any alteration or deterioration in respiratory function is seen to be a key feature. Detection of cardiac failure is vital and initially medical management may be necessary prior to corrective surgery.

Prostaglandin inhibitors may be utilized in pre term infants as a trigger for closing the ductus. Closure of the ductus can be achieved by the use of an umbrella apparatus, during cardiac catherization, which is placed in the ductus to occlude it. Alternatively surgical closure of the ductus may be necessary – the ductus is tied off and the ductus is divided and oversewn (Roberts 1989). All principles in terms of pre and post-operative care apply.

CONGENITAL HEART DISEASE – PARENTAL DISTRESS

Congenital heart disease has a major impact on the child and their family. For babies who are diagnosed early the parents have to come to terms with the shock of finding out that their baby is less than perfect (whatever that may be) and face the challenge of coping with their own feelings, distress and anxieties combined with trying to cope with being 'good parents' and learning to care for their child.

Recent studies have started to address the impact that congenital heart disease has on parental stress and on infant–mother relationships (Goldberg *et al.* 1990; DeMaso *et al.* 1991; Goldberg *et al.* 1991; Lobo 1992). These studies demonstrate the importance of providing effective mother–infant relationships. Goldberg *et al.* (1991) suggest that attention paid to promoting the relationship can improve social development and can have positive outcomes in terms of the infant's physical well-being. DeMaso *et al.*'s (1991) study found that the quality of the mother–child relationship was more influential than the severity of the infant's actual illness in terms of successful adaptation. The importance of good infant–mother relationship/interaction is highlighted by Lobo (1992) in respect to feeding. Lobo (1992) found that infants with congenital heart disease have a different level of behavioural interaction with their care givers during feeding compared with healthy infants, and this may be construed in terms of labelling/identifying the baby as 'difficult to feed'.

Several studies, including Gudersmith (1975), have revealed parents' self reported experiences and difficulties in relation to building up an effective social relationship with their infant. Goldbert *et al.* (1990) recognized that although a number of studies have considered the psychosocial effects on parents caring for infants and children with CHD, very few focused on the initial impact in the early period of adjustment and readjustment and in particular on the stress that parents experience. Interestingly Goldberg *et al.* (1990) found in a comparative study of healthy children, children who had CHD and children with cystic fibrosis, that the parents of infants with CHD experienced relatively more stress than those with either CF or those with healthy infants.

CONGENITAL HEART DISEASE – NEEDS OF THE ADOLESCENT

Increasingly sophisticated technology, techniques and care have resulted in more children with congenital heart disease surviving into adolescence and beyond. For these young adults the pressures of managing the changes of adolescence are often compounded by the restrictions and differences that their cardiac condition imposes on their lives. During a period of growth, development and an increasing need to become independent, adolescents with a cardiac problem are often resentful of their condition. The adolescent survivor of congenital heart disease has special needs, such as information about their condition and lifestyle management, which the nurse should ensure are met appropriately. Uzark (1992) states that:

'specific informational needs include physical activity or exercise allowances and restrictions; sexuality, contraception and pregnancy issues; genetic coun-

selling; vocational guidance; health risks; and stress management'

She concludes that a major role in ensuring that the adolescent has a good quality of life lies in effective and appropriate counselling and in meeting their information needs. A number of studies have demonstrated that adolescents have incomplete understanding of their condition and its implications (Ferencz *et al.* 1980; Manning 1983; Uzark *et al.* 1989; Gantt 1992). Gantt (1992) studied young women who expressed very limited understanding of their actual and potential abilities to conceive, carry and deliver a child.

Body image is also a problem that had been identified by a number of adolescents and this included size, stature, development/bodily maturity and scarring. Adolescents with congenital heart disease are seen to compare themselves unfavourably with their peers or role models (Anderson *et al.* 1986; Uzark 1992).

These ongoing psychosocial needs should be met sensitively by the nurses caring for and supporting the young person, so that the young person is more able to make informed decisions about their lives.

ACQUIRED CARDIOVASCULAR DISEASES

Acquired cardiovascular diseases can occur in children with a previously healthy cardiovascular system as well as in those children with an existing defect(s). They can arise due to infection, autoimmune responses, connective tissue disease, familial characteristics, environmental responses or combinations of these factors (Whaley & Wong 1991; Pitts-Wilhelm 1992). The nurse has a role both in supporting and caring for the child and family during the course of the illness, but just as importantly the role of the nurse as health promoter, health educator and ill health preventer is increasingly being recognized.

The importance of preventing cardiovascular disease is paramount and for children's nurses, their understanding of the child and family and their skills in communicating health related information make them prime people to act positively in improving children's health in the long term. Health promotion can occur in many guises such as in advising and teaching parents (and the child) about complying with treatment regimes. Another role which is important is in screening children with group A streptococci throat infections (possible precursor to rheumatic fever). Other roles may involve screening children for hyperlipidaemia (high cholesterol levels).

In addition, it is important to give health information about diet, lifestyle and exercise to children, even at a very young age, to help them make healthy choices as a means of reducing the risk of acquired cardiovascular disease such as coronary artery disease/atherosclerosis. The crucial importance of health promotion in relation to heart disease is widely recognized (Cowell *et al.* 1989; Scott Brown *et al.* 1989; Watson 1991). The outcome of successful health promotion results in long term benefits for the child which extend into adulthood. It is an investment which must be made.

CARE OF THE CHILD WITH ACUTE RHEUMATIC FEVER/RHEUMATIC HEART DISEASE

Acute rheumatic fever (ARF) is one of the causes of infectious, acquired congenital heart disease. ARF is a self-limited, systemic disease involving the joints, central nervous system, blood vessels, heart and sub-cutaneous tissues (El-Said 1990a; Whaley & Wong 1991). There is an autoimmune response to group A, beta haemolytic streptococcal pharyngitis. El-Said (1990a) cites Lasegue (1884) who stated 'Rheumatic fever is a disease that licks the joints but bites the heart'. This in fact describes the essence of the disease since it is the impact on the heart that makes acute rheumatic fever (ARF) a disease of significance. Although it appears to be diminishing in incidence it is still a common disease in the developing countries (El-Said 1990b; Takahashi 1991) and is said to be associated with poor socio-economic living conditions when it occurs in developed/industrialized countries.

Rheumatic fever can recur but the first attack is usually preceded by a streptococcal upper respiratory tract or throat infection some 10 to 42 days previously (Pitts-Wilhelm 1992). It usually occurs in children aged 5 to 15 years old, affecting boys and girls equally, and may present in more than one member of the family. There is a seasonal incidence with peaks in the winter and spring consistent with normal pattern of streptococcal infection. Often the child will have experienced

recurrent streptococcal infections (El-Said 1990a). The characteristic pathological lesion of ARF is the Aschoff body. These are nodules that are located in the interstitial tissue of the myocardium and as the tissue heals scars are formed and the child experiences problems with valvular disease. The mitral valve is most commonly involved in rheumatic heart disease (85% of cases) with the aortic valve involved in 55% of cases and the pulmonary and tricuspid valves in only 5% (El-Said 1990b).

ARF may present either gradually or suddenly and the child with acute onset most commonly complains of arthralgia (pain) usually of the large joints (knees, elbows, hips, shoulders and wrists). This is the result of oedema, inflammation and effusion into the joint tissue. The pain tends to last a couple of days in one joint before migrating to another, and overall the child may experience up to four weeks of this acute migratory pain. The most significant symptom/effect of ARF is the resultant carditis which is characterized by cardiomegaly, significant murmurs, pericarditis, pronounced tachycardia, precordial pain and congestive heart failure. Assessment may also reveal an erythematous rash (erythema marginatum) which is most often located on the trunk and proximal parts of the limbs. Late on in the course of the disease Sydenham's chorea (St Vitus' dance) may manifest itself. This symptom is more common in girls than boys. Characteristically the child may be observed to have involuntary, purposeless, jerky, uncoordinated movements, muscle weakness, speech disturbances and emotional lability. This is usually much more exaggerated if the child is upset, anxious or fatigued.

For the child and their family the often sudden experience of such a major illness after a seemingly simple infection can be extremely frightening. Unexpected hospitalization for an acute condition in a previously healthy child can provoke a major disturbance within the family and all family members need considerable support from the nurse caring for the child. The child may experience acute pain which requires effective management, and they will also be restricted in their activity level by the impact the disease has on their heart. Whilst medical intervention is a vital part of their care, the psychological support and management of the child and their family is equally important. As with all such illnesses prevention is much better than cure and prophylactic measures and instigation of prompt and appropriate treatment of streptococcal pharyngitis is vital.

Due to the recurrent nature of RF it has been suggested that long term antibiotic therapy is an important way of preventing further damage in these susceptible children (El-Said 1990b). However, there is some debate in the literature about this (Takahashi 1991) and it is important to note that research by Pongpanich & Liamsuwan (1989) found that only 55% of the children who had acquired mitral stenosis had had a history of arthralgia that was suggestive of rheumatic fever. It was proposed that a mild course of rheumatic fever may be associated with progressive, insidious mitral stenosis.

Nursing assessment

Assessment focuses on the impact that the condition is having on the child's cardiovascular status and on the pain that the child experiences. Obviously the other factors will need to be assessed if a holistic approach to the child's needs is taken (Fig. 17.5).

The nurse must carefully observe and document the child's behaviour and needs so that appropriate care can be planned, and it is important due to the potentially slow recovery rate (1–4 months) to be able to evaluate the progress that the child is making and hence the effectiveness of care delivered.

The nurse must carefully assess the child's heart rate and rhythm. A tachycardia disproportionate to the child's pyrexia is often evident. A sleeping pulse should also be taken as this is indicative of the extent of the carditis (Brunner & Suddarth 1991). The nurse should also listen for cardiac murmurs and heart sounds; this, as stated previously, takes great skill and experience but is an important component of nursing assessment. The type and nature of the cardiac murmur should be documented and changes should be recorded appropriately. Other vital signs such as respiratory rate (changes in which could indicate the presence of cardiac failure) should be measured and noted, as should any dyspnoea or changes in the child's colour. It is important to monitor the child's temperature as the child will often be febrile in the initial stages of the disease. A crucial area of assessment lies in relation to the child's pain. The nurse should ensure that a comprehensive assessment of the site, nature, duration and type of pain experienced is recorded, along with information on what pain relief measures work and how the child and their family cope. All this information will help make effective pain

management a realistic and achievable goal. At the same time the nurse must observe the effects that the disease is having on individual joints, and which joint(s) are currently affected.

A holistic assessment requires the nurse to build up a wider picture of the child's problems and needs and this will include gathering information on the child's nutritional input (and any weight loss), and their level of activity/mobility which will be curtailed by both the need for bed rest and their own personal level of fatigue. The child's normal and current sleep patterns should be considered so that an attempt can be made to ensure that the child is able to maintain an adequate level of sleep. Due to the child's immobility/relative immobility it is important to regularly assess their skin so as to detect any signs of potential skin breakdown before they become problematic. If the child develops Sydenham's chorea then the nature, extent, triggering stimuli and effect of the involuntary movements should be recorded so that relief and management measures can be effectively planned.

A vital part of the assessment involves assessing how well the child is coping with the restrictions that the illness places on them, and assessing their compliance/adherence to the treatment regimes and how they are generally coping with the impact of being ill, hospitalized and outside their normal sphere of relationships and activities. Additionally the effect of any medication such as antibiotics and steroids needs to be considered and appropriate observations and assessments made (Fig. 17.6).

Overall the child's health needs and problems and the subsequent needs for assessment will depend on both the nature/extent/severity of the illness itself and the stage along the illness trajectory that the child is at.

Nursing intervention: meeting the child's needs

Of paramount importance in the care of the child is treatment of the streptococcal infection and the limitation of and prevention of further damage. With this in mind the support and management of the other symptoms and needs can be carried out. Obviously for the child and the family, symptom management and supportive care are important, but unless the infection can be controlled the continuing damage can result in a poor

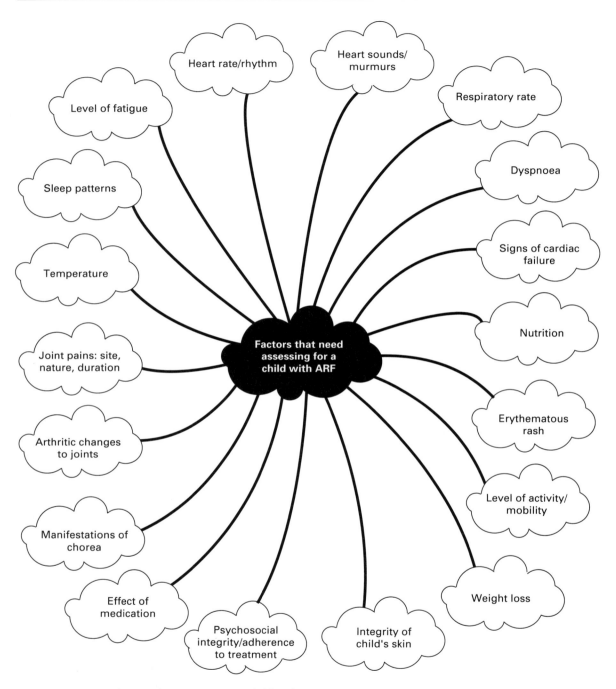

Fig. 17.5 Factors that need assessment in a child with ARF.

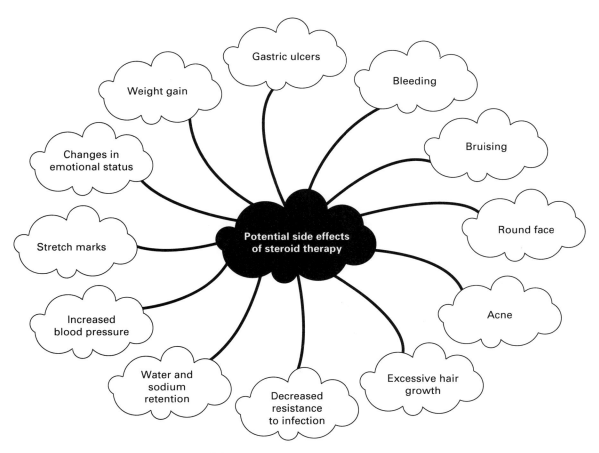

Fig. 7.6 Potential side effects of steroid therapy.

outlook both in the long and short term. Finally, intervention aims to reduce the possibility of future recurrence of the rheumatic fever as this also can result in further damage to an already vulnerable and damaged heart. Nursing care for these children has a long term prospect with not only the physical needs potentially needing to be met acutely over a period of months, but also education, support and advice in respect to prophylactic care needed in the long term. The nursing support both within the hospital and community setting is vital.

Antibiotic therapy is important both in the acute stages of the disease and also long term; monthly IM antibiotics may be prescribed. Alternatively oral medication may be given. Treatment may continue until the age of 21 to 25 years when, if no valvular problems are evident, it can be discontinued (Pitts-Wilhelm 1992).

However, there has always been controversy about the timing of prophylactic treatment (Ayoub 1989). Obviously with such a long term prospect the importance of adhering to the regime needs to be highlighted and any problems that the child has in adhering to the regime should be discussed and, whenever possible, the family involved in reaching an appropriate solution. It must also be stressed by the nurse that special care must be taken and additional prophylactic measures need to be taken if the child needs dental treatment or any invasive procedures.

In the acute phase, where the child is likely to be admitted to hospital, their activity is usually limited to quiet play and rest; this helps both the polyarthritis and the cardiac involvement. However, these limitations on activity are not usually strict and the child generally controls their own level of activity by responding to their own fatigue. Nursing care should be grouped so that the child has sufficient opportunity to rest and sleep. As the child starts to resume normal activities, the nurse should monitor the child's response to increasing levels of activity by checking their pulse rate after the activity to monitor cardiac compensation.

The child's pain from the polyarthritis can generally be managed with mild analgesia such as salicylates, which are also effective in managing the inflammation and the child's pyrexia (the contraindication of salicylate usage in children should be borne in mind). The nurse should be mindful that stronger analgesics may also be required depending on the child's reports of pain. Non-pharmacological strategies such as distraction, touch, massage and imagery can also be employed (Carter 1994).

Throughout the child's care the family should be encouraged to be involved as much as they feel able to. Parents can be particularly helpful in enabling the child to cope with the restrictions of limited activity; quiet play that absorbs the child and reminds them of home can be very helpful as a means both of occupying the child's time and of distracting them from their illness. Play is an important part of the child's life and the nurse should be able to adapt play to suit the child's needs/ desires and limitations. For the child who is fatigued easily, has muscle weakness or Sydenham's chorea, appropriate play must be considered.

Equally important to play is the child's and their family's need for information and education about the child's illness and care. This is especially important as effective communication is a key to relieving the child's anxiety about their condition and what will happen to them. The anxious and stressed child needs time and space to talk to their parents and nursing staff. Listening to their concerns and worries about their heart and the effects the illness is having on them is of prime importance. Relieving their anxiety not only makes them feel better psychologically but it also reduces the demands on the child's energy levels.

The child whilst in bed, and especially during the acute phase of the illness when they are feeling very tired, must be made comfortable and be helped to achieve adequate amounts of sleep. Good support must be provided for the child's inflamed and painful joints. If the child is dyspnoeic then appropriate positioning becomes even more important. Positioning the child carefully, appropriately and safely is vital for the child experiencing chorea. Padded side rails may be seen to be a necessary way of maintaining the child's safety. However, these further restrict the child (in terms of vision) and the reason for them needs to be explained so that the child does not feel imprisoned in bed. The child will need support when walking.

Once the child has recovered from the acute phase their care can be continued at home with the support of the paediatric community nurse. The nurse's role consists of providing ongoing support in ensuring that the child is given an adequate diet and gets plenty of rest. Support in terms of giving advice and help in relation to the child's activity levels during the recovery phase is also needed, as is specific advice in relation to any resultant carditis. The paediatric community nurse also needs to be able to inform parents about the need for prophylactic antibiotic cover for invasive procedures, dental treatment or infection.

Although ARF is rarely seen in children in the UK, it provides an example of how good nursing care can help to prevent further damage occurring and ensure that the child makes a good psychosocial and physical recovery from a sudden onset infection.

CARDIOMYOPATHIES

Cardiomyopathy is a term used to describe/refer to any:

> 'structural and/or functional abnormality of the ventricular myocardium that is not associated with disease of the coronary arteries, high blood pressure, valvular or congenital heart disease, or pulmonary valvular disease.' (Paquet & Hannay 1990)

Myopathies can be classified according to whether the cause is not known (primary) or if it is known (secondary). Additionally they can be classified according to the type of dysfunction and abnormal structure present: dilated cardiomyopathy, hypertrophic cardiomyopathy, and restrictive cardiomyopathy (Paquet & Hanna 1990; Whaley & Wong 1991).

The most commonly seen cardiomyopathy of childhood is dilated cardiomyopathy which is characterized by left ventricular dilation (or both ventricles) and cardiomegaly. The child typically presents with signs and symptoms of congestive heart failure. Treatment is focused on management of the congestive heart failure and is dependent on the severity of the failure. Fluid restriction, drug therapy and restricting the child's activities are key issues in management, as well as meeting the child's psychosocial needs.

Hypertrophic cardiomyopathy is characterized by a disproportionate increase in heart muscle mass without cavity dilation. Again the child may present with congestive failure as well as dysrhythmias and syncope. Drug therapy aimed at reducing left ventricular contractility, heart rate and ventricular wall stress may provide complete relief for the symptomatic child. Additionally any congestive cardiac failure should be treated.

The final type of cardiomyopathy, restrictive cardiopyopathy, is characterized by impaired diastolic filling caused by a scarred endocardium. No specific treatment exists and a poor prognosis is associated with this type of cardiomyopathy. The symptoms are those of congestive heart failure.

With all types of cardiomyopathy, wherever possible the underlying cause is treated as well as treating/managing the dysrhythmias and congestive heart failure. The prognosis tends to be poor and the nurse's main role is that of supporting the child and their family in relation to symptom management, and in dealing/coping with the restriction that the condition imposes on them. Many children with cardiomyopathies are now successfully transplanted although some children still

gement and competence of those involved in delivering basic life support (BLS) and, where appropriate, advanced life support (ALS). A number of writers have highlighted the deficits both in initial training and in updating of skills and knowledge (Wynne 1986; Wynne *et al.* 1987; Collins 1994a, b). BLS is a skill which all nurses should be able to perform at a high standard since ineffective BLS will result in a less than optimal outcome in terms of morbidity and mortality (Collins 1994a; Simpson 1994a). Although paediatric arrest is a rare event (Woodward 1994) the sequelae can be severe. Children most often present with respiratory arrest which can result in extreme tissue hypoxia, severe myocardial compromise and subsequently cardiac arrest. Simpson (1994a) states that:

'Children who survive initial resuscitation commonly die as a result of multi-organ failure caused by tissue damage from extreme tissue hypoxia existing prior to cardiopulmonary arrest.'

The need for prompt recognition of an impending respiratory collapse becomes self evident. Prevention of arrest is a responsibility that all nurses should accept. Woodward (1994) suggests that 'in general, paediatric arrests are preventable'. She further emphasizes the need to be aware of the signs of potential collapse which she

Table 17.9 Potential causes of cardiorespiratory arrest (developed from Woodward 1994).

Circulatory failure	
■ Fluid loss	haemorrhage, gastro-enteritis, burns
■ Fluid maldistribution	septic shock, cardiac disease, anaphylaxis
Respiratory failure	
■ Respiratory distress	foreign body, choking, croup, epiglottitis, asthma
■ Respiratory depression	convulsions, raised intracranial pressure, poisoning

die awaiting a transplant. Psychological support is paramount in helping the family adjust to the fact that their child is dying. All nursing care should be aimed at meeting the child's and family's ongoing needs.

PAEDIATRIC RESUSCITATION: AN OVERVIEW OF ISSUES

Fundamental to the successful management of an infant or child who requires resuscitation are the skills, jud-

classifies as either being respiratory or circulatory in origin (Table 17.9).

The need for not only all nurses to be able to perform basic life support but also for parents and other members of the general public to have this knowledge and skill is becoming increasingly important. Accidents and trauma are still the commonest causes of death in children and as the numbers of chronically ill children increase, the potential for cardiorespiratory arrest to occur also increases. These highly at-risk children are cared for increasingly in the community where the resuscitation environment is less than ideal. For this reason many parents are opting to learn basic resuscitation skills either at antenatal classes or through the British Red Cross (Heath 1994). The opportunity for paediatric nurses to take their skills and knowledge to the public is there – it just needs to be taken. Heath (1994) identifies parental demands for infant resuscitation training and the need to ensure that 'parents feel more prepared to cope with a crisis that everyone hopes will not occur'. The importance of educating and involving lay people as well as professionals is reiterated by Woodward (1994).

In respect to determining actions in BLS, an infant is less than one year of age and a child is one year old to puberty. However a very small child may be most appropriately considered and managed as an infant. The nurse must make an initial assessment in respect to his or her own safety and also should remove the child from any danger. Where possible mouth-to-mouth contact should be avoided by the use of a face shield or clear mask, as this can reduce the risk from infection (Woodward 1994). The infant's/child's responsiveness and level of respiratory difficulty should also be assessed

by gently shaking them and trying to evoke a response. The rescuer should not leave the child but should call for help. If no help is available and cardiopulmonary resuscitation (CPR) is required, the rescuer should perform a full minute of CPR before summoning help and where possible, Simpson (1994a) recommends carrying the child to the telephone. Ongoing assessment and actions are guided by the ABC formula: airway, breathing, circulation (Table 17.10).

CARDIOVASCULAR DISEASE: HEALTH PROMOTION AND RISK ASSESSMENT PERSPECTIVES

This section will focus on the nurse's role as health promoter, health protector and disease preventor (Igoe 1992) in relation to cardiovascular disease (CVD). The importance of this role can be seen from the fact that CVD is the major contributor to morbidity and mortality in the USA and other western countries (Black-

Table 17.10 Child and infant resuscitation (from ERC 1993).

Infant younger than 1 yr		Child older than 1 yr
Shake, pinch gently. Shout for help.	Check conscious level	Shake, pinch gently. Shout for help.
Head tilt. Chin tilt (jaw thrust).	Open airway	Head tilt. Chin tilt (jaw thrust).
Look, listen, feel.	Check breathing	Look, listen, feel.
Five breaths (mouth to mouth and nose).	Breathe	Five breaths (mouth to mouth).
Feel brachial pulse. Start compression if <60/min.	Check pulse	Feel carotid pulse. If no pulse start chest compressions.
Two fingers, over sternum. Rate 100/min, depth 2 cm. Five compressions: one breath.	Chest compressions	Heel of one hand, over sternum. Rate 100/min, depth 3 cm. Five compressions: one breath.

burn & Gillum 1980; Venters 1989). Coronary heart disease kills 150 000 people in England every year (over a quarter of all deaths) and prevention is recognized as needing to have a multifactorial, multi-agency approach if changes are to be achieved and maintained (Health Education Authority 1990). Additionally it should be noted that CHD is more prevalent in certain regions and the nurse should be aware of this so that appropriate strategies can be implemented. Some regions constitute CHD 'blackspots' in relation to morbidity and mortality; Northern Ireland is at the top of the World Health Organisation's CHD mortality league (Uemura & Pisa 1988; Boreham *et al.* 1993). Studies using a variety of methodological approaches have provided new information on risk assessment, health promotion and disease prevention (Boreham *et al.* 1993). Igoe (1992) suggests that children's nurses see health promotion and protection both as a challenge and an opportunity and one in which nurses should be taking a lead in action and research.

Risk assessment of children is an important primary prevention measure for children's nurses to address (Cowell *et al.* 1989). Current risk prevention research is based on health promotion and disease prevention strategies using either an ecological (community targeted delivery of programmes) or an at risk (targeting identified groups/individuals) strategy/approach. Cowell *et al.* (1989) undertook a longitudinal study involving a health education programme in local schools, through producing a newsletter for the families of children and additionally through health screening activities. This programme identified that successful intervention requires that cognitive deficiencies and motivational and affective support be addressed, and it highlighted that a public health approach within the community is vital. A number of factors have been identified as being risk factors in CHD (Fig. 17.7), some of which are deemed to be modifiable (smoking and tobacco use, diet and nutrition, high blood pressure and lack of exercise) (Health Education Authority 1990) and Type A behaviour characteristics (Scott Brown *et al.* 1989; Igoe 1992).

Prevention in childhood may be the key to managing the problem of CHD in adults. Although it is accepted that information from specialists changes and that advice sometimes may seem to conflict, it is important for nurses to increase the family's awareness that they can have a positive effect on their child's future health.

Together parents and children can begin to make sensible choices about lifestyle; for example by ensuring that their diet is not high in saturated fats and sugars and by maximizing opportunities to take part in regular physical activity such as sports, walking, swimming and so on. Nurses need to be involved, along with other professionals such as teachers, youth workers etc., in targeting these messages and in involving the children in health promotion projects at school. So far relatively little work has been undertaken to identify how children perceive and understand heart disease and the factors that can affect them. However, one such study was carried out in Birmingham in three inner city, multiracial primary schools. The findings highlighted the need for the professional health worker to develop a more facilitative role in order to help families identify their own needs and locate appropriate resources (Health Education Authority 1990). It was emphasised that 'child health cannot be divorced from family health and parental involvement is therefore not an option or added extra'.

It could be argued that children and families need to be motivated to change their lifestyle, behaviour and thus their risk factors. Nurses may be in a prime position to provide relevant knowledge, information, resources and support. To do this appropriate communication strategies need to be devised to both disseminate the information throughout the community (ecological) or to specific targeted children/families (at risk). It is vital to consider the ways in which the community, society and government may be persuaded to provide effective support and advice such as antismoking campaigns, good food labelling, access to sports and leisure facilities and availability of screening for health status.

Although some nurses may not see health promotion as a major part of their role it is a part which can no longer be ignored. Paediatric nurses have a responsibility to the children they care for not only in the short term in relation to their current health needs but also as proactive, long term health promoters. Children who grow up aware of their health and the factors which can affect it have greater opportunities for planning healthy lives as young adults and beyond. The current catastrophe of morbidity and mortality associated with coronary heart disease can be reduced providing everyone involved in health care delivery for children acts now.

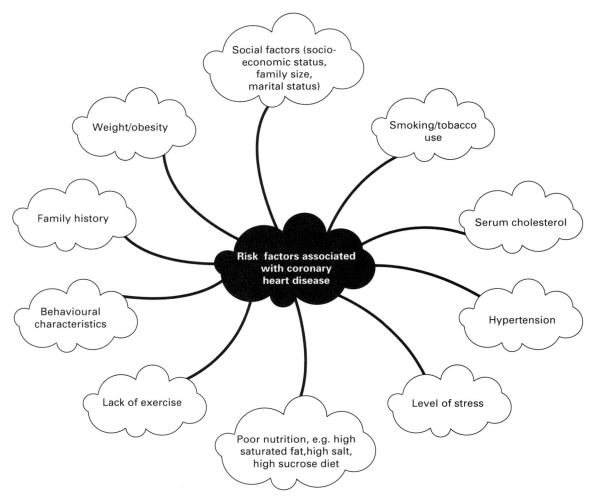

Fig. 17.7 Risk factors associated with coronary heart disease.

ACKNOWLEDGEMENT

Julia Coles Lecturer Practitioner, SDU Manager Children's Cardiac Services, Oxford Radcliffe Hospital, Oxford Brookes University.

REFERENCES AND FURTHER READING

Anderson, F.G., Deynes, M.J. & Altshuler, A. (1986) The adolescent. In *Comprehensive Pediatric Nursing* (eds G.M. Sapion, M. Barnard, M. Chord, J. Howe & P. Phillips). McGraw-Hill, New York.

Ayoub, E.M. (1989) Prophylaxis in patients with rheumatic fever: every three or four weeks? *Journal of Pediatrics*, 115, 89–91.

Behrman, R.E. & Kliegman, R. (eds) (1990) *Nelson Essentials of Paediatrics.* W.B. Saunders, Philadelphia.

Berenson, G.S., Voors, A.W. & Gard, P. (1982) Clinical and anatomic correlates of cardiovascular disease in children: the Bogalusa heart study. In *Proceedings of the Sixth International Symposium on Atherosclerosis* (ed. F.G. Schertler). Springer-Verlag, New York.

Blackburn, H. & Gillum, R. (1980) Heart disease. In *Public Health and Preventative Medicine* (ed. M. Last), p. 1168. Appleton-Century-Crofts, New York.

Boreham, C., Savage, J.M., Primrose, D., Cran, G. & Strain, J. (1993) Coronary risk factors in schoolchildren. *Archives of Disease in Childhood*, 68, 182–6.

Brunner, L.S. & Suddarth, D.S. (1991) *The Lippincott Manual of Paediatric Nursing* (3rd edn) (adapted for UK by B.F. Weller). HarperCollins Nursing, London.

Carter, B. (1994) Child and infant pain. *Principles of Nursing Care and Management*. Chapman and Hall, London.

Collins, P. (1994a) Knowledge and practice of CPR. *Paediatric Nursing*, 6(2), 19–21.

Collins, P. (1994b) Recognizing the need for CPR in children. *Nursing Times*, 90(35), 14.

Cowell, J., Montgomery, A.C. & Talashek, M.L. (1989) Cardiovascular risk assessment in school age children: a school and community partnership in health promotion. *Public Health Nursing*, 6(2), 67–73.

DeMasa, D.R., Campis, L.K., Wypij, D., Bertram, S., Lipshitz, M. & Freed, M. (1991) The impact of maternal perceptions and medical severity on the adjustment of children with congenital heart disease. *Journal of Pediatric Psychology*, 16(2), 137–49.

Douglas, J. (1993) *Psychology and nursing children*. Macmillan BPS Books, London.

Eaton, N. (1993) A play programme. In *Advances in Child Health Nursing* (eds E.A. Glasper & A. Tucker), pp. 15–26. Scutari Press, London.

Eiser, C. & Hanson, L. (1991) Preparing children for hospital: a school based intervention. In *Child Care: Some Nursing Perspectives* (ed. E.A. Glasper) (pp. 215–19). Wolfe Publishing Ltd, London.

El-Said, G.M. (1990a) Rheumatic fever. In *Principles and Practice of Pediatrics* (eds F.A. Oshi, C.D. DeAngelis, R.D. Feigin & J.B. Warshaw), pp. 1486–91. J.B. Lippincott Co, Philadelphia.

El-Said, G.M. (1990b) Rheumatic heart disease. In *Principles and Practice of Pediatrics* (eds F.A. Oshi, C.D. DeAngelis, R.D. Feigin & J.B. Warshaw), pp. 1491–8. J.B. Lippincott Co, Philadelphia.

Engel, J. (1989) *Pocket Guide to Pediatric Assessment*. C.V. Mosby Ltd, St Louis.

ERC (1993) Guidelines for paediatric support. A statement by the paediatric life support working party of the European Resuscitation Council. *Resuscitation* (1994) 27, 91–105.

Ferencz, C. Wiegmann, F.L. & Dunning, R.E. (1980) Medical knowledge of young persons with heart disease. *Journal of School Health*, 50, 133–6.

Gantt, L.T. (1992) Growing up heartsick: the experiences of young women with congenital heart disease. *Health Care for Women International*, 13, 241–8.

Gerraughty, A.B. (1989) Caring for patients with lesions obstructing systemic blood flow. *Critical Care Nursing Clinics of North America*, 1(2), 231–43.

Goldberg, S., Morris, P., Simmons, R.J., Fowler, R.S. & Levinson, H. (1990) Chronic illness in infancy and parenting stress: a comparison of three groups of parents. *Journal of Pediatric Psychology*, 15(3), 347–58.

Goldberg, S., Simons, R.J., Newman, J., Campbell, K. & Fowler, R.S. (1991) Congenital heart disease, parental stress and infant–mother relationships. *Journal of Pediatrics*, 119, 661–6.

Gudersmith, S. (1975) Mothers' reports of early experiences of infants with congenital heart disease. *Maternal–Child Nursing Journal*, 4, 155–64.

Health Education Authority (1990) *Take Heart, Good Practices in Coronary Heart Disease Prevention*. Health Education Authority, London.

Heath, J. (1994) Learning the basics: infant resuscitation training for parents. *Child Health*, Feb/Mar, 181–2, 184, 186.

Higgins, S.S. & Kashani, I.A. (1986) The cyanotic child: heart defects and parental learning needs. *Maternal Child Nursing*, 11, 259–62.

Igoe, J. (1992) Health promotion, health protection and disease prevention in childhood. *Paediatric Nursing*, 18(3), 291–2.

Jordan, S.C. & Scott, O. (1989) *Heart Disease in Paediatrics*. Butterworths, London.

Kulik, L.A. (1989) Caring for patients with lesions decreasing pulmonary blood flow. *Critical Care Nursing Clinics of North America*, 1(2), 215–29.

Lin, A.E. (1990) Etiology of congenital heart defects. *Paediatric Pathology*, 10(3), 305–9.

Lobo, M.L. (1992) Parent–infant interaction during feeding when the infant has congenital heart disease. *Journal of Pediatric Nursing*, 7(2), 97–105.

Lynch, M. & Sweatt, A. (1987) Congenital heart disease: assessment and case-finding by community health nurses. *Home Healthcare Nurse*, 5(4), 32–41.

Manning, J. (1983) Congenital heart disease and the quality of life. In *Congenital Heart Disease after Surgery* (eds M.A. Engle & J.K. Perloft), pp. 347–61. Year Book Medical Books, Chicago.

Moore, K.L. (1988) *The Developing Human – Clinically Oriented Embryology*, 4th edn. W.B. Saunders, Philadelphia.

Moynihan, P.J. & King, R. (1989) Caring for patients with lesions increasing pulmonary blood flow. *Critical Care Nursing Clinics of North America*, 1(2), 195–213.

Mullins, C.E. (1990) Patent Ductus Arteriosus. In *Principles and Practice of Pediatrics* (eds F.A. Oshi, C.D. DeAngelis, R.D. Feigin & J.B. Warshaw), pp. 1428–31. J.B. Lippincott Co, Philadelphia.

Murphy Mayer, D. (1986) Cardiovascular diagnostic techniques. In *Critical Care Nursing, A Holistic Approach* (eds C.M. Hudak, B.M. Gallo & T. Lohr), pp. 92–105. J.B. Lippincott, Co, Philadelphia.

O'Brien, P. & Boisert, J.T. (1989) Discharge planning for children with heart disease. *Critical Nursing Clinics of North America*, 1(2), 297–305.

Paquet, M. & Hanna, B.D. (1990) Cardiomyopathy. In *Principles and Practice of Pediatrics*. (eds F.A. Oshi, C.D. DeAngelis, R.D. Feigin & J.B. Warshaw), pp. 1467–75. J.B. Lippincott Co, Philadelphia.

Petrillo, M. & Sanger, S. (1980) *Emotional Care of Hospitalized Children*, 2nd edn. J.B. Lippincott, Philadelphia.

Pitts-Wilhelm, P.L. (1992) Alterations in cardiovascular function. In *Child Health Care: Process and Practice* (eds P.T. Castiglia & R.E. Harbin), pp. 565–604. J.B. Lippincott Co, Philadelphia.

Pongpanich, B. & Liamsuwan, S. (1989) Acquired mitral stenosis in children under fifteen. *Japan Heart Journal*, 23, 249–52.

Roberts, P.J. (1989) Caring for patients undergoing therapeutic catheterization. *Critical Care Nursing Clinics of North America*, 1(2), 275–88.

Rønholt Hansen, S. & Dørup, I. (1993) Energy and nutrient intakes in congenital heart disease. *Acta Paediatrica*, 82, 116–72.

Scott Brown, M., Gilhooly, J., Nelson, S. & Hildick, N. (1989) Type A behaviour in children: what a paediatric nurse practitioner needs to know. *Journal of Pediatric Health Care*, 3, 131–6.

Simon, K. (1993) Perceived stress of nonhospitalized children during the hospitalization of a sibling. *Journal of Pediatric Nursing*, 8(5), 298–304.

Simpson, S. (1994a) Paediatric basic life support – an update. *Nursing Times*, 90(21), 40–42.

Simpson, S. (1994b) Paediatric advanced life support – an update. *Nursing Times*, 90(27), 37–9.

Stein, R.E.K. & Jones Jessop, D. (1984) Relationship between health status and psychological adjustment among children with chronic conditions. *Pediatrics*, 73(2), 169–74.

Takahashi, M. (1991) Acquired cardiac disease. *Current Opinion in Cardiology*, 6, 129–34.

Talner, N.S. (1990) Cardiovascular disease in the newborn. *Principles and Practice of Pediatrics* (eds F.A. Oshi, C.D. DeAngelis, R.D. Feigin & J.B. Warshaw), pp. 352–69. J.B. Lippincott Co, Philadelphia.

Thompson, R.H. (1988) From questions to answers: approaches to studying play in health care settings. *Children's Health Care*, 16, 188–94.

Tunstill, A. & McCarthy, C. (1993) Care of the child with cardiovascular problems. In *Manual of Paediatric Intensive Care Nursing* (ed. B. Carter), pp. 132–54. Chapman & Hall, London.

Uemura, K. & Pisa, Z. (1988) Trends in cardiovascular disease mortality in industrial countries since 1950. *World Health Statistics Quarterly*, 41, 155–78.

Uzark, K. (1992) Counselling adolescents with congenital heart disease. *Journal of Cardiovascular Nursing*, 6(3), 65–73.

Uzark, K., VonBargen-Mazza, P. & Messiter, E. (1989) Health education needs of adolescents with congenital heart disease. *Journal of Pediatric Health Care*, 3, 137–43.

Venters, M.H. (1989) Family-oriented prevention of cardiovascular disease: a social epidemiological approach. *Social Science Medicine*, 28(4), 309–14.

Watson, M.C. (1991) Working together for Project Health. *Health Visitor*, 64(1), 22.

Whaley, L.F. & Wong, D.L. (1989) *Essentials of Pediatric Nursing*. CV Mosby Co., St Louis.

Whaley, L.F. & Wong, D.L. (1991) *Nursing Care of Infants and Children*. Mosby Year Book, St Louis.

Woodward, S. (1994) A guide to paediatric resuscitation. *Paediatric Nursing*, 6(2), 16–18.

Wynne, G. (1986) ABC of resuscitation: training and retention of skills. *British Medical Journal*, 293(6538), 30–32.

Wynne, G.A. (1987) Inability of trained nurses to perform basic life support. *British Medical Journal*, 294(6581), 1198–9.

Zideman, D. (1986) Paediatric resuscitation. *Care of the Critically Ill*, 2(4), 137–8.

Chapter 18

Nursing Support and Care: Meeting the Needs of the Child and Family with Altered Haematological and Immunological Function

Nicki Mackett and Liz Dyer

INTRODUCTION

The child with a haematological or immunological disorder requires nursing care that is creative, supportive and proactive. The major physiological response of the child will depend upon the component of blood that is deficient. Therefore the nurse needs to be conversant with the composition of blood and the significance of blood tests (Waterworth 1989). This understanding will also be invaluable in explaining the complexities of the disorder to the child and family. The nurse also needs to be aware of the likely progression of such disorders in order to support the child and family through the various reactions which often follow diagnosis.

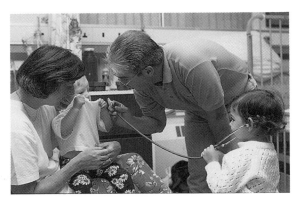

Fig. 18.1 Building relationships with the child and family. (*Photograph reproduced courtesy of Jon Sparks*).

Within this chapter a range of haematological disorders have been selected to illustrate deficits in blood cells, the effects upon the child and the principles of nursing care. Section one of the chapter explores the nurse's role in addressing the needs of the child with iron deficiency anaemia. Section two discusses some of the special considerations when the child has a disorder which has a genetic origin, for example thalassaemia, sickle cell anaemia and haemophilia. Section three considers the needs of the child with immunoedeficiency, including human immunodeficiency virus (HIV). The final section examines ways in which the nurse can provide holistic care for the child with leukaemia.

NURSING CARE OF THE CHILD WITH IRON DEFICIENCY ANAEMIA

Anaemia is a reduction in haemoglobin and hence the oxygen carrying capacity of the blood (Table 18.1). It is the most frequently occurring haematological disorder of childhood. It is not a disease, but the symptom of an underlying problem. There are many types and causes of anaemia (Table 18.2) but commonly it is a late manifestation of iron deficiency (Holmes 1991).

Table 18.1 Range of normal haemoglobin according to age.

Age	Haemoglobin grammes/decilitre
Newborn	15.0–21.0
3 months–1 year	9.5–12.5
1 year–puberty	11.0–13.5
Post-puberty	11.5–17.5

The child is vulnerable to anaemia between six months and two years of life and during adolescence (Seabrook 1993). Iron deficiency anaemia in early childhood is often caused by depletion of iron stores and inadequacy in the weaning diet. In adolescents it may be associated with sporadic eating patterns and a growth spurt (Tanner 1978).

Nursing assessment

The parents often bring their child to the attention of the GP or health visitor because of pallor, fatigue and irritability. There is often enthusiastic drinking associated with a reluctance to eat. The nurse by combining skills of observation, communication and knowledge of development will be able to glean information from the family to complement that obtained by the medical staff. An assessment should be made of the child's usual eating and drinking patterns to ascertain whether current changes are linked to a period of previous ill health.

Fatigue and lethargy due to reduction in oxygen to the muscles, often develop insidiously. The parents may

Table 18.2 Classification of anaemias.

Appearance of erythrocyte	Microcytic Hypochromic	Normocytic Normochromic	Macrocytic
Examples	Iron deficiency	Many haemolytic anaemias	Also megaloblastic: B12 or folate deficiency
	Thalassaemia	Secondary anaemia after acute blood loss	Aplastic anaemia
	Lead poisoning		

mention sleeplessness at night and drowsiness and irritability during the day. It is important to document alteration in sleeping patterns and activity levels for future evaluation of progress. There is also often a loss of interest in toys and friends. The nurse will need to assess the dynamics, communication and relationships within the family because the child's behaviour often becomes the focus of attention and anxiety and this leads to tension between family members.

An assessment of vital signs should be undertaken to provide a baseline. If the child is breathless it may indicate that the cardiorespiratory system is compromised, this is unusual except after rapid blood loss.

Nursing intervention: meeting the child's needs

Nursing interventions will focus on addressing the problems identified in the assessment. There is rarely a need for the child with iron deficiency anaemia to be admitted to hospital, except when blood transfusion is necessary. Care is usually managed in the home with the support of the primary health care team.

The family needs to be supported in their attempts to provide a nutritious diet containing adequate iron (Table 18.3). There may be a lack of awareness of iron rich foods and an unrealistic expectation of the amount of food the child should eat. Parents need to be encouraged to be creative with a wide variety of iron sources rather than create or compound conflict by focusing purely on meat and dark leafy vegetables.

Parents need to experiment in order to discover foods which will stimulate the child's interest and the nurse can offer advice on techniques to encourage

Table 18.3 Nutritional sources of iron.

Animal sources	Vegetable sources
minced beef	chick peas
liver	baked beans
lamb	lentils
pork	tahini (sesame seed paste)
bacon	butter beans
corned beef	ground almonds
beefburgers	tofu (soya bean curd)
sardines	spinach
eggs	prunes and apricots

positive eating habits (Fig. 18.2). Showing the child encouragement and praise for even slight improvement in eating will help to develop a positive behaviour cycle.

Diet alone may be insufficient to increase the iron intake and it will often be supplemented with iron replacement therapy until both haemoglobin and serum ferritin have returned to within normal parameters. This is continued for four to six months as the average life of a erythrocyte is 120 days. The preparations are often unpalatable and if the child is reluctant to take the medicine, play may be used to gain co-operation. Liquid iron preparations may discolour the child's teeth, this can be avoided if the medicine is given through a straw or is immediately followed by teeth cleaning. Parents should be reminded that iron medication is toxic and maybe fatal if consumed in large quantities. Medication should be kept out of the reach of children.

A change in sleeping habit must be felt to be advantageous for the whole family to be successful. Sometimes a deterioration in sleep patterns precedes an

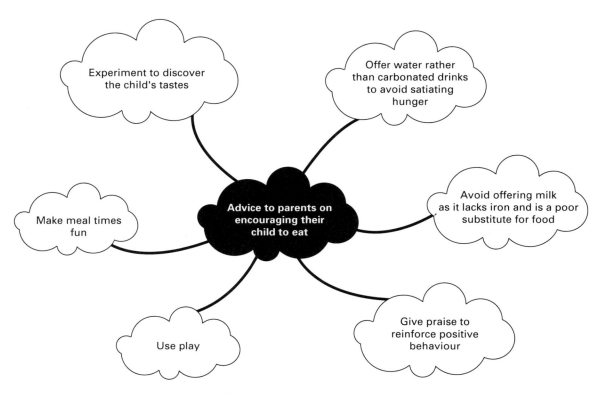

Fig. 18.2   Encouraging the child to eat: advice to parents.

improvement and the community paediatric nurse, in conjunction with the health visitor, has a role in offering support and encouraging persistence with new routines (Black 1993).

As the iron deficiency gradually corrects there will be a slow return to interest in play and physical activities. Encouraging play helps divert attention from meal times to other activities. Joining play groups, nursery and toy libraries helps promote a creative environment.

THE CHILD WITH A DISORDER OF GENETIC ORIGIN

There are many haematological disorders of genetic origin, for example thalassaemia, sickle cell anaemia and haemophilia.

NURSING CARE OF THE CHILD WITH THALASSAEMIA

Thalassaemia is an inherited disorder causing synthesis of abnormal haemoglobin. The reduced ability to synthesize alpha or beta chains results in severe anaemia which if left untreated may be fatal. In 1992 there were 570 children with beta thalassaemia major in the UK and an average of 16 births a year (Anionwu 1992).

Thalassaemia is an autosomal recessive inherited disorder which predominantly affects people of Asian, Far Eastern and South European descent. The diagnosis maybe made by analysing DNA obtained by chorionic villus sampling, amniocentesis or analysis of foetal blood. Where there is no previous history of thalassaemia, diagnosis may not be made until the child is between six months and two years. The child presents with severe anaemia previously undetected because of the persistence of foetal haemoglobin. The nurse needs to be aware of the implications of the diagnosis of this debilitating sometimes fatal disease. Where diagnosis has been made in utero the parents will need to discuss and decide whether they want to continue with the pregnancy. Their decision making may be influenced by their personal and observed experience of people with thalassaemia. Where the diagnosis has been made in infancy personal adjustments and new understanding of the diagnosis will be needed. Linguistically appropriate information which gives details about the disease and outlines the implications for future pregnancies is necessary in conjunction with counselling. It is important, when providing support and screening for the family that there has been consideration to the cultural and social implications of the disorder. Contact with the local haemaglobinopathies group will provide access to helpful resources and counselling.

When interviewed, children perceive some of the worst aspects of the disease as:

> 'needles for blood tests and transfusions, the pump used for chelation therapy and the side effects, coming into hospital, missing a lot of school and the future.' (Jennings 1990)

Maintaining optimum health is dependent upon compliance with invasive and regular therapies. The overall aims are to increase the haemoglobin, to correct anaemia by replacing the deficient erythrocytes, and to minimize the risks associated with blood transfusions. There are many potential problems when receiving all blood products (Fig. 18.3). However, the 'most life threatening transfusion reactions result from incorrect identification, leading to administration of incompatible blood' (Mintz *et al.* 1986, cited in Miller 1989).

The child with thalassaemia requires 3–6 weekly transfusions of packed red blood cells. Frequent transfusions are associated with the slow accumulation of serum iron. Excess iron cannot be absorbed or excreted instead it is deposited in other body structures (Table 18.4). This leads to progressive organ dysfunction and is potentially fatal. To prevent the build up of ferritin iron chelation therapy usually in the form of desferrioxamine is administered approximately six times a week. The infusion is given subcutaneously via a syringe pump over an eight to twelve hour period. The chelated iron is excreted in the urine. Research and

trials continue to search for an oral iron chelating agent (Jennings 1990).

There is disruption associated with admission to hospital. Access to the same ward amongst children with similar problems may enhance peer support and increase feelings of security and confidence. Admission overnight minimizes disruption to education, although it has been discovered that if sleep is disrupted in hospital children are often too tired to attend school the next day (Jennings 1990). This potential problem may be alleviated if the community paediatric nurse can support the parents giving the iron chelation therapy at home.

Nursing intervention: meeting the child's needs

If iron chelation therapy is given at home the nurse has a major educative and support role in helping the parents to take on this aspect of their child's care. There are many factors to consider when formulating a teaching programme (Table 18.5). If the family understands the need for iron chelation therapy they will adhere to treatment regimes more readily. The child will be more co-operative when there is minimal disruption to their usual activities and if they have confidence in their parent's abilities. These prerequisites to effective treatment should be recognized by the nurse when planning care and teaching programmes.

In the long term there is excessive haemolysis associated with this disease, which causes the spleen to enlarge; sometimes a splenectomy is performed. The introduction of bone marrow transplants has introduced another treatment option for some of these children (Sawley 1991, Cao *et al.* 1992) and it is likely that the number of children given this opportunity will increase in the future. The nurse should offer information and support to the family in their decision making.

The nurse should seek opportunities to provide information and health education for the child and family with thalassaemia. Jennings (1990) found that children were usually told about the genetic features of their disease but had limited information about other aspects, for example HIV risk through the blood transfusions. They tended to exchange information with each other whilst in hospital. The thalassaemia society offers comprehensive, language specific, literature about this disease.

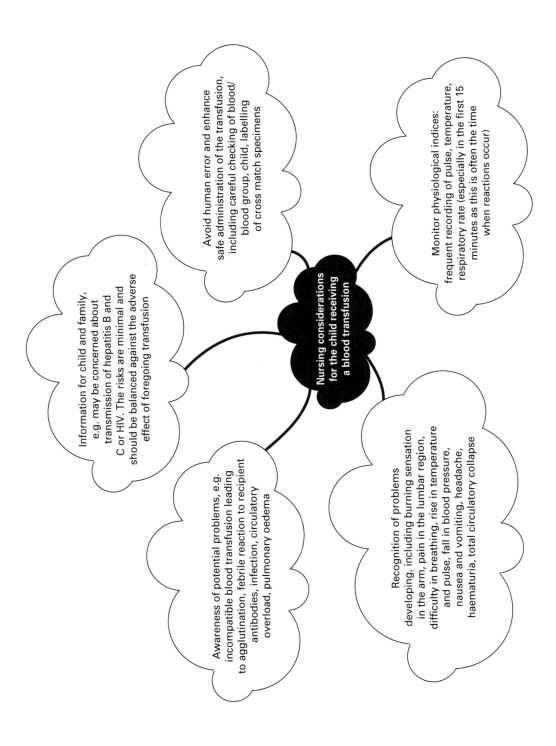

Fig. 18.3   Nursing considerations for the child receiving a blood transfusion.

Table 18.4   Complications of iron overload.

Damaged system or organ	Incidence, effect and management
Endocrine: growth retardation	Usually at puberty. Not always fully defined. Where growth hormone deficiency is diagnosed, replacement therapy is given.
Endocrine: hypothyroidism	If asymptomatic requires monitoring. Replacement therapy necessary if symptomatic.
Endocrine: hypoparathyroidism	Particularly common when heavily iron loaded. Presents as hypocalcemia with itching, tingling and, if untreated, convulsions. Replacement calcium.
Endocrine: diabetes mellitus	Common at puberty or older, particularly those with liver disease and poor compliance with chelation therapy. Always insulin dependent and difficult to keep controlled.
Cardiac	Arrhythmias, pericarditis, and cardiac failure. Managed according to symptoms.
Hepatic	Cirrhosis and hepatitis management according to symptoms.

Table 18.5   Factors to consider when formulating a programme to teach parents/child iron chelation therapy in the home.

- English may not be the first language of the child or family and so it may be necessary to find an interpreter either from within the family or an outside source. There may be language-specific written or taped information.
- It is often very difficult for a family to imagine a 'clinical' area within the home. Preparation and training for home therapy should take place either in the home or after a home visit. During the home visit an appropriate place for carrying out mixing and siting of the infusion can be identified.
- Learning new skills requires maximum concentration; this is difficult when members of the family are making demands for attention. The family should be encouraged to choose a specific time in the day for mixing and setting up the infusion.
- The practical training programme should include theoretical background reinforced by accurate information. Usually about 20 hours' training is necessary. The pace at which the family take on these new skills should be determined and controlled by them.
- Identify at least two family members who would be prepared to administer therapy to avoid the responsibility resting with one person.
- Gaining the child's co-operation for insertion and maintenance of a subcutaneous infusion may be a challenge. Initially there may be reliance on the community nurse but the child should be encouraged to co-operate for relatives.
- Bum bags may be more acceptable as a holder for the syringe pump than the holder supplied by the manufacturers.
- There should be ongoing support once the home therapy is established. Sometimes children have periods of non-cooperation and the nurse should be prepared to give the parents a break.
- Drinking tea with meals is thought to assist in the absorption of iron.

NURSING CARE OF THE CHILD WITH SICKLE CELL ANAEMIA

Sickle cell anaemia is an autosomal recessive disorder which affects approximately 5000 people in the UK (Brozovic 1987). It is predominantly associated with people of African origin but is also seen in Asian and Southern European populations. The presence of abnormal haemoglobin S creates haemoglobin which is particularly sensitive to a reduction in oxygen levels in the blood. If the oxygen concentration is reduced the altered amino acid component in the haemoglobin molecule causes alteration in the definition of the erythrocyte from a round to a crescent shape. This leads to further reduction in oxygenation and precipitates one of the main problems for the child, a physiological crisis.

Ideally women who are aware that they have sickle cell trait, the carrier state of the disease, should have access to genetic counselling. However, often the first encounter with the diagnosis is at the antenatal clinic. If both parents are carriers they may wish to consider the option of chorionic villus sampling, and possible termination of a fetus affected by sickle cell anaemia. This decision will be difficult for the parents because the effects of the disease are unpredictable and vary greatly between individuals. Many children may be less active than their peers but experience very few crisis periods and remain symptom free. On average a child requires three hospital admissions a year for management of painful crises (Franklin 1990).

Diagnosis can be made from birth from a cord sample, in conjunction with other neonatal screening. Although present from the time of conception, problems do not usually manifest until about four to six months of age because the fetal haemoglobin inhibits 'sickling'. Later children develop a haemolytic type of anaemia which is usually asymptomatic because despite the low levels of haemoglobin the sickle haemoglobin is more able to relinquish oxygen to the tissues.

There are a few obvious precursors to a sickle cell crisis (Fig. 18.4 and Table 18.6) and therefore there is an opportunity for proactive intervention. The nurse has an important role in helping the family to recognize these factors in helping them to take proactive steps to avoid a crisis. These may include providing additional warmth in winter, seeking medical intervention at the first sign of infection, and informing teachers, dentist and all

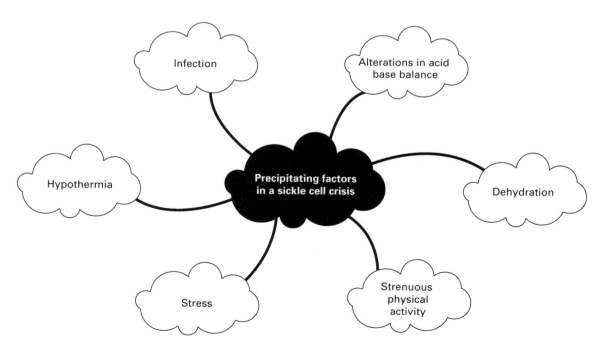

Fig. 18.4 Sickle cell crisis: precipitating factors.

Table 18.6   Crisis in sickle cell disease.

Painful, vascular-occlusive	Precipitated by infection, acidosis, dehydration, deoxygenation circulatory stasis, exposure to cold, violent exercise.	Infarcts may occur in a variety of organs, lungs, spleen, bones: hips, shoulders and vertebrae commonly affected. Most serious is in the brain (stroke occurs in 7%). Infarcts in the fingers and toes may lead to digits of varying sizes.
Visceral sequestration	Sickling within organs and pooling of blood often with severe exacerbation of anaemia.	Severe chest syndrome, hepatic and girdle sequestration crisis and splenic sequestration may all lead to severe illness requiring exchange transfusion.
Anaemic and aplastic crisis	Viral infection, commonly parvovirus. Sometimes folate deficiency.	Sudden fall in haemoglobin usually requiring transfusion, characterized by a fall in reticulocytes as well as haemoglobin.
Haemolytic crisis	Can accompany a painful crisis.	Increased rate of haemolysis with fall in haemoglobin and rise in reticulocytes.

members of the health care team about the child's problem.

Whelan (1991) describes the use of Orem's model to assess, plan and implement care for the child with sickle cell anaemia, and the remainder of this section makes references to the key considerations.

Nursing assessment

Pain caused by a crisis is often acute and severe and therefore the initial assessment will focus on pain to evaluate the effectiveness of pain management. It is also important to identify the possible stressors which may have precipitated the crisis. If the crisis has been induced by exposure to cold it may be relevant to assess the social situation, such as problems with financial constraints and any problems with heating. The child should be assessed for signs of fever, regular monitoring of the temperature may indicate infections.

Other aspects of assessment relate to wider implications of the disease upon the whole family, for example, the level of understanding within the family and the effects upon the siblings when one child attracts parental attention.

Midence *et al.* (1994) undertook a study to ascertain

the knowledge levels amongst patients with sickle cell anaemia. It was found that there was confusion between patients, health care professionals and the general population as to the cause of 'crisis' and the appropriate actions to take. The findings may be significant because as it is an inherited disorder the knowledge and attitudes of the adults and potential parents may have an influence on the management of the child. This may have implications for the development of educational programmes.

Nursing intervention: meeting the child's needs

The nursing interventions are aimed at relieving pain (Carter, 1993, 1994) and giving adequate fluids.

Increasingly morphine is given via patient controlled analgesia providing adequate and consistent pain relief (Schechter *et al.* 1988). Sometimes this is required for a week before it is possible to change to milder analgesia. Limiting the child's mobility may also reduce pain.

As a lack of fluids may have precipitated the crisis, if the child is unwilling or unable to take fluid orally an intravenous infusion will be commenced. If a pathogen is identified, antibiotics will be administered. Children over two years may be given pneumococcal vaccination.

The nurse should identify any problems created by inadequate heating as it may be possible to argue for rehousing on medical grounds. Health education advice about altering activities to minimize prolonged exposure to cold may be beneficial.

Both thalassaemia and sickle cell anaemia are debilitating disorders. Until the 1980s they remained a low priority on the country's health agenda. Prashar (1985) recognized that there were no guidelines for the needs analysis and management of such children. He recommended increasing effective screening, counselling and proactive treatment to reduce complications. In 1993 the Department of Health (Johnson 1993) issued a policy document outlining some strategies to bring the care of these children into the arena.

NURSING CARE OF THE CHILD WITH HAEMOPHILIA

Haemophilia is an X linked chromosomal inherited disorder of haemostasis (Fig. 18.5). To fully understand the required nursing interventions it is necessary to have an appreciation of the normal haemostatic response to injury. Haemophilia A and B are a reduction or absence of coagulation factors VIII and IX respectively and are associated with prolonged bleeding (Fig. 18.6). Although mucosal bleeding can create intermittent difficulties for children, the most significant problems – bleeding into muscles and joints – are discussed here. However, sometimes there is bleeding into the kidneys, or cerebral haemorrhage. The large bruises associated with haemophilia are unsightly and parents have been suspected of nonaccidental injury until diagnosis is confirmed. The following interview with a parent of a child with haemophilia illustrates her feelings about this:

'From when John first started crawling to when he was 11 months old, I was frequently taking him to the doctor with bruising. I was very concerned; all my worries were dismissed though. At one point the health visitor told me that the bruising round his bottom was because I was putting his nappy on too tight.

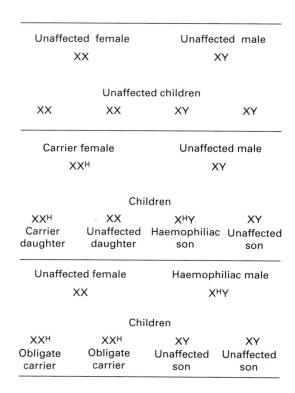

Fig. 18.5   Haemophilia inheritance pattern.

... Eventually he had an enormous bruise which was lumpy as well. This time I saw a locum GP who gave me a form for John to have a blood test. I was frightened; although the doctor didn't say anything to me I was sure he thought there was something seriously wrong.

... Later that day I was at my mum's, with John, when a neighbour rang to say that a social worker was waiting to see me. I went back home with my mum and John and there he was, this social worker with the health visitor wanting me to undress John. They told me they had to see his bruises. They examined him closely. I felt sick; I knew what they were thinking.

... Then, having talked between themselves and checked up whether I was married or "just had a boyfriend", they told me I had to take John to casualty straight away.

... The social worker ended up taking me and John; the health visitor took my mum. On the way to the

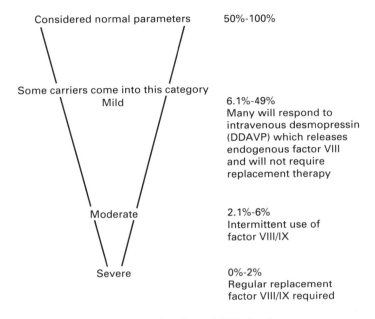

Considered normal parameters 50%-100%

Some carriers come into this category
Mild

6.1%-49%
Many will respond to intravenous desmopressin (DDAVP) which releases endogenous factor VIII and will not require replacement therapy

Moderate

2.1%-6%
Intermittent use of factor VIII/IX

Severe

0%-2%
Regular replacement factor VIII/IX required

Fig. 18.6 Severity pyramid for haemophilia A and B, factor VIII/IX level.

hospital the social worker stopped off at his house to pick up his camera, then he stopped to buy a film . . . to photograph the bruising.

. . . When we got to the hospital I was made to feel more and more guilty. They took John's blood and kept me waiting for ages without telling me what was going on. I was terrified. I kept telling them that I wouldn't let them take John away from me. Eventually . . . late in the afternoon, the blood test results came back.

The social worker came into the cubicle we had been sitting in for hours, with his camera over his shoulder, and said 'Oh, they say that John has got haemphilia and that's the cause of his bruising. A doctor will be in to see you soon. I've got to get back to the office.'

. . . The following day and for three days the health visitor came twice a day to talk to me and seemed surprised that I either yelled at her or wouldn't let her in . . . I didn't then and haven't since had one word of apology from the social worker, health visitor or GP.'

The main disruptions to the child's lifestyle are related to activity and play and this may have psychological and social implications (Markova & Forbes 1979).

Nursing assessment

When the child has a bleed into a joint, acute pain is caused by the accumulation of blood within the joint capsule. The signs of a bleed may have been recognized at the time but sometimes it is not detected until the child is noticed to be reluctant to walk, or move the affected limb.

Learning to assess early symptoms of bleeding is a continual process. The prospect of 'another trip to hospital' or 'another needle' can make it easy to ignore the symptoms, despite the knowledge that an ignored bleed may lead to permanent joint or muscle damage. The nurse should assess the family's knowledge of the signs of an early bleed so that treatment with factor VIII can commence as early as possible.

Nursing intervention: meeting the child's needs

The main aims of care are related to reducing the child's pain and immobilising the affected joint in the optimum position to promote healing and minimize the risk of rebleeding. Rebleeding is a common problem; the sensitive synovium is irritated by the blood, swells and develops tears. Factor VIII is given intravenously to enhance coagulation, reduce pain and reduce risk of rebleeding.

It is also important to provide appropriate education of the family so that bleeds are recognized early (Fig. 18.7). This will help to minimize permanent damage to joints and muscles (Fig. 18.8). There are long term effects of delaying treatment, for example fibrosis of muscles and arthropathy; this can lead to wheelchair dependence in later life. This is often intangible for the child, as illustrated in this statement from a nine year old boy:

'... being in a wheelchair sometimes it is really good fun ... but I wouldn't like it all the time when I am older because I would never make it to the pub on time.'

There is often parental anxiety surrounding the child's schooling and potential employment opportunities. Prior to the availability of replacement clotting factors for treating bleeds in the mid 1970s, long periods were spent at home without education, dealing with the protracted effects of joint and muscle bleeds. The advent

of bolus dose treatment with Factor VIII/IX and home therapy minimises the need for absences from school and encourages involvement in most (except contact sports) sporting activities. The use of prophylactic therapy maintains the deficient factor level at a moderate level (Figure 18.6) reducing the chances of sudden onset bleeding.

With the parents' and child's consent there can be discussion with teachers regarding any perceived need to limit activities. Liaison with the school nurse may establish a suitable storage place for the bottles of replacement therapy. This enables immediate administration of therapy by the child, parent or nurse.

Once the child has reasonably accessible veins and is able to cooperate, from about three years of age, many parents learn to administer home therapy. Children are encouraged to learn self administration before reaching senior school. The nurse usually needs to offer approximately 30 hours of tuition. It is also important to ensure that there is continued support once the home therapy is begun, and that the process is evaluated periodically to ensure that the principles originally learnt are maintained.

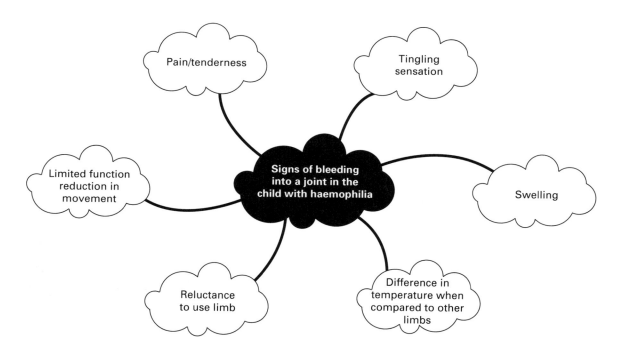

Fig. 18.7 The child with haemophilia: signs of bleeding.

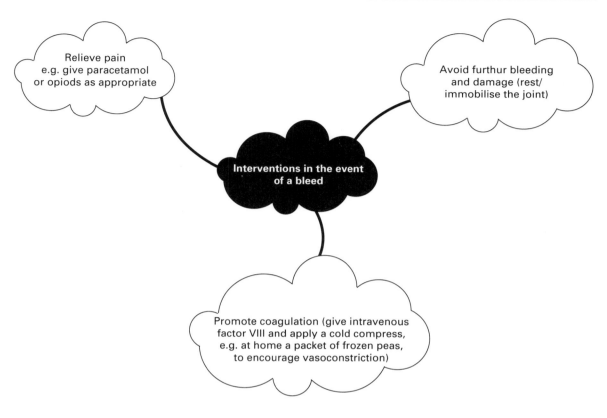

Fig. 18.8 Interventions in the event of a bleed.

CONCLUSION

There are many issues relating to inherited disorders which need consideration. Ideally opportunities for discussion and decision making should be available in pre conceptual planning and through genetic counselling. Counselling is unable to take account of spontaneous genetic mutations, these have occurred, for example, in one third of newly diagnosed cases of haemophilia. Decisions surrounding ante natal screening, investigations, contraception and termination of pregnancy are culturally influenced. Frets (1990) discovered that a couple's desire for children and their familiarity with the disorder often influenced their decisions. Skirton (1994) suggested that clients had to be able to relate the information being given to them to their own experiences and circumstances. Emery & Pullen (1984)

emphasized that genetic counselling should facilitate clients to make informed decisions based upon their own personal and social circumstances. It appears that the most successful schemes have started to make populations at high risk more aware of the implications of the diseases. Community nurses and midwives are ideally placed to lead this campaign (Pallister 1992a).

NURSING CARE OF THE CHILD WITH IMMUNE THROMBOCYTOPENIC PURPURA

Immune thrombocytopenic purpura is a common, acquired, usually transient haemostatic disorder of childhood. In 80% of children there is a history of some form, usually viral, of infection, for example rubella or chickenpox (Eden & Lilleyman 1992). Remission is usual but 5%–10% of children develop a chronic form of the disorder. Simultaneous to the immune response to infection there is an autoimmune destruction of platelets which increases the risk of haemorrhage (McFarlene 1993).

Nursing intervention: meeting the child's needs

The child often presents with a large number of diffusely spread bruises. Frequently bruising or purpura can be elicited by finger tip pressure. There is often a purpuric rash and sometimes mucosal bleeding. This is a worrying time for parents who again may be viewed with suspicion of nonaccidental injury until the diagnosis is confirmed.

Nursing interventions are largely dependent on the nature of the child's presentation and the proposed medical treatment. The nurse, in the community or outpatient department, has a supportive and educative role. For both parent and child the knowledge that a low platelet count increases the tendency for bleeding creates anxiety. This is usually allayed if parents are provided with advice regarding the appropriate action in the event of the child bleeding at home.

Immune thrombocytopenia is only treated medically if symptoms develop. There are usually two treatment options. First, a short course of steroid therapy as it is thought that steroids act by suppressing antibody formation; due to the brief duration of treatment, iatrogenic effects are uncommon. Second, high dose intravenous immunoglobulins (McFarlane 1993), which requires admission to hospital of between two to five days duration and for some children such admissions can be as often as two to three weekly. The intravenous immunoglobulins are thought to prevent antibodies binding to platelets, and transiently blocking receptors on the macrophages (McFarlane 1993). The nurse has an advocacy role in planning with the parents the most convenient time of day for the infusions, as even in an acute form the thrombocytopenia can last for three months and therefore treatment can be potentially disruptive to the child's lifestyle.

Occasionally the child does not respond to treatment and splenectomy is considered necessary. The nurse may provide essential support and advice during this period of stress and uncertainty.

NURSING CARE OF THE CHILD WITH HUMAN IMMUNODEFICIENCY VIRUS

The first group of children to be infected with HIV in the UK were children with haemophilia who had received contaminated pooled plasma products prior to 1985, in the form of factor VIII/IX replacement therapy (AIDS group of Haemophilia Directors 1988). Changes since then have made this method of transmission very rare (Table 18.7).

Vertically transmitted HIV infection, i.e. from mother to infant is increasing. In 1993 in the UK there were approximately 200 children with vertically transmitted HIV infection and there are records of more than 300 infants born to HIV positive women (Communicable Diseases Report 1994). The World Health Organisation estimates that globally by the year 2000 there will be thirteen million women and ten million children infected with HIV (WHO 1993; Yogev & Connor 1992). The majority of these children will have been infected through vertical transmission, from mother to baby.

The human immunodeficiency virus, as its name suggests, gradually attacks the immune system until it is depleted. The virus has a particular affinity with T4 lymphocytes, invading them and so replicating the virus (Pratt 1991). The virus also has an affinity to the glial cells of the central nervous system. As management of opportunistic and other infections improves, an increasing number of children with HIV will have neurological symptoms such as developmental delay and regression and so-called AIDS dementia complex.

Increasingly HIV is being viewed as a new chronic disease of childhood (Meyers & Weitzman 1991).

'After working with several families we realised that we had a chronic illness on our hands, and we now treat it as a chronic illness . . . we find that many of the theories and concepts are applicable to the care of children with AIDS. While HIV is a fatal illness for many children it is a long term process . . . so, we really use the chronic illness approach, and I would recommend it to anyone who is in the process of developing services.' (Boland 1988)

There are considerable medical advances and innovations for the child infected with HIV. The nursing

Table 18.7 Routes of HIV transmission in children and young people.

Route of transmission	Mode of transmission
Vertical from mother to infant	There is approximately a 14.4% risk of transmission from pregnant woman to her child.
Breast feeding	This is thought to increase the risk of transmission from mother to child to about 29%. In areas with good sanitation, breast feeding should not be encouraged. In countries with poor sanitation leading to high morbidity and mortality from enteric disease, breast feeding should be actively encouraged.
Contaminated blood and blood products prior to 1985	The test for HIV antibody only became available in 1985. People with haemophilia were particularly vulnerable as replacement clotting agents are from the pooled plasma of 3000 or more donors. Since 1985 blood has been tested for HIV antibodies and blood products heated to temperatures higher than those tolerated by the virus.
Blood to blood contact	Sharing used needles and syringes. Needlestick injuries.
Under-age penetrative sex	Between consenting partners or in situations of abuse.

management is focused upon enhancing quality of life. Hospital and community based nurses have a multi-faceted role to play in caring for children and families affected by the virus. This ranges from an educational role, providing health promotion for young people and teaching about HIV prevention (Boyer & Kegeles 1991) to the care of the infected mother, child and the wider family.

The diagnosis may be as devastating as the disease. There is a progressive course and poor ultimate prognosis (Duggan 1993). However, perhaps more difficult for the family is the associated stigma and uncertainty.

Nursing assessment

Where a woman is HIV antibody positive prior to pregnancy her new born infant will be shown also to have a positive antibody test result. The significance of this result is uncertain as there is a persistence of maternal HIV antibody in the infant for up to eighteen months. The infant should have access to facilities to assess growth and development and identification of any health problems. This enables a picture to develop indicating whether the child is also infected with the virus. Where the child does develop infections such as candida, otitis media and diarrhoea (Table 18.8), it is important that there is opportunity for radical treat-

ment. There should be evaluation of the child's developmental milestones as these are sometimes compromised. The child's weight and height should be recorded regularly, together with an appraisal of the child's nutritional status.

The nurse should assess the parents' understanding of the illness and if the mother is unwell her needs should be considered with a view to exploring ways of keeping the mother and infant together if they are simultaneously unwell.

Nursing intervention: meeting the child's needs

An adequate support network may influence the process and the outcome of the disease for the child. The mother or whole family may feel isolated. Friends, may feel unable to provide support or may feel daunted by the prospect of watching a friend's mortality, may reject the family. Sometimes, due to the stigma, the mother will place herself in voluntary isolation. The nurse has a key role in helping her to build links, whilst respecting her decision making.

Another major part of nursing intervention will be related to information giving. It is important that there is access to clear, jargon-free information. Although many women appear to be well informed, it is important to

Table 18.8 Some common manifestations of HIV infection in infants.

Manifestation	Definition
Persistent/recurrent oral candida	Persistent for two or more months, or recurrent after a course of treatment.
Persistent diarrhoea	Three or more loose stools a day for more than a month.
Severe/recurrent varicella zoster	Two or more episodes of recurrent zoster or chronic infection for more than 30 days despite treatment.
Severe bacterial infection (not AIDS defining)	Single severe bacterial infection.
Failure to thrive (not AIDS defining)	Failure to thrive, not yet meeting AIDS definition.
Regression of developmental milestones.	Consistent regression over at least three months.

establish the accuracy of their knowledge. It is likely that they only retain limited information, because stress and anxiety are known to inhibit communication. The nurse should recognize when stress levels are lower and use these times to discuss pertinent issues. Any discussion should take place in private to maintain confidentiality. If talking at home it should not be assumed that other family members are aware of another's HIV status and permission should be sought before disclosing it.

Advice should be given about the importance of giving regular prophylactic antibiotics, as these are recommended for all infants until their antibody status is clarified. It is also important to discuss immunization programmes. All immunizations can be given, with the

Table 18.9 Immunizations for infants and children with HIV antibodies.

Vaccine	Age given	Notes
Diphtheria, tetanus, whooping cough, polio, and haemophilus influenzae B	2, 3 and 4 months	Polio vaccine has two forms: live given orally; inactivated given intradermally. It is recommended that the inactivated form is given because of the theoretical risk of infecting an immunocompromised parent.
Diphtheria, tetanus, whooping cough and polio	4–5 years	As above.
Measles, mumps and rubella	Over 12 months	Live vaccine; a child with a damaged immune system is more at risk from the disease than the vaccination.
Rubella	10–14 years	As above
Bacillus Calmette–Guérin (BCG)	10–14 years	Should not be given; there is greater risk from the vaccine than chance of getting the disease.
Hepatitis B	Any age	If parents known to be infected with hepatitis B.

exception of BCG (Table 18.9). Inactive polio vaccine is given rather than live vaccine, as the live polio virus is excreted in the faeces. If the child's immune system is compromised, some immunizations may be less effective (Ridgeway 1989).

The child's development may be inhibited by the state of health of both the child and the carer. If the mother is unsupported and has limited energy herself she is often less able to play with and stimulate her child. Even relatively short periods of ill health can cause a slowing down of the infant's developmental achievement. Access to day nursery should be organized and in some areas voluntary organizations provide a 'baby relief' service and opportunities for mothers to meet together in a supportive environment and discuss issues.

A sudden deceleration in growth marked by a reduction over two centile lines in three months is usually indicative that the infant has AIDS, although it is important to assess whether the child is receiving adequate nutrition. If the mother feels nauseated by the smell of food she may have difficulty in preparing food for her child. Oral candida may make the infant reluctant to eat, and malabsorption from diarrhoea may cause weight loss. The nurse can liaise with the dietitian to explore nutritional supplements.

A unique feature of HIV and AIDS is that frequently the main carer and sometimes other members of the family are chronically unwell simultaneously. Therefore close liaison and co-operation between all health care workers is important. Sometimes both the mother and child may need to be admitted to hospital, and strategies to minimize the separation should be explored.

When providing nursing care for a child with HIV there needs to be an awareness of local infection control policies. In the hospital environment it may be desirable for the child to be admitted for care to a cubicle, as HIV suppresses immune function creating potential risk of infection from other inpatients on the ward.

The infant with HIV commonly spends long periods of time at home in good health, the symptoms of HIV that require nursing intervention occurring infrequently. Over a variable period of time the child will become less well, symptomatic of bacterial or viral infection, and eventually will develop AIDS. The time between the first AIDS descriptor disease and death is unpredictable. Supportive community and hospital nurses help to make episodes of ill health more manageable. Ultimately there

will probably be a need to explore with the mother either her own death and future child care arrangements or feelings about the death of her child. Social workers, psychologists and local organizations may provide useful resources.

Conclusion

Several articles discuss some of the wider implications of caring for a person with HIV/AIDS. Although none of these relate specifically to children, some of the following may provide interesting further reading and some of the principles may still be applied. Burnard (1989) identifies methods for exploring attitudes and feelings. Peate (1989) conducted an examination of nurses' views of patients with AIDS. Stanford (1988b and c) facilitates an exploration of attitudes and reactions and introduces the public health responsibilities of the nurse. Shuttleworth (1988) discusses some of the complex ethical considerations related to HIV testing, and Howe (1989) offers an ethical perspective on the rights of the individual.

NURSING CARE OF THE CHILD WITH LEUKAEMIA

In 1989 in the UK there were 1200 children affected by malignancy (Draper & Stiller 1989). Approximately 500 of these presented with leukaemia, making it one of the most common forms of childhood cancer.

Leukaemia is a proliferation of immature or blast leukocytes. In this immature state the cells are unable to fulfil effective function and the marrow produces additional leukocytes in an attempt to compensate. Gradually the number of blast cells increases at the expense of the mature cells.

Often the parents take the child to the GP because the child is pale and tired and may have a history of frequent infections. At this early stage the diagnosis may be suspected but is subsequently confirmed by the results of a venepuncture, bone marrow aspiration and lumbar puncture. The blood, bone marrow and cerebral spinal fluid will contain blast cells. All these procedures are potentially traumatic for the child and family and as they are the first of many invasive experiences, the nurse's role in offering adequate preparation and support is particularly important. Sedation such as Ketamine or a general anaesthetic is usually given, this may also minimize the trauma.

There are two main types of leukaemia: acute lymphoblastic and acute myeloid; each is determined by the position of error in the leukocyte production. Each has different treatment options and a varied prognosis. To understand the information that will be given to the parents once the diagnosis is disclosed, the nurse needs to be conversant with the production of leukocytes. Acute lymphoblastic leukaemia has a more favourable prognosis, infants of less than a year have a 23% chance of a five year survival, and those over a year a 75% chance.

Optimum treatment is centrally organized within oncology centres where similar treatment protocols are used. In an endeavour to find the most effective combination of cytotoxic drugs, treatment is organized in trials with the same basic drug therapy arranged in different ways.

The parents and, where possible the child, should be asked to give their informed consent prior to a child being admitted to a drug trial. Charles Edwards & Casey (1992) identify criteria which must be satisfied to validate consent for treatment:

■ Competence to understand the information given.
■ Sufficient accurate information supplied.
■ Consent given willingly.

Nursing assessment

It is more common for the child to present with acute lymphoblastic leukaemia (Chessels 1985) so this has been selected to discuss principles of care. The child's problems and needs are generally associated with the dysfunction of the bone marrow and the inappropriate production of blood cells.

An assessment of the child will usually reveal:

■ Breathlessness on exertion, and lethargy, due to anaemia as a result of the deficit in erythrocytes.
■ Bleeding gums or bruising, due to thrombocytopenia and deficient platelet production.
■ Frequent sore throats and fever, indicating infection

which is most likely to be caused by the reduction in mature leukocytes and lymphocytes.
■ Pain in the legs as a result of an overactive bone marrow.

Nursing intervention: meeting the child's needs

Nursing care (Fig. 18.9) should include physical and psychosocial dimensions and will largely focus upon nursing support of the strategies to correct the anaemia and thrombocytopenia. It will also aim to (Forsyth 1992):

■ Minimize the risk of infection.
■ Manage the child's pain.
■ Perhaps most importantly, keep the family informed in order to reduce their anxiety.

The child will probably require little incentive to rest, quiet activities and games should be provided. If the child is lifted or handled this should be done with care to minimize bruising. The child will receive a blood and platelet transfusions. If these are prescribed simultaneously it is important to give the platelets first as this will minimize the loss of newly transfused blood. If there are signs of a raised temperature, blood cultures, stool, urine, and nose and throat swabs will be taken and intravenous antibiotics will be given. Most children require the insertion of a central venous line for administration of drugs, blood products and to enable blood sampling. The nurse should work in partnership with the parents to prepare the child for these procedures and should ensure that the appropriate measures are taken to ensure safety (Fig. 18.3).

Pharmacological and non-pharmacological methods of managing pain should be explored. Adequate analgesia should be given to relieve the pain. By regular assessment of pain levels the dosage or drugs can be altered accordingly. Sometimes story telling, massage, physiotherapy and warm baths are effective (Devine 1990, Carter, 1994) in distracting a child from their pain.

Overall it should be remembered that the diagnosis will create anxiety for the child and family, especially as disease progression varies between individuals and it is not possible to predict the outcome of treatment (Ross

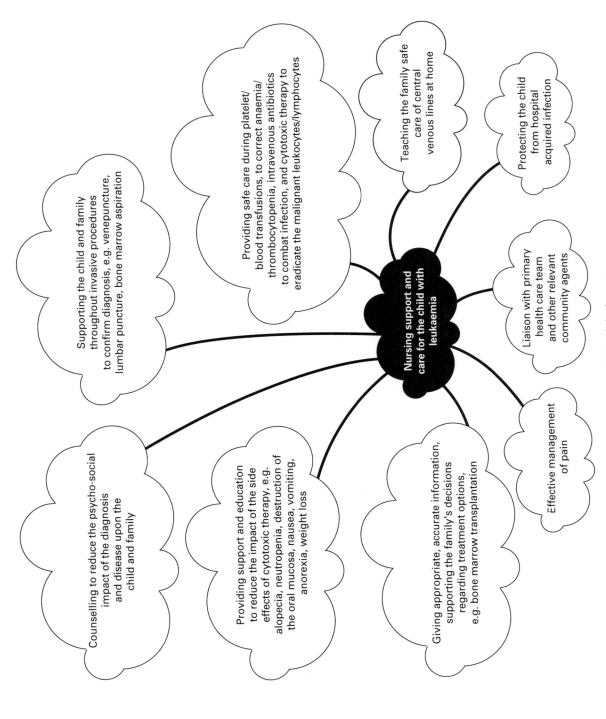

Fig. 18.9 Specific nursing support and care considerations for the child with leukaemia.

1980). The nurse may draw upon a range of resources and by co-ordinating the contributions of the Malcolm Sargent Agency, social workers and child psychologist may encourage a multidisciplinary approach to care and psychological support.

Possible reactions to a diagnosis of leukaemia are illustrated in this interview with a mother of a seven year old:

> My first reaction, although there had been suggestions that Sally has leukaemia, was definitely shock and despair. It really was only a confirmation of what we had thought but it still felt like I had been winded when that word leukaemia hit ... a total disbelief. I remember thinking that I should get to Sally; if she was going to die I wanted to spend every minute, every second with her – ridiculous I know but that is how I felt. The rest of the talk with the doctor is all a blur; I didn't take much in after that word. Then I thought to myself, don't be so stupid, my little girl looks just like Sally, just a bit pale, there must be some mistake ...'

It is important to explain all procedures and allow the family time to ask questions, and by assessing the family's reception information can be offered in measured amounts. Information booklets may be useful and the play specialist can use play therapy to explain the treatment to the child and assist them in expressing their feelings about it.

Nursing intervention: meeting the needs of the child receiving cytotoxic therapy

The treatment for leukaemia involves the administration of cytotoxic agents. During and following cytotoxic therapy the child's health problems increase and are related, in the main, to the iatrogenic effects of therapy caused by the destruction of both healthy and deficient blood cells (Fig. 18.10).

To provide access for drug therapy a central venous catheter is usually inserted under general anaesthetic. The catheter is tunnelled via a major vessel until the tip is positioned in the right atrium where it is held in place by a Dacron cuff. It is important to explain to the child and family that the insertion of this line is to reduce venepunctures by allowing easier access to blood for tests, and to give the drugs required, but it may not eliminate the 'needles' completely. Blood counts are usually recorded about seven days from the start of treatment as this is when neutropenia will become evident.

There are several hazards for the child with a central or Hickman line in situ (Fig. 18.11). The hazard of septicaemia is reduced if the nurses apply the principles of asepsis when handling the line, including hand washing and the use of sterile gloves (Leese 1989). Gillies (1985) suggests it is unnecessary to flush the line regularly but if a Brovia catheter with a lumen of less than 1.0 mm is used, there is a tendency for it to become blocked and therefore a daily heparin flush may be required to keep the line patent.

To reduce the time that the child needs to spend in hospital the parents are taught to care for the line. It is important that responsibility is negotiated with the family so that they do not feel under pressure. Dimond (1990) discusses the legal position when tasks, which were formally undertaken by nurses, are adopted by parents. The implication is that:

> 'professional staff have a duty to ensure that only appropriate tasks are delegated and that there is instruction accompanied by the appropriate level of supervision.'

It is suggested that 'appropriate' is:

> 'what is reasonable given the knowledge, the level of understanding and competence of the parents, the nature and complexity of the treatment.'

Depending on the intensity of the chemotherapy and hence the degree of neutropenia, the child's susceptibility to infection is increased, especially during the time they are in hospital. The child is usually allocated a cubicle, and individualized nursing care with a named or primary nurse. This may reduce the number of nurses unnecessarily having contact with the child. During neutropenic episodes the temperature should be taken at regular intervals and the nurse and parents should be alert to the first signs of infection.

Cytotoxic therapy may affect the child's ability or enthusiasm for eating, one of the most distressing effects is a sore mouth. This is due to the destruction of the oral mucosa and reduction in saliva production. The damage can also admit intestinal flora into the systemic circulation and cause diarrhoea. Other common effects include anorexia, nausea and vomiting, all leading to weight loss.

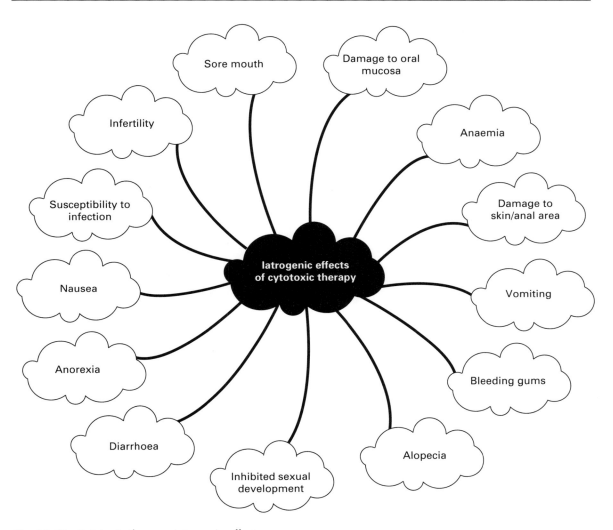

Fig. 18.10 Cytotoxic therapy: iatrogenic effects.

The nurse can provide health education for the parents on the importance of mouth care. It is important to inspect the child's mouth daily, especially in the younger child who may be less able to verbalize their discomfort. The teeth should be cleaned after each meal and before bedtime. Toothpaste has a drying effect and it is important to rinse the mouth after cleaning (Barnett 1991). A soft brush may be used to minimize trauma and bleeding gums.

Mouthwashes are available containing chlorhexidine these have an antiseptic and antifungal action. To enhance the effectiveness of these, the child should not

eat or drink for twenty minutes after the mouthwash has been given (Crosby 1989). Some parents find undertaking mouth care a challenge, and sometimes star charts may offer motivation to the child to co-operate.

Nausea and vomiting are recognized side effects of cytotoxic drugs. Fortunately vomiting is less common due to the effectiveness of the newer anti-emetic drugs. Initially these can be given intravenously one hour before chemotherapy commences and regularly for twelve hours afterwards (Gibson 1989a). In some children distraction or self hypnosis may be helpful in alleviating nausea (Contanch 1985). Anorexia and

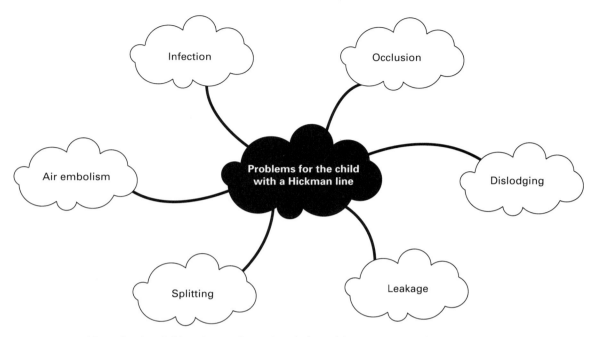

Fig. 18.11 Problems for the child with a Hickman line (adapted from Leese 1989).

weight loss can be potentially dangerous and are of concern to parents. It is important to keep accurate records of the child's weight and height as these are also used for calculating drugs.

A team approach will increase the effectiveness of care and the dietitian can provide advice. The child's calorie intake can be increased by adding flavourless high calorie substances to drinks. While the child is in hospital it is important to ascertain the child's favourite foods so these can be obtained from the diet kitchen or brought in from home. Few children find hospital food appetising (Mills *et al.* 1993) and some children complain that the chemotherapy makes food taste 'metallic'. Red meat seems to create an unpleasant after taste but fish and poultry are more palatable. Sometimes total parenteral nutrition (TPN) is required.

Alopecia creates considerable distress affecting the child's self concept (Horowitz 1983, cited in Price 1993). The nurse needs to support the child during this time by gaining a measure of the child's perception of their body image in order to discuss this issue with them (Price 1993). The child may be reassured that it is not a permanent effect and hair growth will return rapidly after treatment is completed. Caps and hats can be

recommended and it is also possible to provide the child with a wig. Children with long hair may find it less upsetting if they have their hair cut before it begins to fall out (Price 1993).

Leukaemia and chemotherapy have psychosocial effects which should be recognized. The activities and daily life for the whole family may be restricted; for example, holidays and time away from home may be problematic and therefore occur infrequently. Siblings may have to assume additional responsibility for other members of the family (Hewitt 1990). Evans (1993) suggests that for the child the 'developmental tasks' are threatened. The nurse may play a significant role in helping the child to adapt to changes. Often the child will understand their illness and treatment but when they have not refined their coping mechanisms their behaviour may regress.

As treatment becomes more effective and life expectancy increases, the long term effects of the treatment become more evident. Chemotherapy inhibits sexual maturity and may creates infertility. Boys may be offered the facility of a sperm bank (Evans 1993). In addition, there may be muscle wasting, compromised growth and impaired intellectual functioning. Evans

(1993) suggests that the young adult must make four major adaptations:

(1) To the effects of the disease and treatment.
(2) To loss of personal control.
(3) To uncertainty about the future (they may experience problems obtaining employment or insurance).
(4) To changes in social relationships.

Many hospitals employ paediatric community nurses with expertise in the care of children with oncology problems. These nurses are able to bridge the gap between tertiary and primary care. They have a vital role in liaising between all agencies involved with the child to ensure that they receive the relevant information regarding all aspects of care and treatment. They also provide security for the parents who may feel very vulnerable following discharge from the perceived safety of the hospital environment.

There are specific considerations when discharging a child who is immunosuppressed or has leukaemia:

■ Vaccinations should not be given.
■ Chickenpox and measles can be fatal; in the event of contact immunoglobulins should be given within 48 hours.
■ If the child becomes febrile intravenous antibiotics should be given.

When the child returns to school, with the parents' permission, the teachers should be told about the treatment, especially alopecia as the child may wish to wear a hat all day. There may be a tendency to 'over-protect' the child and everyone should be encouraged to treat them like everybody else and not single them out for special privileges or be more lenient. It may be useful to discuss the issue of discipline with the parents as they may feel guilty about reprimanding their 'sick' child.

Providing nursing care for a child with leukaemia may be rewarding when they respond to treatment but particularly distressing when medical interventions prove unsuccessful. It has been suggested that nurses need support and access to counselling 'to enable them to work through their sadness and avoid burn out' (Schroeder 1993). There are schemes where child psychologists are employed and they provide opportunities for nurses to discuss their work and issues related to terminal illness and death.

NURSING CARE OF THE CHILD EXPERIENCING BONE MARROW TRANSPLANTATION

For children with relapses in leukaemia or aplastic anaemia, bone marrow transplantation offers the only real hope of long term survival. This procedure is not without risk and is not the 'magical cure' that it is often perceived to be by the media. The aim of the transplant is to limit the severe bone marrow ablation. The deficient bone marrow is replaced by autologous or allogenic marrow obtained from a donor. The ideal donor is a sibling but a matched unrelated donor may be found through voluntary agencies such as the Anthony Nolan Trust. Compatability between donor and recipient will minimize the problems following the infusion of the bone marrow.

Nursing assessment

An assessment of physiological indices, together with neurological and psychological functions, will be made to provide a baseline from which to monitor future effects of the bone marrow transplantation. The nurse will need to support the family and give them accurate information regarding the medical investigations undertaken. These involve assessment of cardiac, respiratory, renal and liver functions. An infection screen will also be performed to ensure that the child has no underlying infection.

Nursing intervention: meeting the child's needs

All family members require in depth information regarding the expected steps during the transplant and the long term effects. Parents should be warned about 'graft versus host disease' (Garland 1991), in which the T lymphocytes in the donor marrow reject the patient and a reaction is set up. This is manifested by urticuria, skin rashes, jaundice and diarrhoea occurring during the first 84 days; it can be fatal. It is for this reason that drugs are given proactively for up to six months following transplantation to suppress the immune system.

Parents find all this information distressing and need time to assimilate it. Where the donor is a sibling two family members will need to be prepared, it is especially important that the donor appreciates that they are not responsible for the success or failure of the transplant (Williss 1993).

Prior to the transplant the child will undergo 'conditioning' which involves administration of high doses of cytotoxic agents and total body irradiation (the latter is not undertaken in children under the age of three years due to the associated damage to the brain). This creates pancytopenia and potentially problems similar to those discussed earlier in relation to leukaemia and chemotherapy, in particular it leaves the child susceptible to infections. Therefore they need to be isolated from other children, especially when in hospital. They will be confined to a cubicle and reverse barrier nursed for about four weeks (Williss 1993). A relatively new medical innovation in the form of a granulocyte stimulating factor is now available, it elevates the white cell count and reduces the length of time required in isolation (Heron 1992).

As the parents spend extensive periods of time in hospital they often take on extended roles. These include housework and cleaning of the cubicle, caring for their child's hygiene, managing their child's diet and keeping them amused to relieve their boredom. Gibson (1989b) found that generally parents were positive about their involvement but Cole (1991) found that they experienced isolation and needed to take frequent breaks. It was discovered that they experienced guilt every time they left their child but if the family had the opportunity to establish a relationship with a primary or named nurse they felt more confident and less guilty about leaving the child alone with the nurse.

The nurse needs to co-ordinate the range of professionals involved in the care of the child following bone marrow transplantation. They have a prime role in interpreting information and ensuring that the family have an adequate understanding at all stages. The team members may include a transplant co-ordinator and play specialist as well as the ward nurses and haematologist or oncologist who provides physiological checks (Gibson 1989b). Later, as the longer term effects become more evident, endocrinologists, cardiologists and psychologists may also be required.

CONCLUSION

Although this chapter has explored many aspects of care in relation to specific disorders, there are several features that may be common to any child with an altered haematological function.

The nurse's role can be seen to be orientated towards supporting the child and family throughout investigations and treatment by providing accurate relevant information. The diagnosis will rely upon haematological studies from which vital information is gained (Waterworth 1989). These require repeated venepuncture and one of the worst fears of children may be 'needles'. By applying the principles of preparation and enhancing the coping strategies within the family the nurse can reduce the stress for the child (Rodin 1983).

Once a diagnosis is confirmed the family will need further detailed information upon which to base their decisions, and possibly counselling.

The nurse's role in direct care activities is usually related to the provision of supplementary blood products. In many cases the nurse will teach the family the skills of self administration. When this is successful the child will spend a reduced time in hospital and will experience minimal disruption to their lives.

SOCIETIES AND USEFUL RESOURCES

Haemophilia and von Willebrands disease
Haemophilia Society, 123 Westminster Bridge Road, London SE1 7HR. Tel. 0171 928 2020. *Information, advice and support.*
Health Publication Unit, DSS Distribution Centre, Heywood Stores, Manchester Road, Heywood, Lancs OL10 2PZ. *Special medical card: haemorrhagic states.*

HIV and AIDS
Barnardos Positive Options, 154 Goswell Road, London EC1V 7LQ. Tel. 0171 278 5039. *Information, advice and support and future planning for HIV positive parents.*

Black HIV/AIDS Network (BHAN), 111 Devonport Road, London W12 8PB. Tel. 0181 749 2828. *Counselling and information in many dialects.*

Grandma's, PO Box 1392, London SW6 4EJ. Tel. 0171 610 3904. *Practical support in the home for HIV positive children.*

Mildmay Mission Hospital, Hackney Road, London E2 7NA. Tel. 0171 729 5361. *Hospice and respite facilities for parents and children with AIDS.*

Positive Partners and Positively Children, Jan Rebane Centre, 14 Thornton Street, London SW9 0BL. Tel. 0171 738 733 (head office), Tel. 0171 250 1369 (north London office). *Information, advice and support for HIV positive partners and children.*

Terence Higgins Trust, 52–54 Gray's Inn Road, London WC1X 8JU. Tel. 0171 831 0330, Helpline 0171 242 1010 (seven days a week 12 noon to 10pm). *Practical support, welfare rights, buddying and education.*

Primary immune deficiency

The Primary Immunodeficiency Association, Aliance House, 12 Caxton Street, London SW1H 0QS. Tel. 0171 976 7640. *Practical support and advice.*

Sickle cell disease

OSCAR (Organisation for Sickle Cell Anaemia Research), Sickle Cell Community Centre, Tiverton Road, Tottenham, London N15 6RT. Tel. 0181 802 3055/0944. *Research and information.*

Runneymede Trust, 178 Gower Street, London NW1 2ND. Tel. 0171 387 8943.

Share, King's Fund Centre, 126 Albert Street, London NW1 7NF. Tel. 0171 267 6111. *Database of books, articles, projects and services for health and black populations.*

Sickle Cell Society, 54 Station Road, Harlesden, London NW10 4UB. Tel. 0181 961 7795/8346. *Information and advice.*

Thalassaemia

UK Thalassaemia Society, 107 Nightingale Lane, London N8 7QY. Tel. 0181 348 0437. *Information and advice.*

Courses

Genetic counselling in the community

Institute of Child Health, 30 Guildford Street, London WC1N 1EH. Tel. 0171 242 9789, ext. 2610.

Sickle cell and thalassaemia

The George Marsh Sickle Cell and Thalassaemia Centre, St. Ann's Hospital, St. Ann's Road, London N15 3TH. Tel. 0181 442 6230.

Nightingale Institute of Nursing and Midwifery, Normanby Campus, King's College Hospital, London SE5. Tel. 0171 272 6222, ext 3121.

HIV and AIDS

ENB for Nursing, Midwifery and Health Visiting, PO Box 2EN, London W1A 2EN. Tel. 0171 388 4031.

REFERENCES AND FURTHER READING

Ades, A.E. & Newell, M.L. (eds) (1991) Children born to women with HIV-1 infection: natural history and risk of transmission. European Collaborative Study. *Lancet*, **337** (8736), 253–60.

AIDS group of the Haemophilia Centre Directors (1988) Prevalence of antibody to HIV in haemophiliacs in the United Kingdom. *Clinical and Laboratory Haematology*, 10, 187–91.

Anionwu, E.N. (1983) Sickle cell disease: screening and counselling in the antenatal and neonatal period, part 1. *Midwife, Health Visitor and Community Nurse*, 19, 10.

Anionwu, E.N. (1990) Community development approaches to sickle cell anaemia. *Talking Point*, Grindon Lodge, Newcastle upon Tyne.

Anionwu, E.N. (1991) A multi-ethnic approach. *Nursing*, 4(41), 9–12.

Anionwu, E.N. (1991) Teaching community genetics. *Nursing*, 4(42), 37–8.

Anionwu, E.N. (1991) Sickle cell disorders and the school child. *Health Visitor*, 65(4), 120–2.

Anionwu, E.N. (1992) *Sickle Cell Disorders and Thalassaemia*. Highlight No. 115. National Children's Bureau, London.

Aronstam, A. (1985) *Haemophiliac Bleeding – Early Management at Home*. Bailliere Tindall, London.

Bailey, C. (1992) *Leukaemia*, 2nd ed. (ed. J.A. Whittaker). Blackwell Science, Oxford.

Barnett (1991) A reassessment of oral healthcare. *Professional Nurse*, 6(12), 703–4, 706–8.

Berger, M. (1989) *Understanding Haemophilia, a Personal Account and Practical Guide for Parents, Teachers and Caring Professions.* Ashgrove Press, Bath.

Black, P. (1993) Setting a regular pattern: encouraging socially acceptable sleep habits in the young child. *Child Health*, 1(4), 145–57.

Boland, M. (1988) Practical aspects of caring for children with AIDS. In *Aids in Children, Adolescents and Heterosexual Adults* (eds R.F. Schinazi & A.J. Nahmias). Elsevier Science Publishing, New York.

Boyer, C.B. & Kegeles, S.M. (1991) AIDS risk and prevention among adolescents. *Social Science and Medicine*, 33(12), 11–23.

Brozovic, M. (1987) Acute admissions of patients with sickle cell disease who live in Britain. *British Medical Journal*, 294, 1206–8.

Burnard, P. (1989) Exploring nurses' attitudes to AIDS. *Professional Nurse*, 5(20), 84–8.

Buzzard, B.M. & Jones, P.M. (1988) Physiotherapy management of haemophilia: an update. *Physiotherapy*, 74(5), 221–6.

Cao, A., Gabutti, V., Maswera, G., Modell, B., Sarchia, G. & Vullo, C. (1992) *Management Protocol for the Treatment of Thalassaemia Patients.* Tenny Graphics.

Carter, B. (1993) *Pain: perspectives and reflections.* In: Pain, Towards a New Standard. Sickle Cell Trust, Cardiff.

Carter, B. (1994) *Child and Infant Pain: Principles of Nursing Care and Management.* Chapman and Hall, London.

Charles Edwards, I. (1991) Who Decides? *Paediatric Nursing*, 3(10), 6–8.

Charles Edwards, I. & Casey, A. (1992) Parental Involvement and Voluntary Consent. *Paediatric Nursing*, 4(1), 16–18.

Chessells, J.M. (1985) The management of childhood leukaemia. *The Practitioner*, Sept, 229, 803–7.

Choiseul, M., Allen, A. & May, A. (1988) Training and needs of health visitors in the haemoglobinopathies. *Health Visitor*, 61, 205–6.

Claxton, R. & Harrison, T. (ed.) (1991) *Caring for Children with HIV and AIDS.* Edward Arnold, London.

Cluroe, S. (1989) Blood transfusions. *Nursing*, 3(40), 8–11.

Cluroe, S. (1990) Children who won't eat. *Nursing*, 4(5), 11–17.

Cole, S. (1991) Developing Trust. *Paediatric Nursing*, 3(5), 22–3.

Communicable Diseases Report (1994) Public Health Laboratory Service Board, London.

Contanch, S. (1985) Self hypnosis as antiemetic therapy in children receiving chemotherapy. *Oncology Nurses Forum*, 12(4), 41–6.

Crawford, M. (1991) Sickle cell disease in children. *Nursing*, 4(31), 23–5.

Crosby, C. (1989) Methods in Mouth Care. *Nursing Times* Aug 30, 85(35), 38–41.

Dawson-France, M. (1994) Painful crisis in sickle cell conditions. *Nursing Standard*, 8(45), 25–8.

Devine, T. (1990) Pain Management in paediatric oncology. *Paediatric Nursing*, 2(7), 10–12.

Dimond, B. (1990) Parental Acts and Omissions. *Paediatric Nursing*, 2(1), 23–4.

DoH (1991) *Dietary Reference Values for Food Energy and Nutrients for the United Kingdom.* HMSO, London.

Douglas, J. (1987) Coping with sleeping problems in children. *Health Visitor*, 60(2), 52–3.

Draper, G. & Stiller (1989) Cautious optimism. *Paediatric Nursing*, 1(3), 22–4.

Duggan, C. (1993) A family affair: multi disciplinary care for children and families with HIV and AIDS. *Child Health*, 1(1), 33–8.

Eden, O.B. & Lilleyman, J.S. (1992) Guidelines for management of idiopathic thrombocytopenic purpura. *Archives of Disease in Childhood*, 67, 1056–8.

Emery, A.E.H. & Pullen, I. (eds) (1984) *Psychological Aspects of Genetic Counselling.* Academic Press, London.

Evans, M. (1993) Teenagers and cancer. *Paediatric Nursing*, 5(1), 14–15.

Ferguson, M. (1991) Sickle cell anaemia and its effect on the new parent. *Health Visitor*, 64(3), 73–6.

Forsyth, L. (1992) Children with cancer: supporting the family. *Nursing Standard*, 6(15/16), 26–7.

Franklin, I. (1990) *Sickle Cell Disease: A Guide for Patients, Carers and Health Workers.* Faber and Faber, London.

Frets, P.G. (1990) Factors influencing the reproductive decision after genetic counselling. *American Journal of Medical Genetics*, 35, 496–562.

Garland, E. (1991) Paediatric Bone Marrow Transplants. *Nursing Standard*, 5(46), 30–32.

Gibb, D. & Walters, S. (1993) *Guidelines for management of children with HIV infection.* AVERT, Horsham, West Sussex.

Gibson, F. (1989a) Hazards of aggressive therapy. *Paediatric Nursing*, 1(8), 8–9.

Gibson, F. (1989b) Parental involvement in bone marrow transplant. *Paediatric Nursing*, 1(7), 21–2.

Gillies, H. (1985) Is repeated flushing of Hickman catheters necessary? *British Medical Journal*, 290, 1708.

Heiney, S.P. (1991) Helping children through painful procedures. *American Journal of Nursing*, 91(11), 20–24.

Heron, D. (1992) Talking about a revolution: growth factors and peripheral stem cell transplants are set to revolutionise leukaemia and bone marrow treatments. *Nursing Standard*, 3(7), 6.

Hewitt, J. (1990) A sibling's response to hospitalization. *Paediatric Nursing*, 2(9), 12–16.

Hoffbrand, A.V. & Pettit, J.E. (1993) *Essential Haematology*, 3rd edn. Blackwell Science, Oxford.

Holmes, S. (1991) The value of vitamins and minerals. *Nursing*, 3(40), 8–11.

Howe, J. (1989) AIDS: The right approach. *Professional Nurse*, 5(3), 156–9.

Hully, M. & Hyne, J. (1993) Using parent held records in an oncology unit. *Paediatric Nursing*, 5(8), 14–16.

Jennings, P. (1990) Levels of knowledge. *Paediatric Nursing*, 2(7), 22–3.

Johnson, A.G. (1993) *Sickle Cell, Thalassaemia and other Haemoglobinopathies*. Report of a working party of the standing medical advisory committee on sickle cell disease, thalassaemia and other haemoglobinopathies. HMSO, London.

Jolly, J. (1981) *The Other Side of Paediatrics*. Macmillan, London.

Jones, P. (1990) *Living with Haemophilia*, 3rd edn. Castle House Publications, Tunbridge Wells.

Joyce, A. (1989) Bone marrow transplant. *Paediatric Nursing*, 1(6), 21–3.

Kaufert, J.K. (1980) Social and psychological responses to home treatment of haemophilia. *Journal of Epidemiology and Community Health*, 34, 194–200.

Leese, D. (1989) My Friend Wiggly. *Paediatric Nursing*, 1(3), 12–13.

Markova, I. & Forbes, G. (1979) Haemophilia: a study into social and psychological problems. *Health Bulletin*, 37(1), 24–9.

Mayers, A. & Spiegal, L. (1992) A parental support group in a paediatric AIDS clinic: its usefulness and limitations. *Health and Social Work*, 17(3), 183–91.

McFarlane, K. (1993) Idiopathic thrombocytopenic purpura in children. *Paediatric Nursing*, 5(5), 16–18.

Meyers, A. & Weitzman, M. (1991) Paediatric HIV disease: the newest chronic illness of childhood. *Pediatric Clinics of North America*, 38(1), 169–94.

Midence, K., Davies, S. & Fuggle, P. (1992) Courage in the face of crisis ... sickle cell disease. *Nursing Times*, 88(22), 46–8.

Midence, K., Graham, V., Acheampong, C. & Okuyiga, E. (1994) Increasing awareness for higher quality care: measuring knowledge of sickle cell disease in adult patients. *Professional Nurse*, 9(4), 255–6.

Miller, J.A. (1989) Transfusion of blood and blood products. *Professional Nurse*, 4(11), 560–65.

Mills, A., Magill & Allen, S. (1993) Children's dietary habits in hospital. *Paediatric Nursing*, 5(8), 17–19.

Pallister, C.J. (1992a) Thalassaemia: a preventable disease. *Professional Nurse*, 7(10), 66–7.

Pallister, C.J. (1992b) A crisis that can be overcome: management of sickle cell disease. *Professional Nurse*, 7(8), 509–13.

Peate, I. (1989) Do we discriminate against AIDS patients? *Professional Nurse*, 4(4), 177–81.

Pike, S. (1989) Family participation in the care of central venous lines. *Nursing*, 3(38), 22–5.

Pizzo, P.A. & Wilfert, C.M. (ed) (1991) *Pediatric AIDS: The Challenge of HIV Infection in Infants, Children and Adolescents*. Williams and Wilkins, Baltimore.

Prashar, U. (1985) The disease that discriminates. *Nursing Times*, 4 September, 16–17.

Pratt, R. (1991) *AIDS: a Strategy for Nursing Care*, 3rd edn. Edward Arnold, London.

Price, B. (1993) Disease and altered body image in children. *Paediatric Nursing*, 5(6), 18–22.

Rejman, A.S. (1993) *Provision of Haemophilia Treatment and Care*. Health Service Guidelines. Health Publications Unit, Heywood, Lancs.

Ridgeway, G. (1989) Immunising the Sick Child. *Paediatric Nursing*, 1(2), 22–3.

Rodin, J. (1983) *Will it Hurt*. Royal College of Nursing, London.

Ross, J.W. (1980) Childhood cancer: the parents, the patients, the professionals. *Issues in Comprehensive Paediatric Nursing*, 4(1), 7–16.

Sawley, L. (1991) Thalassaemia update. *Paediatric Nursing*, 3(8), 24–5.

Schechter, N.L., Berrien, F.B. & Katz, S.A. (1988) PCA for adolescents in sickle cell crisis. *American Journal of Nursing*, 88(5), 721–2.

Schroeder, I. (1993) Stressbusters. *Nursing Times*, 89(34), 36–7.

Seabrook, N. (1993) A missing element? *Nursing Times*, 89(49), 46–7.

Shuttleworth, A. (1988) Balancing public concern and patients' rights in HIV testing. *Professional Nurse*, 4(1), 29–32.

Skirton H. (1994) More than an information service: should genetic services offer clients counselling? *Professional Nurse*, 9(6), 400–404.

Stanford, J. (1988a) Safe steps in caring for patients with HIV/ AIDS. *Professional Nurse*, 4(2), 77–80.

Stanford, J. (1988b) AIDS/HIV How do you react? *Professional Nurse*, 3(98), 292–4.

Stanford, J. (1988c) Test your reactions to AIDS/HIV. *Professional Nurse*, 3(7), 256–8.

Stiller, C.A. (1988) Centralisation of treatment and survival rates for cancer. *Archives of Diseases of Childhood*, 63, 23–30.

Tanner, J.M. (1978) *Fetus into Man: Physical Growth from Conception to Maturity*. Open Books, Exeter.

Waterworth, S. (1989) Blood investigations. *Nursing*, 3(40), 24–5.

Whelan, J. (1991) Sickle cell disease. *Paediatric Nursing*, 3(4), 24–7.

WHO (1993) *Thirteen million HIV positive women by 2000.* World Health Organisation, Geneva.

Williss, J. (1993) Bone marrow transplantation. *Paediatric Nursing*, 5(7), 28–31.

Yogev, R. & Connor, E. (1992) *HIV infection in Infants and Children.* Mosby Year Book, London.

Chapter 19

Nursing Support and Care: Meeting the Needs of the Child and Family with Altered Cerebral Function

Lindy May and Bernadette Carter

INTRODUCTION

As with many aspects in nursing and medicine today, improved knowledge, facilities and equipment have resulted in longer survival of the child with altered cerebral function than would otherwise have occurred. Antibiotics and appropriate treatment of acute raised intercranial pressure have resulted in the survival of many children with meningitis. Improved ventilation techniques and increased knowledge have resulted in the survival of more children following head injury. Technological and surgical advances have aided in the treatment of the neonate born with congenital abnormalities. Operative techniques and chemotherapy and radiotherapy have led to a longer survival of children with central nervous system neoplasm. Enhancing the recovery of these children is a central goal in all care and intervention although, as Rose & Johnson (1992) state: 'a lack of consensus about how recovery and recovery related processes should be defined persists, and continues to form a fundamental hurdle to advancement.'

Many of the children who survive neurological crisis are left with long-lasting neurological deficits that affect the whole family as well as the child. In the community children with neurological deficits and/or seizures may be stigmatized. Unfortunately this attitude also exists in schools and this compounds difficulties for the child and their family. However, moves have been made in which the government has acknowledged the rights of the disabled child in relation to the care with which they should be provided (DES 1978) (see Table 19.1). In addition the Report also recommends that a named person be made responsible for the holistic care of the child.

There are widely accepted definitions, in relation to describing the brain injured patient, which have

Table 19.1 Main points of the Warnock Report relating to the child who is disabled.

- Anticipating disability and preparing the family for this.
- The prevention of further handicaps.
- The rehabilitation of the child, support of the family, and the prevention of further deterioration.

immediate relevance to clinical objectives. Disability is defined as any restriction or lack (resulting from an impairment) of ability to perform an activity in the manner or within the range considered normal for a human being. Handicap is defined as a disadvantage resulting from an impairment or disability, which limits the fulfilment of a role normal to that individual outcome – the cumulative impact of the condition. Rehabilitation is seen to be the fullest physical, social and mental restoration capacity.

The goal therefore of any nursing intervention in relation to the care of a child with neurological deficits is to ensure that their level of impairment, and their ability to compensate and to recover, are supported. Collaboration between different scientific disciplines and clinicians (neurologists, neurosurgeons, psychologists, psychiatrists, nurses, occupational therapists, physiotherapists and speech therapists) and through them, the patient and relatives, is essential, not only for the individual patients but for research which in the long term will be beneficial. Only when a multi-disciplinary approach is utilized and started early in the injury process, can an improved recovery be realistically achieved. Evaluation is not only a tool with which the clinician can measure the success/failure of treatment, it is also a helpful measurement by which the child and family may gain some optimism if improvement has occurred. Evaluation is also a necessary tool in research, the relevance of which is illustrated as follows:

'Research on recovery is now a multinational, multi-disciplinary and multimillion dollar activity, the progress of which can be charted through numerous conferences, in several major books and more recently in the emergence of journals devoted to this area...' (Rose & Johnson 1992)

The needs of the child with a neurological deficit or challenge are vast and diverse and they require the nurse to have an in-depth knowledge of what is or could be occurring physically as well as a high level of perception as to the psychological and emotional impact on the child and family. This chapter aims to explore both of these issues.

Section one will discuss the specific issues related to anatomy and physiology that impact on the child's developing nervous system and which affect their response to neurological challenge. A knowledge of the underlying principles of anatomy and physiology is assumed. Section two considers a range of neurological investigations and examines them in relation to the preparation of the child and the family and their actual experience of them. Section three explores the nurse's vital role in respect of neurological assessment and examines the rationale behind aspects of assessment. The final section examines a range of neurological deficits and diagnoses which the nurse caring for a child may meet in practice. These have been chosen as being fairly typical of the diversity of both symptoms and needs.

THE HEALTHY BRAIN

Development

The transient period of brain growth in the human fetus is known as the brain growth spurt. Various cellular systems in the brain develop in a definite order and in relation to the growth spurt of the whole brain. Adequate intake of nutrients is essential as the capacity for

their storage is very limited, and thus a continuous supply of nutrients is vital for efficient brain growth, development, and maturation to occur. Two main areas of brain development occur, the first concerning the order in which general areas of the brain develop, and the second, the order in which body localizations advance within these areas.

From early fetal life onwards, the human brain in terms of its gross weight, is nearer to the adult value than any other organ in the body, except the eye. By fifteen weeks gestation, the fetal brain has the adult quotient of neurones; subsequent growth involves the glial cells, and at birth, the human brain has reached its total velocity – about 25% of its adult weight. Two years after birth, the rapidly growing brain weighs about 75% of its adult weight (it reaches 95% by 10 years of age). Different parts of the brain grow at different rates, and reach their maximum velocities at different times.

Absence of required nutrients (Fig. 19.1) results in intellectual impairment, although clearly the only studies available are those based on early infant malnutrition (Richardson 1976). Interestingly, during the first thirty days of life, the baby's brain can withstand a

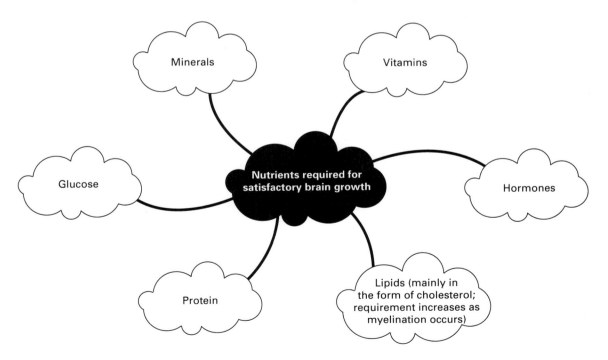

Fig. 19.1 Nutrients required for satisfactory brain growth.

degree of hypoxia and hypoglycaemia, reflecting glycolysis and the ability to function anaerobically. The effects of a young child's social environment also affect this; severe malnutrition in infancy in a positive social environment appears favourable for intellectual functioning. The importance of adequate nutrition and stimulation is this illustrated to be important in the developing brain's ability to reach its true potential.

Processing

The brain receives information from the sense organs and all parts of the body, via the nerves and spinal cord. It analyses this and is ultimately responsible for any purposeful reactions to the information received. The efficiency of this system increases with maturity and is closely associated with the physiology of learning. After maturity is reached, learning ability deteriorates, but continues to a lesser extent in the healthy brain. The most frequently used neuronal pathways become strengthened and preserved and may eventually become well established (Russell & Denver 1975). This process may explain why adaptation and rehabilitation is greater in the young child than in the adult following trauma, illness or congenital abnormalities involving the central nervous system. A young child's recovery from a head injury is greater than that of an adult. A toddler undergoing hemispherectomy for intractable epilepsy for example, is more likely to retain speech than the adult, and has a greater potential to recover partially/ fully from the effects of the resulting hemiperesis.

A basic understanding of how information is processed in the brain is illustrated by examining vision; thus a neurological examination assessing vision will uncover any deficits and hence the probable underlying cause for them, and the areas of damage. Destruction of a tiny area of visual cortex in, for example, the right cerebral hemisphere causes a permanent blind spot to the left of the point of eye fixation in the visual fields of both the left and right eye. Knowledge concerning the speech areas of the brain enhances our understanding in caring for the patient with speech deficits. Expressive or motor aphasia, described as halting, telegraphic speech, is caused by damage to the area known as Brocca; comprehension is intact, but does not include comprehension of 'connecting' vocabulary such as 'but'. Receptive or sensory aphasia is due to damage to

Wernicke's area, and comprises fluent but deviant speech and the inability to word find, with comprehension difficulty.

Language is further controlled by hemisphere dominance. Ninety five percent of those with left sided dominance (and hence right handedness) have language control in the left hemisphere. Of those with right sided dominance, 76% have bilateral hemispheric control of language. The child under three years old has the ability to change dominant hemispheres; for example, the young child with hemimegaencephaly involving a poorly functioning left hemisphere and demonstrating intractable epilepsy, will retain language following a left hemispherectomy. The assumption here is that compensation for the unhealthy hemisphere has already taken place and the child has switched to utilizing the right hemisphere. McManus & Bryden (1991) describe further aspects and issues related to brain lateralization.

Memory comprises registration, storage and retrieval; one theory is that of a module processing information from the senses. Another suggests that recall activates specific areas connected to sensory perceptions, such as smell and vision. Short term memory can process up to seven pieces of information for 10–15 seconds; it is the 'working' memory, bringing thoughts to consciousness. Long term memory is said to be declarative (information about specific facts and events) or procedural (involving motor skills). An understanding of memory and the anatomy involved, will greatly enhance the nurse's care of a child with amnesia. Prosopagnosia (difficulty in recognizing facts) points to occipital lobe damage; the question remains as to whether the problem is one of naming or recognition, and whether the impairment is sensory or intellectual (Squire & Zole-Morgan 1988).

NEUROLOGICAL ASSESSMENT

In the acute stage of an illness resulting in cerebral deficit, the relevant nursing care must be assessed and implemented; this includes airway management, coma scale assessment, safety, nutrition, elimination and rehabilitation (Fig. 19.2).

Any initial assessment should also involve commencement of discharge planning in relation to the above points. With neuroscience patients the services of various health professionals are often necessary because

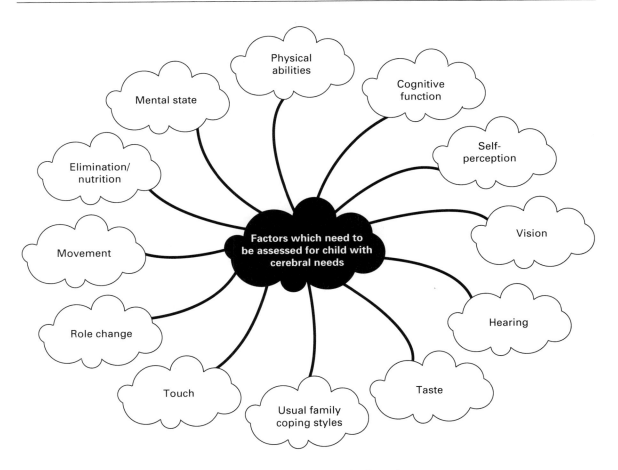

Fig. 19.2 Factors which need to be assessed for child with cerebral needs.

of the complex needs of the patient. This may include nurses, doctors, physiotherapists, speech therapists, social workers, psychologists, school teachers and support agencies. Once formal discharge planning commences, it is usually the nurse who co-ordinates activities and communications.

The nurse is also responsible for planning the management of any unresolved problems, in the next level of care. The knowledge and experience of the skilled children's nurse will help in anticipating the child's needs and projecting implications. Monitoring potential patient and family needs is part of the nurse's assessment, the aim being to meet those needs by exploration of appropriate resources and development of a family teaching plan. Evaluation of the process and outcomes is important.

Awareness of the normal reflexes is an important indication of nervous system maturation or deterioration, and is an easy tool for the nurse to use. The moro reflex is present in all normal full term infants. It is an indicator of the symmetry and intactness of the nervous system and diminishes by about the fifth month. When the position of the head is changed abruptly in relation to the body, sudden abductions of the arms occur together with extensions of the legs and flexions of the hips. Various developmental screening tests exist for children, for example the Denver Developmental Screening Test (Frankenburg & Dodds 1969; Frankenburg *et al.* 1987) which outlines motor performance, language development and so on. Many other tests and assessments exist in relation to assessing neurological damage (Fig. 19.3).

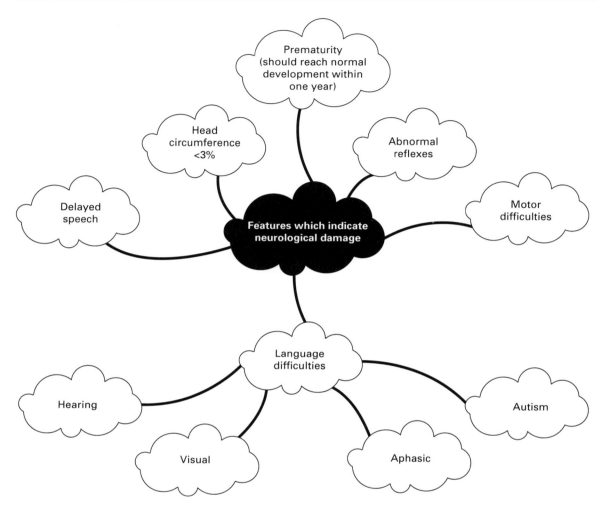

Fig. 19.3   Features which can be used as part of neurological assessment.

Many processes only affect specific areas of the nervous system, and consequently localization of any dysfunction becomes the foundation for diagnosis and treatment. Assessment is supported by technology and a range of investigations including intracranial pressure (ICP) monitoring, MRI scans and CT scans as well as the more routine investigations such as X-ray and blood testing.

Intracranial pressure (ICP) monitoring

ICP monitoring is performed by inserting a probe into the ventricle, subarachnoid space or the epidural/subdural space. The most commonly used probe today is

the fibre optic transducer tipped catheter. Light fibres within the catheter convey light impulses created by movement of a mirrored diaphragm, which reflects pressure changes. The light signal is then converted into electrical signals and displayed on a digital monitor which also displays wave forms. The wave forms are characteristic and the nurse can assess not only the level of ICP but also other factors from the wave form. The child's ICP monitoring must form part of the nurse's role as this may give the earliest sign of any deterioration or improvement.

Only a few of the classic signs of raised ICP occur early and the appearance of plateau waves is a danger sign. These are sudden, transient waves that last five to 20 minutes and begin from a baseline of already raised ICP. As these occur, subtle changes in the patient's level of consciousness also occur, including increased restlessness, disorganized motor behaviour, complaints of headache and disorientation. Changes in vital signs and pupillary and motor signs occur more frequently at sustained peaks of pressure, not as the pressure rises. Any of the above symptoms must be reported promptly, so that early intervention measures can be instigated.

Electroencephalogram (EEG)

An EEG (electroencephalogram) provides a recording of the electrical activity of the brain; neuronal electrical signals from the cerebral cortex are picked up via scalp electrodes and amplified one million times to be displayed on graph paper. In addition to displaying normal patterns, an EEG will demonstrate epileptic activity, abnormalities of amplitude and the slowing of normal rhythms.

Computed tomography (CT)

Computed tomography (CT) produces cross sectional radiographs. An X-ray beam passes through the patient and the intensity of the emerging beam is measured by an electronic detector. The X-ray tube and detector are mounted at opposite ends of a frame, the whole of which can be rotated around the child to make measurements from many different angles. The radiation measurements received are fed into a computer. This records how much of the beam was absorbed, that is the X-ray density in each region of the body. A CT image presents a cross section of the body, the various densities displayed in grey and white.

A contrast agent is usually given intravenously and allows better visualizations of structures and disease processes. A contrast agent absorbs more X-rays, is more easily seen, and is readily taken up by tumour cells. The majority of large hospitals now have a CT scanner, and some specialist units are able to 'fax' CT scans from one unit to another, for advice or prior to referral. A CT scan can be performed out of hours and hence support an efficient emergency service.

Magnetic resonance imaging (MRI) scan

A magnetic resonance imaging (MRI) scan offers a far more complex picture, but is vastly more expensive and not so widely available as the CT scanner. The child is positioned in the machine (basically a magnet). This is a large cylinder that is noisy and claustrophobic for many children, and sedation is usually required for the young child. A radio wave is sent into the magnet, and when it is turned off the body emits a signal which is received and used for reconstruction of the picture. MRI scanning looks at the distribution of hydrogen atoms scattered throughout all living tissues, particularly water and fatty compounds. An atom of hydrogen has one proton for its nucleus and behaves as if it were spinning; since it has an electric charge, this gives it a magnetic axis. When the correct pulse of radio frequency radiation is sent in, relaxation times called T_1 and T_2 can be measured, allowing tissue characterization. MRI images can be obtained on any plane.

MRI is also safe, as ionizing radiation is not used and there are no known biological hazards. Metallic equipment, however, can be affected by the strong magnetic field of the main scanner, hence children with pacemakers and intracranial aneurysm clips, for example, should not be scanned by MRI. The MRI scanner gives very precise pictures of the central nervous system, and can be used to identify abnormalities very early, even before structural changes have occurred.

Paediatric coma scales

The Glasgow Coma Scale (GCS) is widely used to assess a patient's level of consciousness and was devised by Teasdale & Jennet (1974). The scale is divided into three categories: eye opening, best verbal response and best motor response, and each of these categories has further definitions. The resulting graph provides a visual record of deterioration, improvement or stabilization of the child's neurological status/observations. Numerical values are totalled for each category, the higher the score the more conscious and alert the patient, and the lower the score the more deeply comatosed the patient. Vital signs of blood pressure, pulse, respirations and temperature are also performed by the nurse and are used in correlation with the GCS in identifying nursing diagnoses and planning nursing and medical interventions. The nurse's ability to identify change, interpret its significance and act accordingly is vital to the outcome of care.

The GCS is difficult to apply to children, since many of the responses required involve adult neurodevelop-

THE HOSPITALS FOR SICK CHILDREN COMA CHART

Name :   Referring Hospital :   Weight :

D.O.B :   Unit No :   Consultant :

Date :   Ward :

DATE :

TIME :

Eyes Open		Spontaneously	4			C = Eyes closed by swelling
		To speech	3			
		To pain	2			
		None	1			

Best verbal response	Smiles	Orientated	5			T = endotracheal tube or tracheostomy
	Cries	Disorientated	4			
	Inappropriate cries	Monosyllabic response	3			
	Occasional whimper	Incomprehensible sounds	2			D = Dysphasia
	None	None	1			

Best motor response (record best arm)		Obeys/Spontaneous	6			
		Localize pain	5			
		Normal flexion	4			P = Paralysed
		Abnormal flexion	3			
		Extension	2			
		None	1			

COMA SCALE TOTAL

Pupil Diameter Guide

1 mm ·   240   40.0
          230   39.5
2 mm ●   220   39.0
          210   38.5
3 mm ●   200   38.0
          190   37.5
4 mm ●   180   37.0
          170   36.5
          160   36.0
5 mm ●   150   35.5
          140   35.0
          130   34.5
6 mm ●   120   34.0
          110   33.5
          100   33.0
7 mm ●   90   32.5
          80   32.0
8 mm ●   70
          60
          50
          40
          35
          30
          25
Respiration ●   20
          15
ICP X   10
          5

Blood Pressure and Pulse   **Temperature °C**

PUPILS	Right	Size (mm)			+ = reacts
		Reaction			− = no reaction
	Left	Size (mm)			SL = sluggish
		Reaction			

LIMB MOVEMENT	ARMS	Normal Power			Record right (R) and left (L) seperately if there is a difference between the two sides
		Mild weakness			
		Severe weakness			
		Flexion			
		Extension			
		No response			
	LEGS	Normal Power			
		Mild weakness			
		Severe weakness			P = Paralysed
		Flexion			# = Fracture
		Extension			
		No response			

THE HOSPITALS FOR SICK CHILDREN, LONDON
COMA SCALE

The coma scale is scored on a total of 15 points. A total of less than 12 should give rise for concern. This is a universally accepted tool for measuring coma. A decrease in coma scale will be associated with a decreased level of consciousness. This needs to be considered along with the patient's vital signs.

A **Eyes Open**

If eyes closed by swelling, please write 'C' in relevant column, in red biro, thus indicating reason for lower score.

B. **Best verbal response**

In the left hand margin are two separate scales: the far left is the scale for babies and infants, and on the right is the scale for older children.

The following section gives an explanation of the best verbal response of infants.

a) **Smiles**

This can be used to describe an alert contented infant, as not all will smile at a stranger. The interaction between parents and infant should therefore be taken into account.

b) **Appropriate Cries**

The infant may be unable to settle.

c) **Inappropriate Cries**

The infant may have periods of being drowsy, but at times is heard to cry out. This is not always associated with being disturbed. The cry maybe high pitched.

d) **Occasional Whimper**

Less frequent than above and may be associated when deep painful stimuli is required to gain motor response.

e) **None**

No verbal response.

C. **Best Motor Response to Stimuli**

The age and cognitive abilities of the child must be taken into account.

D. **Pupils**

When recording pupils size it is important to remember the effects of drugs; eg morphine will cause pinpoint pupils, and atropine drops will dilate pupils for up to 6 hours.

E. **Limb Movememts**

a) If a child has a permanent hemiparesis, please indicate such in the relevant column - eg weakness, even though it is normal for this child.

b) A child with a severe developmental delay, may score lower on the coma scale, as his motor response may be poor.

Fig. 19.4   Great Ormond Street Hospital for Children NHS Trust Coma Chart 1993.

mental function and are consequently difficult to grade in the child under ten years old. The verbal response, for example, is impossible on the existing GCS if the baby has no vocalization at all, and the motor component of the GCS is applicable only after the first few months of life. The child may not comply with the command; and the difference between an agitated toddler missing his mother and one who is agitated due to an increase in intercranial pressure challenges the skills of the children's nurse.

Throughout the assessment an awareness of the child's developmental and not chronological age must be taken into consideration. In addition, further difficulties arise in neurologically assessing a young child as regression may occur due to hospitalization, separation from their parents and home environment and the impact of the illness itself. It should be borne in mind that regardless of what may appear to be a superficial challenge to neurological integrity, the nurse must regularly assess neurological status. The GCS is a central means of achieving this type of assessment. Children's neurological status can change very rapidly and may only be picked up if frequent and comprehensive assessment can be made. Simpson & Reilly (1982), Morray *et al.* (1984), Raimondi & Hirschener (1984) and Neatherlin & Brillhart (1988) all provide a commentary on paediatric coma scales. Due to the difficulties encountered with the original GCS, revisions have been deemed necessary in order to develop an effective and useful tool (Fig. 19.4).

NURSING CARE OF THE CHILD WITH RAISED INTRACRANIAL PRESSURE

The Monro-Kellie doctrine states that the craniospinal intradural space is nearly constant in volume and its contents are almost incompressible. The volume of the adult brain is approximately 1400 ml, cerebrospinal fluid (CSF) volume is approximately 150 ml and blood volume 150 ml (Adams & Victor 1989). The rigid skull is filled with essentially non-compressible contents – 80% brain matter, 10% intravascular blood and 10% CSF – therefore if the volume of one of these three components rises, another component must decrease and with this an increase in ICP must occur. Infants or

very young children whose skull sutures have not yet fused allow, at least initially, for an increase in contents without a reciprocal rise in intracranial pressure.

An understanding of cerebral blood flow (CBF), cerebral blood volume (CBV), cerebral perfusion pressure (CPP) and ICP is fundamental to the nurse since these parameters are closely monitored, assessed and reported when caring for the child with raised intracranial pressure. CBF is normally maintained at a rate that matches the metabolic needs of the brain. During times of increased cerebral metabolism, vasodilatation occurs with a subsequent increase in CBF and CBV to the area. Metabolic factors affecting the CBF include CO_2 concentration, hydrogen ion concentration, and O_2 concentration (Guyton 1986). CBV is affected by the autoregulatory mechanisms that control CBF. A limited compensatory mechanism is operational when ICP begins to rise. However, as the rate of CBF does decline, ischaemeia and cerebral infarction occurs.

CPP is defined as the blood pressure gradient across the brain. It is calculated as the difference between the mean arterial pressure (MAP) entering the brain and the opposing ICP on the arteries. CPP is an estimate of the adequacy of cerebral circulation. CPP, CBF, CBV, and ICP are all closely interrelated (Fig. 19.5) and it is crucial that the nurse understands how they relate and respond to each other. CPP is represented by the formula:

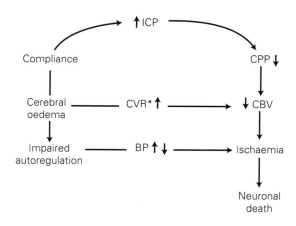

Fig. 19.5   Relationship between ICP, CPP, CBF and CBV.

* compliance represents the ratio of change in volume to the resulting change in pressure; thus compliance is the ratio of change in ICP – a result of change in intracranial volume.

CPP = MAP – ICP.

CBF can be represented as:

CBF = $\frac{CPP}{CVR}$ (CVR is cerebrovascular resistance).

ICP will become raised due to mass effect, cytotoxic oedema, vasogenic oedema, and hydrocephalus.

Nursing assessment

Nursing assessment focuses on both the physical and emotional/psychological needs of the child, and crucially on the nurse's understanding of the signs and symptoms of raised intracranial pressure. The signs and symptoms depend on the degree of brain compliance, the specific location of any mass and the compartmental location of any lesion. They are best considered in terms of early and later findings (Table 19.2).

eventually stop. Alterations in respiratory pattern relate to the level of brain dysfunction. An acute rise in ICP can cause acute neurogenic pulmonary oedema. Pyrexia is usually due to hypothalamic dysfunction.

Cerebral ischaemia and infarction occur as intracranial pressure increases. Herniation will occur if the situation continues untreated, and is defined as the abnormal protrusion of a body structure from one compartment to another. Brain herniations consist of supratentorial herniation and intratentorial herniation. Herniation syndromes are life threatening and early recognition of signs and symptoms is essential, although deterioration is often rapid and frequently irreversible.

Nursing intervention: meeting the child's needs

Meeting the child's needs is vital in respect of the care of the child with raised intracranial pressure, and they

Table 19.2 Findings associated with raised intracranial presssure.

Early findings	Later findings
■ pupillary dysfunction ■ deterioration in level of consciousness ■ cranial nerve palsy ■ headache ■ vomiting ■ seizures ■ motor deficits	■ further deterioration in level of consciousness ■ impaired brain stem responses (cornea, gag) ■ respiratory irregularities ■ alterations in vital signs ■ hemiplegia, decortication or decerebration

The nurse must regularly assess the child's vital signs as these provide another source of information about the child's progress or deterioration. Blood pressure and pulse remain relatively stable in the early stages of rising ICP, although once pressure on the brain stem occurs the blood pressure rises. In order for cerebral blood flow to be maintained the pressure on the cerebral arterial vessels must be in excess of the ICP. An elevation of blood pressure increases cardiac output which thus increases systemic blood pressure with a widening pulse during the compensatory phase of increasing ICP. The decreased pulse rate is the result of an attempt by the heart to pump blood upwards into vessels on which pressure is being exerted from the intracranial bulk. If the situation continues and the ICP rises, the heart will

require the nurse to display a wide range of skills. The nurse must ensure that the child's physical and psychological needs are met. Both aspects of care are vital, although emphasis may be placed on ensuring that the child's intracranial pressure is reduced to within normal limits (Fig. 19.6). ICP needs monitoring regularly and maintaining the integrity of the equipment is part of the nurse's role; this includes ensuring that the site of entry of the monitoring line is kept clean and that all due care is given.

Often the child is fluid restricted, thus limited in their oral and intravenous fluid intake. Fluid restrictions aid in decreasing extra cellular fluid from the body, so it is also important to monitor the child's urinary output. In addition, the nurse should be aware that either diabetes

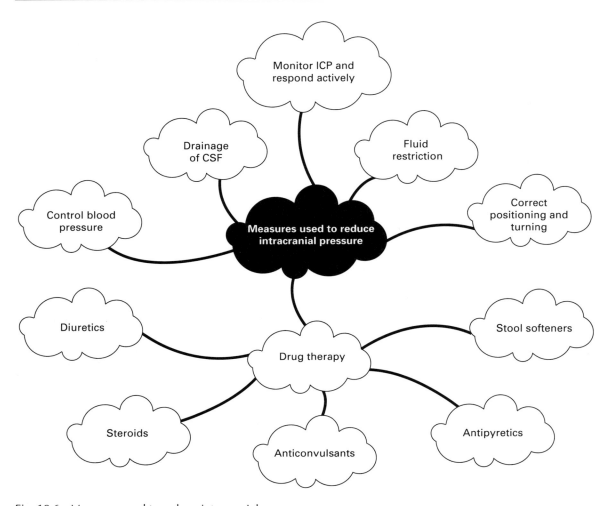

Fig. 19.6 Measures used to reduce intracranial pressure.

insipidus or insufficient ADH (antidiuretic hormone) secretion may develop in response to trauma. Skin care and regular turning is necessary to avoid skin break-down, and changing the child's position may also prevent chest infections. The head of the bed should be elevated to 30°–45°, avoiding a prone position as this facilitates venous return from the brain (Hickey 1992).

A range of drugs may be used in the management of raised intracranial pressure and their use is dependent on the nature/cause of the rise. Osmotic diuretics will reduce cerebral oedema and thus ICP. Steroids are also given to reduce cerebral oedema. Anticonvulsants are prescribed to reduce seizure activity and antipyretics to control pyrexia. Stool softeners prevent straining at stool as this is

known to result in a rise in ICP. The nurse needs to be aware of drug administration protocols, side effects, contra-indications and interactions (UKCC 1992).

Rapid reporting of a change in blood pressure by the nurse may aid in avoiding cerebral ischaemia. In order to maintain an adequate CPP the arterial blood pressure may need to be artificially maintained at a higher than usual level to compensate for an elevated ICP. Another means of attempting to reduce ICP is through external CSF drainage. A burr hole is made in the skull and under strict asepsis a catheter is inserted into a ventricle. CSF is drained into a closed drainage circuit with the amount drained being ordered by the physician. Drainage of CSF is dependent on gravity and if the drainage system is placed too high this may result in little drainage, and if placed too low will result in excessive drainage of CSF. Neither is acceptable and the nurse must ensure that the drainage rate is appropriate and that the child is tolerating it.

In ICP monitoring it remains the nurse's responsibility to maintain a sterile dressing around the probe entry site and to interpret the data for signs of increasing ICP. It is also important that the nurse ensures that the probe remains in situ. This can be problematic when caring for an agitated or active child where there is the potential for the probe to be unintentionally pulled out. The doctor needs to be informed as soon as the nurse is concerned about the readings and the child's condition.

NURSING CARE OF THE CHILD WITH HEAD INJURY

Improvement in the delivery of trauma care has increased survival from injury and thus it has become essential to assess the resulting morbidity and to plan for medical and psychosocial services to support the child and family. This is particularly so in children whose needs may be many, long term and involving the whole family. One of the major issues that must be considered is the impact that head injury may have on the whole family. Severe head injury places long term strains on the family and after care is vitally important. After severe head injury many children continue to experience major behavioural and cognitive problems in addition to emotional difficulties, even following good physical recovery. Scott-Jupp *et al.* (1992) illustrated that 42% of head injured children in their study had persistent neurological impairment and 35% had an identified need for special educational support at a median interval of 13 months following severe head injury. A need for improved support and training of staff who teach head injured children was identified.

Rivara *et al.* (1992) looked at family functioning one year following traumatic brain injury in children and found that over 50% of families interviewed exhibited high levels of stress and at-risk family relationships. This was greatest amongst the more severely injured group. However, pre-injury family global functioning was also strongly predictive of twelve month family functioning rather than purely the injury severity. Pre-injury coping

was found to be the best predictor of stress in this study, and hence the need for identification of the families most at risk and the need for ongoing support for optimal functioning, were recognized.

Clearly then, one of the aims of assessment in the early stages of these children is for the nurse to enquire into the family dynamics and functioning, to identify those families with an increased risk of reduced coping abilities.

Nursing assessment

Head injury occurs from either penetration or impact and the consequent damage will result from the direct injury itself, or from the resulting phenomena of cerebral oedema or ischaemia (Table 19.3). The end result is an increase in intercranial pressure, further complicating the child's management.

A systemic approach to assessment is vital and the initial assessment provides both baseline observations and a means of prioritizing essential care. The nurse should assess and ensure that the child has a patent airway and adequate respiratory effort. The nurse should also ensure that the child is positioned appropriately and carefully. It is vital to ensure that the child's airway is maintained, although due consideration of potential or actual cervical injury must be made. The nurse also needs to generate a comprehensive nursing history in respect to the injury itself, such as the timing, response to injury and other circumstances. A neurological assessment by the nurse and accurate documentation are essential. Specific details ensure accurate data comparisons later, particularly when performed by others.

The child's level of consciousness and pupillary and motor responses are a crucial part of the assessment and the nurse must be aware that signs of increasing raised intercranial pressure should be noted and immediately reported. Hypovolaemia and shock, which often occur following multiple trauma, must be noted, documented and reported promptly. The smaller the child the less their ability to cope with rapid blood loss. However, it must be acknowledged that a rapid infusion of blood or colloids can further complicate the problems of raised intercranial pressure.

Michaud *et al.* (1992) examined the predictors of survival and disability in children following severe head injury. Their findings suggest that the GCS score 72

Table 19.3   Types of head injury.

■ Skull fracture (open or closed)	Fracture of the base of the skull is less easily observed and often fatal. Due to the highly vascular nature of the child's scalp, the young child can suffer severe blood loss from a comparatively minor injury.
■ Laceration	
■ Contusion	
■ Epidural haematoma	This haemorrhage occurring in the space between the dura and the inner table of the skull is a neurosurgical emergency.
■ Subdural haematoma	
■ Intracerebral haematoma	
■ Concussion	Described as a transient state of unconsciousness following trauma.

hours following injury, especially the motor component, was a significantly better predictor of quality of survival than was the initial assessment either in the community or the emergency room. The severity of the brain injury and the presence and severity of extra-cranial injuries, especially chest injuries associated with oxygen desaturation, were associated with increased mortality and morbidity. Factors most significantly predictive of survival were severity of total injuries, and pupillary responses in the emergency room. Factors most predictive of disability were GCS motor responses 72 hours following injury and their level of oxygenation whilst in the emergency room.

The main initial assessment by the nurse must then be that of airway and oxygenation. Promoting and maintaining adequate oxygenation is a prime concern. Ongoing, responsive assessment of the child's neurological status, intracranial pressure measurements, fluid balance and seizure status (Fig. 19.7) are all of vital importance.

Nursing intervention: meeting the child's needs

The nurse's role in maintaining a clear airway and promoting adequate oxygenation is vital. Suction may be required to maintain the patency of the airway and artificial airway management may be indicated. The child's head must be positioned carefully to maintain appropriate cerebral blood flow. An adequate oxygen supply must be provided and supplemental oxygen may be required in the form of a head box or face mask oxygen or respiratory support with a ventilator. The child's oxygenation status must be checked carefully and oxygen saturation monitors are ideal, although arterial blood gases will be needed to supplement the readings.

The nurse must be able to perform neurological observations competently and effectively so that any changes can result in an appropriate response. Any deterioration should be immediately reported so that appropriate medical intervention can occur. All recordings should be carefully documented. Intracranial pressure is a vital part of monitoring the child and the nurse must be sure that if the ICP approaches or exceeds the mean systemic arterial pressure, the brain cannot be adequately perfused, the cells become hypoxic and this results in brain damage or death. Sudden rises in ICP can be prevented or the risk reduced by judicious nursing care strategies (Fig. 19.8).

The child's other injuries must also be considered and appropriate care decided upon and implemented. In the early stages of injury intravenous blood products may be essential and the observation of central venous pressures and intracranial pressure will help assess the child. Fluid restriction is an important component of the child's management. Early nutrition is essential due to the metabolic requirements of the injured brain, although

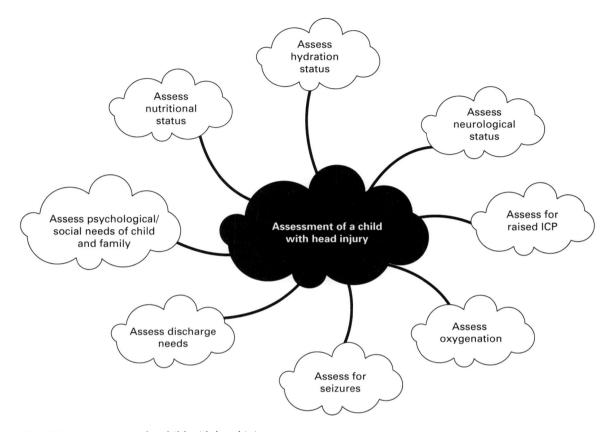

Fig. 19.7 Assessment of a child with head injury.

there are a number of perspectives on what is the most suitable nutrition (Anderson 1987).

For those children who develop epilepsy as a consequence of their head injury the impact on the family is enormous as this comes on top of the primary injury itself. It is vital that the parents and the child, where appropriate, are fully cognisant of the crucial role that drug therapy plays in treating the seizures.

Rehabilitation of the head injured child and discharge planning should commence almost on admission. Involvement of the family unit in assisting nursing care, assessing daily needs, stimulation, physiotherapy and forward planning are vital. Early identification of potential difficulties in coping by the family can be reduced by early intervention of the psychologist and social worker. Involvement of the multi-disciplinary team in the hospital and the community can be initiated by the nurse in the early stages of the child's treatment.

The expected outcomes for this group of children will be that they can maintain their own respiration and nutrition, with appropriate help in the young child, and that they become as responsive and oriented as their condition enables. It is also expected that their development and rehabilitation progresses and that goals set in conjunction and participation with their family are realistic and achievable. It is also important that the community is able to continue the child's programme of rehabilitation.

The head injured child, regardless of the degree of injury, presents a nursing challenge. Reassurance, support, constant reassessment, encouragement, and an excellent standard of nursing care which involves the family unit, are what each of these children has a right to receive and which they definitely deserve.

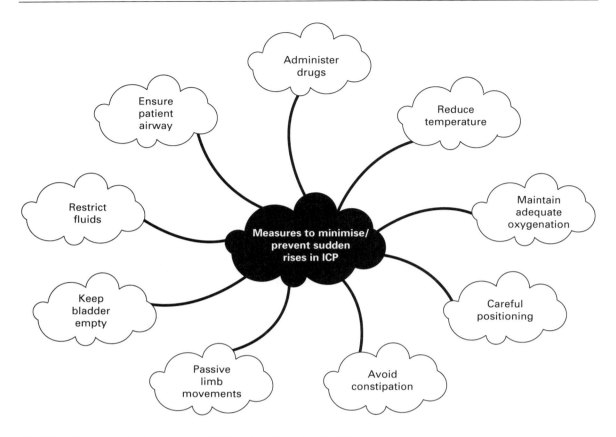

Fig. 19.8   Measures to decrease possibility of sudden rises in ICP.

NURSING CARE OF THE CHILD WITH EPILEPSY

Epilepsy is a chronic disorder characterized by recurrent outbursts of electrical activity from abnormal neurons in the brain, and resulting from a variety of causes (Table 19.4). The result is a disturbance in behaviour, consciousness, sensations and skeletal motor function. It is a symptom rather than a disease in itself. The clinical presentation varies according to the patient's age and brain maturation. Ninety per cent of all epileptic patients experience the onset of epilepsy before the age of 20 years, and the highest incidence of epilepsy occurs in children (Shorvon 1988). From age one to five the incidence is approximately 0.5 per 1000 per year (Gunnet 1984). If a child suffers a single seizure from pyrexia, trauma or hypoglycaemia, for example, they are

not epileptic since seizure recurrence is a requisite for such a diagnosis. Any individual can suffer seizures, but some individuals have an inborn genetic prevalence to seizure activity, the seizure threshold of the brain being lower than normal. Seizures can be classified into two main groups and then further subdivided (Fig. 19.9).

Nursing assessment

The nurse's prime aim when assessing a child's seizures is to ensure the child's safety in regards to oxygenation, and prevent further injury. Another important aspect of assessment relates to confirming the epileptic nature of the fit from a clinical viewpoint. Assessment of the type of epilepsy is also important, and accurate and detailed documentation of the events is important. The charts used for documentation should allow the characteristics

Table 19.4   Causes of epilepsy.

Idiopathic	No identifiable cause.
Post traumatic	Following birth trauma, infection or head injury. Seizures may occur from 2 months to 5 years following cerebral insult.
Biochemical	Biochemical disorders often include epilepsy.
Cerebral epilepsy	Due to a cerebral lesion.
Congenital abnormalities	Such as hemimegaencephalopathy and Sturge-Webber syndrome.

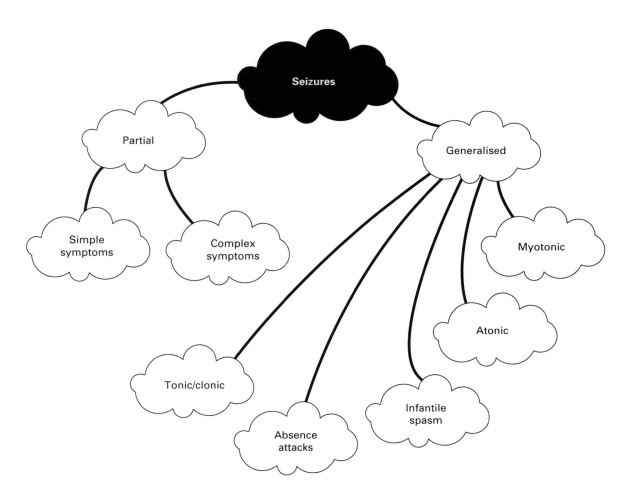

Fig. 19.9   Classification of seizures.

of the fit, its duration, type, the response of the child and interventions required, if any, to be noted. The nurse also needs to assess for any predisposing factors that were associated with the onset or triggering of the fit. Finally, assessment must focus on the child and family's coping ability both in hospital and in the community.

Additionally the nurse will be involved in supporting and preparing the child for diagnostic assessments, including intellectual assessment and behavioural assessment as well as computerized tomography (CT) scan, if indicated, and electroencephalogram (EEG).

Nursing intervention: meeting the child's needs

The child's airway remains a prime concern throughout their care and suction may be required to maintain its patency. The child's head should be positioned so that pharyngeal secretions are readily drained, although this may not be feasible. If appropriate the nurse should monitor the child's oxygen saturation and administer oxygen if it is needed and available. Cerebral blood flow is increased by 250% during a seizure and cerebral oxygen consumption is increased by approximately 60%. The nurse also needs to be involved with managing the child's drug therapy, and rectal diazepam may be used as part of the management strategy. Parents will often continue with this part of the treatment if it is still required when the child is at home.

The nurse must also ensure that the child does not incur any secondary injury as a result of the seizure and should stay with the child until the seizure has passed. Restrictive clothing can be removed or loosened and any potentially dangerous items should be moved from the child's immediate vicinity. However, the nurse should not attempt to restrain the child in any way. Part of the nurse's role in keeping the child safe lies in teaching the parents how to recognize the signs of an imminent seizure, such as auras. The parents may need to be advised to encourage the child to wear a safety helmet to maximize the child's protection from head injury.

All of the child's seizures should be documented so that an accurate picture of the nature, frequency, duration and response can be established. Some parents continue to document their child's seizures at home; this is often prevalent during the transition phase following

adjustment to the child's diagnosis. As the child and the parents become more expert in their understanding and management of the child's seizures, the nurse should increasingly rely on their reports of the child's condition. Once the seizure has stopped the child should be placed in the recovery position and should be gently reassured (Kempthorne 1994).

Another major aspect of care lies in encouraging the child and their family to cope with the devastation that epilepsy can initially impose on the family. The nurse should encourage the family to verbalize their concerns and the aim of care should be to facilitate the family in mobilizing effective coping mechanisms and clarifying any misconceptions that they hold. Often several interviews are required to ensure that adequate understanding has been achieved and that the family appreciate the foreseeable course of the disorder. Only once this has been achieved can the fears and prejudices associated with seizures be addressed. The nurse must also ensure that the parents understand the importance of, and therefore the need for, adherence to the regular and prolonged treatment and the possible complications/side effects of the drugs.

The impact on the family and child is enormous; much social prejudice still exists and remains difficult to overcome. A normal lifestyle needs to be encouraged whenever possible and personal restriction limited to a reasonable minimum; most sporting activity can be allowed, except in severe cases, including swimming with proper supervision. The slight increase in risk resulting from a liberal policy is compensated for by the avoidance of overprotection and isolation – but clearly individualization is essential. Children with intractable epilepsy may benefit from the multidisciplinary approach provided by special schools. Children with uncomplicated epilepsy generally attend normal schools. Learning difficulties are often related to attentional deficits. Difficulties with language and abstract thinking are more common in children with epilepsy (Voeller & Rothenberg 1973). Behaviour problems are also quite commonly seen.

Self administration of drugs under careful administration can be a starting point for self responsibility and an increase in self esteem by the patient. Sleep deprivation and alcohol use in the adolescent should be avoided, along with any other recognized precipitant factor. Prohibitions and the need for taking antiepileptic drugs need to be accepted and followed. The choice of a career needs to be considered in relation to the need for a driving licence, the handling of machinery and the young person's own individual needs or deficits.

NURSING CARE OF THE CHILD WITH A CEREBRAL INFECTION

The child with a cerebral infection provides a real challenge to the nurse in respect of care and management. The nurse is responsible for not only ensuring that the child's infection is monitored and cared for appropriately, but also in terms of containing the infection and minimizing the risk to other children. Although many infectious diseases/agents can impact on the nervous system, those most commonly seen include meningitis, encephalitis and the parameningeal infections of the brain (abscess, subdural empyema, and extradural abscess). All cerebral infections require urgent attention and responsive treatment in order to minimize the damage/morbidity and in some cases prevent death.

Nursing assessment

A number of core assessments must be made by the nurse caring for the child with a suspected or actual cerebral infection. These assessments are vital and must be ongoing in order to detect signs of deterioration or response to treatment. The prime focus of assessment must as always be related to airway and oxygenation and the child's neurological status. It is also important to establish and assess the route of the pathogen's entry (Fig. 19.10). It is advisable to isolate the child initially to prevent the spread of infection.

The child's level of consciousness must be observed, as should signs of raised intracranial pressure. Evidence of increasing meningeal irritation should be assessed for, such as by the presence of Brudzinski's sign and Kernig's sign (Table 19.5).

Nursing intervention: meeting the child's needs

Although the underlying pathology may differ and the response of the child will always be individual, some of

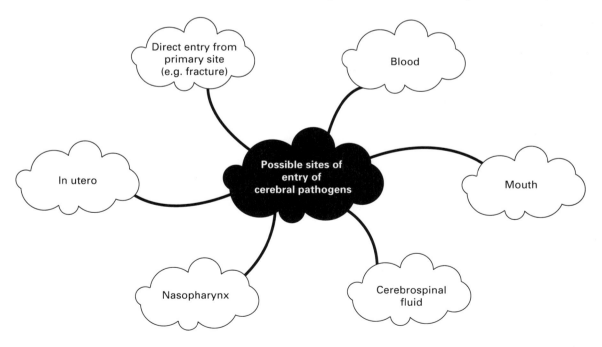

Fig. 19.10 Possible sites of entry of cerebral pathogens.

Table 19.5 Neurological signs.

Brudzinski's sign	The child is placed in a dorsal recumbent position. The nurse's hand is placed behind the head and the neck is flexed forward. Signs of pain or resistance indicate meningeal irritation, neck injury, or arthritis. If the hips and knees are flexed in response to the manoeuvre, meningeal inflammation is likely.
Kernig's sign	The child is placed in the supine position and the leg flexed and the hip and knee are then straightened. Signs of pain or resistance indicate meningeal inflammation.

the nursing care and support required is broadly similar. Fluid management, administration of antibiotic therapy, airway and oxygenation support, pyrexia management and sleep, rest and comfort are all vital. Prompt diagnosis and treatment are essential for children with a cerebral infection. Nursing care must be directed to the relevant areas and drug treatment prompt. Despite all medical and nursing skills, these patients may be left with long term cerebral deficits. Pomeroy *et al.* (1990) demonstrated that 14% of the 185 infants he followed after bacterial meningitis, had persistent cerebral deficits, including seizures. Feferbaum *et al.* (1993) found that 62% of babies in his study had gross neurological deficits following neonatal bacterial meningitis, including hydrocephalus and cerebral infarction. The need for counselling and community help is of real importance if the family is to cope with the continuing care for their child after discharge. Some of the special nursing considerations related to specific conditions are briefly discussed here.

Meningitis

Meningitis results in an elevated temperature and increases the brain's metabolic and oxygen needs, and also increases the likelihood of fits, therefore measures to reduce a pyrexia must be implemented. This will include administering paracetamol and, where appropriate, tepid sponging. The child will have a severe headache and the nurse has much to offer in terms of minimizing this by ensuring that the child is cared for in a quiet, darkened environment (to reduce noxious stimuli). Additionally assessment of the child's pain should be made and analgesia administered appropriately. Once diagnosis has been established by CT scan and lumbar puncture, the nurse will be involved in the administration of the appropriate antibiotics. The child's more routine needs must also assume a level of importance and the nurse must ensure that the child's fluid and

nutritional needs are being met. Throughout the child's care psychological support must be seen to be paramount.

Encephalitis

Meningitis and encephalitis may initially present with similar signs and symptoms, but the diagnosis of encephalitis is often difficult to establish at its early stage. By the time a diagnosis is established, brain damage or death may have occurred. In addition to a CT scan, lumbar puncture and EEG, a brain biopsy may be performed. The child with encephalitis does not normally need to be isolated and good hand washing technique is an appropriate means of minimizing the risk of cross infection. Some additional nursing interventions are important to consider for the child with encephalitis. The main focus of nursing management relates to the control of a rapidly rising ICP which can result in herniation. The child must be closely assessed and monitored to detect any changes in conscious level as normally a coma indicates a poor outlook. If the child survives, neurological defects, including dysphagia, then seizures, motor defects, personality changes and a wide range of cognitive deficits are common.

Extradural and subdural empyema; cerebral abscess

The signs of cerebral irritation initially described also apply here and further signs and symptoms depend on the location of the infection. The infection is often associated with primary infections of the middle ear, sinuses and mastoids. The nursing management of a patient with a parameningeal infection can be viewed in two stages:

(1) The initial invasion stage when the patient experiences symptoms that correspond to a general systemic infection.

(2) The second stage when the infection may behave more like a space occupying lesion.

Nursing management includes assessing the patient's condition, managing any presenting symptoms, providing supportive care and administering any drug treatment. Any neurological deficit must be reported as it will aid with diagnosis and location of the abscess. Surgery may be necessary (Hickey 1992). The impact that cerebral abscess has on the family is described in the following case study.

Case study –
Joseph aged eight, cerebral abscess

Joseph was eight years old when he was admitted to the neurosurgical ward with a coma scale of 10. His CT scan showed a cerebral abscess and the need for imminent surgery was explained to his mother, who at that stage was on her own with Joseph. This was the beginning of a month's stay for Joseph, following which he was returned to his local hospital for rehabilitation and completion of a course of intravenous antibiotics. He required two operations for drainage of his cerebral abscess and exploration by the team; he also had insertion of a Hickman's line for his drugs, following initial peripheral installations.

Post-operatively he had a dense right hemiperesis, which with time and physiotherapy (and much determination on Joseph's part) has largely resolved. Fortunately, he is left handed; he now walks 'with a very slight wobble'. He was dysphasic following surgery and now (seven weeks later) is only slightly slow in speech. He had seizures initially, which were effectively controlled with anticonvulsants.

His parents' views
Despite explanation of the situation, it was not until Joseph was in theatre (about two hours following admission) that shock and fear set in. Joseph's mother says comfort was given by a nurse, who waited until dad arrived, and who she describes as a 'friendly companion – who listened as well as talked'. Both parents stated that it 'was reassuring and essential to have the nurse present'. They describe feelings of lack of control, shock, the speed of the situation, and the need for explanation of all eventualities – enabling them to mentally face the future (short and long

term). They faced many ups and downs, but by then felt that they were part of the process, not visitors; they required knowledge and explanation as to what was happening to their child.

Continuity of care by the same nurses was important to Joseph and his parents; it was also reassuring to hear their views on his progress, which often they themselves could not see. Joseph's parents are aware that he will be a bit fragile for a while and will have some social and learning problems; they feel he was helped so much by the positive attitudes of the staff, and his own determination (and their own, I would add). They describe the difficulties arising from Joseph's illness and hospitalization, including the effect on the family as a whole, the difficulties of hospital visits (Joseph's brother was at school during the week and visited at weekends) and the jealousy and occasional arguments that arose. They described a feeling of isolation whilst in the hospital, and were much helped in finding support and sympathy from their family and friends at home. They feel Joseph's illness has changed their view of life, and that life itself is now the most important thing to them as a family.

Joseph's view
Joseph initially thought he had fallen off his bike, and hence his headache. He now describes what happened as: 'A sinus infection got in my brain. It caused my right hand and leg to stop working and my speech is slow. It is hard to think sometimes'. He described the nurses as friendly, and although sometimes he missed home he enjoyed being spoiled, and liked his friends in hospital; he hated needles. With regard to his future, Joseph says that he knows he will get better and that it will take a long time; he enjoys his physiotherapy, sees the benefits, and enjoys helping in his own rehabilitation. His family do not envisage him returning to school until three months following his surgery. Joseph himself says he does not want his friends to see him in a wheelchair, and that he does not intend to return to school until he is better.

His parents reiterate that the positive attitude of all concerned with his care was reflected in the single mindedness and determined way in which Joseph coped with and overcame this condition. Joseph's case gives numerous examples where the nurse's presence, skills, attitudes, encouragement and friendship were felt to be highly beneficial in his coping and recovery. Honesty was appreciated by the family; the parents' involvement in Joseph's care and rehabilitation was encouraged and evidently effective. In addition, they felt more able to face the future with a knowledge of what that might entail.

NURSING CARE OF THE CHILD WITH HYDROCEPHALUS

Hydrocephalus is a clinical symptom rather than a disease and refers to dilatation of the ventricular system because the production of CSF (cerebrospinal fluid) exceeds its absorption. Hydrocephalus can be defined as communicating or noncommunicating. In communicating hydrocephalus the arachnoid villi are unable to absorb CSF in the normal manner, resulting in a 'backlog' of CSF. In noncommunicating hydrocephalus there is an obstruction in the ventricular system which prevents outflow of CSF and there is a resultant build-up of CSF. Hydrocephalus may be caused by a wide range of reasons (Fig. 19.11). Hydrocephalus is diagnosed by clinical examinations and by CT scan. It is treated by insertion of a shunt system to divert the CSF elsewhere, and normally a ventricular-peritoneal shunt is used. Shunt malfunction occurs in some cases and involves blockage, disconnection, infection, overdrainage and subdural haematomas (Table 19.6).

Nursing assessment

Assessment involves considering the child's neurological status and paying particular attention to the assessment for raised intracranial pressure. In addition, when assessing a baby the nurse should assess the child's head circumference, eyes and fontanelles. The baby with hydrocephalus can be diagnosed by an increase in head circumference (the suture spaces widen), characteristic sunset eyes and a tense bulging fontanelle. As the child progresses with treatment the need to assess the family's coping abilities becomes increasingly important.

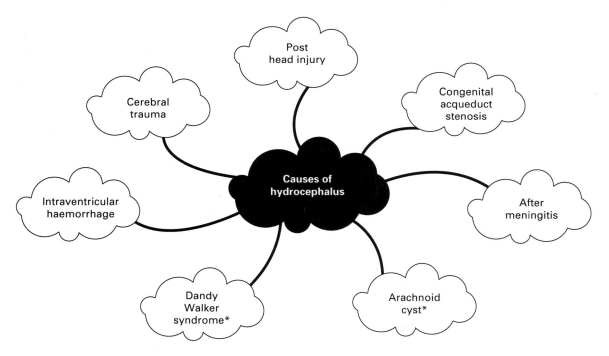

Fig. 19.11 Causes of hydrocephalus (* less common causes).

Table 19.6 Shunt malfunctions and possible actions.

Blockage or disconnection	This requires a shunt revision and may present as a neurosurgical emergency.
Infection	Generally occurs following shunt surgery and normally requires shunt system removal during a course of IV and intrathecal antibiotics, shunt is then replaced.
Rarer complications (over-drainage)	The treatment is to change the pressure of the valve, and to treat a subdural haematoma if necessary.

Nursing intervention: meeting the child's needs

Throughout the child's care the nurse must ensure that the family is fully cognisant of their child's prognosis, progress and care. Parents need to be given full information about the care of their child's shunt and what symptoms they should be aware of in relation to shunt malfunction. It is paramount that they contact a physician if they suspect any problems with the shunt or with their child generally. Additionally, families in the community can be vulnerable and isolated and the need to help the family make contact with local support groups is essential. Effective communication between all members of the multidisciplinary team, both in the hospital and the community, is essential.

It is important for the nurse to encourage the parents to allow their child to mature and develop. Many children with hydrocephalus have normal intelligence, physical development and co-ordination, but are often slower in acquiring such skills as eye–hand co-ordination and learning to walk. Each child is different and the levels of attainment of skills depends on many factors. The child's developmental progress will be influenced by the nature of the problem causing the hydrocephalus, by the degree of any brain damage, and by any other complications such as infection. However, the individual child's overall development and adaptations to the world are greatly influenced by the attitude afforded him by his parents and the environment (Derechin 1987).

NURSING THE CHILD WITH CEREBRAL DEFICITS DUE TO BIRTH TRAUMA

Govaert & Vanhaesbouk (1992) found that 50% of infants suffering supratentorial damage after traumatic forceps or vacuum delivery suffered long term neurological damage. This was due to haemorrhage, vasospasm, and cerebral ischaemia, the degree of neurological damage being directly related to the degree and location of the insult. Birth asphyxia causing hypoxic ischaemic encephalopathy resulted in cerebral atrophy in a significant number of children (Knave & Merchant 1990). Brain damage acquired in utero or at birth secondary to anoxia, acidosis or hypotension may not immediately present, as with the spastic diplegia associated with cerebral palsy. Idiopathic respiratory distress syndrome and convulsions during the first few days of life following a traumatic delivery, may also be followed by a 'silent period' of several months without any symptoms of brain damage (Gordon & McKinlay 1986). Early diagnosis can be established by following up infants who have been exposed to harmful events in utero or at birth. This follow-up needs to go on for at least the first two years of life in order to identify signs of a neurological handicap (Nelson & Ellennberg 1982).

Cerebral palsy is a description not a diagnosis, and elimination of progressive processes as diagnostic possibilities is essential. Despite the nonprogressive nature of the damage the clinical expression of cerebral palsy may change as the child matures. Severely affected children with cerebral palsy may be quadriplegic and developmentally delayed with difficulty in speaking and swallowing. Less affected children may have normal intelligence and only mild motor deficits.

It is important, however, for the nurse to report and

document any birth trauma and to be aware of the normal developmental milestones and any deviations a child may have from these. Early involvement of a multidisciplinary team can then be instigated and the child's potential can be optimized. Honest information must be given to the parents and in a setting where time, empathy and support can be offered.

NURSING CARE OF THE CHILD WITH A BRAIN TUMOUR

For the family with a child diagnosed as having a brain tumour, the uncertainty about their child's future is intense and the nurse can play a part in supporting them through the investigations and treatment. Not only is the brain tumour seen to be invasive and aggressive but the subsequent treatment such as surgery, radiotherapy and chemotherapy can also be seen as equally invasive. Brain tumours are the second most common form of childhood malignancy (leukaemia being the most common) and the majority of brain tumours in children are primary tumours.

One of the difficulties in terms of diagnosing the child with a brain tumour is the relative rarity of the condition. Most GPs only encounter one child with a brain tumour during their entire career and since the early symptoms may actually be confused with other childhood illnesses, there is often a delay in referral and diagnosis. The effects of brain tumours depend on their nature, location and other characteristics. Children present with a range of tumours including astrocytoma, ependymona, medulloblastoma, primitive neuro-ectodermal tumour, craniopharyngioma, and brain stem tumours (see Table 19.7).

Nursing assessment

The clinical manifestations of a brain tumour cover a wide range of signs and symptoms, depending on the location, size and tumour. Headache, vomiting and lethargy are common symptoms of many childhood illnesses, and it is often not until the tumour is causing a significant increase in intercranial pressure, identified by papilloedema, that the child is referred to a specialist. The occurrence of hydrocephalus secondary to the tumour often results in a decline in the child's neurological status, and consequently a referral is made.

Once the child is admitted to hospital, a neurological examination is made and the tumour may be localized by some of the presenting symptoms. The presence of ataxia in a young child, for example, is indicative of a posterior fossa tumour, whereas visual disturbance and diabetes insipidus is indicative of a probable craniopharyngioma. A comprehensive picture is obtained by using other investigative techniques, such as computed tomography (CT) and/or a magnetic resonance imaging (MRI) scan.

Small children generally require sedation for a CT scan, although if this proves unsuccessful or is inadvisable due to the child's condition, a general anaesthetic will be required. Many children, if adequately prepared by either the nurse or play specialist, can be scanned without the need for either sedation or anaesthesia. The use of photographs and simple, appropriate explanations is useful and increases the chance of success in scanning the unsedated child.

Once the diagnosis of a brain tumour has been made, three general methods for treatment are available: surgery, irradiation and chemotherapy. The variable selected depends on the tumour type, location, size, related symptoms, and the general condition and age of the patient. The nurse's assessment of the child and family must be made in relation to the above, and must reflect the changing needs of the child. In addition to the physical needs, the family unit have an ongoing need for information and emotional support. This will be further discussed in the following section.

Nursing intervention: meeting the child's needs

Although physical care is important, children must have their psychological and emotional needs met. Many children will feel anxious and frightened and their altered level of consciousness may affect their ability to grasp the essentials. For the child, fantasy and imagined fears are often worse than the reality of the situation. Therefore it is crucial to communicate effectively with children as this can minimize many of their fears and allow them to express themselves openly and honesty.

The importance of good communication which is age and cognitive appropriate can be highlighted by some of

Table 19.7 Childhood cerebral tumours.

Astrocytoma	Most common brain tumours and can be benign or malignant. Often contain a cyst with a solid tissue surrounding and found in all areas of the brain. Treatment depends on the area of the brain involved and the grade of tumour. Surgery is performed in the majority of cases and radiotherapy/chemotherapy if the tumour is malignant. Cure is achievable if complete removal of a benign astrocytoma has occurred and prognosis is good. With incomplete removal of a benign astrocytoma tumour, re-growth is possible and regular follow up is necessary. Long term cure from malignant astrocytoma is difficult to achieve.
Ependymona	These tumours arise from the ependymal cells lining the ventricles and account for a small number of childhood brain tumours. Can be benign or malignant. Normally occur in the posterior fossa region and involve surgical removal followed by radiotherapy/chemotherapy. Tumours may metastasize down the spine and radiation is given to both brain and spine. It is difficult to achieve a long term cure for malignant ependymona.
Medulloblastoma	Second most common childhood brain tumour and arises from primitive cells in the cerebellum. It is malignant and may spread within the brain and spinal cord. Surgery is followed by chemotherapy and radiotherapy to both the head and spine. A long term cure is difficult to achieve.
Primitive neuroectodermal tumour (PNET)	A rare tumour occurring in the younger child, and a highly malignant tumour. Surgery is followed by chemotherapy/radiotherapy to both head and spine.
Craniopharyngioma	This tumour is found in the region of the pituitary gland and consequently may involve the optic pathways, pituitary and hypothalamus. Surgery may be followed by radiotherapy if removal is incomplete. Long term follow up also involves the endrocrinologist.
Brain stem tumours	Surgery is usually impossible due to the tumour's location, although a biopsy may sometimes be performed, for histology. Radiotherapy and/or chemotherapy is given, but the long term prognosis remains poor, particularly for the malignant tumours.

the misconceptions that occur when communication goes wrong. For example, when talking to an eight year old, preparing him for surgery for a tumour the nurse explained 'this is the anaesthetist; she's the lady I told you about, who's going to put you to sleep for your operation'. The child, who had been calm, now became agitated. In trying to find out why this had happened the nurse found out that the child's dog had been 'put to sleep' the previous week. After realising why the child had become frightened the nurse was able to allay his fears.

Another example highlights the shock instilled by a four year old running round the ward singing 'I've got a brain tumour' at the top of his voice. Although he had no fear or understanding of the terminology he was using, it had a devastating effect on his relatives and friends. Specialized psychological care for these families is discussed by Hickey (1992).

In addition, the child's present physical and mental disabilities need to be addressed and their future needs prepared for. Community requirements such as physiotherapy, assessment and reassessment of educational needs, and addressing the altered family processes, need to be considered and catered for. The nurse must work alongside the family, allowing the parent a feeling of control of the situation. The nurse is an essential part of the multidisciplinary team, working with the child and their family. In addition to providing for the child's physical needs it is equally important to provide continual sensitive, supportive care. This can be followed through in the community by effective liaison between the hospital and community nurses.

Radiotherapy

Radiotherapy remains, with surgery, the cornerstone in management of paediatric brain tumours (Hebrand *et al.* 1990). The objective of radiotherapy is to destroy tumour cells without injuring the normal ones, and thus increase the child's likelihood of survival. The amount of radiation given depends on histology and location of the tumour and the tolerance of the patient. Cerebral oedema is a temporary side effect of treatment which must be considered when utilizing radiotherapy.

An individual shell or mask is made for each child, to ensure radiotherapy is directed to the desired area only.

nursing care so that the child has plenty of opportunities to sleep and rest. Skin care is important and appropriate lotions can be used to help ensure that the problem of dry skin does not distress the child. Hair loss can be distressing for the child and family, although it is often more difficult for the parents to accept than the child. Body image problems associated with alopecia can be helped by offering the child an appropriate wig, although baseball caps, hats and scarves can help to boost the child's confidence. The nurse also needs to be aware of the possible long term effects of radiotherapy which include cerebral necrosis and endocrine damage (Table 19.8).

Table 19.8   Long term effects of cerebral radiotherapy.

Cerebral necrosis	The likelihood of this is decreased by limiting and spreading out the doses of radiation. However, educational and behavioural changes may occur some months after treatment has finished. Educational psychologists must be involved to assess and monitor the child's educational ability and to offer help and advice when needed.
Endocrine damage	Radiation damage to the pituitary gland may result in the child needing growth hormone replacement therapy.

Sedation or anaesthesia may be necessary to enable the treatment to be performed, although generally children quickly learn what is required of them and co-operate with the treatment. An intercom system, and a favourite tape, make it easier for the child to stay unattended in the radiotherapy room. The treatment itself only takes about two to four minutes. The treatment is given daily for five days a week and for between five and eight weeks in total.

The nurse should be aware of the side effects of the radiotherapy so that he or she can adequately prepare the child and family and be proactive in the child's care. Side effects include nausea, vomiting, headache, lethargy, loss of appetite, changes in the sense of taste, and cold symptoms. Local hair loss occurs and it may take three to four months to regrow. Additionally the skin where the radiotherapy is directed may become sore, so skin assessment and care is vital. Bone marrow suppression may also occur.

The nurse's role in helping the child receiving radiotherapy involves proactive management in order to minimize the symptoms and decrease the overall impact of the treatment. This will involve judicious use of medications to ease/relieve the nausea, and managing

Chemotherapy

Chemotherapy is a relatively new treatment for brain tumours in children under three years old. Radiotherapy is not given to children under the age of three due to the high risk of damage to the developing brain. Consequently chemotherapy is the treatment given following surgery. Combined chemotherapy and radiotherapy may be the treatment of choice for some children over three years old.

Chemotherapy is given via a Hickmann line or a Portacath and those children on the baby brain protocol (that is those under three years of age) require chemotherapy over a period of a year. Side effects include nausea and vomiting, alopecia and bone marrow suppression (affecting red and white blood cells and platelets). The nurse must consider all these side effects when caring for the child undergoing chemotherapy, and should ensure that proactive care is given. Once again, the nurse can be a huge help in the role of counsellor, advocate and educator. A familiar face is important during the repeated hospitalization these families endure.

Follow up consists of regular brain scans at various times, and examinations by the medical teams caring for that child. A liaison nurse, based in the hospital and community, is a great advantage, forming a vital link for the family. It is difficult for parents to relax about their child's health following such a serious illness and with an uncertain future still ahead of them. Liaison sisters, ward nurses and social workers need to work within the available sources of help in the community, offering constructive emotional help and practical advice whenever possible.

REHABILITATION AND RECOVERY

Research continues in the field of recovery from brain damage, in an effort to determine the nature of the changes that have occurred after an insult and the kinds of therapeutic interventions that might help the individual.

> 'No physically restricted lesion of the brain should ever lead to an absolute impairment of any particular specific mental or behavioural capacity, since every function is multiply represented in the brain at different hierarchical levels.' (Levere *et al.* 1988).

This idea that changes within the brain may not be absolute is reinforced in the same article. Recovery of function following a cerebral insult is more frequent when goal achievement is the major criterion for a recovery determination. The ability to establish whether compensation or recovery have occurred is difficult. Behavioural 'sparing' also occurs; for example, if subjects with slow growing lesions do not exhibit symptoms, when subjects with matching lesions show functional deficits one must assume that behavioural sparing has occurred. The three suggested stages of recovery following brain damage are discussed in the same paper and consist of:

- Restitution of the damaged substrates.
- Simplifying the environment.
- Relearning, by using those systems that remain functional following brain damage.

Brain damage can affect not only the neurological–physiological body systems but also the cognitive functions, personality, individuality, behaviour and identity. Patients may often lack self-awareness of any change in themselves due to alteration of their cognitive abilities. The normal patterns of family interactions and family structure are changed, and family members find that physiological changes are easier to accept than personality or behavioural changes in their child (Hickey 1992).

A parents' adaptation and coping in relation to their child's changed needs, are complex. An understanding of their attitudes, and of the child's, is essential for the nurse to understand, and so to improve, the quality of care for this family.

REFERENCES AND FURTHER READING

Adams, R.D. & Victor, M. (1989) *Principles of Neurology*, 4th edn, p. 501. McGraw-Hill, New York.

Anderson, B. (1987) The metabolic needs of head trauma victims. *Journal of Neuroscience Nursing*, 19, 211–15.

Basser, L.S. (1962) Hemiplegia of early onset and the faculty of speech with special reference to the effects of hemispherectomy. *Brain*, 85, 427–60.

Callanan, M. (1988) Epilepsy: putting the patient back in control. *Registered Nurse*, 51, 48–55.

Chudley, S. (1994) The effect of nursing activities on intracranial pressure. *British Journal of Nursing*, 3(9), 454–9.

Derechin, M.E. (1987) Paediatric head injury. *Critical Care Nursing Quarterly*, 10(3), 12–24.

DES (1978) *Special Educational Needs*. Report of the committee of enquiry into the education of handicapped children and young people (Warnock Report). HMSO, London.

Feferbaum, R., Vaz, F.A., Krabs, V-L., Diniz, E.M., Ramez, S.R. & Manissadjia, A. (1993) Bacterial meningitis in the neonatal period. *Archives in Neurophysiology*, 51(1), 72–9.

Frankenburg, W.K. & Dodds, J.B. (1969) *Denver Developmental Screening Test*. University of Colorado Medical Centre, Colorado.

Frankenburg, W.K., Fandal, A. & Thornton, S. (1987) Revision of Denver Prescreening Development Questionnaire. *Journal of Paediatrics*, 110(4), 633–7.

Gordon, N. & McKinlay, I. (1986) *Neurologically Handicapped Children*, 62. Blackwell Science, Oxford.

Govaert, P. & Vanhaesbouk, P. (1992) Traumatic neonatal intra-cranial bleeding and stroke. *Archives of Disability in Childhood*, July, 67, 840–51.

Griffiths, M. & Russell, P. (1985) *Working Together with Handicapped Children*. Souvenir Press, London.

Gunnet, R.J. (1984) *The Epilepsy Handbook*. Raven Press, New York.

Guyton, A. (1986) *Textbook of Medical Physiology*, 7th edn., pp. 338–40. W.B. Saunders, Philadelphia.

Harrison, M. (1991) The minor head injury. *Paediatric Nursing*, 3(10), 15–19.

Hebrand, J.L., Benk, V., Bouhnik, H., Teisser, E., Kalifa, C. & Sarrazaz, D. (1990) Modern technology of radiotherapy for brain tumours in children. *Bull-Cancer*, Paris, 77(7), 725–36.

Hickey, J.V. (1992) *The Clinical Practice of Neurological and Neurosurgical Nursing*, 3rd edn. J. Lippincott & Co.

Jennet, B. & Teasdale, G. (1981) *Management of Head Injuries*. F.A. Davis, Philadelphia.

Johnson, D.A., Uttley, D. & Wyke, M. (1989) *Children's Head Injury – Who Cares?* Taylor & Francis Ltd, London.

Kempthorne, A. (1994) Epilepsy in Childhood. *Paediatric Nursing*, 6(2), 30–33.

Khave, M.D. & Merchant, R.M. (1990) Diagnostic and prognostic value of CT brain scan in term neonates with moderate birth asphyxia. *Indian Pediatrics*, March 27(3), 267–71.

Lee, A. (1994) Hats off to Angela. *Nursing Standard*, 9(4), 21–3.

Levere, T., Almic, T. & Stein, D. (1988) *Brain Injury and Recovery* (ed. Stanley Flnger). Plenum Press, New York.

Levin, A. (1977) *Neurosurgery*, 1(3), 266–71.

McManus, J.C. & Bryden, M.P. (1991) Geschwind's theory of cerebral lateralisation. Developing a formal causal model. *Psychological Bulletin*, 110, 237–51.

Michaud, L.J., Rivara, F.P., Grady, M.S. & Reay, D.T. (1992) Predictors of survival and severity of disablement after severe brain injury. *Neurosurgery*, August 31(2), 254–64.

Millard, D.M. (1984) *Daily Living with a Handicapped Child*, pp. 12–15, 39–47, 55–56. Croom-Helm, London.

Mitchell, P. Ozuna, J. & Lipe, H. (1981) *Nursing Research*, 30(4), 212.

Morray, J., Tyler, D., Jones, T., Stuntz, J. & Lemire, R. (1984) Coma scale for brain injured children. *Critical Care Medicine*, 12, 1018–20.

Neatherlin, J. & Brillhart, B. (1988) Glasgow coma scale scores in the patient post cardiopulmonary resuscitation. *Journal of Neuroscience Nursing*, 20, 104–9.

Nelson, K.B. & Ellenberg, J.H. (1982) Children who outgrew cerebral palsy. *Paediatrics*, 69, 529–36.

Pomeroy, S.L., Holmes, S.J., Dodge, P.R. & Feigin, R.D. (1990) *Journal of Medicine*, Dec. 13, 323(24), 1651–7.

Raimondi, A. & Hirschener, J. (1984) Head injury in the infant and toddler. *Child Brain*, 11, 12–35.

Richardson, S.A. (1976) The influence of severe malnutrition in infancy on the intelligence of children at school: an ecological perspective. *Environmental Therapy for Brain Dysfunction* (eds R.N. Walsh & W.T. Greenborough), pp. 256–75. Plenum Press, New York.

Rivara, J.B., Fay, G.C., Jaffe, K.M., Polissar, N.L., Shurtleff, H.A. & Martin, K.M. (1992) Predictors of family functioning one year following traumatic brain injury in children. *Archives of Physical Medical Rehabilitation*, 73(10), 899–910.

Robinson, M. (1989) Care of the child with a head injury. *Paediatric Nursing*, 1(9), 13–15.

Roffe, J. (1989) Head injury rehabilitation. *Paediatric Nursing*, 1(9), 13–15.

Rose, F.D. & Johnson, D.A. (1990) *Recovery from brain damage – reflections and directions. Advances in Experimental Medicine and Biology*, 235, 188. Plenum Press, New York.

Rose, F.D. & Johnson, D.A. (1992) Progress in understanding recovery of function after brain damage: the need for collaboration. *Restorative Neurology and Neuroscience*, 4, 241–4.

Russell, W.R. & Denver, A.J. (1975) *Explaining the Brain*, 15. Oxford University Press, London.

Sadler, C. (1994) Seen but not heard. *Nursing Times*, 90(21), 23.

Scherer, P. (1986) Assessment: the logic of coma. *American Journal of Nursing*, 86, 541–50.

Scott-Jupp, R., Marlow, N., Seddon, N., Rosenbloom, L. (1992) Rehabilitation and outcome following severe head injury. *Archives of Disability in Childhood*, 67(2), 222–6.

Shorvon, S.D. (1988) Late onset of seizures and dementia: a revival of epidemiology and aetiology. In *Epilepsy, Behaviour and Cognitive Functions* (eds M.R. Trimble et al.), pp. 189–207. John Wiley & Sons, New York.

Simpson, D.A. & Reilly, P.L. (1982) Paediatric Coma Scale. *Lancet*, ii. 450 (letter).

Squire, L.R. & Zole-Morgan, S. (1988) Memory: brain systems and behaviour. *Journal of International Nursing Studies*, 11(4), 170–5.

Teasdale, G. & Jennet, A. (1974) Assessment of coma and impaired consciousness. *Lancet*, 2181.

UKCC (1992) *Standards for the Administration of Medicines*. United Kingdom Central Council, London.

Voeller, K. & Rothenberg, M. (1973) Psychological aspects of the management of seizures in children. *Paediatrics*, 51(6), 1072–82.

Volpe, J. (1981) *Neurology of the newborn*. Major Problems in Clinical Paediatrics, vol. 12. W.B. Saunders, Philadelphia.

Weiner, H., Urion, D. & Levitt, L. (1982) *Paediatric Neurology*. Williams & Wilkins, Baltimore.

Williams, J. (1992) Assessment of head injured children. *British Journal of Nursing*, 1(2), 82–4.

Chapter 20

Nursing Support and Care: Meeting the Needs of the Child and Family with Altered Endocrine and Metabolic Function

Adele McEvilly, Beryl Holmes and Lynne Styles

INTRODUCTION

Parent: 'To be told your child has a chronic condition is one of the most devastating experiences in the world.'

Endocrine or metabolic dysfunction gives rise to a wide variety of acute and long term effects. Even minor variations from the normal limits can result in marked behavioural and developmental changes. Children and their families need to be helped to adjust to the restrictions that such a dysfunction imposes, and to deal with the impact that the disease has on their lives. For some families diagnosis not only brings the grief of being told that their child is ill, but implicit in the diagnosis is the tragic realization that their child has a limited life expectancy.

As with many other chronic childhood illnesses, the role of the nurse must be one that is both dynamic and responsive. Hands-on care, support, education, advocacy and friendship are all required in what is often a long term relationship. Paediatric community nurses can and do play a major part in supporting the family in the community and ensuring that problems are addressed and needs met within the child's usual environment.

Endocrine and metabolic problems are complex and provide a challenge to the nurse. An adequate knowledge of the underlying disease process is vital, although in some cases of rare diagnosis this information may be difficult to access. The importance of liaising with specialist nurses working specifically within the field must be stressed.

This chapter will explore the effects on children of disorders related to altered endocrine and metabolic activity. Some prior knowledge of endocrine and metabolic function is assumed but a brief overview will be given; more in-depth knowledge should be obtained from an appropriate physiology text.

Within this chapter emphasis will be placed on meeting the information needs of the parents (and child where appropriate), therefore a description of the aetiology and particular features of each of the disorders is provided. Based on this knowledge the nurse will be able to identify the specific problems that may arise from overactivity or insufficiency. This in turn will assist them in planning comprehensive care based upon sound rationale. Providing appropriate information and edu-

cation for the child and family enables them to manage their child who may be experiencing complex, chronic problems.

In looking at endocrine dysfunction a number of key issues/conditions are considered as these help to illuminate the role of the nurse and the needs of the children. Diabetes is explored as this is one of the most common endocrine disorders affecting children, and the effect on the child of disorders of the thyroid are also discussed. Disorders of the pituitary, growth hormone insufficiency and dysfunctions of the adrenal glands are addressed. Several of the many complex metabolic dysfunctions are described. Although these occur infrequently, particular examples have been selected to illustrate different facets of the nurse's role. This may range from screening, dietary and health education in phenylketonuria, to recognizing the acute onset in medium chain acetyl CoA dehydrogenase deficiency and to supporting the family through care of the terminally ill child in Tay Sach's disease. Since many of these disorders are comparatively rare, the nurse may need to draw on the resources available from specialist centres where there is an increased level of expertise within the area.

An overview of the endocrine system and function

The endocrine system consists of a series of glandular structures which often depend on each other for optimal balance in health. Understanding the system will enable the nurse to comprehend the way in which altered functions may affect the child in the short or long term. The system is divided into three components:

(1) The cell – sends messages via hormones.
(2) The target organ/tissue – receives messages.
(3) The transfer medium by which messages are transported, for example blood, extracellular fluid.

The endocrine system is responsible for controlling and regulating metabolic processes, resulting in growth, energy production, fluid and electrolyte balance, stress response, sexual development, maturation, and reproduction. Table 20.1 provides a summary and identifies the location and function of the different glands of the endocrine system and the ways in which under or over activity will affect the child's body.

NURSING CARE OF THE CHILD WITH INSULIN DEPENDENT DIABETES

It is relevant to discuss some of the significant features of the aetiology of diabetes because the nurse who is aware of these will be able to provide appropriate and comprehensive information to parents. It is a disorder of carbohydrate metabolism which occurs when the pancreas fails to produce sufficient insulin to oxidize glucose for energy. It is estimated that 1:5000 children are affected and therefore it is classified as the most common endocrine disorder. There is evidence that this incidence is increasing, particularly in children of school age (Metcalf & Baum 1991), and there are peaks of onset which seem to become apparent at the times of starting or changing schools. This correlation may be significant because by providing community support and thereby avoiding admission to hospital, the nurse may be able to minimize any additional stresses associated with these critical periods. There is a genetic pre disposition, but this factor alone is not sufficient to induce the disease. Usually a catalyst is required. These 'triggers' may be viral or environmental. A common sequence of events and physiological changes, together with the child's likely behavioural changes, generally occurs (Table 20.2).

Nursing assessment

The nurse must assess the child through the use of a nursing history, observations, assessment and investigations. A nursing assessment will be based largely upon the information provided by the child and parents. They usually mention the child's poor weight gain and growth, hunger, excessive thirst, polyuria, nocturia, changed personality, persistent infections (largely due to a raised blood glucose which impedes the immune system and ability to fight off infection), and blurred vision brought about by a change in the shape of the lens of the eye.

The overall main aim of care is to achieve optimum metabolic control as this is essential to prevent complications (DCCT 1993). If this is achieved in childhood it will prevent poor growth, delayed puberty and other problems including disability in the longer term.

Nursing intervention: meeting the child's needs

Dietary intake and insulin therapy

In some areas children are admitted to hospital regardless of their medical needs, for initiation of insulin therapy and dietary management (McEvilly 1991). However, the child with nonketotic diabetes may be managed at home where adequate community support is available to assist the family as they come to terms with the diagnosis and begin to learn about its management (McEvilly 1991). The initial aims of this holistic care are to alleviate symptoms, begin to develop optimal metabolic control and establish a rapport with the family. This will enable the child to return to their normal routine as soon as possible. All newly diagnosed children require a nursing care plan which includes emotional support for the child and family, with an educational programme, provided at a rate and time to suit the individual. This programme will include the information shown in Fig. 20.1, as recommended by the British Diabetic Association (BDA 1989). The nurse will need to assess the most appropriate way to teach each child and family, taking into account their individual differences and needs.

Children with diabetes have the same nutritional requirements as other children of similar age (Magrath 1992). However, the diet requires some modification in order to reduce the risks of hypoglycaemia, hyperglycaemia and other long term complications. The changes involve ensuring the child eats regular meals and snacks which include unrefined carbohydrate. Sometimes this is managed by the introduction of an exchange system represented by 10 g of carbohydrate per exchange or portion. An alternative approach is the 'free' diet, which involves ensuring each meal contains some starchy (unrefined carbohydrate) foods, but the amounts are not measured. Recent recommendations produced by the BDA Nutritional Sub-committee (1989) include those shown in Table 20.3.

The British Diabetic Association actively discourages the use of diabetic food products. Dietary requirements must be regularly reviewed by a paediatric dietitian who has a specific interest in childhood diabetes. Whenever possible this should be carried out within the home, enabling the dietary recommendations to be translated into foods and a meal pattern acceptable to the child and family.

Table 20.1

Gland	Position	Hormone	Target organs	Function	Underactivity	Overactivity
Islets of Langerhans	Group of cells within the pancreas which is situated behind the stomach.	Insulin.	Many metabolic effects.	Regulates sugar metabolism. Ensures complete fat combustion.	Diabetes mellitus.	Hyperinsulinism, i.e. hypoglycaemia.
Thyroid	In the neck two lateral lobes each side of the trachea immediately behind the larynx.	T3 T4	Many metabolic effects.	Increases metabolic rate. Promotes normal physical growth maturation and mental development.	Hypothyroidism, (cretinism). Delayed epiphyseal closure.	Thyrotoxicosis goitre. Accelerated linear growth.
Parathyroid	Usually four small oval bodies attached to the posterior surface of the thyroid gland.	Parathormone.	Kidney, Bones.	Controls concentration of calcium and inorganic phosphate in the blood.	Hypocalcaemia. Tetany.	Hypercalcaemia. (Bone demineralisation). Hypophosphataemia.
Anterior Pituitary	Suspended from the base of the brain. Protected by the sellsa turcica in the sphenoid bone. Two lobes. Anterior and posterior.	Growth hormone.	Bone. Body tissues.	Promotes growth of bone and soft tissue. Main effect on linear growth. Essential for proliferation of cartilage cells at epiphyseal plate. Has hyperglycaemic effect.	Growth retardation. Hypoglycaemia	Pre-pubertal gigantism. Hypoproteinaemia. Diabetes mellitus.
		T.S.H.	Thyroid gland.	Promotes and maintains growth and development of thyroid gland. Stimulates thyroid hormone secretion.	Hypothyroidism.	Often secondary to hypothyroidism.
		A.C.T.H.	Adrenal cortex.	Promotes and maintains growth and development of adrenal cortex. Stimulates adrenal cortex to secrete adrenocorticoids.	Primary: adrenal insufficiency. Secondary to hypopituitarism. Hypoglycaemia.	Cushing's syndrome.
		Gonadotrophins	Gonads.	Stimulates gonads to mature and produce sex hormones and germ cells.	Absent or incomplete spontaneous puberty.	Precocious puberty.
		F.S.H.	Ovaries.	Stimulates follicles to mature and secrete oestrogen.	Ovarian failure – loss of secondary sexual characteristics.	Precocious puberty.
			Testes.	Stimulates development of seminiferous tubules. Initiates spermatogeneses.	Hypogonadism – loss of secondary sexual characteristics.	Precocious puberty.
		L.H.	Ovaries.	Causes follicle to rupture with discharge of mature ova. Stimulates secretion of progesterone.	Ovarian failure – loss of secondary sexual characteristics.	Precocious puberty.
			Testes.	Stimulates differentiation of Leydig cells which secrete androgens. Testosterone.	Hypogonadism – loss or failure of secondary sexual characteristics.	Precocious puberty.
		Prolactin.	Breasts.	Stimulates secretion of milk.	—	Hyperprolactinaemia, e.g. inappropriate lactation.

Table 20.1 (cont.)

Gland	Position	Hormone	Target organs	Function	Underactivity	Overactivity
Posterior pituitary	(See anterior pituitary).	Antidiuretic (Vasopressin).	Renal tubules.	Controls re-absorption of water and concentration of urine.	Diabetes insipidus.	—
		Oxytocin.	Uterus. Breasts.	Stimulates contraction of uterus. Causes excretion of milk from alveoli into breast duct.		
Adrenal cortex	Two glands situated above the kidneys, each one enclosed with a capsule and consisting of two parts.	Mineralcorticoids. Aldosterone.	Renal tubules.	Stimulates tubules to reabsorb sodium therefore promoting water retention but potassium loss.	Adrenocortical insufficiency.	Electrolyte imbalance. Hyperaldosteronism.
	Cortex outer	Sex hormones.		Influence development of bone. Secondary sexual characteristics.	Rare enzyme deficiency.	Adrenogenital syndrome. Precocious pseudopuberty.
		Glucocorticoids.		Promotes fat, protein and carbohydrate metabolism.		Cushing's disease. Impairment of growth.
		Cortisol.		Organises body's defence system during periods of stress. Suppresses inflammatory reaction.	Addison's disease. Increased skin pigmentation.	Delayed bone maturation.
Adrenal medulla	Medulla inner	Adrenalin. (Catecholamines). Noradrenalin.	Many metabolic effects.	Produces vasoconstriction of heart and smooth muscle (↑ BP). Increases blood sugars. Metabolic rate increases. Causes generalized vasoconstriction. Raises both systemic and diastolic blood pressure.	Impaired response to hypoglycaemia.	Phaeochromocytoma episode. Episodic hypertension.

Table 20.2 Sequence of events and likely behavioural changes.

Physiological changes	Behavioural manifestations in the child
A trigger factor initiates changes in the beta cells of the pancreas which produce insulin. These are gradually destroyed reducing the amount of insulin produced.	
↓	
Reduction in insulin levels leads to a rise in the blood glucose as the sugar cannot pass into the cells to be used for energy.	
↓	
Raised blood glucose levels cause an increase in the volume of urine excreted as the hyperglycaemia exceeds the renal threshold.	Polyuria, nocturia, sugary deposits around toilet, bed wetting.
↓	
Inability to utilise glucose for energy.	Lethargy.
↓	
Lipolysis (breakdown of fats) and gluconeogenesis (glucose synthesised from carbohydrate sources) occurs.	Weight loss, unsatisfied hunger.
↓	
Dehydration and metabolic imbalance develop.	Excessive thirst (small children may drink the toilet water).
↓	
Ketones appear in the urine as fat is oxidized at an abnormal rate.	Abdominal pain, nausea, vomiting.
↓	
Untreated severe ketosis will lead to acidosis and diabetic coma.	Kussmaul breathing (deep sighing), drowsiness.

Almost all children in the UK are treated with genetically engineered insulin which is produced to replicate human insulin and is available in a strength of 100 international units per ml. The aim is to keep the preprandial blood glucose maintained at less than 10 mmol/l. The way that insulin is administered affects both the way that it works and people's lifestyles (Burden 1994). Most children are initially given two injections a day with a combination of short and medium acting insulins (Table 20.4). These may be mixed in the syringe after withdrawing from two bottles; however, this is a difficult procedure, particularly for children, and therefore ready mixed preparations are being more frequently used. Many of these mixtures are now available for use in pen injectors, which are becoming increasingly popular. When introducing a pen device

the nurse must consider whether the child is able to handle the pen or whether its size will limit their ability to undertake self-injection.

Insulin injections should be administered 20 to 30 minutes prior to food. Given subcutaneously, the angle of injection should be adapted to between 60° and 90°, depending on the size and weight of the child. There are devices to aid with injections, available for children and parents who are having problems (Monoject/Inject Aid). The nurse must ensure that the child's injection sites are rotated but should also remember that absorption varies depending on the site used and therefore a routine should be established; for example, the upper arm and stomach in the mornings and thigh and buttocks in the evenings. This rotation not only changes the location but also the area within the site, and prevents hyper-

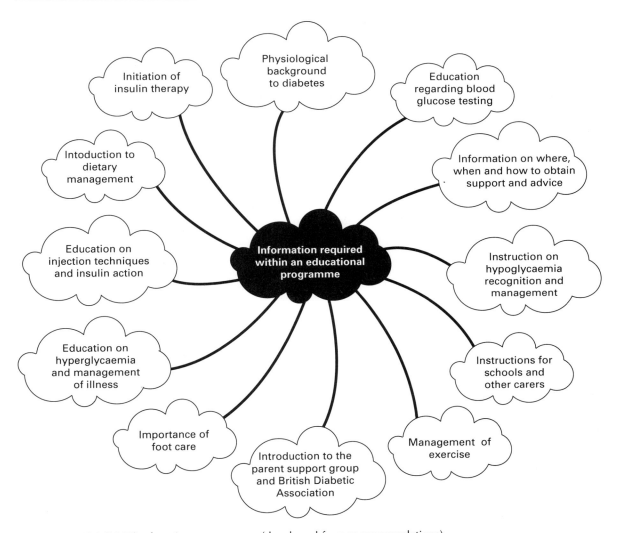

Fig. 20.1 BDA (1989) education programmes (developed from recommendations).

trophy which leads to poor absorption of the insulin. Education about the safe disposal of sharps should also be provided to the child and their parents to reduce the chance of needle stick injury (needle clippers are available on prescription).

Maintaining metabolic control

It can be seen that the management of diabetes involves maintaining blood glucose levels as near normal as possible and coping with day to day problems which may affect control. Quality of life is most important and must be a major consideration when evaluating the effectiveness of any interventions. The nurse must enable the family to adapt the management to fit into their routine. This will minimize effects on the lifestyle of the child and family. There are three ways in which metabolic control can be evaluated: blood glucose monitoring, urine glucose monitoring, and glycated haemoglobin or fructosamine.

One of the most significant technology advances in the past ten years has been the introduction of self blood glucose monitoring using portable machines (Cox 1989). Normal blood glucose level is between 4 and 8 mmol/1. This is the preferred method of routinely

Table 20.3   Recommended intakes of foodstuffs (BDA 1989).

Carbohydrates	Carbohydrates (CHO) when digested provide the body with sugar for energy. Fibre rich, unrefined CHO should provide: (1) 50–55% of energy requirements for adolescents and adults. (2) 40–45% of energy requirements for younger children, particularly under five years. A high consumption of bulky fibre rich foods may lead to a reduced intake of the high energy foods containing fat which they require.
Fibre	Fibre should gradually be increased as soluble and leguminous fibre help in achieving better blood glucose control. A suggested target for fibre in school age children is 2 g/100 kcal per day.
Refined carbohydrates	Refined carbohydrates (sugar) will cause a rapid rise in blood glucose levels but when taken as part of a high fibre meal this will be minimal and makes the meal more palatable. Recommendations state that up to 25 g of refined CHO may be taken per day as part of a high fibre diet. Refined CHO is necessary for the management of exercise and the treatment of hypoglycaemia.
Fats	Fats, particularly saturated fats, are associated with the risk of cardiovascular complications, but in children a vast reduction may lead to energy deficit and failure to thrive. In adolescents the larger amounts of fats in convenience foods may lead to obesity. Children over five years of age should obtain 35–40% of energy from fat.
Proteins	Protein intake should not exceed that of other children. The risk of renal complications may be heightened when large amounts of protein are taken in the diet.

Table 20.4   The three main groups of insulin action.

Insulin type	Duration of insulin action	Peak of insulin action
Soluble/short acting e.g. Humulin S, actrapid	30 mins to 6 hrs	2–4 hrs
Isophane/medium acting e.g. Humulin I, insulatard	2–12 to 14 hrs	4–8 hrs
Lente (zinc suspensions)/long acting e.g. Monotard, Ultratard	4–14 to 48 hrs	12–24 hrs

assessing control. The nurse must be responsible for the education and regular assessment of techniques and for ensuring that the child/parents understand the meaning of the results. The side or end of all fingers should be used to avoid long term damage to the pad of the fingers, and lancets must be disposed of safely to avoid injury to others. Tests should be performed at varying times, in a routine to suit the individual child and

family. Reflectant meters may be used but usually have to be purchased by the families.

Urine testing is of minimal benefit when assessing control because the result does not reflect the blood glucose level at the time of testing, and its significance depends on the individual renal threshold (Reading 1968a). Testing for ketones, however, is important and should be done at times of illness or poor control as this may demonstrate early ketoacidosis. The nurse should advise the families to obtain advice when ketones are found in the urine.

Glycated haemoglobin and fructosamine are laboratory assessments of long term control. Fructosamine measures control over the preceding two to three week period. Glycated haemoglobin measures control over the preceding six to eight week period and gives a more satisfactory measure of control for children. Normal ranges of these tests depend on the individual laboratory techniques.

terns, which may be of particular concern in the pre-school and young adult age groups. Considerations when taking exercise, and of growth and puberty and the importance of liaison with the nursery or school also need to be discussed at length. Parents who have been provided with a good level of information which they understand, can use effectively and are happy with, are more likely to be able to take positive, preemptive action with/on behalf of their child. Equally important is the need to discuss and develop strategies to avoid recurrence of swings in blood sugar (Table 20.5).

Table 20.5 Hypoglycaemia and hyperglycaemia: causes, interventions and strategies.

Child's problem	Causes	Interventions	Strategies to avoid recurrence
Hypoglycaemia Over a short period of time the child will become pale, sweaty, unsteady, aggressive and may complain of abdominal pain, headache, tingling, hunger	Missing a meal, exercise, altered provision of/ absorption of insulin, stress.	Give refined carbohydrate, Dextrosol, Lucozade, or fruit juice followed by unrefined carbohydrate such as a biscuit or sandwich.	Isolate a cause, ensure that there is correct carbohydrate intake, discuss insulin dose and absorption.
Hyperglycaemia The child will gradually complain of excessive thirst and nausea, and pass large volumes of urine leading to nocturia and enuresis; they may vomit.	Insufficient insulin, rapid growth, puberty, no recent appraisal of insulin needs, illness, intake of additional food, stress, poor rotation of injection sites leading to poor absorption.	Adjust insulin therapy, obtain appropriate treatment for underlying illness, check sites for features which may inhibit absorption.	Regularly monitor blood glucose to maintain effective control, assess dietary management and assess insulin administration.

Advice to parents regarding the management of potential problems

This advice needs to be comprehensive but acceptable. Parents need to be aware of what will happen if their child experiences hypoglycaemia or hyperglycaemia. This is important so that they are aware of the predisposing factors, and will be able to recognize it developing and take appropriate action. There should be a discussion on the management of erratic eating pat-

Many toddlers have erratic eating patterns and varying likes and dislikes. They often eat different amounts from day to day, causing increased parental anxiety, particularly in diabetes, because of the risk of hypoglycaemia. Advice must be available to support the parents at this very difficult time and to prevent the child learning to manipulate the situation. It is important that children do not learn to control their parents through their eating habits.

Exercise management varies depending on the level of exercise both in terms of activity and duration. Refined carbohydrate should be taken before activity and for prolonged spells; extra unrefined carbohydrate may be required afterwards. This is not always as simple as it seems as it is important to consider energy expended during training and competitions. The nurse can support the child and parents by building up a profile of the child's sports and leisure interests, and can give advice as to how to handle this aspect of their life.

School and nursery staff also need to be involved as they need to understand possible problems and their management. Education should be provided for carers, with continuing support and education for the child to increase their independence. There are increased problems when children commence senior school because of the large numbers of staff and pupils; these make education of all those involved a particular challenge. However, the paediatric community nurse, specialist liaison nurse and school nurse can work together in a partnership to meet the child's and the school community's needs.

During growth spurts and puberty, hormonal interaction will inhibit insulin action, causing the blood glucose to rise. Adolescents and parents require knowledge of these possible problems and guidance on their management, as the adolescent's insulin requirements will increase rapidly.

Adolescence is a difficult time in all families, when dynamics may change and adolescent conflicts and rebellion add to the stress. Parents and adolescents need support at this time to prevent major problems being manifested in the control of diabetes. Baum & Kinmouth (1985) noted that 'effective care of the adolescent with diabetes must involve attention to emotional and social factors as well as to insulin, diet and exercise'. The adolescent must be encouraged to carry identification cards and glucose tablets in case of hypoglycaemia, to keep alcohol consumption to a reasonable level, and to eat sensibly – things which few of their peer group may seem to have to do. Many adolescents with a chronic medical problem have low self esteem and this is aggravated if there is a major problem with management. Weight gain because of inappropriate insulin management may lead to a poor body image. Parental concerns reflect the anxieties of all families, but the parents of the adolescent with diabetes have extra considerations at these times. It may be useful to consider

introducing them to the Youth Diabetes Group, part of the BDA.

Conclusion

All children and families living with a chronic condition such as diabetes need continuing emotional support, as it is with them daily. They may experience all the usual stresses and strains of life and these can affect metabolic control. The overall aim is to provide care which will enable the child to gain increasing independence and become a secure, stable, young adult who has learned to live to the full, with their diabetes. To achieve this the nurse must work closely with the family and must highlight resources that are available to provide suitable support (Fig. 20.2), including that offered by the BDA which has specific sections for its younger members such as Tadpoles for toddlers, YD for adolescents.

NURSING CARE OF THE CHILD WITH A THYROID GLAND DISORDER

Thyroid gland disorder may be congenital due to failure in the development of the thyroid gland in utero, or it may be acquired in later childhood as a result of an abnormality of the immune system resulting in enlargement of the gland (goitre) and loss of thyroid function. Secondary hypothyroidism may be caused by failure of the pituitary gland to secrete thyroid stimulating hormones necessary for the production of thyroxine.

Nursing assessment

Early diagnosis of congenital hypothyroidism is provided by a national screening programme which measures thyroxine and thyroid stimulating hormones by a heel prick taken when babies are 4–6 days old. If undetected parents may report the baby is excessively sleepy, a poor feeder, constipated or jaundiced. They may also have noticed jaundice. If it occurs later in life the onset is gradual and may only be noticed on routine screening and evidence of diminishing yearly growth. This slow progress makes the diagnosis particularly difficult and

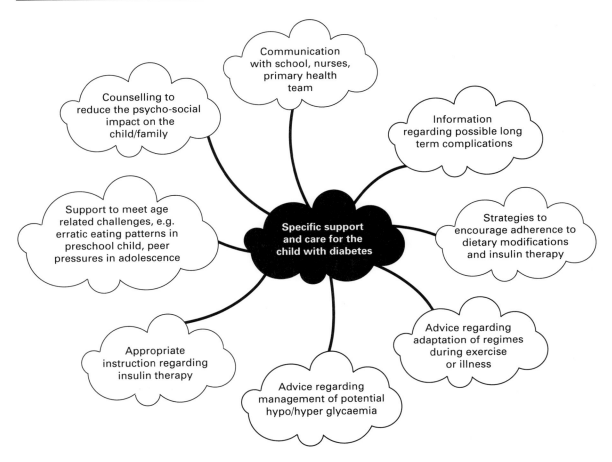

Fig. 20.2 Specific support and care considerations for the child with diabetes.

results in frustration for the family. Other features include lethargy, weight gain, poor tolerance to the cold, dry skin, coarse hair, and reduced mental ability.

Nursing intervention: meeting the child's needs

The main aim of care is to achieve an optimal level of thyroxine whilst encouraging compliance with oral therapy. The expected outcomes of successful intervention will encourage optimal growth, intelligence and independent life. The nurse should offer reassurance to parents and children who may find the diagnosis difficult to understand, especially if there are no tangible signs. Explanatory literature highlighting the aims of

treatment should be provided for the family and this can be supported by giving the family opportunities to discuss their fears and anxieties with nursing and medical staff. Families may wish to meet other families who have coped with the condition, and they should be made aware of possible changes in behaviour after commencement of the treatment.

Both parents and children require a clear understanding of the medication that their child needs; this is important in terms of dosage and repeat prescriptions. Effective liaison with the GP reduces the risks associated with over and underprescription/medication. The nurse needs to discuss the signs of over and undertreatment with the parents; this is vital if early detection of problems is to occur. Overtreatment presents an increased irritability, weight loss and tremors, and undertreatment is demonstrated by constipation, dry skin and lethargy and poor school performance.

Follow up is essential and treatment will be adjusted as necessary according to the clinical response and blood levels. If there are problems of adherence, these may be minimized by education and the encouragement of self management of medication. It is important to ensure that children are aware of the need to inform other carers of the problems associated with this disorder. The child's long term prognosis is generally good but much will depend on the age at onset and advances to treatment, and as this is a lifelong condition the importance of this cannot be overemphasized. Hypothyroidism used to result in mental deficiency but due to early detection through the national screening programmes, children can grow to achieve optimal physical and mental development.

NURSING CARE FOR THE CHILD WITH PRECOCIOUS PUBERTY

Precocious puberty is a disorder of the pituitary gland and the hormonal changes which occur at puberty are the key to understanding the altered function (Tanner 1978). Precocious puberty is indicated by the onset of sexual characteristics such as breast development and growth of pubic hair in girls less than 8 years old and boys less than nine years old (Fry & Stanhope 1992). This occurs due to early stimulation of the ovaries and testes. True precocious puberty occurs when there is excessive stimulation from the hypothalamus/pituitary glands, whereas precocious pseudopuberty occurs when there is excessive sex steroid secretion, for example as a result of a cyst or adrenal gland tumour.

Nursing assessment

The nurse needs to be particularly sensitive when conducting an assessment, to avoid distressing or embarrassing the child. The nurse may also need to adopt an advocacy role and ensure all staff involved in caring for and particularly those involved in examining the child are scrupulous in maintaining the child's dignity. Photographs are often taken for medical records and permission for this potentially intrusive act should be negotiated with the child and family. Overall the child will show evidence of rapid growth (advanced bone age), pubic hair, breast development and development of genitalia. Confirmation of the suspected diagnosis is made by comprehensive assessment and investigations. Bone age is determined by radiography which shows the bones as having an advanced appearance. The luteinising hormone releasing hormone (LHRH) test assesses if there is excessive production of luteinising hormone (LH) and follicle stimulating hormone (FSH). Additionally, an ultrasound of uterus and ovaries is performed, as is a brain CT scan.

Nursing intervention: meeting the child's needs

One of the main nursing aims will be to provide psychological support whilst the child accepts medical treatment to arrest puberty and decrease the rate of bone maturation until a more appropriate time. Many of these children feel alone and are teased by their peers because of their height. They may become prone to mood swings and may use their physical strength to gain attention, culminating in furthering their isolation.

Oral medication such as cyproterone acetate will be given to prevent the oestrogen and testosterone stimulating the tissues. Children with severe bone advancement may be prescribed Zoladex (Goserelin), a long acting gonadotrophin analogue to prevent stimulation of the hypothalmus. This in turn prevents the pituitary secretion of gonadotrophins. These products are not formally licensed for use in children, but are the preferred treatment and are well established in most paediatric endocrine centres. There are few documented side effects, but parents should be warned that compliance with the subcutaneous depot injection schedule must be achieved otherwise a stimulation rather than a suppressive effect may result. The injections are administered every three to four weeks. Trials are currently being carried out to ascertain whether giving growth hormone will increase the final height attained in adulthood.

A careful explanation should be given to parents, and children should be encouraged not to think of themselves as abnormal but rather that their 'body clock has been turned on too soon'. Time should be spent with the parents so they can express their worries. They should be informed of their child's predicted height, which after being extremely tall for a child may be surprisingly small for an adult. Normal fertility is usually achieved and side effects of treatment may include headaches, acne and menstrual spotting.

The nurse's role in the community should include education of the GP and practice nurse on the administration of the subcutaneous implant. The nurse must emphasize to the parents, school teachers and others that they should remember to treat the child to age not size. Parents and children should be advised to select clothes which do not emphasize the child's development. The nurse has a major role in maintaining contact with the child and their family and being involved in the child's follow up. Frequent follow up must be maintained to assess the progress of development, hormone levels, bone age, psychological problems and the family's coping ability.

NURSING CARE OF THE CHILD WITH GROWTH HORMONE DEFICIENCY

A consistent growth pattern is recognized as a reliable indicator of good health in children, but the range of normality for both height and weight is wide so it should not be assumed that children of short stature have abnormal growth. Growth is a complex process influenced by many factors including: heredity, constitutional growth delay, medication, congenital disorders, delayed puberty, nutrition, childhood illness, psychosocial factors, and endocrine disorders. Growth is most dramatic during the first year of life and should continue at a steady but declining rate until the child reaches puberty (Table 20.6) (Tanner 1978). Following a rapid pubertal growth spurt and sexual maturity, adult height will be attained.

Growth hormone may be completely absent or pro-

Table 20.6 Average growth rates: birth–puberty.

Age	cm per year
Birth to 1 year	18 to 25 cm per year
1 to 2 years	10 to 13 cm per year
2 years to puberty	5 to 6 cm per year
Puberty	
girls average age 11 years	6 to 15 cm per year
boys average age 13 years	6 to 15 cm per year

duced in inadequate amounts, and deficiency may result from a number of causes (Table 20.7). This may be an isolated deficit due to deficiencies of thyroid stimulating hormone, adrenocorticotrophic hormone, luteinising hormone, and follicle stimulating hormone.

Nursing assessment

The child may have a height velocity of less than 5 cm per year, delayed bone age, normal body proportions, increased skin fold thickness, small penis/genitalia, and fat around the waistline.

Children's nurses have an important role to play in routine monitoring of growth and assessment of growth disorders (Henry 1992). They also provide an important link between parents and endocrinologists when children need referral for growth evaluation. As mentioned previously, not all short children have hypopituitarism and growth needs to be assessed by looking at the child's height, the parents' height, medical history, social history, physical examination, bone age, chromosomal analysis (to exclude Turner's syndrome), and routine blood screening, e.g. haemoglobin, urea and creatinine.

Table 20.7 Some causes of growth hormone deficiency.

Congenital	Acquired	Transient
Hereditary, midline developmental defects	Primary tumours of hypothalamus, e.g. craniopharyngioma, irradiation, injury	Psychosocial, hypothyroidism Prepubertal

Testing for growth hormone deficiency will be carried out when other possible causes of short stature have been eliminated. Growth hormone secretion varies during the day and levels increase in 'spurts' throughout the night while the child is asleep. Sometimes investigations are carried out at night. However these tests are potentially hazardous and therefore it is recommended they are undertaken in centres where experienced staff and emergency resuscitation equipment are available in case of hypoglycaemia.

Stimulation of pituitary secretion may be assessed following the administration of insulin, glucagon, clonidine or arginine (Hughes 1986) (Insley 1992). When panhypopituitarism is suspected, provided there is no adrenocorticotrophic hormone (ACTH) deficiency, combined pituitary function tests will be performed using the above, as well as thyroid releasing hormone and luteinising release hormone. The child and family should be given full explanations of these tests as they involve venepuncture which can be very distressing for the child. The aim is for the child to reach acceptable adult height and achieve sexual development. In order to achieve this aim the nurse has a role in supporting and educating the family to aid compliance with treatment. Compliance reflects how well the child accepts the treatment and their level of understanding (Smith *et al.*, 1993).

Nursing intervention: meeting the child's needs

Relevant literature must be provided for the child and family and recommended sources include the Child Growth Foundation, specialist endocrine growth centres and drug companies. The nurses should provide emotional support and advice for the family and child. All carers can be encouraged to treat the child according to their age and not their height. Growth hormone is given weekly or in divided doses daily, subcutaneously using one of the many different devices available. Each child and family should be assessed individually, by a suitably qualified nurse, to enable them to develop the necessary skills. Sometimes specialist endocrine nurses are available to support and train others in the management of the care, including community staff, ward staff and practice nurses. If thyroxine and cortisol replacements are necessary both the parents and child must be provided with information about management. Lamont (1992) discussed considerations during holiday times,

including equipment and refrigeration of the growth hormones.

Gondatrophin deficiency may require the induction of puberty and this should be co-ordinated so as to be as close as possible to the usual time of puberty. The natural process should be initiated by a gradual build up of oestrogen and testosterone and should be continued to maintain sexual development and function. Fertility may be possible and it is important that teenagers are referred to adult endocrinologists so this can be discussed fully and other referrals made. It is important that parents feel confident that advice is readily available. Children often have dental problems and should be seen regularly by the dentist, who must be aware of the possible problems associated with the condition. Appropriate support must be provided for the parents, children and siblings and this should demonstrate an understanding of their specific problems.

Children and families need advice and support to facilitate their adjustment to the child's short stature. Advice needs to be available to the families so that they do not feel isolated or different and it should be supportive and practical for their individual needs. Some principles can be applied in terms of what parents and their child may want to know (Table 20.8).

Growth disorders can be associated with a low self esteem and under achievement. During the first year, three-monthly assessments of height and weight are required. Subsequent follow up should be six-monthly as the replacement therapy dosage is calculated on body weight and therefore it increases with growth and development. Paediatric growth centres usually facilitate shared care with GPs, paediatric community nurses, and district nurses.

NURSING CARE OF THE CHILD WITH ADDISON'S DISEASE

This is a disorder of the adrenal cortex which results in a deficiency of glucocorticoids and aldosterone. Primary failure of the cortices may be the result of atrophy of the glands, of infection, or of neoplasm. Secondary hypofunction occurs as a consequence of hypopituitarism due to a deficiency of adrenocorticotrophic hormone (ACTH). Table 20.9 summarizes the child's problems associated with deficiency of glucocorticoids and aldosterone.

Table 20.8   Issues that may need discussing with the child with short stature and their family.

- Being short does not mean a child is less intelligent than their peers.
- Listen to the fears and worries of your child and avoid conveying your own anxieties. Short stature may not be affecting their lives as much as you think.
- Encourage your child to ask their own questions in clinic. This will help others to treat him/her according to age not size.
- A short child often behaves more appropriately for their apparent age than for their actual age. This must be discouraged and they should be expected to perform tasks within the home appropriate to their age.
- Reduce the impact of short stature by having a lower bed or positioning the mirrors at a suitable level.
- Being small often means your child may have difficulty finding suitable clothes. Suggest they buy clothes that their friends might wear, and alter them to fit. Allow them to choose.
- Encourage the young person to follow the 'fads' which their friends are following, so they do not feel isolated.
- Dressing themselves may be difficult but they should be encouraged to try even if it takes longer, although a helping hand is fine.
- Be aware of problems such as lack of friends, preference to mix with younger children, destructive behaviour, isolation, immature behaviour and reluctance to go to school. Sometimes parents may feel they have failed if the problems do not improve and they may need to be reminded that time is available if they wish to discuss their concerns.
- Teachers and siblings can be very helpful and supportive. Teachers need to be made aware of the diagnosis and should then encourage the child to join in as much as possible. Sport is an area when they are seen to be too small but they should still be encouraged to take part. The teacher should also be alert to bullying.
- Sibling rivalry may occur but generally children of short stature find their brothers and sisters very supportive. It is important to involve and encourage the siblings so they do not become jealous of the attention their short brother or sister may receive.
- Ask your child to identify their personal qualities, e.g. humour, kindness, good looks, and enable them to realise inner development is more important than outer growth.

Table 20.9   Problems associated with Addison's disease.

The child's problems associated with	
Deficiency of glucocorticoids	Deficiency of aldosterone
Hypoglycaemia between meals	Reduced reabsorption of sodium by renal tubules leading to loss of water and sodium
Anorexia, vomiting and diarrhoea	
Hyperpigmentation (ACTH)	Increased reabsorption of potassium by renal tubules leading to hyperkalaemia
Lack of energy	
Reduced ability to cope with mild stress, slight injury, extreme temperatures and emotional problems	Acidosis may occur because of abnormal exchange of hydrogen and sodium ions in the kidneys

Nursing assessment

The nurse needs to assess not only the physical effects of the problem but also the emotional and mental impact that it has on the child and their family. The nurse will aim to provide education and support for the family and encourage compliance with oral medication of cortisol and fludrocortisone in order to alleviate the problems. Assessment of the degree of compliance/adherence and/ or the reasons for nonadherence is an important aspect of the nurse's role.

Nursing intervention: meeting the child's needs

The nurse should be responsible for the holistic care of the child. It is important that the family understand the need for maintaining treatment with cortisol and flu- drocortisone; these should be taken at mealtimes to avoid gastric irritation. The family need to be informed about the adverse effects of treatment, e.g. increased fat or oedema, hyperglycaemia and increased risk of infec- tion, as well as signs of inadequate treatment, e.g. nausea, vomiting, anxiety, weakness and gastric upset.

They must be aware of the need for a high carbohydrate diet, including snacks, to prevent hypoglycaemia, and should discuss management of illness and stress, when medication may need to be increased. Other carers should be informed of the diagnosis and the child should wear a medic alert necklace or bracelet outlining the treatment. Body image is often poor and emotional support is required (Paton & Brown 1991).

Regular follow up in outpatients is required to assess the effect of treatment by blood analysis and bone age, and to reinforce information and give education and advice where needed. Ongoing education and support needs to be available from the nurse.

NURSING CARE OF THE CHILD WITH CUSHING'S DISEASE

Excessive production of adrenal corticosteroids may be caused by primary dysfunction of the adrenal cortex (neoplasm or adenoma) or by hypersecretion of ACTH due to pituitary tumour (Table 20.10).

Table 20.10 Child's problems associated with Cushing's disease.

Child's problems associated with		
Increased glucocorticoids	**Increased mineral corticoids**	**Increased sexual development**
hyperglycaemia	electrolyte and fluid imbalance	precocious sexual development
muscle wasting	hypernatraemia	
weakness	water retention	
increased deposition of fat on face and trunk	hypokalaemia	
round, bloated face	hypertension	
purple striae on thigh, abdomen, buttocks	alkalosis	
osteoporosis		
recurrent infections (suppressed lymphocytes)		

Nursing intervention: meeting the child's needs

The main aims of care are associated with education and support of the child and family to reduce anxiety, and preparation for any surgery, minimizing the problems. The family must be given the opportunity to discuss the diagnosis and treatment, which includes surgery. The child must be provided with the opportunity to discuss their feelings about their body image and the diagnosis.

Preparation for surgery should include correction of electrolyte imbalance, assessment of normal blood pressure, physiotherapy, reduction in sodium intake, and explanation of aftercare including possible side affects – Addison's disease.

The child must be encouraged to carry identification and notification of treatment.

NURSING CARE OF THE CHILD WITH CONGENITAL ADRENAL HYPERPLASIA

This is an inherited disorder which causes an enzyme deficiency (commonly 21-hydroxylase), resulting in the inability of the adrenal glands to produce cortisol in the desired amounts. This leads to increased ACTH secretion and excessive production of androgens. There are two types, both caused by an autosomal recessive gene: nonsodium losers with cortisol deficiency, and sodium losers with cortisol and aldosterone deficiency.

Nursing assessment

Before birth the excess androgens stimulate the growth of genitalia. This is more obvious in females, as it causes the external genitalia to look male in appearance. Males do not have distinctive signs of raised androgen levels and therefore they may not be detected at birth, although increased pigmentation of the genitalia may be evident. A newborn male who is losing sodium may present with vomiting, poor weight gain, poor feeding and electrolyte imbalance; it can be life threatening. Older male children who are not losing sodium may present with rapid growth and precocious sexual

development. Diagnosis is made by measuring 17-hydroxy progesterone and androgens in the blood and steroids in the urine.

The idea of replacing adrenal hormones is to provide the body with the ability to maintain normal energy and electrolyte balance, and to produce maximum growth potential, sexual maturation at the normal time and fertility in later life.

Nursing intervention: meeting the child's needs

Early diagnosis and treatment is crucial for both girls and boys. Those not losing sodium require cortisol replacement (hydrocortisone). Those losing sodium need cortisol replacement and a synthetic form of aldosterone (fludrocortisone). A careful explanation should be given to parents, including reassurance that the steroid therapy is only to replace the body's deficit.

Abnormal female genitalia will require surgery as an infant, usually once the child is out of nappies, and possibly reconstruction in later life. The seriousness of cortisol therapy must be explained to the parents, making them aware of side effects, signs of under-dosage, requirements during illness, need for compliance and carrying identification. There is a one in four chance of future babies being affected and antenatal diagnosis is available. Parents should be offered genetic counselling. Blood cortisol levels need to be monitored regularly to assess the effectiveness of care in order to identify the need for adjustment of treatment; additionally bone age needs to be monitored to evaluate progress.

NURSING CARE OF THE CHILD WITH A METABOLIC DISORDER

Metabolism describes the numerous complex chemical reactions which occur continuously within the body. A metabolic disorder results when the balance of one of these reactions is disturbed, and causes observable symptoms. This happens when there is an insufficiency or malfunction of an enzyme. The defect or block in the metabolic pathway causes an accumulation of some chemicals on one side and a lack of others.

There are many inherited metabolic disorders (IMD) and the presentation, age of onset, treatment and outcome of the individual disorders vary considerably (Table 20.11). Awareness and research into IMD is expanding on a worldwide basis and those children affected form a large group requiring paediatric care. Each disorder is comparatively rare (some very rare) and when a child is diagnosed it is important to provide current information about the specific diagnosis. Nurses must identify if they have sufficient knowledge to support the family (Fig. 20.3) and if not, must recognize where to get help and advice, such as from a regional screening advice service.

Parent support groups

Rare disorders leave parents feeling isolated and anxious. The nurse has a part to play in introducing them to relevant support groups, which will present an opportunity for the child and family to meet others with similar problems. These include the Research Trust for Metabolic Diseases, and the National Society for Phenylketonuria. Groups provide social support and a forum for the exchange of ideas to overcome difficulties. Many groups are now organized on a national and international basis, and arrange educational conferences for families and health professionals, while others are involved with the organization and funding of research projects.

Table 20.11 Inherited metabolic diseases, presentation and age of onset.

Detection	Inherited metabolic disease	Age
Screening (presymptomatic)	Phenylketonuria, cystic fibrosis, sickle cell anaemia	first two weeks of life
Acute presentation	Galactosaemia, methylmalonic aciduria, medium chain acetyl CoA dehydrogenase deficiency, tyrosinaemia type 1	usually first two years of life
Chronic presentation	Batten's disease, Niemann Pick C disease, metachromatic leucodystrophy, Tay Sach's disease	infancy to adolescence

Implications for the family of a child with an inherited metabolic disorder (IMD)

As these are inherited disorders families should be referred to a consultant geneticist for counselling (Harper 1993). There are many other implications for the family and nurses should encourage them to discuss their anxieties. A number of specific aspects need to be considered (Fig. 20.4).

Decisions about future children will be affected by a number of considerations including the personal, ethical and religious views of individual families. The severity of the disorder, the treatment, its outcome and the problems of caring for another affected child should also be discussed with parents to help them make informed decisions about future pregnancies.

NURSING CARE OF THE CHILD WITH PHENYLKETONURIA

Phenylketonuria (PKU) is an autosomal recessively inherited metabolic disorder in which there is a deficiency of the liver enzyme phenylalanine hydroxylase. This leads to a build up of phenylalanine and without treatment the high levels of phenylalanine lead to irreversible neurological damage. This adverse effect is prevented by limiting the intake of phenylalanine, using lifelong dietary therapy.

In the UK, since the Department of Health recommendations (1969) screening for PKU is provided as part of a national screening programme. All babies are offered the Guthrie test on the sixth to tenth day of life to check for PKU and congenital hypothyroidism. The

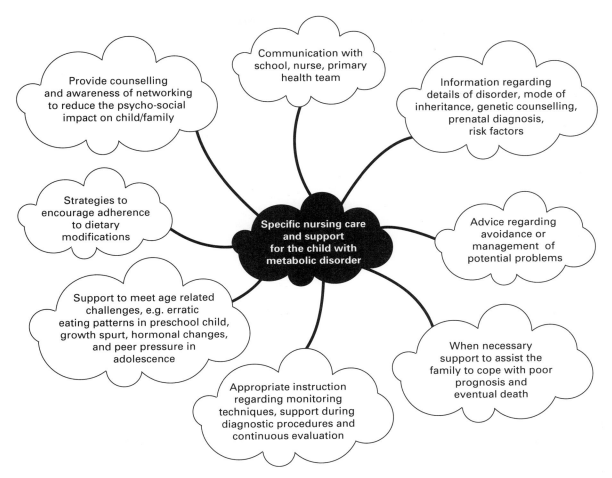

Fig. 20.3 Specific nursing support and care considerations for the child with a metabolic disorder.

tests are done from a simple heel prick capillary blood sample, usually taken by the community midwife. The baby should have been on full milk feeds for 72 hours prior to the test. If not on milk feeds a sample should still be taken to test for congenital hypothyroidism and a repeat specimen taken for PKU when appropriate feeding has been established. A positive screening test will show a greatly elevated level of phenylalanine > 1200 µmol/l (normal range 30–70 µmol/l), an essential amino acid present in all natural protein. The result is available within a few days of sampling. Early diagnosis is dependent on the blood test because there are no signs in the first few weeks of life. Following a positive blood test, a repeat sample is taken to confirm diagnosis and establish the current plasma phenylala-

nine level. This will have risen and may be as high as 2000–3000 µmol/l.

During pregnancy phenylalanine is transported to the fetus via the placenta. Therefore it is important for the mother to have a low plasma phenylalanine of 50–200 µmol/l preconceptually and during pregnancy to optimize outcome (MRL 1993). It is unlikely that her children would have PKU unless her partner is a carrier, but a high concentration of plasma phenylananine could harm the developing fetus.

Priority must be given to parental and family support, which in this case will include genetic counselling. The nurse's role involves education and support within the home and community. Dietary changes are required to reduce the plasma phenylalanine levels and maintain

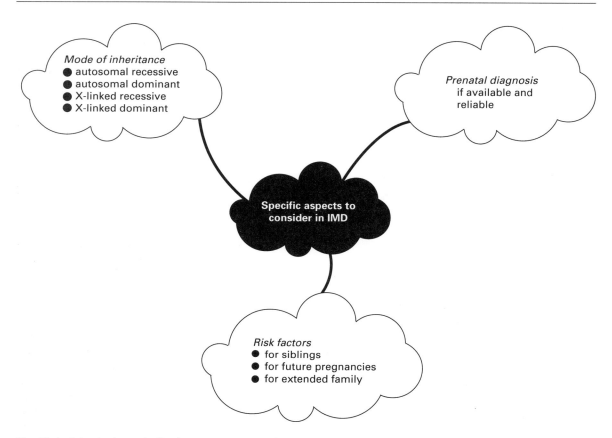

Fig. 20.4   Inherited metabolic diseases: aspects to be considered.

them at 100–250 μmol/l (Table 20.12). Parents are taught to take capillary blood samples to monitor phenylalanine levels and must be reassured of the efficacy of the treatment. Compliance with long term treatment is always a challenge and the nurse must be responsible for the education of the children as they get older, ensuring that they understand the importance of the management of their condition. Adolescent girls must also be informed of the importance of correct management pre conceptually and during pregnancy.

Nursing intervention: meeting the child's needs

Parents will need a careful explanation about the blood tests leading to diagnosis as often there are no obvious clinical signs. The provisional diagnosis may be explained by the community midwife, health visitor or a clinical nurse specialist, where available. The nurse must have a clear understanding of the implications, to reassure parents and to answer questions. Parents will often be concerned and aspects will be related to poor knowledge of the condition, perceptions that untreated the disorder causes mental retardation, alterations in their baby's feeding regime, anxieties about effectiveness of treatment, the need to carry out frequent blood tests and risks to future children.

Ideally a multiprofessional team is involved in the care of the child with PKU, consisting of a consultant paediatrician, paediatric dietician, clinical nurse specialist (CNS) and biochemist. This may obviate the need for admission to hospital, with the baby being seen as an outpatient and home visits being undertaken by the clinical nurse specialist.

Table 20.12 provides guidelines on phenylalanine

Table 20.12 Blood phenylalanine monitoring.

Age	Frequency	Recommended levels μmols/l
Until level stable	2–3 times weekly	100–350
up to 5 years	weekly	100–350
5–10 years	fortnightly	100–450
10 years +	monthly	ideally 100–450 and up to 700
Preconception	weekly	50–200
During pregnancy	twice weekly	50–200

levels (Medical Research Council 1993). More frequent sampling is necessary if unacceptably high or low levels are detected. Sampling more than three times weekly is generally unhelpful as phenylalanine levels need one to two days to stabilize after dietetic changes. Ideally they should be done in the early morning or, if this is not possible, at the same time every day.

Carrying out the blood tests is usually stressful for parents and requires a planned teaching programme. This should be provided at a rate and time to suit the individual family and should include discussing the parents' wishes, and encouraging parents to observe the technique on several occasions. Providing parents with clear written instructions, support with setting up the equipment, and collecting samples under the supervision of the nurse are all vital in the early stages of the programme. On-going support and advice for problems and anxieties, and information regarding changing to thumb or finger pricks when the child is one to two years old, are important. Nurses should ensure that a record sheet is provided to record phenylalanine levels.

The dietician will advise the parents of the immediate dietary changes and will discuss the principles of the lifelong low protein diet. The following factors are involved in reducing the plasma phenylalanine level and ensuring a nutritionally complete diet.

Meat, fish, cheese, eggs and nuts are rich in protein and are omitted from the diet. Phenylalanine, an essential amino acid, is provided using small amounts of natural protein. A 50 mg phenylalanine exchange system is introduced, initially using breast or formula milk. After weaning, the exchanges are given as precisely weighed amounts of certain foods, e.g. cereals, potatoes, sprouts, and baked beans. Dietary scales

which weigh in 5 g increments must be used. A protein substitute is given providing all the other amino acids essential to growth and development, e.g. Analog XP, and Minafen.

It is important to ensure that vitamin and mineral intake, and calorie intake, are adequate, although some protein supplements include added vitamins and minerals. In babies this is achieved by breast or formula milk and the protein supplement. After weaning, other foods will include permitted fruit and vegetables, prescribable low protein foods such as bread, biscuits and flour, and prescribable high calorie products such as Duocal, Calogen and Maxijul. A child's tolerance to phenylalanine varies and the dietician will adjust the intake until the plasma phenylalanine level is acceptable and stable.

Although the nurse must be aware of the dietary implications when providing advice and support to the family, the precise regime is the responsibility of the dietician.

There may be difficulties in supervising the child with PKU because the low protein diet is very restrictive and it may not be immediately obvious when the child has deviated from the strict regime (Table 20.13). It is important that all family members, carers and school staff understand the dietary principles and that permitted foods are readily available. Food refusal is common in the toddler age group and they may use this as a weapon, compounding the anxiety for the parents. It is important that the older child is allowed to feel as much like their peers as possible. Current recommendations are for lifelong dietary therapy (MRC 1993). The nurse should be aware that expert advice is available from specialist centres and should develop good links with them.

Table 20.13 Management of problems.

Factors that lead to high phenylalanine levels	Strategies to increase compliance
Eating incorrect foods	
in error	Educate child/parents/carers.
child's curiosity about other foods	Educate child, keep unsuitable foods out of reach.
adolescent rebellion	Continue education and counselling.
Eating an excess of exchange foods	
in error	As above.
easily accessible	Educate and keep foods out of reach of young children.
scales (broken or not used)	Replace broken scales, remind child/parents of need for accurate weighing of exchanges.
Not drinking sufficient protein supplement	Supplement is unpleasant to taste; advise on flavouring, temperature, fun cups and straws.
Insufficient calories	Introduce new low protein foods, recipes, cookery advice. Calorie supplements.
Illness – causing catabolism	Small, high calorie protein free drinks. Exchanges as milk. Return to diet as soon as possible. Consult dietician if illness persists more than a few days.
Factors that lead to low phenylalanine levels	**Strategies to increase compliance**
During growth spurts	Increase exchanges only under instruction of dietician.
Not taking all exchanges	Advise on variety of foods.

NURSING CARE OF THE CHILD WITH MEDIUM CHAIN ACETYL CoA DEHYDROGENASE (MCAD) DEFICIENCY

MCAD is the enzyme which is deficient in this inborn error of fatty acid oxidation, and it affects fasting tolerance. It is a disorder of acute metabolic onset. It is an autosomal recessively inherited disorder and potentially life threatening. Fatty acids, present in muscle and other tissues, are long term energy sources. They are utilized when glucose supplies are depleted, and ketosis occurs when they are in excess. Ketones are necessary to provide the brain with its only nonglucose energy source. In MCAD deficiency the lack of enzyme prevents the utilization of fatty acids as an energy source. Symptoms present after a period of fasting, often characteristically associated with an intercurrent illness.

Nursing assessment

The child may experience problems any time between birth and adulthood, but usually before two years of age. Prior to this diagnosis parents may report episodes of lethargy with persistent vomiting, often occurring after periods of fasting. There may also be a history of neonatal deaths or unexplained illnesses. More significant symptoms may be precipitated by an intercurrent illness, which is associated with a limited calorie intake. These include nonketotic hypoglycaemia, with symptoms of poor feeding, sweating, tremors, lethargy, hypotonia, tachypnoea or apnoea. Hypoglycaemia may lead to convulsions or coma. Presentation may be associated with signs of encephalopathy.

Low blood glucose on BM stix (< 4 mmol/1) should be checked by laboratory tests; urine tests for ketones are likely to be negative. All checks should be done at a time of illness as they may return to normal when the child is well. Additionally specific laboratory based investigations are undertaken (Green *et al.* 1994).

Nursing intervention: meeting the child's needs

Aims of care include a rapid correction of hypoglycaemia to avoid neurological complications. A regular eating pattern must be introduced to avoid periods of fasting and prevent hypoglycaemia. An essential part of the nursing care includes the appropriate education of the child who must understand the importance of crisis prevention, and of the parents who must seek early medical advice when the child is unwell.

Children in a coma or with encephalopathic signs will require intensive therapy management and care. On admission intravenous dextrose will be given to correct the hypoglycaemia. Parental support is important as they see their child acutely ill and will be anxious about possible neurological complications of hypoglycaemia. These concerns may be exacerbated because of a family history of unexplained infant deaths.

After the initial crisis the care required to avoid further hypoglycaemia should be discussed with the family. A feeding pattern should be introduced to prevent periods of fasting. The nurse must be able to provide guidance and education about the recognition, management and treatment of hypoglycaemia, so that appropriate action can be taken when the child is unwell. The parents should be advised that if the blood glucose is less than 4 mmol/1 the child should be given a glucose drink and the test repeated after 30 minutes. If the level is still below 4 mmol/1 then urgent medical advice must be sought. Although initially distressing for the family, the parents may be taught to monitor blood glucose using a planned teaching programme which includes written instructions and advice. The nurse must be confident that parents are able to carry out the procedure competently and that they know the significance of the results and the actions to take.

The successful management of MCAD deficiency is dependent on the child developing a lifelong eating pattern which avoids long periods of fasting, and an ability to self-monitor blood glucose. Parental anxiety about further episodes of hypoglycaemia may cause them to become overprotective of their child and to give them food in excessive amounts and/or frequency. The same anxiety may lead parents to undertake unnecessary blood glucose monitoring to reassure themselves, even though the child appears well; or during periods of illness, when a child may require carbohydrate supplements due to low blood glucose, parents may be overzealous in their testing. Advice and reassurance can help the family overcome these problems.

NURSING THE CHILD WITH TAY SACH'S DISEASE – INFANTILE FORM

This is a neurometabolic storage disorder of chronic onset caused by a deficiency of the enzyme hexosaminidase A (hexA). It is a progressive disorder and the child usually dies by three to five years of age. No curative treatment is currently available. Lipid molecules are found in all body cells. The deficiency of the enzyme (hexA) causes a breakdown in the metabolism of part of the lipid molecule. This leads to an accumulation of the lipid GM(2) ganglioside within nerve cells, predominantly in the grey matter of the brain, damaging them irreparably.

Tay Sach's is an autosomal recessively inherited disorder. There is a high incidence in the Ashkenazi Jewish population, where one in 30 people are estimated to be carriers. About one in 250 of the general population are carriers. Testing is available for carrier status and prenatal diagnosis (Harper 1993).

Although the storage of GM(2) ganglioside begins in the fetus during pregnancy, babies usually develop normally in the early months; the onset of symptoms occurs between four and 12 months of age. An excessive auditory startle reflex may be present for several months before other symptoms develop, but this may often only be noted as part of the history taken, when more significant problems arise.

First indications of these are the slowing down in achieving expected milestones, followed by a loss of previously acquired intellectual and motor skills. As the disease progresses dementia, inappropriate laughter (gelastic fits) and subsequently spastic tetraparesis develop. Blindness occurs due to shortage of the gangliosides within the optic fundus. Seizures are common from the second year of life. An ophthalmic examination reveals the cherry red spot in both macular areas of the optic fundi. This is a characteristic finding in Tay Sach's disease. A blood sample is taken to measure the activity of the enzyme hexosaminidase A. An electroencephalogram (EEG) will be performed if the child is having seizures.

The child's early normal development, with the gradual onset of symptoms, may mean that parents have spent several weeks or months seeking advice and reassurance before being referred to the hospital. They are usually devastated when the seriousness of the diagnosis is explained to them. Unless there is a family history of Tay Sach's disease they will be unprepared for the bleak prognosis. Parents must be told of the diagnosis in privacy and the nurse must provide support and respond sensitively to the needs and questions of parents. The reactions of parents vary and can include shock, anger, disbelief, denial, guilt and grief.

Nursing intervention: meeting the child's needs

The main aim will be to adjust the care in accordance with the child's individual needs to maximize the effects on the child's development and provide a support system for parents and family. The care required will vary according to the child's individual needs so regular assessment of their independence in activities of living may provide a baseline from which to plan a comprehensive care package. The nurse will co-ordinate a multiprofessional approach.

If the child's mobility is limited by hypotonia and spasticity, physiotherapy may be required to prevent contractures and to maximize mobility for as long as possible. The parents can be taught to continue the exercises whilst at home. In order to maximize stimulation and developmental potential, the play specialist will be able to advise on suitable toys. Bright reflective toys will maximize the visual abilities but gradually the child's sight will deteriorate and then toys with sound, texture and smell will be more appropriate.

Often the child will have seizures and medication will be required to control these. Parents should be taught how to calculate the correct dose, the timing of administration and routine of emergency drug techniques to ensure that the drugs prescribed are given safely and competently.

As the blindness, hypotonia and eventual spasticity begin to affect the child they may need special equipment to position them comfortably and safely to allow them to eat, sleep and play. As generation of the child's condition leads to difficulties in eating and drinking, the parents will need advice on the management of feeds and referral to a dietician for nutritional advice. Speech therapists may also be in a prime position to give advice on techniques to promote oral feeding for as long as possible. Eventually feeding by nasogastric tube may be required and the parent will be taught new skills in order to carry out this aspect of care.

In addition to the more physical aspects of care the parents will need support and resources from a range of voluntary and statutory agencies including social services. Parents should be made aware of the various benefits and care allowance available. Effective liaison between the community and hospital services is essential because for the majority of the time the child will be at home. The community nurses need to be aware of adjustments to medication and in turn should discuss with hospital colleagues any problems occurring at home.

Eventually it may be appropriate to raise the option of hospice care. This idea may be emotive for the parents and care should be taken when introducing the concept. The nurse can help the parents discuss their feelings and can refer them for counselling if necessary. It is also important to recognise their spiritual needs and ethical principles or religious practices in order to support them in their decision making.

The care for a child with Tay Sach's disease is complex as no one can predict the duration of the child's life or the full extent of the problems they will encounter. Throughout this episode in their lives the parents should have access to clear written information, the addresses and telephone numbers of support groups who may be able to supply appropriate literature, and the opportunity to contact other parents in a similar situation. Siblings may need counselling as they become aware of the irreversible changes in their brother or sister. They may feel responsible for the illness and may fear that they will develop it later. The nurse has an important role in making the parents aware of the range of resources and support available to them and in co-ordinating care to enable the child and family to maximize independence.

CONCLUSION

A range of dysfunctions have been selected to illustrate the diversity of the problems encountered by a child with altered function of the endocrine and metabolic systems. However, although they are very different and some are extremely rare, they have certain common features. First, they are usually present throughout life and therefore compliance with treatment is essential in order to alleviate or minimize the disabling effects. Second, the aims of care relate to promoting the growth of the child so that they are able to make the transition into young adulthood with the opportunity to live life to the full potential.

Children who experience chronic illness often have a poor self-esteem; hormonal dysfunctions are often obvious and this may alter the child's appearance leading to poor body image. The children require specific skills from their carers (Paton & Brown 1991). This aspect of care is an important part of the nurse's role as educator, supporter and carer. Through the utilization of interpersonal and counselling skills, integrated with knowledge of a child's usual developmental patterns and the psychological impact of illness, the nurse can support the parents through the early stages following diagnosis and can assist the child in coming to terms with their situation and adjusting to adulthood (Scammell 1992).

RESOURCES

Support groups

British Diabetic Association, 10 Queen Anne Street, London WIM OBD. Tel. 0171 323 1531.

Child Growth Foundation, 2 Mayfield Avenue, Chiswick, London W4 1PW. Tel 0181 884 7625.

Thyroid Aplasmia Support Group, Mrs Worthington, 3 Kay Street, Atherton, Manchester M29 9FH. Tel. 01942 874740.

National Society for Phenylketonuria, Mr G. Goff, Worth Cottage, Pickles Hill, Keighley, West Yorkshire BD22 0RR.

Research Fund for Metabolic Diseases in Childhood, Lesley Greene, Golden Gate Lodge, Weston Road, Crewe, Cheshire CW1 1XN. Tel. 01270 250221.

Videos

Neonatal Screening – for general use. *National Screening* – for health professionals. *Phenylketonuria: The Facts* – for parents and children. All produced by the Metabolic Team, Clinical Chemistry Department, Birmingham Children's Hospital, B16 8ET.

Taming the Dragon – for children with diabetes. Available from Novo Nordisk Pharmacy Ltd, Novo Nordisk House, Broadfield Park, Brighton Road, Pease Pottage, Crawley, West Sussex RH11 9RT.

Being Frank – for adolescents with diabetes. Available from Eli Lilley & Co Ltd, Kingsclere Road, Basingstoke, Hampshire RG21 2XA.

Leaflets

Blood Screening Tests for Babies in the United Kingdom. Produced by Metabolic Team, Clinical Chemistry Department, Birmingham Children's Hospital B16 8ET.

Growth Insufficiency and Growth Hormone Therapy – An information booklet for parents and children. Corbi Pharmacia Peptide Hormones DW, Davy Avenue, Knowle Hill, Milton Keynes, Bucks MB5 8PH.

I Have Diabetes – a booklet for children. Dinosaur publication (1992). HarperCollins, London.

What Professional Supervision Should Children with Diabetes and their Families Expect? (1989) British Diabetic Association, 10 Queen Anne Street, London WIM OBD. Tel. 0171 323 1531.

The Child with PKU. National Society for Phenylketonuria, Mr G. Goff, Worth Cottage, Pickles Hill, Keighley, West Yorkshire BD22 0RR.

REFERENCES AND FURTHER READING

Baum, J.D. & Kinmouth, A-L, (1985) *Care of the Child with Diabetes*, pp. 165–9. Churchill Livingstone, Edinburgh.

BDA (1989) *What Professional Support Should Children with*

Diabetes and Their Families Expect? British Diabetic Association, London.

Burden, M. (1994) A practical guide to insulin injections. *Nursing Standard*, 8(29), 25–9.

Cox, S. (1989) Equipped to cope. *Paediatric Nursing*, 1(4), 6–9.

DCCT (1993) The effect of intensive treatment of diabetes on the development and progression of long term complications in insulin-dependent diabetes mellitus. The Diabetes Control and Complications Trial Research Group. *New England Journal of Medicine*, 329, 977–86.

Erikson, E.H. (1980) *Identity and the Life Cycle*. Norton, New York.

Fry, T. (1993) Charting growth: developments in the assessment and measurement of child growth. *Child Health*, 1(3), 104–9.

Fry, V. & Stanhope, R. (1992) *Premature Sexual Maturation*. Child Growth Foundation, London.

Green, A. & Morgan, I. (1994) *Neonatology and Clinical Biochemistry*. ABC Venture Pub, 182–6.

Harper, P.S. (1993) *Practical Genetic Counselling*, 4th edn. Butterworth, London.

Hatcher, T. (1990) Learning is fun. *Paediatric Nursing*, 2(2), 10–12.

Henry, J.H. (1992) Routine monitoring and assessment of growth disorders. *Journal of Paediatric Health Care*, 6(5), 291–301.

Hughes, I.A. (1986) *Handbook of Endocrine Tests in Children*. Wright, Bristol.

Insley, J. (ed) (1992) *A Paediatric Vade-Mecum*. Edward Arnold, London.

Krans, H.M.J., Posta, M. & Keen, H. (ed) (1992 *Diabetes Care and Research in Europe*. The St Vincent Declaration action programme. World Health Organisation, Geneva.

Lamont, G. (1992) Growth disorders and the role of the specialist nurse. *Paediatric Nursing*, 4(8), 23–25.

Mcgrath, G. (1992) Normal diet and diabetes in childhood. *Paediatric Nursing*, 4(20), 19–21.

McEvilly, A. (1991) Home management on diagnosis. *Paediatric Nursing*, 3(5), 16–18.

McEvilly, A. (1993) Childhood diabetes. *Paediatric Nursing*, 5(9), 25–30.

Medical Research Council (1993) Working party report on phenylketonuria. *Archives of Disease in Childhood*, 68, 426–7.

Metcalf, M.A. & Baum, J.D. (1991) Incidence of insulin dependent diabetes in children under 15 years in the British Isles during 1988. *British Medical Journal*, 302, 443–7.

Newton Young, C. (1990) Children with diabetes. *Nursing*, 4(16), 16–19.

Nuffield Council on Bioethics (1993) *Genetic Screening, Ethical Issues*. The Nuffield Foundation, London.

Nutritional sub-committee, British Diabetic Association (1989) Dietary recommendations for children and adolescents with diabetes. *Diabetic Medicine*, 6, 537–47.

Orem, D.E. (1991) *Nursing: Concepts of Practice*, 4th edn. McGraw Hill, New York.

Paton, D. & Brown, R. (1991) *Lifespan Health Psychology*, pp. 127–30. Harper Collins Nursing, London.

Price, B. (1993) Diseases and altered body image in children. *Paediatric Nursing*, 5(6), 18–21.

RCN (1993) The Role and Qualifications of the Nurse Specialising in Childhood Diabetes. Working party report. Royal College of Nursing, London.

Reading, S. (1986a) Blood glucose monitoring: teaching effective techniques. *Professional Nurse*, 2(2), 55–58.

Reading, S. (1986b) Blood glucose monitoring: a tool in managing diabetes. *The Professional Nurse*, 2(1), 9–11.

Scammell, Barbara (1992) *Communication Skills*. Macmillan Press, London.

Smith, S., Hindmarsh, P., Brook, C. (1993) Compliance with Growth Hormone Treatment – Are They Getting It? *Archives of Diseases in Childhood*, 68, 91–3.

Stephenson, A. (1992) Learning for life. *Paediatric Nursing*, 4(3), 6–7.

Swanwick, M. (1990) Development and chronic illness. *Nursing*, 4(16), 24–7.

Tanner, J.M. (1978) *Fetus into Man: Physical Growth from Conception to Maturity*. Open Books, Exeter.

Tomalin, D.A. & Moyer, A. (1990) Diabetic children's skill in blood glucose monitoring. *Practical Diabetes*, 7(6), 262–4.

Worswick, J. (1993) *A House called Helen: the Story of the First Hospice for Children*. Harper Collins, London.

Chapter 21

Nursing Support and Care: Meeting the Needs of the Child and Family with Altered Genito-urinary Function

Maggie Hicklin and Marcelle De Sousa

'I went to a party last night and didn't stop dancing. I usually sit at the side because I am tired, but I joined in for the entire party. I didn't know you could feel like this. I didn't realise that I felt ill until I was better. I used to be the last person in my family to get up every morning and now I am the first. My mum says she can't believe how much energy I've got.'

This extract is from a 10 year old boy who after four years of dialysis finally received a successful renal transplant.

INTRODUCTION

This chapter describes the nursing roles and care of children presenting with common renal problems and will attempt to dispel some of the myths surrounding nephrology. An understanding of renal anatomy and physiology is assumed, although some altered states are briefly described. To appreciate the considerable impact of a renal or urological deficit on the child and family, the nurse must understand the many functions of the kidney particularly in relation to maintaining homeostasis in fluid and electrolyte balance and blood pressure.

In nursing such children the nurse requires the skills of assessment. The ability to assess accurately is critical and the observations necessary and reasons for them are described in detail.

The first section outlines the investigations that the child may experience in order to confirm the diagnosis. An in depth understanding of these will enable the nurse to give accurate advice and preparation to the child and family regarding the processes involved and their role in supporting their child.

The second section discusses the care of a child with a urinary tract infection and considers the role of the nurse in health education. Section three considers the principles of care for the child following renal surgery. The fourth section explores the experience of the child with nephrotic syndrome. The final sections address both acute and chronic renal failure and the principles of dialysis. The latter is less common and usually requires referral to a specialist centre, of which there are thirteen in the UK.

A particular feature of care for many of these children is the close long term relationship between the nurse and the family, and the multi-professional liaison. This involves, not least, dieticians, play specialists, school teachers, psychologists, social workers and pharmacists working together to enhance collaborative care for the family. Communication between home, school, hospital and community is also important to ensure that there is consistency in often complex care regimes.

Overall a major aim of the nurse looking after a child with a renal deficit must be to prevent harm to the child and their kidneys.

NURSING SUPPORT OF THE CHILD REQUIRING INVESTIGATIONS OF THE GENITO-URINARY TRACT

This section outlines many of the investigations which may be performed to assist in the diagnosis of a urinary tract or renal deficit. These 'tests' are potentially distressing for the child and family and it is important that they know what to expect. A nurse who understands the rationale for, and process of, these is better able to provide information for the family, thus reducing the fear, embarrassment, unpleasantness and discomfort.

Apart from the psychological preparation most of the investigations require little direct nursing care and are often performed in an outpatient department (Swallow 1990). The exception is renal biopsy which is discussed in some detail.

Preparing the child and parents for investigations

(Heiney 1991) identifies some strategies which may be employed to enable a child to retain mastery and control. This is of particular relevance when a child has a chronic illness, requiring repeated investigations or invasive procedures. It is suggested that an invasive experience often comprises four aspects: anticipation, preparation, the procedure itself and the aftermath. An assessment which incorporates age and stage of development, language skills, imaginative abilities, the child's personality, attention span and anxiety levels, previous experiences and family situation will provide a sound basis upon which to plan appropriate nursing interventions to support the child and family at each stage of the event. There is an emphasis upon providing information and education to enable the child to make choices, and offering positive reinforcement and relaxation techniques.

Before the investigation it may be helpful to show the child pictures of the equipment and provide opportunities for preparation play. During the investigation, distraction with music or story cassettes can help the younger child, whilst an older child often responds well

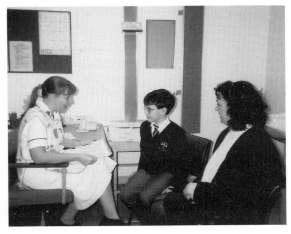

Fig. 21.1 The role of the nurse in providing information for the parents and child.

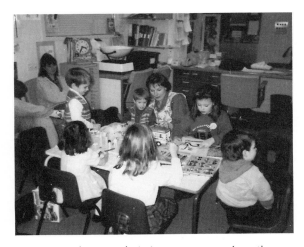

Fig. 21.2 The pre-admission programme in action.

to distracting conversation or to being involved in the procedures; for example, being given a running commentary and being able to identify their own kidneys on the ultrasound screen. The presence of parents is also beneficial.

INVESTIGATIONS OF THE GENITO-URINARY TRACT

Urine specimens

The collection of urine specimens is often an essential part of the assessment of a child with renal or urological deficit. There are three main types of urine specimen needed:

A *spot urine* – for ward testing for blood and protein, for laboratory analysis of chemistry, to identify some tumours and some poisons.

A *timed urine collection* – The bladder must be emptied and the urine discarded. The subsequent urine is then collected and the time of the last specimen noted. The most important factor in collecting a timed urine is that the collection is complete. An accurate 12 hour sample collection may be more useful than a 24 hour collection with a sample missing. The only way to achieve a successful timed urine is to gain the co-operation and understanding of the child and family. An older child may prefer to collect the urine at home rather than in hospital: a notice by the toilet may be helpful to remind the child. In a smaller child, who is not toilet trained, an indwelling urethral catheter may be the only way to achieve an accurate complete timed urine collection. These are important to aid the diagnosis of renal tubular disorders, to aid stone analysis, and to quantify elements such as protein.

A *clean urine specimen* – to enable the diagnosis of a urinary tract infection to be made. A successful clean urine for culture and microscopy is not easy to obtain and can be time consuming. The appropriate method of collection depends on the age of the child. To achieve reliable results the specimen must not be contaminated by the skin or faeces. Sometimes sitting a baby over a dish during feeding is effective.

Supra-pubic aspiration (SPA)

This is the most reliable method of collecting an uncontaminated specimen in a child who is not toilet trained. A needle is inserted through the skin into the bladder and urine aspirated via the syringe. It is traumatic though no more so than venepuncture, and can be aided by ultrasound to ensure the bladder is full and to minimize failed attempts. Careful explanation is required to the parents of the necessity of the test, and gentle, calm but firm handling of the child is needed during the procedure. The parents should be warned that slight haematuria may follow SPA.

Clean catch urine

The vulval area or penis is cleaned with cotton wool or saline. The child is then left without a nappy until micturition when the urine is caught in a sterile pot. This is time consuming but most parents are willing to undertake the responsibility for collecting urine in this manner. A clean catch urine gives reliable results (though not quite as reliable as SPA) and is non-traumatic

Bag urine

This is probably the most common type of urine specimen taken on a children's ward and the most unreliable. There is a high risk of the urine becoming contaminated by the skin flora or faeces. To minimize this risk the skin should be washed and dried with saline and cotton wool, and the bag then carefully applied keeping the urethral meatus and anal region separate. The child should then be left without a nappy so that the bag can be removed the moment urine is passed, minimizing the risk of contamination. However, most children immediately want to play with, or pull off, the bag, and skilful distraction is required.

Midstream urine (MSU)

In a co-operative toilet trained child this is usually successful. The child needs a careful explanation of how to clean the area with cotton wool and saline, to gently retract the foreskin or hold the labia apart during micturition, and to catch the middle of the stream of urine. A younger child will need assistance from a nurse or parent.

Catheter urine

If a child passes urine through a stoma such as a vesicostomy or ileal conduit, the stoma should be catheterized to collect a specimen.

Ultrasound

This is a simple noninvasive examination of the structure of the urinary tract, and can be described to parents as 'like the scan you had in pregnancy'. Ultrasound will help to identify structural abnormality and obstruction of the kidneys and urinary tract.

Micturating cystourethrogram (MCUG)

MCUG is an unpleasant invasive investigation. A urethral catheter is inserted into the child's bladder in the X-ray department, and radio opaque dye instilled via the catheter. The dye is then observed by X-ray during micturition. This will outline the shape of the bladder, show any reflux into the urethra during micturition, and any urethral obstruction. MCUG should be performed under antibiotic cover to minimize the possibility of a subsequent urinary tract infection (e.g. a single dose of gentamycin prior to catheterization).

Urodynamic studies

This is similar to a MCUG but measures pressures within the bladder before, during and after micturition. A pressure probe is inserted into the rectum. Two separate urethral catheters are used.

Diethylalanine triaminepenta acetic acid (DTPA) scan

This is a scan which demonstrates the perfusion of the kidneys. A radioactive isotope is injected intravenously and the kidneys are scanned immediately. The uptake of the isotope is recorded and the perfusion index calculated by computer.

Dimercaptosuccinic acid (DMSA) scan

This is a scan which demonstrates the anatomy and

effective excretion of the kidney. The radioactive isotope is injected and the child is scanned four hours later.

Plain abdominal X-ray

A straight abdominal X-ray is carried out to discover either an abnormality of the spine, e.g. spina bifida, which can affect bladder function, or to look for stones.

X-ray of the hand and wrist

This is done in the case of chronic renal failure to determine bone age and detect any signs of renal osteodystrophy.

The child undergoing a renal biopsy

This usually requires admission to hospital either for the day or overnight. As it is an invasive procedure a consent is required from the parents.

Although the idea of the biopsy is often frightening for the child, parents can be reassured that their child will be sedated and therefore will remember little about the actual procedure. It may be helpful to introduce the family to another who has already undergone a biopsy.

An image of the renal tract will be undertaken to establish the position of the kidney. The kidney is a vascular organ and hence there will be a risk of haemorrhage. Blood will be taken for clotting times and grouping and cross matching. EMLA cream should be applied for an hour and a half prior to venepuncture and over the proposed biopsy site. After taking blood, the intravenous cannula may be secured and used later to administer the sedation thus avoiding the need for successive venepunctures. To minimize the risk of inhalation of gastric contents whilst under sedation, fluids and food will be withheld for two to four hours prior to the investigation.

Pethidine compound is often the drug of choice for sedation. Once drowsy the child is encouraged to lie prone with a roll under the hips to ensure correct positioning. It may be important at this point to reassure the child that they will be given further medication to help them sleep. This is usually in the form of midazolam and diazemols and parents are encouraged to be present until the sedation takes full effect. The sedation may inhibit the effective functioning of the medulla, causing respiratory depression, so oxygen saturation monitoring, oxygen, resuscitation equipment and drugs to reverse the effects of the sedation should be readily available. An intravenous infusion is also commenced.

The biopsy site is infiltrated with lignocaine, the EMLA cream removed, and a trucut biopsy needle is inserted under X-ray and a specimen of renal tissue is obtained for histology.

Whilst post procedure the nurse should decide the frequency of observations, in particular pulse, respirations and biopsy site, based on the child's physiological status, it should be remembered that the kidney is a particularly vascular organ and thus the risk of haemorrhage is great. To minimize this risk bed rest is usually encouraged for about 18–24 hours. Parents should also be forewarned about the risk of haematuria. The maintenance fluids prescribed intravenously are usually continued until the child is drinking and has passed urine.

The biopsy results are generally available 24–48 hours later but some parents, especially if they live a long distance away, may prefer to wait for the result before they go home. It should be remembered that this waiting may seem more traumatic than the biopsy itself as they will often be aware of the possibility of serious disease.

The results should be discussed with the parents by both the doctor and nurse in a quiet and private environment with plenty of time for questions. The decision as to when to involve the child, at the same time as the parents or later, and who should be the first to talk to the child, can only be decided individually. The parents know their child better than anyone else but many ask for advice, not having encountered the situation before. Factors to be considered are the child's age, personality, and previous experience.

NURSING CARE OF THE CHILD WITH A URINARY TRACT INFECTION

Urinary tract infection (UTI) is common, affecting 7% of girls and 1% of boys during childhood (Berry & Chantler 1986). However, approximately 50% of children with UTI who are investigated are found to have a normal urinary tract. The diagnosis of a UTI is made by microscopy and culture of a clean urine specimen. More than 20–30 white cells and a pure growth of more than 100 000 (10s) microlitres of organisms following 24–48 hours culture is regarded as a proven UTI. If the urine specimen was a supra pubic aspiration (SPA) any pure growth of organisms should be regarded as a UTI.

Nursing assessment

Careful nursing assessment of the child is invaluable. The parents may describe the child as 'not quite right' and particular consideration should be given to presence of fever or reports of febrile convulsions or rigors (Lee & Jones 1991). As the hypothalamus is immature in the younger child this is a common response to a rise in temperature. There may also be evidence of irritability, vomiting, poor feeding, failure to thrive, offensive cloudy urine, frequency of miturition or dysuria, lower abdominal pain and groin pain (although the younger the child the greater the challenge of isolating the position of the pain) general malaise/lethargy; babies may draw their knees up to their chest.

An older child may be able to articulate the problem by saying 'it stings when I go to the toilet'. Any child with a serious UTI may be significantly unwell. However, the assessment of a sick baby is not always quantifiable, and the instinct of the mother combined with the observation and handling of the baby by an experienced children's nurse or paediatrician are as important as any other investigation. Urgent attention is needed if a baby or young child is peripherally cold, mottled, pale, tachycardic, hypotensive, and with poor muscle tone, as this may indicate septicaemia.

The aims of care will be related to supporting the child and family during investigations and treatment and providing health education regarding managing the child's temperature and avoiding the reoccurrence of the infection.

Nursing intervention: meeting the child's needs

The care of a child with a UTI is similar as for any other infection. Antipyretic drugs, such as paracetamol, are important, and loose cotton clothing will help to keep the child comfortable. Febrile convulsions do sometimes occur and may be the presenting problem.

Hardman (1990) discovered that parents had limited knowledge of how to cope with a febrile convulsion and 54 out of 89 parents were frightened and brought their child to the Accident and Emergency Department. Educating the parents on the reasons for taking prompt action in the event of pyrexia is essential (Hardman 1990) as this will reduce the incidence. They should be given advice on how to recognize a pyrexia and the steps to take, for example ventilating the room, removing their child's excess clothing, giving additional fluids and paracetamol and monitoring the progress of the temperature to ensure that the child does not become hypothermic. If a fit occurs they should be advised to place their child on its side to maintain a clear airway.

The child may need intravenous antibiotics to treat the infection. An increased fluid intake is advisable if the child is pyrexial to 'flush' the urinary tract and ensure the kidneys remain perfused. If the child is vomiting, or is unable/unwilling to drink, intravenous fluids should be given. The fluid requirement for a six month old baby is 100ml/kg/day. A two year old would require 60ml/kg/day. The child will often look and feel better within 24 hours after starting antibiotics. If the child is not vomiting and able to drink, they can be given oral antibiotics and they should be cared for at home.

Every child with a proven UTI will be investigated for abnormality of the urinary tract. This is done when the child is in optimum health, and can be undertaken as an outpatient. Many families turn this into a treat: a visit to hospital for an unpleasant test, combined with a visit to see the nurses they know, and a trip afterwards into town for a MacDonalds would make it seem like a positive day out.

The frequency of urinary tract infections may be reduced by adequate health education. The nurse can advise on hygiene needs, for example frequent baths and the avoidance of bubble bath and strong soap, and elimination needs especially, allowing adequate time for miturition and cleaning the perineum from front to back afterwards. Finally, the nurse can give advice on fluid intake. Encouraging extra fluids may encourage frequent miturition and reduce stasis of urine in the bladder. Rogers (1991) advocates the drinking of cranberry juice although there is limited scientific basis for this.

NURSING CARE OF THE CHILD UNDERGOING SURGERY OF THE GENITO-URINARY TRACT

A medical diagnosis requiring surgery is often shocking for both the child and parents and the psychological impact should not be underestimated. A sound knowledge of the anatomy of the urinary tract and kidney will enable the nurse to explain the necessity for the surgery and this will often compliment or clarify the information offered by the medical staff. Many parents and children respond well to the suggestion that the problem can be corrected and they can understand that many of these abnormalities may cause stasis of urine which predisposes to infection; this coupled with reflux may increase the risk of impaired renal function.

Although there are many different abnormalities of the renal tract, the principles of nursing before and after surgery are broadly similar. Sometimes, as in post urethral valves, the diagnosis is made antenatally and intra uterine surgery is performed, but usually the surgery is elective and performed later in life.

Nursing intervention: meeting the child's needs

Preparation of the child and the family will begin before admission so that they know what to expect. Pre-operative admission days are useful, as is written information sent to the home. All parents need to know what facilities are available and what to bring on admission (Glasper & Straddling 1989).

When admitted to the ward it is important that the named nurse familiarizes the child and family with the environment and introduces them to other families. A play specialist can be invaluable in using play techniques to explain to the child the expected sequence of events.

Ideas for play preparation
- Books and stories about children in hospital.
- A photo album following a child from admission to discharge showing a theatre gown, anaesthetic room etc., combined with a simple explanation.
- Play box containing equipment such as syringes, bandages, charts, plastic cannula, stethoscope, theatre caps and masks for supervised play.

- Colouring books.
- Videos.
- Playmobile hospital.

Prior to surgery
Prior to surgery it will be important to collect a urine specimen in order to establish that the child does not have a current urine infection, as surgery in such circumstances could lead to septicaemia. Action for Sick Children (Hogg 1994) recently issued standards for children undergoing surgery and reference to these will provide a more detailed account of the pre and post operative care required. Aspects related to pre operative starving, minimizing the stress of the anaesthetic room experience and the parental role are briefly highlighted here.

Children are usually denied food and drink for up to four hours prior to surgery to ensure that they do not vomit during anaesthesia. However, there is evidence that clear fluids can be given up to two hours prior to anaesthetic and this results in less gastric fluid (Agarwal, cited in Radford 1990).

It is a good idea to keep a child occupied in school or in a playgroup prior to theatre. If the child objects to a theatre gown, there is no reason why they should not go to theatre in their nightdress or pyjamas and be changed whilst asleep; older children often prefer to keep their underpants on until they are asleep. Once the usual pre-operative checks have been made, the child is taken to theatre. Here distress can be prevented by sending the child in their buggy, their parent's arms, or even 'driving a train', if this keeps them happy. If they go to theatre with an IV cannula already in place they can be anaesthetized quickly and efficiently. Parents should be encouraged to be present until their child is asleep (Sherwood 1990).

On return from theatre, the named nurse usually takes the parents to collect the child from recovery. It is important, however, to remember some parents find this very difficult and they should be given the choice rather than presuming that they wish to accompany the child at all times.

Following surgical intervention
In general, some of the nursing responsibilities relate to maintenance of the child's airway, monitoring changes in physiological indices which may be indicative of pain or haemorrhage, management of pain, maintenance

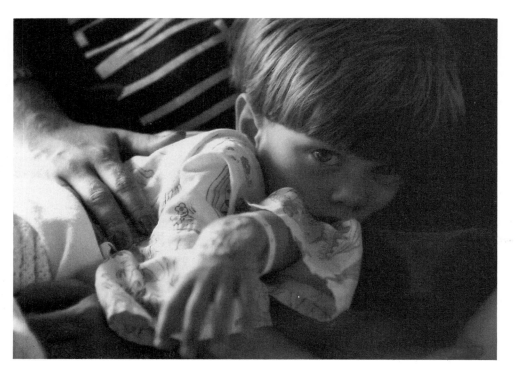

Fig. 21.3 Children need their parents with them in the pre-operative period to provide cuddles and reassurance. (*Reproduced by permission of Jon Sparks.*)

of the child's fluid balance and promotion of wound healing.

Some of these are particularly relevant to a child experiencing surgery to the genito-urinary tract and will now be discussed in further detail.

Recording physiological indices is very important as the kidney is a vascular organ and any surgery involving the kidney has a potential for haemorrhage. Therefore the appropriate observations of BP, pulse, temperature, and colour at frequent intervals are essential. Blood pressure measurements can be inaccurate because sedation may cause hypotension, and hypertension may occur in the presence of pain, or the cuff may be of an inappropriate size. The cuff should be two thirds of the upper arm in width and length; if the cuff is too small it will give a false high reading. It has also been found that inaccurate readings may occur when using ambulatory blood pressure machines because they cause arousal from sleep; this should be taken into account when interpreting readings (Davis 1994).

The preferred form of analgesia is a morphine infu-

sion, which can be adjusted to provide pain control; the older child can do this themselves with a patient controlled unit. It is important to assess the child regularly with a pain score to ensure adequate analgesia is being given, and with a sedation score to ensure the child is not oversedated.

In order to ensure perfusion through the kidneys, fluid balance should be maintained. The child will return from theatre with an IV infusion which will continue until they are drinking, which is usually the following day unless they have undergone complex urological surgery resulting in post-operative ileus.

Post-operatively the child may have a catheter to drain the urine until swelling has subsided and wounds have healed; for example, following reimplant of ureters a suprapubic catheter, or following a pyloplasty, a nephrostomy tube. Haematuria is not unusual and the parents and child should be told to expect this and reassured that it is to be expected as children may become frightened by the sight of blood. The catheter should be checked hourly initially to ensure that urine is draining freely and the tubing 'milked' at regular intervals to maintain patency. If the catheter does block it can be *very gently* flushed with normal saline using an aseptic technique. The minimal acceptable urine output is one to two ml per kilogram per hour.

The catheter bag should be lower than the child and the tubing. The catheter should be secured to the child with hypo-allergenic tape to prevent pulling at the exit site. The parents are often frightened of pulling the tubes and are therefore reluctant to hold the child. The way to overcome this is to show the parents how the catheter is taped to prevent this happening, and to help the parents lift the child until they gain confidence. Eventually most children, given the opportunity, will run around trailing their catheter bags behind them.

The haematuria will lessen, and many children can be encouraged to drink by showing them the relationship between fluid intake and the colour of their urine.

Wound infections are generally rare in children as most wounds heal by primary intention (Foale 1989). If the wound is closed with subcutaneous dissolving sutures the dressing, when removed at 48 hours, will probably not require replacing. However, the catheter site will need a dry dressing until the catheter is removed, often five to seven days post-operatively.

If the parents can be taught to empty and change the catheter bags and undertake redressing of the site to keep it clean and dry, and the catheter secure, the child may be nursed at home from about four days post-operatively until the tube is removed. Most children will eat and drink more readily at home and most families prefer a shorter hospital stay. However, if they are particularly anxious about taking their child home with a tube in-situ, it may be preferable to keep the child in hospital.

An effective way to remove a dressing is often in a bath: if the child is distracted by water play the dressing can usually be removed before they even notice it, resulting in a happy child and a wet bathroom! Suprapubic catheters can cause painful bladder spasm which is very distressing for the child. Regular doses of oxybutinin can help to relieve this but in some cases the only way to relieve this unpleasant pain is to remove the catheter earlier than intended.

The child may experience specific complications. If an obstruction of the urinary tract is relieved the child may become polyuric, and excessive urine output will need to be replaced with intravenous fluids. Urinary tract infections can occur when a child has a catheter and regular urine specimens should be sent for microscopy and culture. Renal tract obstruction is unusual, but if present the child usually complains of pain, may be disinterested in food and drink, may vomit, and their blood pressure will become raised (hypertensive). All these observations should be reported to the appropriate medical staff.

CONCLUSION

The early diagnosis of a genito-urinary deficit and surgical intervention can prevent frequent hospital admissions due to urinary tract infections, and, in severe cases, can prevent renal damage causing end stage renal failure. Admission to hospital can be traumatic but skilled nursing care can make a child's stay in hospital pleasant rather than frightening (Colliss 1990). Small gestures such as a Mickey Mouse plaster, or a bravery certificate, can mean the child remembers the plaster or the certificate rather than the procedures.

NURSING CARE OF THE CHILD WITH NEPHROTIC SYNDROME

To fully appreciate the rationale for care of these children the nurse needs to be familiar with the principles of osmosis and diffusion, the physiological processes associated with oedema, hypovolaemia and hypervolaemia, and the influence of the kidneys in the maintenance of optimal blood pressure. Some of these processes are described briefly here but referral to a physiology text book will be needed to provide additional information.

The term 'nephrotic syndrome' is not the name of a disease but is used to describe a triad of symptoms: proteinuria, hypoalbuminaemia and peripheral oedema (Jeffries 1979). To plan the nursing care of a child with nephrotic syndrome it is necessary to understand these symptoms. This section therefore explains the problems and needs and nursing interventions related to these aspects.

Nursing assessment

The following physiological explanation (Fig. 21.4) will

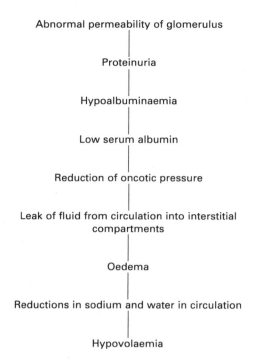

Abnormal permeability of glomerulus

Proteinuria

Hypoalbuminaemia

Low serum albumin

Reduction of oncotic pressure

Leak of fluid from circulation into interstitial
compartments

Oedema

Reductions in sodium and water in circulation

Hypovolaemia

Fig. 21.4 Development of oedema in the child with
nephrotic syndrome.

aid an understanding of the child's appearance and
provide rationale for assessment. The child will experience protein losses which can be massive; this is called
proteinuria. As the glomerulus has an abnormal
permeability to macromolecules, plasma proteins, predominantly albumin, are filtered into the urine. The
presence of protein can be detected by urine testing with
a Labstix, and when large amounts of protein are present
the urine will appear frothy. The loss can be up to 3.5 g/
hour (Trompeter & Barratt 1988).

Due to the loss of albumin in the urine exceeding the
rate at which the liver can synthesize it, the child
develops a low serum albumin and consequently a low
oncotic pressure in the intravascular space. This is
referred to as hypoalbuminaemia. This low oncotic
pressure in the intravascular space causes fluid, normally
held in by the pressure, to leak out into the interstitial
compartment causing oedema. It is usually at this point
that the parents notice the changes in their child.

The most common age for presentation is below five
years old. This in itself has implications for the child's
understanding of their illness. They are usually taken to

the GP when the parents notice oedema, especially
around the eyes on waking. On admission to hospital it
is a matter of urgency to assess the child's fluid status,
general appearance and behaviour.

In addition to the proteinuria and oedema, other
major features of nephrotic syndrome include hypovolaemia, hyponatraemia and hypervolaemia. The nurse
should understand the principles of these in order to
conduct a comprehensive assessment and understand the
rationale for care prescribed.

As the child's plasma protein is low, sodium and
water leak into the tissues and this can lead to hyponatraemia and hypovolaemia. If the child has considerable oedema this presents difficulties with assessment as
the child may appear on the surface to be well hydrated
and thus hypovolaemia may not be immediately
obvious.

A discussion with the parents may reveal that the
child has been vomiting and complaining of abdominal pain; this information is significant as they are
both signs of hypovolaemia. The blood pressure, pulse
and respiratory rate should be monitored frequently
and the difference between the core and peripheral
temperature should be recorded. A discrepancy of
more than 2°C may be indicative of physiological
shock. It is also important to determine whether the
child is passing urine and to measure accurately the
amount.

It is very often the nurse who first notices these subtle
changes in the child's condition and in recognizing the
significance of these is able to be proactive and prevent
further deterioration and complications. Hypovolaemia
causes hyperviscosity and sluggish circulation and this,
coupled with increased synthesis of clotting factors by
the liver, leads to a potential risk of thromboembolism
resulting in deep vein thrombosis, pulmonary embolism,
renal vein thrombosis and neurological consequences
due to cerebral embolism.

Further investigations of blood and urine will reveal a
raised haemoglobin and reduced urinary sodium. This
latter sign is due to reabsorption of sodium and water
initiated by the decrease in plasma volume and hence
renal blood flow. This stimulates the renin angiotensin
mechanism which in turn increases aldosterone secretion
and therefore the reabsorption of sodium and water in an
attempt to maintain blood pressure.

Nursing intervention: meeting the child's needs

In an emergency situation the child will be oedematous and peripherally cold and it will be very difficult to find an appropriate vein. A central line may be inserted to administer the plasma until the vital signs indicate an improvement in homeostatic fluid balance. A plasma albumin infusion will be prescribed because normal saline will only exacerbate the oedema because it will leak into the tissues. Equally children should not be fluid restricted because this only serves to increase the hypovolaemia.

It is also important for the nurse to be alert to the risk of causing hypervolaemia when administering plasma albumin infusions. If this is developing the child will become breathless, indicating pulmonary oedema. This is because the albumin increases the plasma albumin which increases the oncotic pressure in the circulation; this causes extravascular fluid (oedema) to be pulled back into the circulation, increasing the intravascular fluid. Frusemide may be given to increase diuresis. To prevent fluid overload causing pulmonary oedema, the child should be encouraged to sit up during the infusion. Frequent observations of the circulation, including respiratory rate, should be undertaken.

Body image

The oedema is one of the most distressing aspect for the child and family. The child can be so oedematous as to be almost unrecognisable, gaining kilos of fluid in days, changing from a pretty toddler to one with a very abnormal appearance in a short space of time. The oedema is uncomfortable; the eyes may be so swollen as to be hardly open; clothes do not fit; socks leave deep dents in the legs; shoes will not fit on the feet; the scrotum can become so swollen that the child can hardly walk. Oedema will be dependent, therefore the eyes look worse in the morning and the feet look worse at the end of the day. Severe oedema can leave residual stretch marks. Bed rest is generally contra-indicated because of the risk of pressure sores, chest infection and thrombus formation. It may, however, be difficult to mobilize initially, due to the massive oedema causing great discomfort. In this case the child will need incentives to encourage them to move around the bed as much as possible or sit in an armchair. The skin should be kept clean and dry, particularly the scrotal area as it is a potential site for candida infection. If the skin is broken, oedematous fluid may leak for many days and healing will be delayed.

Nutritional needs

Whilst in theory, as the child is losing protein in the urine a high protein diet should be encouraged, in reality the urinary protein losses are so massive that in the acute phase even the infusions of albumin do little to alter the serum albumin levels; consequently a high protein diet has little benefit. Instead, the child is encouraged to eat small regular meals of whatever they would like. However, avoiding a high sodium diet does seem to help minimize oedema formation. A sodium free diet is unpalatable so parents are just asked to avoid obviously salty food. Again, because the protein losses are great, the child can lose real weight despite enormous fluid gains. Junk food containing calories, sweets, Coca-Cola and cakes can be encouraged. When the oedema disappears the child is often surprisingly thin.

Involving the parents is the best way to get a young child to eat. They can cook on the ward, bring in food, or even take the child out to a local MacDonalds.

Susceptibility to infection

Children are susceptible to infection. This is due to a reduction in IgG levels, possibly lost through the glomerulus. They are hypoalbinaemic, often anorexic and generally unwell, and the treatment with steroids is immunosuppressive. (Prophylactic penicillin may be given whilst the child is in an active phase). Infection may manifest itself as septicaemia, cellulitis, primary peritonitis, or pneumonia. The nurse must be alert to the first signs of infection so it can be treated quickly and aggressively. The herpes group of viruses are particularly dangerous to the child who is immunosuppressed. Contact with chickenpox requires a ZIG (zoster immunoglobulin) injection in an attempt to prevent the disease. Development of chickenpox requires immediate treatment with intravenous Acyclovir. It is important to involve the school, to gain their co-operation in informing the parents when the child has been in contact with this virus. When a child is in remission, common infections such as colds, sore throats and influenza can cause relapse. The parents have to balance the needs of the child and the family to socialize, with the risk of infection to the child.

Considerations for home care

Parents will be given advice regarding the continuation of weight and urine testing at home and the administration of medication. The nurse will teach the child and parents necessary skills, will provide information regarding the maintenance of accurate records, and will discuss the side effects of drug treatments.

The nurse will advise them to contact the hospital in the event of an increase in weight and presence of protein in the urine which may indicate a 'relapse'. Parents may have heard about the side effects of steroids, which include mood swings, irritability, aggression, increased susceptibility to infection, growth disturbances, increased appetite, striae, glycosuria, diabetes and Cushingoid features. If they are concerned about these this may affect their compliance with treatment, therefore the nurse should discuss their concerns with them and help them to put them into perspective.

Psychological support

This will be a stressful time for both the child and parents. As mentioned previously the child is likely to be under five years of age and the effects of hospitalization, the illness and procedures may be especially distressing at a time when they may be mixing with peers at nursery or school.

Parents need help to understand the prognosis. They can be reassured that if compliance with treatment regimes can be achieved their child will have long periods of remission either without steroids or on low doses, during which time they should be able to lead an active life, and some children 'grow out of it' altogether. However, they should be prepared for the fact that frequent relapse occurs in 40% of children (Holliday *et al.* 1993) and this will necessitate frequent hospital admission, disruption of schooling and family life, and may even lead to end stage renal failure, requiring dialysis or a renal transplant.

The child and family will also have to cope with changes in both appearance and behaviour. The child's appearance alters first because of the oedema and later due to the iatrogenic effects of the steroids; the side effects may also influence behaviour. Coupled with the impact of the illness and frequent hospitalization, the parents may feel that they have a 'different' child. Overall the parents require considerable support during this challenging time and providing comprehensive information regarding the disease process, and opportunities to talk to other parents in a similar situation, may be immensely helpful.

NURSING CARE OF THE CHILD IN ACUTE RENAL FAILURE (ARF)

This section sets out to explore principles of care for acute renal failure rather than offer detailed descriptions of disease processes; these can be found in Holliday *et al.* (1993). Some of the general causes of renal failure are outlined, as this knowledge can help in understanding the likely progression or prognosis of the child.

Acute renal failure is a sudden reversible reduction in renal function. There are several causes including obstruction within the renal system, reaction to anaesthetic or hypotensive agents during surgery, hypovolaemia and fluid loss as a result of haemorrhage, diarrhoea or burns. There are also some underlying diseases which have a direct effect upon kidney function, for example haemolytic uraemic syndrome or acute glomerulonephritis. Whatever the cause, at the time of admission to hospital the child and the parents will usually be distressed by the sudden and serious nature of the disease and will require considerable support. The prognosis for any child requiring dialysis has been shown to be better if the child is transferred to a specialist paediatric renal unit (EDTA Registry). The fact that the child needs to be transferred often many miles from home causes further anxiety and stress to the family.

The parents and child need time spent with them, and careful explanation and understanding. Often little of this initial explanation is taken in, and they need frequent repetition and reassurance from the nursing staff, especially if the child is so unwell that emergency dialysis is instigated.

Nursing assessment

The first priority of the nurse is to contribute to the assessment of renal function. Appropriate observations include accurate measurement of fluid intake and urine output; measurement of blood pressure, pulse and respiratory rate, central and peripheral temperatures; monitoring of central venous pressure (CVP) or observation of the jugular venous pressure; and accurate record of weight. The combination of all these initial assessments will provide a comprehensive record of the child's physiological status, in particular that pertaining to fluid balance and renal function.

It is important to remember that collective observations are more useful, as a single observation can be misleading. It is possible for the child to be hypovolaemic and hypertensive: blood pressure is to a large extent controlled by the kidneys and renal disease therefore often interferes with normal blood pressure control mechanisms.

Nursing intervention: meeting the child's needs

It may be necessary to catheterize the child to measure the urine output accurately. This can be distressing and adequate preparation should be given to both child and parents. If blood tests reveal raised creatinine or potassium levels and the child shows evidence of fluid overload and fails to pass urine at the rate of 1 millilitre per kilogram per hour, this will usually indicate a need to instigate dialysis. The aim of this is to provide technological support and take over the function of the kidneys until there is evidence of recovery of the kidney. An in-depth discussion of dialysis can be found later in the chapter. The success of this therapy can be measured by improvement in the child's general appearance and behaviour and their ability to pass urine. During dialysis the nurse should record regular observations of the blood pressure, jugular venous pressure, core and peripheral temperatures, weight, respiratory rate, pulse and fluid intake and output.

Diet is important in renal failure. In ARF a high calorie intake is essential to prevent catabolism. If the child becomes catabolic, recovery is delayed and the child becomes hyperkalaemic and uraemic. Renal failure causes anorexia and dietary supplements are therefore needed to ensure an adequate dietary intake.

Parents can play an important role in gaining the co-operation of the child, which also helps them to feel they are contributing to their child's care as well as helping the child. The diet should be low fluid, low electrolyte, low phosphate, low protein and high calorie. There are three ways to achieve this, depending to some extent on the age of the child and their response to the illness.

Nutrition in renal failure

The child should be encouraged to eat more or less what they choose, but with salt and potassium limited as necessary. The child should also drink supplements such as Hycal, Fortical or Fortisip. An ingenious parent can be a great help in encouraging cream on puddings and buying sweets, cakes and biscuits, and all the 'junk' food that they would normally frown upon.

If the child is too sick to eat and drink enough calories it is often kinder to pass a nasogastric tube and feed them slowly, via a pump, with a feed such as Nutrisan or SMA with Duocal. Most children simply do not eat enough calories and after the initial horror of the idea of a nasogastric tube, it may be a more acceptable option than the parents battling and failing with the child at mealtimes. It is important to make sure the child and the parents do not see tube feeding as a failure or a fault on their behalf.

In the case of a smaller or sick child on admission, tube feeding should be predicted as inevitable and the tube should be passed when the child is sedated for insertion of dialysis access. A child who is tube fed will usually eat so little that dietary restrictions are not necessary.

Finally, if the child's gastro intestinal tract will not tolerate enteral feeding, a central line should be inserted and total parenteral nutrition (TPN) commenced.

Fluids

A fluid restriction will usually be necessary, particularly if the child is anuric; they may only be allowed 200–300 mls of free fluid per day with a similar amount of fluid in the nasogastric feed. This is probably the most distressing aspect of treatment for most children and their families. It is therefore important that the parents, and the child if they are old enough, understand the reasons for it. Drinks are best spaced throughout the day and given in a small cup to give the illusion of more fluid; ice cubes and ice lollies can be used to make a little fluid last a long time. Distraction is probably the best way to achieve a fluid restriction; a child who is kept occupied with a video, an inspired play-therapist or a school teacher, will ask for fewer drinks than a child who is bored.

Salt

Sodium should be restricted. Parents are advised to avoid salt at the table and avoid giving obviously salty foods. Salt is allowed in cooking as a salt-free diet is unpalatable. It is very difficult to adhere to a fluid restriction without a salt restriction, e.g. eating a packet of crisps or a Chinese meal without a drink.

Blood transfusions may be necessary to correct anaemia. The transfusion should be given slowly; if the child needs dialysis the blood should be transfused during dialysis so the extra fluid and potassium can be dialysed off as the blood is transfused. Older blood has a higher potassium content. Many parents and children worry that a blood transfusion carries the risk of AIDS, and they may need reassurance.

Medications

Prescribing drugs to a child in renal failure requires particular consideration. Some drugs, such as Brufen and Diclofenac, are nephrotoxic or affect renal function and can worsen or prolong the renal failure. Other drugs are excreted renally and in the absence of normal renal function may only be removed by dialysis. These drugs should be prescribed in smaller doses or with a longer interval between doses, depending on the level of renal function or the amount of dialysis. Information on alterations of doses in renal failure can be found in the manufacturer's information leaflet or a good paediatric formulary. Drug levels may be necessary to monitor dosage and prevent toxicity, e.g. gentamycin, vancomycin. Drugs designed to act on the kidneys may have to be given in larger doses if renal function is poor. Some drugs can be added to dialysate and delivered via the peritoneum; this is a good way to ensure safe levels of drugs such as gentamycin, vancomycin and potassium.

Check the paediatric formulary before administering any drug to a child in ARF for contraindications and dose alterations.

After care

Children are often very sick but in hospital for only a short period of time as recovery can be rapid. Both the child and the parents are shocked by the severity of the illness and may lose confidence; often siblings may also be frightened that they too could become ill (Hewitt 1990). It is important to address these fears and discuss them. Sometimes you have to tell a mother to let the child go out and ride a bike again like other children do, because they are so protective. They need to know they can telephone the unit after discharge to voice any

worries they inevitably have at the first sign of a common childhood illness. Sometimes the parents may perceive that diagnosis was delayed and they may have lost confidence in their GP. This has to be recognized and they should be encouraged to make an appointment to talk over the issues; if the relationship is beyond repair then they will need to change the child's GP. Direct nursing care is not usually needed after discharge but it is important that any healthcare team involved with the family should be aware of their experiences; communication between the hospital and community is very important.

NURSING CARE OF THE CHILD WITH CHRONIC RENAL FAILURE

Chronic renal failure (CRF) is irreversible and eventually leads to end stage renal failure where the only options for maintaining quality of life are regular dialysis or renal transplantation.

Medical advice is often not sought until the disease process is well established. An in-depth interview will be used to build up a full history and during this parents repeatedly talk about their child as being 'not quite right for a long time'. There is an insidious onset and the parents of such children may feel guilty because they have not noticed the slowly developing problems. It may be important to reassure them that it is difficult to attach significance to the changes in their child's behaviour, for example enuresis or truanting, and they have not been neglectful. Parents may be frustrated in their attempts to obtain what they perceive to be the right treatment at the right time, and there is often guilt following admission to hospital which is quite profound and will need to be addressed by the team.

Nursing assessment

The child may exhibit any combination of the following deficits:

Poor growth – This is due to the effect of renal failure on bone development, many of these children appearing shorter than their peers or siblings.

Poor appetite – Gradually increasing uraemia and rising

creatinine often suppress the appetite which results in poor nutrition. This also contributes to poor growth.

Nausea and vomiting – Increasing uraemia makes the child nauseated and unwell, so appetite becomes non-existent. Any food or drink that is offered is usually vomited back quite soon after ingestion.

Lethargy – Lack of energy with pallor and anaemia, associated with the depleted production of erythropoetin, means the child feels tired and listless and not wanting to participate in activities.

Headaches – Many children complain of headaches. This is due to hypertension.

Acidosis – Renal acidosis causes many problems with growth and homeostasis in renal failure. Acidosis also affects growth.

Accurate measurement of height, weight and head circumference is essential, to provide a baseline from which to measure growth. Temperature, pulse, respiration and, most importantly, blood pressure must be recorded correctly using the correct-sized blood pressure cuff. Urine must be tested for microscopy and electrolyte content, as deviation from the normal range may be an indicator of an underlying renal pathology. A DTPA or DMSA scan and a micturating cystogram, together with an X-ray of the hand and wrist to determine bone age and detect any signs of renal osteodystrophy, will be performed.

Once all investigations have been completed, usually a nephrologist will make a diagnosis. This is often a traumatic interview where parents are faced with a life-threatening disease which can only be alleviated by a successful renal transplant.

The nurse will need to reiterate the diagnosis, treatment and prognosis and offer time to talk through the options for treatment and listen to the views of the child and parents. At this point parents often question whether it is desirable or fair to their child to start a long and often painful treatment. If the parents make the decision to terminate treatment they should be given access to all available support. It may be helpful to begin to view death as a third option rather than a totally negative end result of the failure of treatment. Ellis (1992) offers a debate on who should make the decisions in this complex issue.

As with other chronic illness, there are effects on both the child and the whole family unit. Chronic renal failure is life threatening unless there is adherence to an aggressive, conservative, treatment regime which includes regular medication, nutritional limitations and frequent venepunctures to assess serum levels.

Nursing intervention: meeting the child's needs

Nursing interventions should be aimed at minimizing the potentially disruptive effects on life associated with treatment, enhancing the coping abilities of the child and family and encouraging compliance with treatment to delay the onset of end stage renal failure (Fig. 21.5).

The nurse can provide support for the child and family whilst treatment is instigated both to manage the underlying disease causing the chronic renal failure, renal acidosis and anaemia, and to promote optimal development of bones, preventing renal osteodystrophy and thus encouraging normal and accelerated growth. In addition, the nurse is often in a position to initiate and plan care episodes to maintain regular attendance at school, provide psychological and social support networks and prepare the child for possible dialysis and transplantation.

Some of the specific aspects of care will now be discussed in more detail, in particular medication regimes, nutritional needs and dialysis.

Adherence to medication regime

Table 21.1 illustrates the range of drugs that the child will be required to take, often daily. It may be seen that attaining adherence may be a challenge for the child and family.

Nutritional needs

Nutrition is almost as important as the administration of medication. The diet has to be high in calories to prevent catabolism and enhance growth (Rigden cited in Naylor 1989), adequate in protein (essential for muscle growth development) and low in phosphate (i.e. all dairy products, to prevent or stop renal osteodystrophy).

Try telling a child that he/she cannot have cheese (high in PO_4), chocolate (high in PO_4 and K^+), yoghurts (high in PO_4) and they will immediately crave them and cheat on the diet. Calorie intake for children in CRF can range from 1100 calories at the lower end to 3000 calories at the upper limit. The protein intake, which is never forbidden or restricted, ranges from 18 g at the lower end to 85 g at the top of the range (Fig. 21.6).

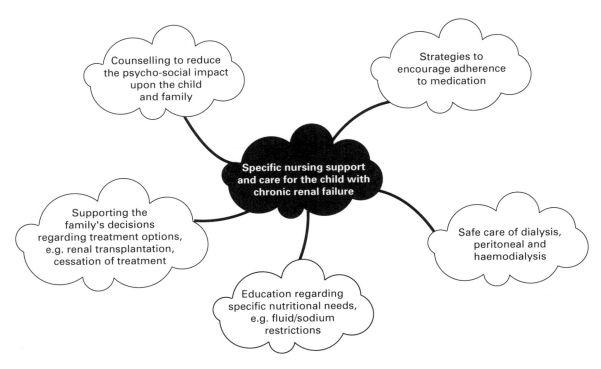

Fig. 21.5 Specific nursing support and care considerations for the child with chronic renal failure.

Sometimes nasogastric feeding is recommended to alleviate progressive uremia, anorexia, nausea and vomiting. When this is first discussed with parents they may be resistant (Naylor 1989). It is important that they realize that the need to tube feed is not a reflection on their abilities to sustain optimal oral feeding regimes. Once accepted, parents are taught to administer bolus and continuous feeds via a pump. When the child is discharged home the parents often increase in confidence and request that they be taught additional skills to enable them to re-pass the nasogastric tube themselves.

Peritoneal dialysis

This is a harmless and relatively safe technique which can be carried out at home or in the hospital. This treatment is achieved by inserting a soft silastic tube into the peritoneal cavity.

The peritoneum is a semi-permeable membrane whose inner layer is covered with numerous villi providing a large surface area with an excellent blood supply. Dialysate (usually between 30–40 mls/kg) is inserted via the catheter into the peritoneal cavity. Dialysis occurs across the peritoneum. The waste pro-

ducts of metabolism, such as potassium, urea and solutes, move across the membrane by osmosis and diffusion.

Both parents and child can be trained efficiently to be operators of the four exchanges required daily. It is painless, safe, and a relatively easy technique to learn. If parents agree to undertake responsibility for care at home, it is important to explain the principles of dialysis to both the child and their family, particularly the need for adherence to a strict aseptic technique.

The parents should be given advice regarding the care of the catheter. The dressing of the 'exit site' is usually replaced daily so that the site can be assessed for signs of inflammation or infection and pain. An inflamed site indicates infection and requires prompt action. A swab should be taken and oral and local antibiotics will usually be prescribed. The child should be discouraged from picking their nose because *staphylococcus aureus* is a bacteria commonly isolated and may be transmitted from the child's nose on their fingers to the exit site. Comprehensive written advice should be given regarding medication, diet and asepsis when connecting the systems.

Table 21.1 Drugs taken by child with chronic renal failure.

- Sodium chloride (tablets/liquid) to supplement Na loss.
- Sodium bicarbonate (tablets/liquid) to correct acidosis.
- Vitamin D supplements (Calciferol for the prevention of renal bone disease)
- Calcium carbonate – widely used for the control of phosphate present in diet, in the treatment of renal osteodystrophy.
- Anti-hypertensives – used if there is hypertension due to underlying cause of CRF.
- Multi-vitamins and iron supplements.
- Synthetic EPO (erythropoetin) injected subcutaneously twice or three times weekly to treat renal anaemia.
- Calorie supplements – such as Hycal, Fortisip, Fortical, Maxijule, Calogen, etc. to provide calories for growth.
- Growth hormone – still in its infancy regarding efficacy of inducing growth in children with CRF without exacerbating progress of renal failure. This treatment is expensive.

Before discharge parents should also be given advice about the common problems associated with peritoneal dialysis; for example, if the child complains of shoulder or abdominal pain or there is cloudy dialysis fluid and a fever, this may be indicative of peritonitis and medical intervention should be sought. This infection may have been introduced as a result of nonadherence with the aseptic technique and the principles will need to be reiterated.

The peritoneal catheter may become misplaced or occluded and nonfunctioning, in which case the parents

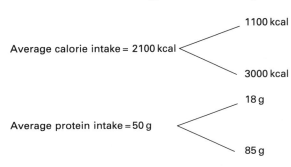

Fig. 21.6 Calorie and protein intake.

should refer to professional advice. An apperient or fruit in the diet, if allowed, may avoid severe constipation which contributes to poor efficacy of the dialysis. Non-compliance with dietary and fluid regulations may lead to ineffective dialysis.

Haemodialysis (HD)

HD is carried out when access to the circulation is possible (Wright 1989). Access is by one of three ways:

(1) Fistula – surgical joining of an artery and vein, usually in the wrist or elbow, so that a resulting hypertrophied vessel can be cannulated using large bore fistula needles.
(2) Shunt – rarely used now, where silastic tubing is inserted into artery and vein and joined externally to a teflon connector.
(3) Gortex graft – synthetic tubing inserted into vessels in the arm or thigh creating a conduit for cannulation.

Access is vital in order to haemodialyse a child. Once the circulatory system is accessed via the methods listed above, the blood is pumped using a machine through an 'artificial kidney' where dialysis occurs across an artificial membrane. The dialysate (cleaning fluid) is provided by the machine.

The child may experience problems with haemodyalasis and these may be physical, associated with coagulation or infection, or psychological, related to the distress of canulation. If the distress experienced by the child is severe the nurse may need to liaise with the psychologists or psychiatrists.

Non-adherence with dialysis

Children having dialysis have a severely limited dietary and fluid intake daily. Here is scope for non-adherence, which is the most important and serious problem in dialysis. Parents may need counselling from dieticians and pharmacists. Nurses can provide information and education and involve the parents in evaluation. Life becomes peppered by frequent clinic visits, where serum electrolyte levels can be measured, blood pressure and weight monitored, and most importantly, support given to the parents and child.

During dialysis the child can continue their usual activities, for example playing, school work, or even taking examinations.

Psychosocial impacts on the family

There are financial and social implications for those families who opt for rigorous treatment regimes for their child from birth or later in life. The frequent visits to the hospital incur travelling costs (Shelley 1992), and there may be loss of earnings due to inability to engage in regular paid work as a result of considerable periods spent in hospital, often in a regional centre away from home.

The psychosocial impact of this illness affects the whole family. The child's education, school attendance and ability to maintain friends with peers will be affected. The parents will need to adjust to life with a child with a chronic illness. Siblings may feel neglected as a result of the attention given to the sick child (Hewitt 1990) and this may result in behavioural problems such as truancy from school, enuresis and sibling rivalry.

The experience of transplantation

As a result of current medical advances many children with chronic renal failure have healthy growth patterns, virtually no bone disease and can be transplanted before they require dialysis. Transplantation is a viable form of treatment for children with end stage renal failure although it can be emotive and expensive for those directly concerned and a subject that arouses controversy (Maynard 1993; Castledine 1993).

Prior to being entered for transplant call (Tx) it has to be established that the child is in optimal health in order to cope with the risk of infection associated with the immunosuppression therapy. To that end certain criteria must be fulfilled, including a review of the immunization records to ensure that all have been given, because the live vaccine cannot be given once therapy is started (Hicklin 1989), and an evaluation of dental hygiene to ensure that there is no infection.

There are considerable stresses on the family waiting for a suitable donor. They have to be available 24 hours per day and the waiting time is about one month (Hicklin 1989). As the waiting period lengthens parents may experience myriad complex feelings; these are described by Gold (1986, cited in Maynard 1993).

When a child is provided with a functioning kidney there is an immediate improvement in physical health and if they have been on dialysis, they are released from the strict regimes of treatment. They no longer have to connect themselves up to the dialysis system – freedom indeed! Between 60 and 70% of transplants are successful (Hicklin 1989); however, in order to maintain a healthy transplant the child will be required to take immunosuppressant drugs, usually steroids. The child and parents may be unprepared for the psychosocial problems associated with this therapy, including altered physical appearance. These drugs have many physical side effects such as obesity, acne and hirsutism. During puberty there may be difficulty coping with these problems. Changing body image can become the single most important problem to these children/adolescents. Many of these problems can be addressed by the use of topical creams and facial scrubs to help the acne, and depilatory products to lessen the hirsutism. Dietary advice may minimize the problem of obesity.

Maynard (1993) suggested that quality of life or psychosocial factors have received little attention in the literature and some parents reported that they felt as if they 'traded one disease for another' (Gold 1986, cited in Maynard 1993). This may lead to non compliance with treatment and may become a particular concern during adolescence to young adulthood. Hudson & Hiott (1986, cited in Maynard 1991) suggest 'that compliance is enhanced by strong family support'. It seemed that families who exhibited most stress had fewer resources to deal with it (Maynard 1993).

Nurses should be aware of the psychosocial issues and should provide support or counselling themselves, facilitate support groups or draw on the available resources, for example psychologists.

The need for research into these aspects of care has been recognized by psychologists, nurse counsellors and pharmacists. Some of the problems may be heightened when the young adult is transferred to the care of an adult unit, as this is a critical time when there may be a sense of loss, of being parted from a 'family' with whom they have felt a part for many years. There may also be a realization that they are now responsible for their own care. Some will welcome this phase in their lives; in fact despite minor difficulties most children showed favourable social adjustment (Reynolds 1991, cited in Maynard 1993). But for others it can be traumatic and requires sensitive handling by the family and health professionals.

CONCLUSION

This chapter has explored several aspects of care but many of the principles are common to all. Nurses need to possess a range of knowledge and skills, for example:

- Observational skills in order to assess accurately changes in the child's fluid balance and understand the significance of the observations.
- Interpersonal skills to assist the family with their concerns regarding changes in body image.
- Teaching skills to promote the self care abilities of the child and family and enhance compliance with treatment regimes.

Nursing a child with a renal or urological deficit is both challenging and rewarding. These children are often both seriously ill and frequent visitors to hospital. It is important that the nurse is not only able to focus on the child's unique needs but also enables and encourages them to enjoy as much normality as possible (Frauman & Gilman 1985).

Nursing care should be flexible to meet the needs of the different client groups. Their approach to a child with a urinary tract infection who may experience one hospital admission of short duration will need to be different from that of the child who may spend many long periods in receipt of health care with chronic renal failure.

The nursing intervention is only one element of the care these children need, albeit a significant one. The skills of the entire multi-professional team are equally important and the nurse has a major role in co-ordinating all those involved and ensuring effective communication.

Although eventually many of the children with chronic illness will be transferred to the care of an adult unit, often they maintain their contacts with the children's unit throughout their adult life. To see a sick, frightened child slowly become a confident, well-adjusted young adult is one of the most rewarding aspects.

ACKNOWLEDGEMENTS

The following people also contributed to the contents of this chapter.

Sarah Haywood, *RSCN, RGN*, Senior Staff Nurse, Paediatric Renal Unit, Guy's Hospital.

Natalie Maughan, *RSCN, RGN*, Senior Staff Nurse, Paediatric Renal Unit, Guy's Hospital.

SUPPORT GROUPS

British Kidney Patient Association (BKPA), Bordon, Hants. Tel. 01420 472021/2.

Nursing and multidisciplinary groups

European Dialysis and Transplant Nurses Association/ European Renal Care Association (EDTNA/ERCA), 6 Chemin du Clos, 1212 Grand Lancy, Geneva, Switzerland.

Royal College of Nursing Dialysis and Transplant Forum, Royal College of Nursing, 20 Cavendish Square, London W1M 0AB Tel. 0171 409 3333.

British Renal Symposium (BRS), 26 Oriental Road, Woking, Surrey GU22 7AN.

REFERENCES AND FURTHER READING

Acharya, S. (1992) Assessing the need for pre-admission visits. *Paediatric Nursing*, 4(8), 20–22.

Berry, A.C. & Chantler, C. (1986) Urogenital malformations and disease. *British Medical Bulletin*, 42(2), 181–6.

Castledine, G. (1993) Laura Davis: should children always get the treatment they need. *British Journal of Nursing*, 2(921), 1077–8.

Colliss, V. (1990) Pre and postoperative management. *Paediatric Nursing*, 2(5), 16–17.

Davis, R.J.O. *et al.* (1994) Effect of measuring blood, ambulatory blood pressure on sleep and on blood pressure during sleep. *British Medical Journal*, **308**(6932), 820–23.

De Sousa, M. (1989) Renal tract problems. *Paediatric Nursing*, **1**(7), 11–13.

Doverty, N. (1992) Therapeutic use of play in hospital. *British Journal of Nursing*, **1**(2), 77–81.

Ellis, P. (1992) A child's right to die: who should decide? *British Journal of Nursing*, **1**(8), 406–8.

Foale, H. (1989) Healing the wound. *Paediatric Nursing*, **1**(5), 10–12.

Frank, J.D. (1988) Antenatal diagnosis of urological abnormalities. In *Controversies and Innovations in Urological Surgery* (eds C. Gingell & P. Abrams). Springer-Verlag, Berlin.

Frauman, A.C. & Gilman, C. (1985) 'Normal life': a goal for the child with chronic renal failure. *American Nephrology Nurses Association Journal*, **12**(3), 192–5.

Gallo, A.M. (1992) Description of the illness experience of adolescents with chronic renal disease. *American Nephrology Nurses Association Journal*, **19**(2), 190–93.

Gartland, C. (1993) Partners in care. How families are taught to care for their child on peritoneal dialysis. *Nursing Times*, **89**(30), 34–6.

Geller, M. (1990) Multisystem failure in a child with haemolytic uraemic syndrome. *Critical Care Nurse*, **10**(4), 56–64.

Glasper, A. & Straddling, P. (1989) Preparing the Child for Admission. *Paediatric Nursing*, **1**(5), 18–20.

Griffiths, C. Renal Holidays. *Paediatric Nursing*, **1**(5), 21.

Guy's, Lewisham & St Thomas' Hospitals (1993) *Paediatric Formulary*, 3rd ed. Includes guidelines for pain relief in childhood. Guy's Hospital, London.

Hardman, M. (1990) Febrile convulsions. *Paediatric Nursing*, **2**(4), 12–13.

Heiney, S.P. (1991) Helping children through painful procedures. *American Journal of Nursing*, **91**(11), 20–24.

Hewitt, J. (1990) The siblings' response to hospitalisation. *Paediatric Nursing*, **2**(9), 12–13.

Hicklin, M. (1989) Renal transplants. *Paediatric Nursing*, **1**(7), 8–10.

Hicklin, M. (1993) Urinary tract infection in children. *Paediatric Nursing*, **5**(10), 24–27.

Hogg, S. (1994) *Setting Standards for Children Undergoing Surgery*. Action for Sick Children, London.

Holliday, M., Barrett, T.M. & Avener, E.D. (eds) (1993) *Paediatric Nephrology*, 3rd edn. Williams & Wilkins, Baltimore.

Jadresic, L. (1993) Investigation of urinary tract infection in childhood. *British Medical Journal*, 307, 25 Sept, pp. 761–4.

Jeffries, P.M. (1979) *Ballieres Nursing Directory*, 19th edn. Balliere Tindall, London.

Jenner, D.A., Vandongen, R. & Beilin, L.J. Blood pressures and body composition in children: importance for allowing for cuff size. *Journal of Human Hypertension*, **6**(5), 367–74.

Jepson, S. (1989) Peritoneal dialysis. *Paediatric Nursing*, **1**(5), 22–3.

Jerrum, C. (1991) Continuous peritoneal dialysis: The State of the Art. *Nursing*, **4**(30), 28–30.

Johnson, D. (1989) *Heart and Lung*, **18**, January, 87.

Kieley, T. (1989) Preparing children for admission to hospital. *Nursing*, **3**(33), 42–4.

Kinmonth, A.L., Fulton, Y. & Campbell, M.J. (1992) Management of feverish children at home. *British Medical Journal*, **305**(6862), 1134–6.

Lee, P. & Jones, K.V. (1991) Urinary tract infection in febrile convulsions. *Archives of Diseases in Childhood*, **66**(11), 1287–90.

Liebermann, Ellin (1976) *Clinical paediatric nephrology*.

MacFarlane, K. (1993) Primary vesicouretic reflux in childhood. *Paediatric Nursing*, **5**(8), 20–22.

Maughann, N. (1994) Care of the child with nephrotic syndrome. *Paediatric Nursing*, **6**(3), 20–21.

Maynard, L. (1993) Transplantation in children: psychosocial issues. *Paediatric Nursing*, **5**(10), 20–23.

McInerney, P.D. (1993) Primary diurnal and nocturnal enuresis. *International Urogynecology Journal*, 4, 157–9.

McKenzie, J. (1989) Haemolytic uraemic syndrome. *Paediatric Nursing*, **1**(9), 14–15.

Naylor, D. (1989) Chronic renal failure. *Paediatric Nursing*, **1**(4), 22–4.

Radford, P. (1990) Physical and emotional care. *Paediatric Nursing*, **2**(5), 12–13.

Ransley, P.G. & Risdon, R.A. (1978) Reflux and renal scarring. *British Journal of Radiology*, supplement 14.

RCP (1991) Guidelines for the management of acute urinary tract infection in childhood. Report of working group of the research unit, Royal College of Physicians. *Journal of the Royal College of Physicians of London*, 25, 36–42.

Rogers, G. (1991) Pass the cranberry juice – herbal remedy for treatment of urinary tract infection. *Nursing Times*, **87**(48), 36–7.

Rogers, M. (1993) Febrile convulsions. *Paediatric Nursing*, **5**(8), 24–7.

Scholtmeijer, R.J. (1993) Treatment of vesico ureteric reflux, results of prospective study. *British Journal of Urology*, 71, 346–9.

Shelley, P. (1992) Too dear to visit. *Paediatric Nursing*, **4**(10), 8–10.

Sherwood, P. (1990) Why can't mummy stay until I am asleep? *Paediatric Nursing*, **2**(3), 18–21.

Swallow, V. (1990) The children's outpatient department. *Paediatric Nursing*, **2**(9), 17–20.

Tan, L. (1994) Nursing care of a child with acute glomerulonephritis. *British Journal of Nursing*, **3**(4), 175–9.

Trompeter, R. & Barratt, T.M. (1988) *The Nephrotic Syndrome* (eds J. Stewart Cameron, R.J. Glassock), p. 423. Marcel Dekker Inc., New York and Basel.

Wilson, L. (1990) Story telling for a child with chronic illness. *Paediatric Nursing*, 2(7), 6–7.

Wright, L. (1989) Haemodialysis. *Paediatric Nursing*, 1(6), 12–13.

Young, H.H., Frontz, W.A. & Baldwin, J.C. (1919) Congenital obstruction of the posterior urethra. *Journal of Urology*, 3, 289–365.

Chapter 22

Nursing Support and Care: Meeting the Needs of the Child and Family with Altered Gastro-intestinal Function

Annette K. Dearmun, Steve Campbell and Jan Barlow

'We expect the nurses to know what is wrong with our child. They explain to us about what the doctor has told us, so that we can understand.'

'I expect the nurse to be able to help me to ask the questions I need to ask the doctor in the clinic. If I do not ask the doctor the questions, then I ask the nurse after I have seen the doctor. The nurse is good because she is on the same level as us and I see her each time I come to the hospital.'

'I wanted to do as much as possible for my child when she was in hospital and it was the nurses who showed me and encouraged me to be involved. Not too much, only when I was ready . . . I did not want to touch her stoma, but they really helped me and now I do everything [at home] and help other mothers as well.'

These are extracts of interviews with parents of children with altered gastro-intestinal function.

INTRODUCTION

This chapter will focus on some of the problems that the child may encounter as a result of alterations to usual patterns of eating, drinking and elimination. It is not the intention to examine in detail all dysfunctions which create alterations in gastro-intestinal function, but those selected for discussion are justified either because of their prevalence on children's wards in the UK or because the principles of care can be generalized to other groups of children.

Eating, drinking and elimination are important behaviours that pervade all aspects of life on physiological, psychological and social levels. In health, when there is optimum functioning, it is as if this idea did not exist at all. In dysfunction problems are created which have a profound effect upon the life of both the child and family; for example, even before birth there may be discussion about the manner of feeding the new-born infant.

New mothers are often encouraged to breast-feed; however, due to prematurity or anatomical abnormalities, oral or enteral feeding may be delayed, sometimes for months. It has been suggested 'that of mothers who initially express a wish to breast-feed their infants in special care nursery, only few are successful' (Pettit 1992). As there is general acceptance that breast milk is nutritionally superior and has protective benefits, a failure to breast-feed can be the source of great guilt.

For other families bowel function can become a preoccupation, for example if the child has encopresis

Table 22.1 Possible causes of constipation (adapted from Keating 1990).

Causes	Examples
Nutritional	Insufficient fluid intake, poor diet. Overfeeding with excessive milk rather than introducing an appropriate weaning diet.
Information source	Conflicting advice from health care professionals.
Organic	Anal fissure, pain on defecation.
Lifestyle induced	Lack of exercise (lifestyle or enforced bed rest, e.g. fractured femur). Child is preoccupied with other activities – ignores the urge to defecate. Lack of available facilities (especially when in an unfamiliar environment).
Behavioural	Manipulative behaviour. Problems with toilet training.
Drug induced	Opiates given as analgesia.
Systemic disorder	Hypothyroidism.
Disorder	Hirschsprung's disease.

(Turner 1991) or constipation (Keating 1990, Table 22.1). It may be seen that even from birth the child and family may be introduced to a pattern of either taking eating, drinking and elimination for granted, or of associating these functions with physiological and social discomfort.

A family centred approach to care (Campbell *et al.* 1993) is inherent in this chapter. The specific principles of care are highlighted as the children's nurse requires such knowledge in order to disseminate appropriate information to the family. Knowledge enables the family to be involved in all aspects of the care of the child, from initial assessment to discharge (Cady & Yoshioka 1991).

A basic understanding of relevant anatomy and physiology is assumed, although some of the altered states are briefly described. To fully appreciate the impact of alterations in gastro-intestinal function the nurse should understand the structure and function of the gut, the process of digestion, absorption and elimination, including the mechanisms of defecation, and the homeostatic mechanisms involved in fluid, electrolyte and acid base balance (Campbell 1993). In most situations care will be focused upon maintaining the above physiological processes within optimal range.

The first section of the chapter briefly outlines some specific anatomical or physiological considerations relating to the immaturity of the gastro-intestinal tract. The second section addresses some general aspects of the assessment of the gastro-intestinal function, including some of the investigations which may be employed to establish a diagnosis.

Section three considers the most common disorder of the gastrointestinal tract, diarrhoea and vomiting. The principles of care may be applied to the child with chronic or acute diarrhoea (DeBenham *et al.* 1985; Ellett *et al.* 1993) and other situations where there is loss of fluids and electrolytes, for example pyloric stenosis.

Section four identifies problems associated with disorders of gut motility. The major dysfunction which has been selected for discussion is Hirschsprung's disease with its consequent reduction in motility. Similarly, constipation (Clayden 1991) may be classified under this heading along with encopresis (soiling) (Younger & Hughes 1983; Coleman Statler 1989; Statler 1989; Ellett 1990).

Section five explores problems associated with inflammatory dysfunction and identifies the principles

of care for the child receiving total parenteral nutrition. Inflammation can occur secondary to all of the other major dysfunctions associated with the gastro-intestinal tract. However, there are several specific problems in which the primary problem is that of inflammation. These include necrotising enterocolitis (NEC), appendicitis, colic, gastro-enteritis, inflammatory bowel disease (Joachum and Hassal 1992; Sutton 1992), Crohn's disease, pancreatitis and Meckel's diverticulum. Ulcerative colitis, Crohn's disease and appendicitis have been selected as examples to illustrate aspects of care.

The sixth section explores the problems associated with absorption disorders. The most often considered malabsorption syndrome is that of coeliac disease. However, other absorption disorders, such as formula milk intolerance and lactose intolerance, are becoming more common. Rare, but no less difficult for the child and family, are short bowel syndrome, following small bowel resection and reconstructive surgery.

The final section identifies some of the problems associated with anatomical anomalies and obstructive disorders, namely tracheo-oesophageal fistula and oesophageal atresia, imperforate anus and intussusception. The principles of care can be applied to other anatomical anomalies of the gastro-intestinal tract. The principles of gastrostomy and stoma care have also been outlined within this section.

Table 22.2 shows the problems divided by age group.

While it is accepted that the liver is a vital part of the gastro-intestinal tract, hepatic problems have not been specifically addressed in this chapter as they are considered to be a specialist area of care.

THE PRINCIPLES OF DIGESTIVE FUNCTION

The gastrointestinal tract extending from the mouth to the anus also includes the accessory organs, the liver, gall bladder and pancreas. It should be remembered that the main role of these systems is to ingest food and digest the constituents of food into glucose, amino acids, fatty acids and glycerol, which can be absorbed into the bloodstream. However, the tract also protects the child from infection through lymphatic tissue in the gut, the Peyer's patches, in addition to secretions which contain

Table 22.2   Age-related gastrointestinal problems.

Birth to four weeks	Toddler	School aged children
Pyloric stenosis	Appendicitis	Appendicitis
Incarcerated hernia	Gastro-enteritis	Chronic and acute diarrhoea
Malrotation and volvulus	Gastro-oesophageal	Constipation:
Hirschsprung's disease	reflux	soiling and encopresis
Meconium ileus	Intussusception	Irritable bowel syndrome
Necrotising enterocolitis	Sepsis and infection (UTI,	Inflammatory bowel syndrome,
Biliary atresia	rotavirus, etc.)	Crohn's disease and ulcerative
Colic	Adhesions	colitis
Formula intolerance	Malrotation, volvulus	Gastroenteritis
Diarrhoea – infective	Pancreatitis	Gastro-oesophageal
Vomiting, gastro-oesophageal	Colic	reflux
reflux	Meckel's diverticulum or volvulus	Henoch Schonlein
Pneumonia leading to abdominal	Incarcerated hernia	purpura
pain and dysfunction	Sickle cell crisis	Pneumonia leading to abdominal
Atresias and fistulas	Acute diarrhoea	pain
Colic	Coeliac disease	Sickle cell crisis
	Short bowel syndrome	Pharyngitis (streptococcal) leading
		to abdominal pain
		Peptic ulcer
		Diabetic keto-acidosis
		Cystic fibrosis
		Recurrent abdominal pain
		Coeliac disease
		Hepatitis

immunoglobulins as well as acid. In this way alteration in the function may not only lead to a failure to absorb important nutrients but may leave the child more susceptible to infection.

In early life there are a number of differences which affect the function of the gastro-intestinal tract, in particular absorption, cell permeability, liver function and gastric secretions. Overall, compared with the adult, the new-born infant has a relatively inefficient digestive tract, largely due to immaturity.

Under three months infants have poorly co-ordinated swallowing reflex and often exhibit a protrusion reflex with the tongue; this leads to a tendency to swallow air when feeding and thus increases the risk of vomiting. The salivary glands are not operative and therefore amylase, an enzyme required for digestion of starch, is not produced. Furthermore, as the immature gut is more vulnerable to allergy, it is generally inadvisable to introduce solid foods before three months (OPCS 1992, cited in Watling 1994).

There is also a limited stomach capacity which ranges from thirty millilitres in the new-born to three hundred and sixty millilitres at the age of one year. The limited absorption of the new born's digestive tract, the large surface area relative to size, and increased gut motility lead to characteristic stools of loose consistency. There are also many secretory glands and few 'normal' intestinal flora. These factors increase the risk of loss of fluid and electrolytes and an imbalance associated with diarrhoea.

There is inefficient production of lactase and thus lactose is poorly absorbed during the first three months of life. Similarly there is incomplete absorption of fat in the diet because of inadequate bile salts. Little is understood about this phenomenon, which seems to place the infant at a disadvantage. The infant has a comparatively high energy requirement of 100 kcal/kg, compared with 30–40 kcal/kg for the adult (Hunsberger & Issenman 1989). An efficient system for the absorption of fat may redress this need and the answer may lie in the properties of breast milk; fat is more easily absorbed because of the presence of lipase.

Breast milk also helps to compensate for the immunological incompetence of the infant. Lactoferrin, an iron binding protein which limits bacterial growth, immunoglobulin A (IgA) and lysozyme all have an antimicrobial effect.

The gut of the infant is porous to high molecular weight proteins which are generally beneficial for growth. However, this permeability is not selective and other proteins such as cow's milk can cross into the bloodstream. This accounts for the greater potential for formula fed infants to suffer from digestive allergic problems.

The new-born infant has many of the secretions of the gastro-intestinal tract present, but in smaller quantities than the adult. This situation is slowly redressed with age. There are exceptions in the case of serum gastrin and gastric acid; both of these are present in higher levels at birth and it has been hypothesized that this is a mechanism which helps to eradicate ingested bacteria. Infants under great stress, such as those in the special care baby unit, can suffer the ill effects of excess gastric acid and can develop stomach ulcers (Hunsberger & Issenman 1989).

Assessment of the child with gastrointestinal dysfunction

It is important that a child with a problem related to gastro-intestinal function is assessed in a holistic manner, using a model which reflects their developmental differences and the variation in the form and function of the child's family. Such an assessment needs to include an appropriate overall history, and should be related to the child's individual health record.

While there may be a need to focus in some detail on the particular gut problem which has led the child and family to seek assistance, there are many factors contained in the child's overall history which may assist in evaluating the nature and severity of the child's current problem. An example is the use of growth charts to establish whether there has been a sudden alteration in growth pattern which may indicate failure to thrive (Fry 1993). These charts are relatively simple for families to understand and the nurse may be able to build upon information provided by other community health professionals. Such engagement of the families in the principles involved in the assessment of the child's overall health is an important aspect of family centred care.

When focusing on the specific gastro-intestinal problem there are several areas of inquiry which should be examined in depth. First, it will be necessary to ascertain whether there are any associated changes in food or fluid intake that are exacerbating the problem. If the child has been away from their usual environment changes in diet may have occurred unnoticed. Second, the circumstances need to be analysed in relation to the family experience. It may also be relevant to explore the family history to discover any familial tendencies. For some families gut problems are accepted as part of life, particularly for those in poor housing. This may make it more difficult for the nurse to elicit relevant information and then introduce interventions and health education to alter established family practices.

The specific nature of gut problems is often difficult to ascertain, especially in young children. As a result and because many of these problems are associated with other anatomical systems, there are many diagnostic tests which are used to make a final diagnosis. Many of these tests are unpleasant and unnatural for children, involving fasting for considerable periods of time or the insertion of tubes. The fear, pain, embarrassment and indignity of such procedures should not be underestimated. As a result it is especially important to give the family appropriate information. If the family understand or appreciate the relevance of such investigations they may be more effective when working with the team to gain the child's co-operation. Many hospitals provide information leaflets and video tapes, the most highly developed of which draw on the experiences of families to shape the information.

The nurse has a clear role in ensuring that any procedures are handled in a sensitive and professional manner in order to avoid undue distress to the child. Strategies should be employed to enhance continuity of care by enabling the nurse who has been providing preparation for the child to support the child during the procedure, thus offering additional security. Some children may be more reassured by this role being performed by the parent with the support of the nurse. Some procedures, for example oesophagoscopy, barium enema or sigmoidoscopy, are especially uncomfortable and therefore may require the use of general anaesthesia, sedation and analgesia.

NURSING CARE OF THE CHILD WITH DIARRHOEA AND VOMITING

One of the most common problems experienced by the young child is that of diarrhoea and vomiting. Some health care workers regard this phenomenon as merely part of normal life (Whaley & Wong 1991). Diarrhoea is usually defined as an increase in the number of stools or a decrease in the consistency which leads to fluid loss. The effect upon this aspect of the child's physiology can be profound and potentially life threatening (Smith 1986, 1988). Candy (1987) reports that the 'first landmark in the treatment of diarrhoea was the recognition that death was due to loss of fluid and electrolytes'. This is most clearly seen in the third world where the mortality rate of young children with diarrhoea and vomiting remains extremely high.

Many children are nursed at home, and in the UK it is likely that a child who is admitted to hospital will be under two years of age, have progressive diarrhoea and vomiting and be unable to tolerate oral fluids. They may be admitted via the GP if there is a limited response to conservative treatment or there may be a self referral by the family via the accident and emergency department. The reasons for such an admission, given that it is such a common life experience for the child, are to correct the dehydration and the alteration in acid-base balance, as well as prevent hypovolaemic shock.

Nursing assessment

Initial assessment of the child focuses upon determining the extent of dehydration and the disturbance of electrolyte balance and monitoring the effects of treatment (Fig. 22.1). By taking an accurate history from the parents the nurse can gauge the success of previous interventions, in particular the amount and nature of recent drinking. The older child who continues to have diarrhoea and vomiting, but has been able to drink clear fluid over the previous 24 hours, is less a cause for speedy intervention than the younger child who has refused or been unable to tolerate oral fluids.

Aspects of assessment are shared between the nursing and medical staff. The medical staff undertake venepuncture to estimate serum levels of electrolytes and this complements the observations made by the nurse relating to the child's behaviour, skin colour, temperature, pulse, respiration and, where appropriate, blood pressure. Assessment of the child's general behaviour may indicate alterations in electrolyte levels.

The key electrolytes involved are sodium, present in gastric mucus and lost through vomiting, and potassium lost through diarrhoea. The loss of these electrolytes creates a major shift of fluid from intracellular to extracellular fluid compartments and ultimately there are also alterations in acid base balance and acidosis or, in the case of prolonged vomiting and loss, of gastric acid and potential alkalosis.

The physiological principles relating to maintenance of fluid balance and dehydration are described in detail in other texts (Metheny 1987; Herbert 1984; Adomat 1992; Campbell 1993). The dehydrated infant often appears listless, possibly due to the effects of electrolyte imbalance and ensuing acidosis. They may have sunken eyes due to loss of intra-occular fluid, and a sunken fontanelle due to reduction in cerebral spinal fluid volume. The skin will lack elasticity due largely to loss of intracellular fluid into the extracellular fluid compartment in order to maintain blood volume. In severe dehydration the child's extremities seem cold to the touch due to peripheral vasoconstriction. The child may not pass urine as antidiuretic hormone is produced in response to changes in plasma osmolarity, and urine output will be reduced in an attempt to conserve fluid.

All the above are adaptive mechanisms which come into play in an attempt to compensate for the effects of fluid loss. Eventually if there is inadequate intervention the pulse rate will be raised and in the latter stages of dehydration, there may be hypotension as a result of hypovolaemic shock (Adomat 1992). Fortunately, this scenario is rare in the UK, but is still sufficiently common to lead to children being admitted to hospital to prevent further deterioration.

Parents need to understand the cause of the diarrhoea and vomiting in order to prevent a recurrence (Table 22.3). The cause, some of which may never be fully understood, may include infections, more common in bottle fed babies, introduced through poor feeding and sterilizing techniques (Khatib 1986), contaminated food, allergy or food sensitivity. The age of the child may be a clue to the likely cause, for example diarrhoea coinciding with the introduction of new foods to the infant may indicate a food sensitivity, or a child starting school may be exposed to greater person to person

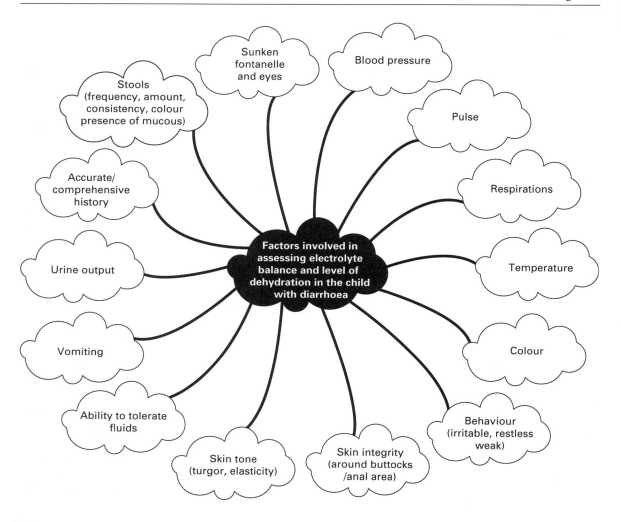

Fig. 22.1 Nursing assessment of electrolyte balance and level of dehydration in the child with diarrhoea.

contact with subsequent risk of infection (Whaley & Wong 1991).

Specific tests to confirm diagnosis will involve the collection of specimens of stool for laboratory examination. More important for the nurse and family is the assessment of the frequency and nature of these stools. Such information should be maintained in a systematic manner, using recognized descriptors and including the consistency, mucous and colour of the stools. Nurses may test the stool for reducing substances, sugars, using a modified urine testing technique with the Clinitest tablet. The presence of sugars is indicative of a gut that is failing to absorb vital substances.

Another critical aspect of the assessment is the capacity of the major carer, in many cases the mother, to continue to be involved in care. The mother is likely to have had little sleep during the illness and, in addition, she may have responsibility for siblings. Sometimes this is a criterion for admission to hospital. The nurse needs to ensure that the parents' need for rest and sleep, and the potential upset of the child, are balanced. A tired parent is likely to become increasingly exhausted and stressed; this anxiety may be transmitted to the child. The family should be actively involved in all decisions and assessed individually. It is important to ensure that the perceived imperative of the parent being resident

Table 22.3   Possible causes of diarrhoea and vomiting.

Cause	Example
Feeding problem	Allergy to cows milk, gluten, food (MacDonald 1989). Poor feeding technique, more common in bottle fed babies (Long (1989).
Infection	Directly related due to ingestion of bacteria, virus. Symptom of other infection, otitis media, tonsillitis.
Drug induced	Anaesthetic agents.
Result of a disorder	Crohn's disease, pyloric stenosis.
Mechanical obstruction	Small bowel atresia, intussusception.

does not lead to judgements and subsequent guilt if this is not possible.

Nursing intervention: meeting the child's needs

As suggested previously, the child with mild and moderate diarrhoea is often treated at home by simple non-invasive techniques. If there is no dehydration their usual feeds are continued. If there is evidence of dehydration oral rehydration fluids, such as Rehydrat or Dioralyte, are prescribed (Emergency Medicine 1992; Evans 1990). Indeed, these are also effective in the third world as well as in western paediatric tertiary care centres. The frequency and volume of the rehydration therapy is varied according to the weight of the child and the extent and frequency of the diarrhoea.

These fluids are not unpleasant to taste, but are unfamiliar to the child and so can present a major difficulty for the carer to actually get the child to take adequate quantities (Tucker & Sussman-Karter 1987) and thus they may need the support of the paediatric community nurse when taking on responsibility for this aspect of care at home. Parents who appreciate the importance of encouraging their child to take adequate fluid are likely to be well motivated, but it can be frustrating for the parent who is unable to gain the child's co-operation. If the child refuses the rehydration fluid parents may be tempted to give milk or formula feed. This practice should be discouraged as it often prolongs the diarrhoea and vomiting and thus the nurse may need to offer the parents advice and suggestions

regarding alternative strategies to encourage optimal intake of fluids.

Severe or intractable diarrhoea and vomiting leading to dehydration and hypovolaemic shock is a source of concern and needs prompt action, especially in the young child or infant; admission to hospital is usually unavoidable. An intravenous infusion will be initiated to replace the fluid deficit, to compensate for the ongoing losses and to replace electrolytes to maintain optimal balance (Whaley & Wong 1991). The overall fluid and electrolyte requirements may be adjusted in response to alterations in the child's weight and plasma concentrations of urea, sodium, potassium and other electrolytes. The intravenous fluid volume should be monitored and recorded hourly, even if an electronic pump is being used, to avoid too little or too much fluid being given. The nurse should be conversant with the precautions necessary when administering intravenous fluids (Livesley 1993), including frequent observations of the cannula site for extravasation (Table 22.4).

Regardless of the setting in which care takes place, the goals of care will need to be realistic and achieved in partnership with the family (Casey 1988; Casey & Mobbs 1988); for example, if the child is still able to tolerate oral fluids the parents can be involved in recording the fluid balance. When goals are measurable and include statements about the volume of fluid which will be taken during a specific period, parents can calculate the amount of fluid to be offered and taken and record the frequency of urine output. When there is a need for increased precision, in the child who is incontinent, nappies may be weighed. Through these activities parents may make a nondirect but considerable

Table 22.4   Potential problems for the child receiving intravenous fluids (adapted from Livesley 1993, 1994).

Problems for the child receiving fluids intravenously	Nursing actions and rationale for care
Trauma of the insertion of the cannula	Use play and preparation strategies. Apply EMLA cream. Enlist the support of parents during the procedure.
Fluid overload, cardiac congestion: children have more fluid per body weight than adults, a higher turnover of fluids and a smaller cardiovascular system	Administer fluids accurately via electronic pump. Observe for engorged neck veins, increase in heart rate and blood pressure; this may indicate cardiac failure.
Extravasation	Record pressure settings: an increase in pressure may indicate a thickening of the internal epithelium which may herald phlebitis. Inspect the cannula site hourly; initially the site may be cool, hard or swollen, later there may be heat and pain, suggestive of phlebitis.
Septic phlebitis: contamination of the cannula with skin flora during cannulation	Undertake effective skin cleansing. Secure the cannula with a sterile dressing. Transparent dressings should be selected to enable moisture transmission from the skin to avoid proliferation of skin flora. Disinfect hubs prior to changing the giving set. *NB* It is suggested that there is a reduced complication in peripheral sites after 72 hours, thus rotation of cannula sites is unnecessary. Filters may be effective in removing microbial contaminants (Bennion and Martin 1991).
Chemical phlebitis: associated with infusion of fluids with high osmolarity	Select the most appropriate cannulation site, for example basilic and cephalic veins in the forearm, antecubital fossa and dorsal veins in the hands or feet. In infants sometimes the saphenous vein or scalp veins are used. Dilute infusions with appropriate volumes.
Mechanical phlebitis: caused by movement of the cannula within the vein	Secure and splint the cannula site effectively. Use extension sets to enable maximum movement without dislodging the cannula. NB When bandages are used the digits should be visible.
Limited mobility	Select the nondominant hand or arm for access.

contribution to the care of their child and in many cases they will maintain more reliable records than a nurse caring for a number of children.

There should be continuous monitoring and evaluation of the child's progress, particularly in relation to the overall fluid and electrolyte balance. Improved hydration may be evident by a reduction in the frequency of diarrhoea and vomiting and an increase in weight; thus

children are usually weighed daily. At this point oral fluids will be reviewed and, when appropriate, the usual drinking and eating patterns will be re-established.

There is some controversy regarding the 'fasting' of children with diarrhoea. This practice is generally 'based on the assumption that whilst fluid is being lost from the bowel it is illogical to overload the bowel with more fluid' (Candy 1987). However, the conclusions drawn from a study undertaken in Birmingham were that there were advantages, on the grounds of safety, simplicity and economy, in using oral sodium and glucose to replace fluid losses (Candy 1987).

If the cause of the diarrhoea and vomiting is known to be an infection there will be a need for the family and nurse to plan remedial action and develop health promotion strategies to minimize a repetition of the illness for that child and/or any siblings, including adherence to regimes for disposal of excreta and hand washing. Most effective health promotion is carried out in combination with the family, community paediatric nurse and health visitor.

THE CHILD WITH DECREASED OR ABSENT GUT MOTILITY

There are many problems associated with a gastro-intestinal tract which has little or no motility and these are well exemplified by children who have constipation or Hirschsprung's disease (Milla 1988). In infancy there may be serious physiological consequences.

Nursing care of the child with Hirschsprung's disease

Hirschsprung's disease is a congenital problem derived from an arrest in embryonic development before the twelfth week. There is absence or reduction in parasympathetic ganglion cells, typically in the bowel, which results in the characteristic aganglionic megacolon and lack of peristalsis. This is responsible for 25% of all neonatal obstruction (Whaley & Wong 1991).

The impact on the infant depends upon both the severity of the defect, that is the length of bowel affected, and the extent to which this inhibits the child's ability to defecate. The failure of peristalsis results in constipation, obstruction and accumulation of faecal contents proximal to the affected part of the bowel.

When a large proportion of the bowel is affected the problems of constipation, obstruction or, in some instances, the passage of watery stools become apparent soon after birth. Immediate palliative surgery is required; this usually involves the formation of a colostomy proximal to the aganglionic bowel.

If only a small segment of the bowel is aganglionic, the child is often noted, by the parents, to be constipated in early life. However, constipation is a relatively common problem to many infants and often the diagnosis of Hirschsprung's disease is not made until much later (Landman 1987). This can lead to frustration if health care professionals do not appear to take the parental concerns seriously.

There are two options of treatment for these children: conservative, using washouts or enemas to evacuate the bowel, or the formation of a colostomy and reconstructive surgery which involves resection of the aganglionic segment and anastomosis. This is usually referred to as a 'pull through'.

Initially the parent may recognize that their child is constipated and appreciate that there is a need for interventions to maintain regular defecation. Suppositories, enema and washouts may provide temporary relief but may not be adequate in the long term.

When conservative measures are ineffective and a colostomy is required it is often at this stage that the family actually realize the full gravity and implications of the diagnosis.

Nursing assessment

The assessment of the child with Hirschsprung's disease can be considered on two levels. The first relates to physiological processes (Fig. 22.2) and the second to the effects of the diagnosis on the functioning of the family. Both of these aspects differ and depend upon the age at which the child is diagnosed and the treatment regimes, for example whether there is conservative or surgical intervention. There may be differences in the ways in which the problems manifest between age groups and, as a result of differences in the nature of relationships, coping strategies within the family.

At any age a major feature of assessment is related to abdominal distension. Abdominal girth measurements will assist in monitoring the degree of distension and to ensure the accuracy and reliability of these measurement marks should be made on the child's abdomen. Parents should be given consistent and accurate explanations regarding the nature of their child's problem, the assessment methods and the ways in which the problem will ultimately be resolved.

If enemas are prescribed an accurate fluid balance chart

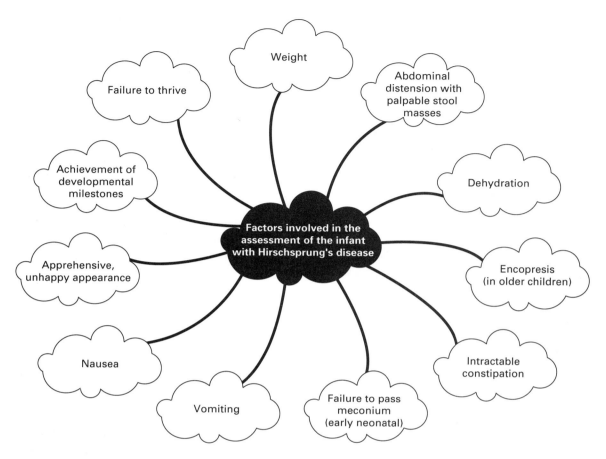

Fig. 22.2   Nursing assessment of a child with Hirschsprungs disease.

will be maintained. This is relatively simple to do, in contrast to the estimation of the quantity of evacuant after an enema, which is notoriously difficult. This makes the regular recording of the infant's girth an even more important assessment of the efficacy of the enema procedure and whether the frequency needs to be altered.

Nursing intervention: meeting the child's needs

If problems are evident in the new-born, immediate surgical intervention is necessary. Ultimately, when the infant is in optimal health and weight to withstand the effects of anaesthesia the complex surgery, outlined previously, is performed, usually at nine months of age.

The formation of a colostomy involves a laparotomy and therefore potentially there will be paralytic ileus, or an overall lack of peristalsis following the procedure. Under such circumstances, the child may have an intravenous infusion and nasogastric tube inserted whilst in the operating theatre. The former will be used to keep the child hydrated, and the latter will remain in place to drain gastric contents to minimize nausea, vomiting and the risk of aspiration. Once paralytic ileus resolves, as evidenced by resumption of bowel sounds or the passage of flatus, appropriate feeding patterns are gradually re-established.

If the conservative option of treatment is selected, initially the infants with Hirschsprung's disease tend to be poorly nourished, disinterested in life and may be uncomfortable, largely due to the distension and nausea (Martin & Torres 1985). To alleviate some of these problems these children are given small volumes of low residue feeds frequently and encouraged to sit up after feeds. This has several implications; first, low residue feeds reduce the need for frequent enemas, and second provision of small frequent feeds and nursing the child in a sitting position reduces the accompanying respiratory embarrassment and restricted diaphragmatic movement associated with abdominal distension.

One of the main aims of care is to ensure that the family appreciate the importance of an adequate diet to maintain optimal growth, whilst limiting the adverse effects on the compromised bowel. The parents, with community nursing support, may be involved in implementing these specific feeding patterns and assessing the resultant effect upon abdominal girth and bowel residue.

It may be relevant at this point to note that these principles of feeding for the child with Hirschsprung's disease are contrary to those which are usually encouraged for constipated children. If the child is constipated they are generally encouraged to consume a diet which is high in fibre and therefore high in residue.

In order to avoid admission to hospital the parents will usually take responsibility for giving regular enemas at home to remove faecal matter as it accumulates. If this becomes the routine form of evacuation, there will be a need for the parents to become skilled in the technique. They require advice on the appropriate temperature of fluid and the use of isotonic solutions to avoid dehydrating or overhydrating the child, and they may need support in gaining the child's co-operation. The timing of inclusion of parents in this care should be led by the family.

Surgery is not necessary for all children and some may outgrow the problem and behavioural management may be effective (Kenner & Breuggemeyer 1984). However, flatus can be a recurrent problem, which may become more difficult and embarrassing particularly during young adulthood.

THE CHILD WITH PROBLEMS ASSOCIATED WITH INFLAMMATORY DYSFUNCTION

Unlike many gastro-intestinal problems, inflammatory dysfunctions can occur at any time in a child's development. Some are associated with a known disease, whilst others are of unknown aetiology. Included in this category are Crohn's disease, ulcerative colitis, necrotizing enterocolitis, peptic ulcer, Meckel's diverticulum, appendicitis and gastroenteritis.

Nursing care of the child with ulcerative colitis and Crohn's disease

Ulcerative colitis (Winch & Ouverson 1992) and Crohn's disease are two inflammatory dysfunctions which can be grouped together as inflammatory bowel disease (McWade 1992). It has been suggested that heredity, environmental, immunological and psychological factors may be implicated (Hunsberger & Issenman 1989). Although these two forms of inflammatory bowel disease differ markedly in their clinical features, they both involve chronic inflammation of the mucosa and submucosa of the large intestine.

Nursing assessment

Diagnostic tests include barium enema, endoscopy and biopsy and it should be recognized that sometimes the parents may have unspoken anxieties regarding these as their only experience may be in relation to investigation for cancer (Hunsberger & Issenman 1989). The nurse needs to be aware of this potential anxiety and where possible create opportunities for parents to discuss their feelings.

Again the nursing assessment (Fig. 22.3) includes estimation of the extent of the diarrhoea, caused by the intestinal inflammation, and the subsequent potential for disturbance of fluid and electrolyte balance. Corticosteroids are among a number of potential chemotherapeutic agents which may be prescribed to reduce inflammation, and the iatrogenic effects should be assessed.

The child may complain of pain and discomfort from a variety of causes, including cramps from the intestinal inflammation and general discomfort due to breakdown of the skin around the anus with the frequency of bowel actions. Prolonged contact with faeces affects skin integrity.

Sometimes the child's overall nutritional status is poor and they may appear to tire easily, lacking energy to cope with activity. This lethargy may be due to

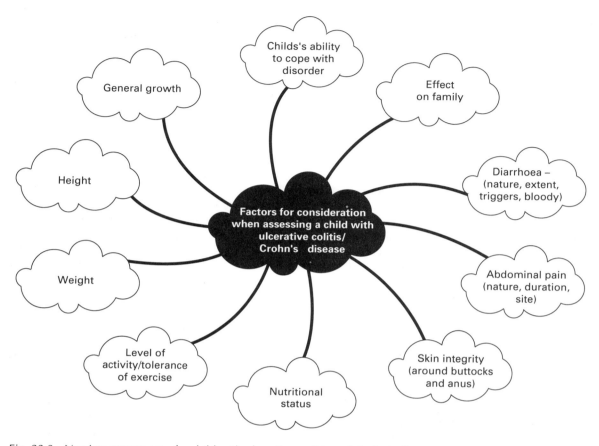

Fig. 22.3 Nursing assessment of a child with ulcerative colitis and Crohn's disease.

limited absorption of iron and other nutrients as a result of chronic inflammation and increased gastro-intestinal motility. There may be sufficient inflammation to cause bleeding into the bowel, so stools need to be assessed for blood.

It is important to assess the child's weight, height and general growth together with a review of the dietary intake and requirements. Additional supplements may be needed to compensate for the inadequate absorption. The nurse may draw upon the knowledge and skills of the dietician who may contribute to a comprehensive appraisal of these nutritional aspects.

It is recognized that chronic and intractable problems affect both the child and family and it is pertinent to assess the family's dynamics and coping ability. The child may experience difficulty in coping with the problems of a chronic inflammatory disease and the nurse

who is aware of this is able to enlist the assistance of the clinical paediatric psychologist.

Nursing intervention: meeting the child's needs

The nature of the nursing interventions is specifically focused on minimizing the detrimental effects of the diarrhoea. This is achieved, medically, to some extent with the use of drugs such as diphenoxylate or anticholinergic drugs, in conjunction with some self-imposed dietary restrictions.

Encouraging an appropriate diet, including essential nutrients, is an important aspect of nursing interventions. Sometimes the child is encouraged to take a low residue diet, or a diet free of restrictions is supplemented with vitamins and other essential nutrients. Sometimes, by recording the nature and extent of the diarrhoea in tandem with records of diet, a correlation between particular foods and increased diarrhoea may be discovered. If the child is malnourished over a prolonged period, total parenteral nutrition (TPN) may be the intervention of choice to provide electrolytes, minerals and zinc and essential nutrients such as protein, in the form of amino acids, carbohydrate, supplied as glucose, and fat in a lipid emulsion.

As mentioned previously, pain and excoriated skin are features of inflammatory bowel disease; such problems are internal to the child. However, problems caused by the odour from excessive diarrhoea are external and a source of great embarrassment. The nurse needs to be sensitive to all of these problems. Advice on skin care – washing with soap and water, careful drying and application of barrier creams – may be effective in reducing discomfort around the anal area. Aerosols are available to combat odour.

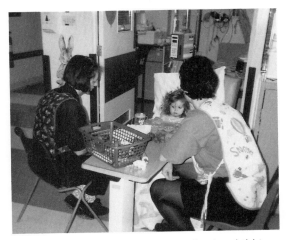

Fig. 22.4　Using play as distraction for the child in pain.

Occasionally, even with careful management, there may be an exacerbation of the disease. During these times the child may need to be restricted in its physical activity, because exercise has been found to further exacerbate the condition.

The principles identified previously can be applied to Crohn's disease but additional problems are those of fistulae and fissures. Skin care for these children is

particularly important such as careful washing and drying and the use of stoma adhesive around such fistulae (Simmons 1984). Promoting psychological adjustment of the family and child to these chronic diseases requires skilled intervention. Counselling is often carried out in a largely informal manner, but there is an increasing awareness that nurses may need preparation for this role and that they should be appropriately supported.

Maintaining a sense of control of their lives is important to children of all ages and particularly those entering adolescence. Strategies which increase the child's and family's ability to cope may promote the self-concept of these children and their families. 'Acting out' is a common expression of older children who are exasperated by the loss of control and they often need to be able to express frustration and anger; this, although potentially distressing, may also be cathartic and help the child adjust to their problems. It is particularly important therefore that strategies are developed to enable the child to maximize their personal and educational development and where possible self care at home should be encouraged.

Quality of life is at the essence of quality care for these children. It is unlikely that initial treatment will induce remission and thus treatment regimes may need to be adhered to over a number of years. Sometimes if the frequency of bowel actions becomes unacceptable to the child they may elect to have an ileostomy created.

Total parenteral nutrition

General principles relating to the use of total parenteral nutrition (TPN) are identified by Ball *et al.* (1994). They suggest 'the use of an expensive and potentially hazardous form of nutritional support, is inappropriate until it is clear that the enteral route, is entirely precluded. There is usually little clinical or nutritional justification for parenteral nutrition which lasts less than five days'. Candidates for TPN include neonates post gastrointestinal surgery and older children with protracted diarrhoea or post abdominal surgery (Stapleford 1990).

As there is a risk of thrombosis or phlebitis of the vein when peripheral access is used, usually a Hickman or Broviac catheter is inserted. If children require TPN over a long period the feeding can be given overnight, the catheter flushed with heparinised saline and the infusion discontinued during the day. In this way the child can maintain its usual daily activities.

To ensure accuracy of delivery a volumetric pump should always be used (Auty 1989). Some have comprehensive alarms which protect against air embolism (Rennie 1992).

As the presence of glucose may indicate sepsis (Stapleford 1990) and the reduction of glucose, hypoglycaemia, the nurse should teach the family about blood glucose monitoring, including testing of the urine. This is initially undertaken daily, then less frequently as the feeding regimes become established. The child will be weighed weekly and the solutions calculated accordingly.

The parents are often educated to provide TPN and the number of children receiving parenteral nutrition at home is increasing (Holden 1991). There are a number of benefits for the child – not least that their usual activities of living can be maintained by minimizing the amount of time which needs to be spent in hospital – and there may be economic advantages for the hospital.

Criteria are established to assess those candidates suitable for home TPN (Holden 1991). These include physiological and psychosocial considerations. The child should be in a state of metabolic stability and be able to tolerate the infusions over a 12 hour period so feeds can be given overnight. Where possible two family members are taught the principles of care to ensure that there is a consistent approach to the management of the central venous catheter. Once the family have completed the teaching programme they are encouraged to spend a limited time at home, perhaps for one night, and this is gradually extended as they become more confident.

Prior to going home the family should be conversant with all aspects of care of the intravenous catheter and where to obtain supplies. Holden (1991) reports that commercial companies can deliver feeds, together with disposable equipment, to the home or other temporary address if the family is on holiday. The family are also provided with a fridge to store the solutions, and a pump with which to administer the fluids.

NURSING CARE OF THE CHILD WITH APPENDICITIS

Abdominal pain is common amongst children of all ages. In the school age child the most common cause

may be appendicitis. Indeed this is the most frequent cause of emergency admission of children for surgery (Peck & Bushby 1992). Currently the average length of stay for a child following removal of the appendix is three days, but despite the improvement in rates of survival for children, there still remains a possibility of death. This will be minimized by recognizing the potential seriousness of the problem.

Appendicitis is caused by an obstruction of the lumen of the appendix. This may be due to impacted faeces, or as a result of inflammatory changes caused by infection. Initially the obstruction blocks the outflow for mucus secretions. Oedema of the gastro-intestinal tract can compromise the blood supply, leading to ischaemia and ulceration of the epithelial lining, which allows bacterial invasion. Finally, if treatment is not given there will be necrosis and perforation, or peritonitis. In children peritonitis is more common because the appendiceal wall is thinner and the omentum is not fully developed. This loss of fluid into the peritoneal cavity leads to hypovolaemic shock. Classically the pain is not localized in the right lower abdominal quadrant until the inflammation has become persistent. Surgical removal of the appendix is usually undertaken.

Nursing assessment

Children with appendicitis often present with pain, vomiting and fever (Fig. 22.5). This may be first noticed by the parents or teachers who are confronted with a child with severe abdominal pain, who may not be able to stand upright (Finelli 1991; Gartner *et al.* 1992). Assessing and locating the pain and making an ultimate diagnosis can be a challenge as the young child is usually less able to describe the exact nature and location of the pain. They are also likely to be irritable and listless and may have diarrhoea (Leape 1987).

The pain engenders fear and stress in the child and this may be exacerbated if the child is referred directly from school to hospital, especially as they may not have immediate access to their parents (Sharrer & Ryan Wegner 1991). Once initial medical assessment has been undertaken appropriate analgesia should be given.

Prior to surgery a comprehensive assessment of health status should be undertaken to ascertain potential anaesthetic risks. This should include a record of temperature, pulse rate and respiration, information

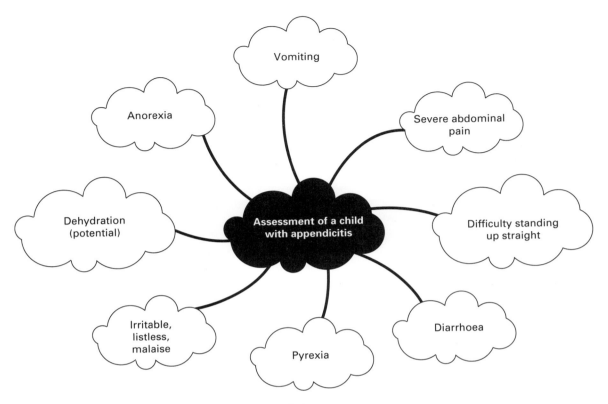

Fig. 22.5 Nursing assessment of a child with appendicitis.

regarding allergies and the time of last intake of fluid and food.

Nursing intervention: meeting the child's needs

In this emergency situation there may be little time for detailed preparation but all events should be explained to child and family prior to consent being obtained. Preoperative intervention includes the application of anaesthetic (EMLA) cream, assessment of health status and measurement of the child's weight to calculate anaesthetic agents, analgesia and antibiotics if required.

Sometimes the diagnosis is inconclusive; in such circumstances, if the child is able to tolerate fluid they will be allowed small amounts to drink until decisions can be made about the appropriateness of surgical intervention. If the child is vomiting an intravenous infusion will be commenced. In common with all children requiring

surgical intervention, oral fluids and food will be withheld for several hours prior to surgery.

Assessment post operatively is related to the identification of immediate problems including anaesthetic complications, haemorrhage, fluid balance deficit and pain, and later problems associated with chest or wound infection (Fig. 22.6). There should be frequent monitoring of pulse, respiration and pulse rate to detect haemorrhage and hypovolaemic shock.

During the initial period following surgery the child remains without fluids and food, and hydration will be maintained via an intravenous line. If vomiting persists antiemetics may be administered. Once nausea and vomiting cease and peristalsis returns, clear fluids are slowly introduced followed by solids.

As the integrity of the abdominal muscles is compromised after appendectomy, particular attention should be paid to pain management. Pain should be assessed and regular analgesia provided. Early mobility is encouraged and this is more likely to be successful if

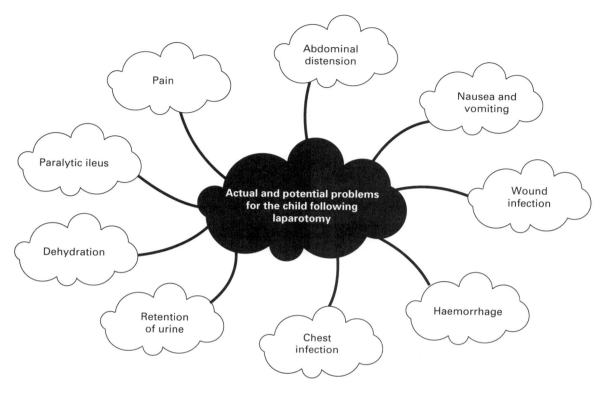

Fig. 22.6   Post operative assessment of the child following laparotomy.

the child receives adequate analgesia. Inspiration, coughing, vomiting and sitting up are likely to be especially painful and the nurse can offer the child and parents assistance and advice about supporting the abdomen during these activities.

There is limited research into wound care of surgical wounds in relation to children; thus nurses, unless they are fully conversant with the principles of wound healing, tend to adopt practices which may be based on ritual rather than scientific principles (Walsh & Ford 1989). The phases and types of wound healing are outlined by Bale *et al.* (1994) and care should be based upon these principles.

Surgical wounds heal by primary intention, which is usually rapid without complications (Bale *et al.* 1994). Initially a dressing is applied over the wound site and if there are signs of infection this should be removed to inspect the suture line. Research has shown that the ritual of daily dressings increases the rate of wound infections (Foale 1989) and cleansing is only necessary if there is infection; if undertaken repeatedly it will trau-

matize new tissue, thereby inhibiting the healing process. Once the dressing is removed the wound may be exposed to air and sprayed with Opsite spray (Foale 1989). If redressing is required, an adhesive airstrip with Melonin or occlusive film, or Opsite dressings can be applied. If the latter dressings are used the child can have a shower two to three days post operatively. Sutures, if not dissolvable, are removed by the GP or community nurse after seven to ten days, when primary intention healing has occurred.

If the child has a perforated appendix, resulting in peritonitis, the recovery period is likely to be extended and pain, vomiting and fever will be more prevalent.

NURSING CARE OF THE CHILD WITH ABSORPTION DISORDERS

These disorders all have one or all of the following aspects: failure of digestion, failure of absorption and lymphatic obstruction (Auricchio *et al.* 1988). These forms of malabsorption can be further subdivided (Table 22.5). Digestive failure can be ascribed to insufficient or absent pancreatic enzymes, poor quality bile salts, or insufficient lactase. Failure of absorption may be attributed to problems with the gastro-intestinal mucosa. This may be due to a lack or reduction in gastro-intestinal surface, either by length or by reduction in the microscopic surface, such as microvilli. It is also possible that such a failure is a result of an infection.

Table 22.5 Types of absorption disorder.

Failure of digestion	▪ insufficient/absent pancreatic enzymes ▪ poor quality bile salts ▪ insufficient lactase
Failure of absorption	▪ lack/reduction in gut surface by length of microsurface area ▪ result of inflammatory infection/disorder

Whaley & Wong (1991) have noted a number of common manifestations of chronic malabsorption. One of these is the wasting of subcutaneous fat, which is especially obvious in the gluteal area of children who are failing to thrive. Children with protein deficiency are often oedematous. Children with insufficient vitamin C or vitamin K may also be noted to be more prone to bruising.

Coeliac disease (gluten-sensitive disease) is the second most common cause of malabsorption in children, cystic fibrosis being the most common cause. Silverman & Roy (1983) have reported the varying prevalence of this disease throughout the world, with the highest incidence reported in Ireland.

Coeliac disease

Commonly the child develops this disease between six months and two years. There is thought to be a correlation between the onset and the age of weaning. There has been a small decline in the incidence, possibly as a result of the tendency to introduce mixed feeding at an older age.

Gluten, which is a protein found in wheat, barley, oats and rye, damages the mucosa of the small bowel. When exposed to gluten, villi become flattened and the surface area for absorption is reduced. In particular, the child will have difficulty in absorbing fats and to a lesser degree carbohydrate and vitamins. Such children tend to have bulky stools with a characteristically foul odour, and chronic diarrhoea which contains unabsorbed digested fat.

Nursing assessment

The parents will bring their child to the attention of health care professionals because they seem smaller than their peers, are not growing or are 'failing to thrive' (Heubi 1992). History often reveals that the problems coincided with the commencement of solids, particularly those containing grains. Some children may also have exhibited a change in behaviour, becoming irritable and uncooperative, although this is not common to all children (Hamilton 1983). It is thought that coeliac disease has familial tendencies and thus other members of the family may also have a history of similar problems.

A child who is failing to thrive will need a comprehensive assessment of growth as this will provide a baseline from which to evaluate the effectiveness of treatment. The child's weight will be recorded on a centile chart. An assessment will also be made of the child's distribution of subcutaneous fat. Various diagnostic tests may be performed to establish whether the child does indeed have coeliac disease; foremost are the D-Xylose test and the jejunal biopsy.

Nursing intervention: meeting the child's needs

Appropriate and achievable goals need to be set for the child around two major areas: appropriate nutrition and the support of the family, recognizing the additional extra stress associated with diagnosis and management.

The child's dietary requirements need to be reviewed and this will usually be undertaken in conjunction with the dietician. The goal is to offer a balanced diet which avoids gluten toxicity. By eliminating gluten from the diet the villi rejuvenate and hence the ability to absorb

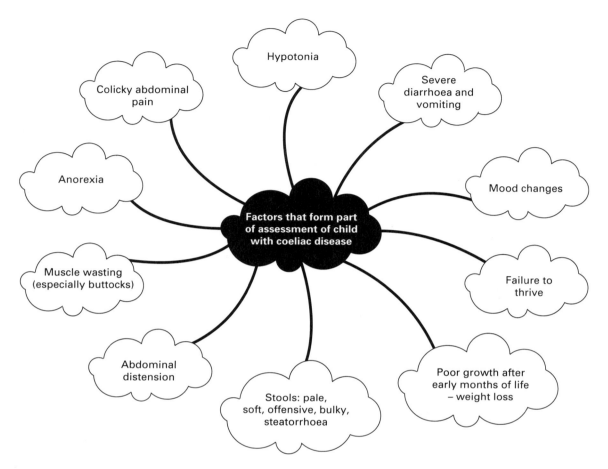

Fig. 22.7 Assessment of child with coeliac disease; some factors will vary according to the age at which coeliac disease presents/ is diagnosed.

nutrients increases. The nurse may help the family to take responsibility for supervising the child's diet.

In order to motivate and encourage the family it may be appropriate to underestimate rather than over-estimate planned weight gain. Hunsberger & Issenman (1989) suggest that the goal should be to progress towards the 50th centile by six months of treatment, and reach average percentile level for height by the end of the two years. These goals have great merit in that they are interpretable as well as achievable. If clear targets are identified in this way they may reassure the families, especially when they are achieved.

Coeliac disease requires the child to maintain a gluten free diet for life. In this respect the family and the older child need to be educated about gluten-containing foods

and these should be substituted with corn, rice, or soya bean flour. As the purchase of specific gluten-free foods is potentially expensive, the cost may be reduced by encouraging the family to explore the gluten-free foods available in the supermarket rather than the chemist. This, therefore, also requires a lifetime of inspecting the product labels, for example to ensure that gluten in the form of other flours has not been used as a thickener in soups and sauces.

As the world of nutrition is not designed for the family of a child with coeliac disease it is likely that at some stage the child will receive a product containing gluten in error. The parents may need to be prepared for this eventuality and reassured that an isolated incident will not result in long lasting effects.

As mentioned previously, centile charts are an important means of assessing the success of the new diet, but it cannot always be assumed that failure to meet centile targets is due to lack of adherence to the diet. If the stools remain frequent and offensive there may still be inadequate growth and weight gain.

The nurse has a particular role in accessing support and information for the family. Once the child is able to understand the implications of their disease they should be involved in decisions and educated about their disease and the rationale for the dietary restrictions. Although coeliac disease is not life threatening, the implications of these restrictions may be significant. Being able to eat freely is usually taken for granted by most children and having to adhere to a different diet may lead to exclusion from usual social interaction at mealtimes.

The planning of the diet needs to be realistic but flexible for both the individual child and family. The family may require additional support from health care professionals during an exacerbation of the disease, when the child can become highly irritable and have a short attention span affecting concentration and educational ability and leading to challenging behaviour. The effect of the child being diagnosed as having coeliac disease, and providing care for a child who fails to thrive over a series of months or years, is a challenge for the whole family and family dynamics are often put under great strain; this is sometimes underestimated.

NURSING CARE OF THE CHILD WITH CONGENITAL ANATOMICAL ANOMALIES AND OBSTRUCTIVE DISORDERS

One in 40 infants has a major defect and gastrointestinal abnormalities account for two in one thousand live births. Obstruction of the gastro-intestinal tract leads to a number of physiological responses (Peck 1992). The nurse should be able to recognize the relevance of alterations in the colour or amount of vomit or gastric secretions, presence or absence of bowel sounds, abdominal distension, pain, and the nature and frequency or absence of bowel actions.

Many of the gastro-intestinal anatomical anomalies occur during the first three months of embryological development and commonly more than one system is affected; for example, Filston & Izant (1985) noted that 30% of children with tracheo-oesophageal fistula also have a further abnormality, often cardiac. The specific problems become evident soon after birth and in order to sustain life immediate palliative surgical intervention is required. Any complex reconstructive surgery is undertaken later when the infant is in optimum health.

Surgery should be performed in regional centres where there is access to specialist surgeons and anaesthetists. This has particular implications for both the baby and mother. During transfer the baby requires adequate ventilation, warmth to avoid hypothermia, and an intravenous infusion, usually glucose, to minimize potential hypoglycaemia. The mother and baby are often separated at birth. The main principles of care and physiological rationale for these are identified in Table 22.6.

This section offers two examples of gastro-intestinal neonatal anatomical problems. The principles of care identified can be applied to infants with other structural defects.

Neonate requiring surgery to correct an upper gastro-intestinal anatomical anomaly

Examples of structural defects of the upper gastro-intestinal tract include tracheo-oesophageal fistula and oesophageal atresia. These often occur together but are two distinct problems and there are different variations of the anomaly. The most frequently seen is atresia with a distal fistula (Ashcraft & Holder 1976), due to a failure in the development of the lumen of the oesophagus. There is a 'blind pouch' and although the baby swallows the secretions they accumulate in the oesophagus and spill over into the trachea. The infant's main problem is aspiration of these secretions.

Nursing assessment

Coupled with a history of polyhydramnious in pregnancy the excessive secretions may be the first indication of this diagnosis. There is confirmation when there is failure to pass a naso-gastric tube into the stomach, and on X-ray it is seen lodging in the proximal pouch. If there is a fistula without atresia some babies are not diagnosed until repeated episodes of pneumonia indicate

Table 22.6   Principles of care for the neonate requiring gastro-intestinal surgery (Dearmun, using adapted Roy's model). P = potential problem

Potential problem (physiological mode)	Principles of care	Rationale
Breathing and circulation Difficulty with breathing/apnoea/ hyaline membrane disease Adverse response to anaesthesia	Monitor respirations, use apnoea alarm Physiotherapy and suction to maintain patency of the airway	Increased respiratory rate in response to stress acidosis High metabolic rate, therefore respiratory rate 35–40 bpm
(P) Chest infections		Immature medulla
	Positioning to maximize diaphragmatic function Minimize handling as this may lead to fall in oxygen tension and hypoxia	Poor stability of chest wall, smaller reactive airways, fewer smaller alveoli, poor development of accessory muscles Diaphragmatic breathing inhibited by abdominal distension Poor cough and gag reflex
(P) Haemorrhage	Ensure vitamin K has been given	Insufficient clotting factor
(P) Anaemia	Ensure safe administration of blood transfusion	Blood volume 80 ml per kg, blood removed for diagnostic tests
Nutrition (P) Hypoglycaemia	Monitor blood glucose regularly Provide adequate calories Daily weight May require phototherapy	Liver immature, poor stores of glycogen (exhausted by the effects of surgery) Reduced ability to produce plasma proteins may lead to a greater risk of oedema Metabolic rate increased by surgery and additional glucose required for energy
(P) Jaundice		Poor conjugation of bilirubin leads to jaundice and kernicterus
Elimination/fluid and electrolyte balance (P) Dehydration	Assess for signs of dehydration or circulatory overload	Immature kidney function Poor tolerance to rapid alterations in fluid balance
(P) Circulatory overload	Record input and output accurately including drainage from nasogastric tubes, wound drains etc. Weigh infant daily Weigh nappies	

Table 22.6 Principles of care for the neonate requiring gastro-intestinal surgery (Dearmun, using adapted Roy's model). P = potential problem (cont.)

Potential problem (physiological mode)	Principles of care	Rationale
(P) Adverse response to blood transfusion (see anaemia)	Assess for adverse reaction by frequently monitoring vital signs	Immunologic response minimized by minimizing donors, irradiating blood and giving packed cells
Immunity (P) Infection	Maintain strategies to minimize cross infection, e.g. handwashing and asepsis when changing IV lines or wound dressings	Immune system – major defence mechanisms cellular and humoral are immature Immunoglobin G passed transplacentally, IgM + IgA absent Unable to generate a rapid effective defence against bacteria → vulnerability Leukocytes limited and phagocytis ineffective
	Provide umbilical cord care with sterets and Ster-zac powder (Bain 1994)	Umbilical cord locus for infection
Temperature (P) Hypothermia	Nurse in thermoneutral environment, e.g. incubator Ensure adequate nutrition and oxygen Ensure that the infant is well 'swaddled' when removed from the incubator	Larger surface area leads to heat loss Heat lost by radiation, convection, evaporation and conduction Temperature regulating mechanism in hypothalamus present but not very effective Maintains temperature within a limited range (compromised by environmental temperature) Produce heat nonshivering thermogenesis involving metabolism of brown fat (this fat has a high enzyme content and is capable of rapid conversion to energy and heat) Heat production is adequate but relies on high metabolic rate which needs oxygen Hypothermia will increase oxygen consumption
Rest and activity handling (P) Deprivation of sleep	Organise care to minimize handling (Sparshott 1991a; Redman 1994) Assess the infant for the effects of environmental noise and light	Infants in a neonatal unit are handled 130 times/24 hrs (Wolke 1987) Found to cause disruption in sleeping patterns, intra ventricular haemorrhage

Table 22.6 Principles of care for the neonate requiring gastro-intestinal surgery (Dearmun, using adapted Roy's model). P = potential problem (cont.)

Potential problem (physiological mode)	Principles of care	Rationale
(P) Trauma to the skin	Handle gently to avoid friction (Polden & Beadshee 1990)	Dermis and epidermis thin Friction may cause blistering Eccrine glands nonfunctional → infection
Pain	Assess pain Use appropriate pharmacological and nonpharmacological methods and monitor effect Use baby massage unless contra-indicated	Massage (Field & Scafidi 1987; White-Taut & Carnier Goldman 1988; Paterson 1990; Russell 1993)

repeated aspiration. The initial assessment of the neonate focuses upon the respiratory system. This is especially pertinent in order to establish the extent of aspiration prior to diagnosis. Any respiratory distress is noted, paying particular attention to the rate, sternal recession and tugging. Note should also be made of any episodes of cyanosis or apnoea and the frequency with which the infant requires suction.

Nursing intervention: meeting the child's needs

Pre-operatively one of the main aims of care is to minimize the potential problem of aspiration. A replogle tube is inserted into the oesophagus and attached to low pressure continuous suction. Replogle tubes are notoriously difficult to maintain and the infant requires frequent supervision. By sitting the infant up the risk of gastric regurgitation will be reduced. If the infant is distressed and crying it may be more likely to experience reflux. In some units the use of the dummy to reduce crying is discouraged because of the increased production of saliva. However, if the replogle tube is correctly placed, the additional secretions will drain.

Where possible a primary anastomosis of the oesophagus is performed and a transanastomotic tube is inserted. This tube remains in place for approximately ten days and provides a splint whilst healing takes

place, and later in the post operative period it may be used for feeding. The transanastomotic tube needs to be secured to ensure that the infant is not able to inadvertently remove it, because unlike many other tubes, it is not possible to replace it without further surgery.

There is a particular need to ensure appropriate airway maintenance. While this is a common goal following any surgical intervention, it is significant because of increased risk of aspiration of secretions, and oedema to the oesophagus associated with surgery. Additionally general principles of post operative recovery can be applied when caring for these infants (Fig. 22.6).

After ten days a contrast study is often performed to assess the healing; if the oesophagus is found to be intact oral feeding will commence. The maintenance of adequate nutrition can be assessed through regular weighing. After an initial weight loss the infant usually gains 200 g per day until they have regained their birth weight.

Longer term problems associated with anomalies of the upper gastro-intestinal tract

Wallis (1993) identified several long term problems common to these infants. First the establishment of feeding for the infant may present a challenge. The oesophagus may not support swallowing and often other temporary methods are required to maintain nutrition, for example a nasogastric tube, a gastrostomy tube or total parenteral nutrition. When oral feeding is not possible it is important that the infant maintains an oral experience and the speech therapist can be asked to provide appropriate advice.

Once feeding has been established, if the infant has difficulty swallowing this may herald the presence of a stricture at the site of the anastomosis and further surgery is required to dilate the oesophagus. The anastomosis may leak, which may require further extensive surgery at a later date; to maintain nutrition a temporary gastrostomy is performed.

Some infants experience gastro-oesophageal reflux and require a Nissen's fundoplication. This involves an abdominal incision to mobilize the fundus of the stomach and wrap it around the lower oesophagus to prevent the reflux of gastric contents (Wright 1990).

The child with a gastrostomy

A gastrostomy allows nutritional access through the abdominal wall directly into the stomach through a tube, a Foley catheter kept in place with an inflated balloon, or a gastrostomy button/peg device. The latter is gaining in popularity and there are several different devices available on the market. An anti-reflux valve minimizes leakage of the gastric contents on to the skin (Taylor & Watson 1990).

There are several reasons for the creation of a gastrostomy:

(1) Because a child is unable to swallow effectively.
(2) To bypass an obstruction.
(3) It may be more aesthetically acceptable than a nasogastric tube for the child who requires long term enteral therapy.

Whether the child has a gastrostomy tube or button the aims of care relate to maintaining optimal nutritional intake, minimizing pain, leakage, infection and trauma, and maximizing opportunities for the family to be able to undertake safe self care at home. A comprehensive home care teaching programme should include information on feeding techniques, care of the skin around the stoma site, and changing the tubes, usually undertaken monthly, or the button, every six months.

Feeds should be at room temperature and can be given manually or via a pump. When using the for-

mer method a syringe is attached to the tube/button. During feeding extension tubes are used to assist with gravity feeding. When feeding is complete the tube should be flushed with water to ensure patency, and the tube spigotted. A blockage, which may be caused by viscous feeds or medications, can be relieved with pineapple juice or fizzy drinks. The feeding equipment if not for single use should be cleaned with soap and water and immersed in Milton between feeds. If the child experiences reflux or abdominal distension after feeding, this may indicate that the feed was too cold or was given too rapidly. The syringe and tube can remain in situ at the height of the oesophagus for an hour after feeds.

If leakage occurs barrier cream can be applied to the skin, although petroleum based creams may damage the tubes (Sidey 1991). Leakage may be minimized by giving frequent feeds of a reduced volume and positioning after feeds with the head of the bed raised and with the child on their right side to facilitate gastric emptying (Huddleston and Ferraro 1991).

Usual bathing routines will keep the skin around the site clean. When a button peg is in place it should be rotated through 360° to prevent adhesion of the button and to ensure that all areas of the stoma are cleaned (Steele 1991). This sometimes creates discomfort and diversional tactics may need to be employed. As soon as the child is able they can learn the technique themselves. Sofradex eye drops have been found effective in treating granulosis.

If the tube becomes dislodged it should be replaced as soon as possible as the stoma may close or reduce in size an hour after removal of the tube. If the child experiences diarrhoea this may indicate that the tube has passed through the pyloric sphincter; the balloon should be deflated, the tube drawn back into the stomach and the balloon re-inflated.

The family should be encouraged to maintain both the child's usual activities and their own; for example, mealtimes should take place with the rest of the family and the child should receive oral stimulation during feeds (Huddleston & Ferraro 1991). If the child wishes to go swimming an occlusive dressing can be applied.

NURSING CARE OF THE CHILD WITH A LOWER GASTRO-INTESTINAL TRACT ANOMALY

Examples of structural defects of the lower gastro-intestinal tract include malformations of the rectum and anus, which can occur as a single entity or with a fistula. Essentially, these defects occur as a result of the abnormal separation of the caudal hindgut during embryological development. There are four main types of imperforate anus: anal stenosis, imperforate anal membrane, anal agenesis and rectal atresia (Hunsberger & Issenman 1989).

Anal agenesis is described as 'high' if there is a considerable gap between the blind pouch of rectum and the skin surface where the anus should be. There is a gender difference in anal agenesis where males tend to have high lesions and therefore poor pelvic muscle control and hence incontinence problems later, whereas females tend to have lower lesions.

Nursing assessment

Sometimes neonates fail to pass meconium, and present with bile stained vomiting and abdominal distension. There are several reasons for this and these include small bowel atresia, meconium ileus, and most commonly imperforate anus. Usually a systematic mid line inspection should be carried out by the midwife to ensure that the anus is patent and is not covered by a membrane. The main specific problems if surgical intervention is delayed relate to loss of fluid and electrolytes and subsequent fluid imbalance.

Nursing intervention: meeting the child's needs

The care following surgery for these infants depends upon the extent of the surgery. There are two likely surgical procedures, either anoplasty or colostomy.

If the infant has an anoplasty performed, care is focused upon maintaining optimum conditions for the perineum to heal. Above all, the incision line needs to be kept clean at all times to promote healing by first intention. This may be achieved by keeping the child without a nappy with the skin exposed to the air. Prior to publicity regarding sudden infant death syndrome, the practice was to nurse the child prone. This is no longer recommended (Stewart & Fleming 1992) and current practice is to nurse the baby from side to side.

If a colostomy is the temporary solution the parents will almost inevitably need time to adjust to their baby with a stoma, particularly if they are grieving the loss of perfection in their new baby. They need to be supported so that they can come to terms with it. The principles of stoma care are identified in Table 22.7.

When the infant is older, generally before they are a year old and prior to the age at which toilet training would commence, reconstructive surgery is performed and an anal opening fashioned. There are a number of specific considerations following this surgery. First, the parents need to be aware of the importance of skin care of the anal area. As the child's skin will not have been in contact with stools there is a potential for it to become excoriated very quickly. It is important to be proactive and barrier cream should be applied before the first bowel action and at every nappy change. Second, the refashioned anus may become stenosed and therefore the parents should be taught to undertake daily anal dilatations. Many parents find this distasteful and the child is often distressed, but the importance of it to maintain patency of the anal opening should be stressed.

In some children, especially those with high lesions, incontinence of faeces may be very likely and, rather than cope with encopresis or adherence to a regime of high retrograde anal washouts, they may elect to have the colostomy replaced or an antegrade colonic enema (ACE) (Hancock 1994).

The child with a colostomy or ileostomy

An ileostomy or colostomy is often created, in children, as a temporary measure to divert the flow of faeces from a distal part of the bowel until reconstructive surgery can be performed, or to protect an anastomosis or promote healing of the peri-anal area. This is generally a 'loop' ostomy which has two openings, proximal and distal. Occasionally, as in the child with ulcerative colitis the colostomy may be permanent.

Children who have experienced ostomy surgery have special needs. Nurses need to provide the family with a comprehensive service, including specific instructions, as well as pre and post operative care (Adams & Selekof 1986).

Table 22.7 Principles of care for the child with a stoma.

Initial assessment: in the post operative period
- Apply transparent bags to allow for observation of the stoma for viability, colour. The stoma should be red or pink; if it is blue or black this may indicate necrosis.

Stomal functioning
- Empty the bag frequently, monitor and record the output, colour, consistency and amount of stools.

After care
- Assess the implications of culture/ethnic origin.
- Encourage self care abilities of the child and family; success may depend on education and support to maintain effective appliance management.
- Ensure privacy and dignity when changing appliances.
- Assess the child and family response to change in body image.

Hygiene and skin integrity
- Bath with the bag off or in situ.
- Assess the skin for inflammation and excoriation when changing the appliance. The area around this is particularly important when the child has an ileostomy as the stools can cause excoriation of the skin.
- Wash the perineum with soap and water and dry thoroughly with a soft tissue.
- Restriction on clothing is not usually required.

Eating and drinking
- Restrictions are not usually necessary unless medically indicated.

Advise parents regarding potential problems, e.g.:
- Leakage from appliance (seek advice re the size of the appliance).
- Prolapse, stenosis of the stoma, retraction of the stoma.
- Bleeding from the stoma (this is common and does not indicate a complication, unless excessive).
- Odour may be due to poor fitting of appliance.
- Flatus – avoid carbonated drinks, experiment with diet, use areosols.
- Changes in bowel function, e.g. if the child has diarrhoea, find cause, offer additional fluids; if the child has constipation, increase roughage in the diet.

Disposal/storage of bags
- Empty into the toilet, wrap the bag in newspaper in a plastic bag in the dustbin.
- Store appliances in a cool dry place as the quality deteriorates if the bags are stored incorrectly.

Post operatively, in addition to usual physiological assessment specific observations of the stoma should be performed.

There seem to be few research studies pertaining to stoma care or the effects of stoma surgery on the child and family. Johnson (1992) found that often the support and information given to children and families were inadequate. The nurse will be required to help the child and family adjust to the stoma and to teach them the principles of stoma care. Many parents have a limited knowledge of the results of stoma surgery and may experience anxiety (Webster 1989). The following extracts illustrate some of the key concerns of parents.

'Lots of things worried me, both before and especially after the colostomy. Questions like, how on earth do you put the bags etc. on the baby? Can you still bath him, with or without the bag on? How often to change, clean them out? Will I be hurting him when I change them? Worst of all, how do I cope with him, his colostomy and all the other children?'

The parents may need to be prepared when they first see the colostomy.

'My feelings when he came back from theatre were very mixed. I was very scared (I didn't quite know what to expect) and also at the same time I was excited, relieved and all I wanted to do was see his stoma. I think mainly to see if I would feel like passing out. I was not sure I would be sick if it looked really sore. What I was not prepared to see was that I thought it looked quite neat and not ugly.'

The team may draw on the expertise of a stoma therapist to advise on the size of the stoma bag, on skin care, the application of the bag, disposal of contents and the provision of resources.

'He had a mucus fistula about half an inch below his stoma and this made fitting the bags difficult.'

Leakage around the appliance or allergies to adhesives may cause skin irritation (Adams & Selekof 1986). The aim of care should be to keep the skin around the stoma clean and dry; however, sometimes barrier creams are required to protect the skin, especially if the child has an ileostomy. This is a particular consideration in those children with an ileostomy or stoma for meconium ileus, a symptom of cystic fibrosis. These children are given pancreatic supplements to aid digestion of fats and this is excreted into stools. This substance can digest skin and thus excoriation of the skin is more problematic.

The parents will also need information regarding potential problems, including the risk of prolapse and the potential for dehydration, particularly if the child has an ileostomy.

'The second worst problem was prolapsing. I was terrified of this after I was told in hospital by a mother whose little boy had had quite a few of those.'

Parents should be advised to give additional fluids in hot weather and to seek advice if their child with an ileostomy has diarrhoea as the risk of loss of fluid and electrolytes and dehydration is exacerbated.

If the child has a colostomy the parents are taught to carry out distal loop washouts. These are undertaken regularly to evacuate faeces and mucus from the distal bowel to minimize infection and keep the bowel in optimal condition for later surgery (Adams & Selekof 1986).

If the colostomy is likely to become a permanent feature the child should be taught to undertake their own care.

'I thought if I continued to care for my child's ostomy because it is faster or easier it may give them the message that he/she can't do it. Tying a shoe lace may be a challenge when one is five, so is changing an appliance – but well worth it.'

Innovations in long term treatment for children with faecal incontinence

Recent innovations have provided a further option, rather than the fashioning of a colostomy, for those children in whom conservative measures have been ineffective. Hancock (1994) described the ACE procedure which involves 'the creation of a non-refluxing catheterizationable channel by which antegrade irrigation can be performed'. A conduit is created between the caecum and abdominal wall to enable irrigation of the bowel. The child and family are taught to perform the washouts which are carried out on a daily basis to evacuate the bowel and hence minimize incontinence.

The nurse has a valuable role in ensuring that the family have access to accurate appropriate information upon which to base their decisions regarding treatment options. It is important to be truthful and not engender false hope in the family (Adams & Selekof 1986).

The infant with intussusception

Intussusception is one of the most common causes of abdominal obstruction in the post neonatal period. There is 'telescoping' of one portion of the bowel into another, commonly at the ileo-caecal valve. Obstruction occurs beyond the deficit and this leads to inflammation, reduced blood flow and necrosis of the bowel. Characteristically the infant has a history of 'good' health and there is a sudden onset of colicky abdominal pain, during which time the infant cries and draws their knees up to their chest. They may be dehydrated due to vomiting caused by the obstruction. The infant's stools may contain blood and mucus and are often referred to as 'redcurrant jelly stools'.

The diagnosis is usually confirmed by a contrast enema and sometimes this has the effect of reducing the intussusception. If conservative measures are ineffective a laparotomy to resect or reduce the obstruction is required. The principles of care have been identified previously and a comprehensive care plan for these infants is offered by Lau (1992).

Table 22.8 summarizes common gastro-intestinal problems.

Table 22.8 Summary of common gastro-intestinal problems in neonates (© Dearmun). P = potential problem

Congenital abnormality	Infant's main actual/potential problems	Physiological rationale for problem
Diaphragmatic hernia	Compromised breathing	Diaphragm develops 8–10 weeks gestation Herniation of abdominal contents into the thorax inhibits lung development Diaphragmatic breathing inhibited
Necrotising enterocolitis	Weight loss due to inability to absorb nutrients	Lack of perfusion to small bowel is thought to lead to ischaemia and compromises the absorptive ability of the ileum
Hirschsprung's disease	(1) Constipation (2) Abdominal distension (3) Vomiting	Aganglionic cells in the colon Lack of nerve impulses to move faeces forward (i.e. peristalisis) creates constipation
Rectal/vaginal urethral fistula	Pyrexia or septicaemia due to ascending infection	Tract between the rectum and vagina or urethra Bacterial infection from faeces
Imperforate anus	(1) Constipation (2) Abdominal distension (3) Vomiting (4) (P) Incontinence of faeces in later life	Atresia of the anus, no exit for faeces If atresia occurs above internal spincter muscle will not be fully developed
Ileal atresia	(1) Constipation (2) Abdominal distension (breathing difficulties) (3) Vomiting (dehydration and acid base imbalance and hypoglycaemia)	Atresia of the small bowel Dilation of bowel above the obstruction, no passage of faeces
Tracheo-oesophageal atresia with/without fistula	(1) Breathing due to (p) aspiration (2) Dehydration due to inability to take oral fluids	Atresia of the oesophagus fistula from oesophagus to trachea. Lungs develop from the foregut
Duodenal atresia	(1) Constipation (2) Vomiting (3) Abdominal distension	Atresia of the duodenum (commonly seen as duodenal web) associated with other abnormalities
Gastroschisis development 2–4 weeks	(1) Constipation (2) Vomiting (3) Infection (4) Hypothermia	Failure of the lateral folds to fuse, midline abdominal contents develop outside the body including liver Membrane covering sometimes damaged during birth Heat loss from exposed surface area of the bowel
Volvulus	(1) Vomiting (2) Constipation (3) Abdominal distension	Malfixation of the bowel which twists on itself

Table 22.8   Summary of common gastro-intestinal problems in neonates (© Dearmun). P = potential problem (cont.)

Congenital abnormality	Infant's main actual/potential problems	Physiological rationale for problem
Meconuim ileus	(1) Constipation (2) Abdominal distension (3) Vomiting	Obstruction due to viscid meconium due to abnormal secretions from the pancreas, associated with cystic fibrosis
Exomphalus	(1) Constipation (2) Vomiting (3) Dehydration	Herniation of abdominal contents outside the body covered with skin

CONCLUSION

This chapter has explored a range of problems associated with eating, drinking and elimination. Common features within all these problems are their potential to inhibit nutrition, alter the homeostatic mechanisms involved in the maintenance of fluid and electrolyte balance and/or adversely influence optimal growth and development. Furthermore it has been suggested that inadequate nutrition in infancy can influence the development of disease in later life (Watling 1994). Although many children can be successfully managed at home, the Audit Commission (1993) identified babies under one year as the major age group in children's wards in England and Wales. The length of stay is often brief and many of these are admitted with diarrhoea and vomiting.

It may be seen that it is very likely that the children's nurse will be required to assess, plan and implement care for children with gastro-intestinal problems because they are major consumers of healthcare.

SUPPORT GROUPS

British Colostomy Association, 15 Station Road, Reading, Berkshire, RG1 1LG. Tel. 01734 391537.

The Ileostomy and Internal Pouch Support Group, Amblehurst House, PO Box 23, Mansfield, Nottingham NG18 4TT. Tel. 01623 28099.

The Urostomy Association, Buckland, Beaumont Park, Danbury, Essex CM3 4DE. Tel. 01245 224294.

REFERENCES AND FURTHER READING

Adams, D.A. & Selekof, J.L. (1986) Children with ostomies: comprehensive care planning. *Pediatric Nursing*, 12(6), 429–33.

Adomat, R. (1992) Understanding shock. *British Journal of Nursing*, 1(93), 124–8.

Ashcraft, K.W., Holder, T.M. (1976) Esophageal atresia and tracheo-esophageal fistula malformations. *Surgical Clinics of North America*, 56, 299.

Audit Commission (1993) *Children First*. HMSO, London.

Auricchio, S., Greco, L. & Troncone, R. (1988) Gluten-sensitive enteropathy in childhood. *Pediatric Clinics of North America*, 35, 157–87.

Auty, B. (1989) Choice of instrumentation of controlled IV infusion. *Intensive Therapy and Clinical Monitoring*, 10, 117–22.

Bain, J. (1994) Umbilical cord care in pre term babies. *Nursing Standard*, 8(15), 32–5.

Bale, S., Jones, V., Richardson, J. (1994) Wound management in children. *Paediatric Nursing*, 6(1), 12–14.

Ball, P.A., Booth, I.W. & Holden, C.E. (1994) *Paediatric Parenteral Nutrition*, p. 9. Pharmacia, Birmingham.

Bennion, D. & Martin, K (1991) In-line infiltration. *Paediatric Nursing*, 3(5), 20–22.

BPA (1993) *The Transfer of Infants and Children for Surgery*. BPA, London.

Cady, C. & Yoshioka, R.S. (1991) Using a learning contract to successfully discharge an infant on home total parenteral nutrition. *Pediatric Nursing*, 17(1), 67–71.

Campbell, S.J. & Summersgill, P. (1993) Keeping it in the family: defining and developing family centred care. *Child Health*, 1, 17–20.

Campbell, S.J., Kelly, P.J. & Summersgill, P. (1993) Putting the family first: interpreting a framework for family centred care. *Child Health*, 1, 59–63.

Campbell, J. (1993) Making sense of shock *Nursing Times*, 89(5), 34–6.

Candy, C.E. (1987) Recent advances in the care of children with acute diarrhoea: giving responsibility to the nurse and parents. *Journal of Advanced Nursing*, 12, 95–9.

Casey, A. (1988) A partnership with child and family. *Senior Nurse*, 8, 8–9.

Casey, A., Mobbs, S. (1988) Partnership in practice: spotlight on children. *Nursing Times*, 84, 67–8.

Clayden, G. (1991) Managing the child with constipation. *Professional Care of Mother and Child*, 1(2), 64–6.

Coleman Stadtler, A. (1989) Preventing encopresis. *Pediatric Nursing*, 15(3), 282–4.

De Benham, B., Ellett, M., Perez, R. *et al.* (1985) Initial assessment and management of chronic diarrhoea in toddlers. *Pediatric Nursing*, 11(4), 281–5.

Ellett, M.A. (1990) Constipation/encopresis: a nursing perspective. *Journal of Pediatric Health Care*, 4, 141–6.

Ellett, M.L., Fitzgerald, J.F. & Winchester, M. (1993) Dietary management of chronic diarrhoea. *Society of Gastroenterology Nurses and Associates*, 15(4), 170–7.

Emergency Medicine (1992) Rehydrating the infant with acute diarrhoea. *Emergency Medicine*, 24(16), 123–7.

Evans, K. (1990) Pediatric management problems. *Pediatric Nursing*, 16(6), 590–91.

Field, T. & Scafidi, F. (1987) Massage of the pre term newborns to improve growth and development. *Pediatric Nursing*, 13(6), 385–7.

Filston, H.C., Izant, R.J. (1985) *The Surgical Neonate*, 2nd edn. Appleton Century Crofts, New York.

Finelli, L. (1991) Evaluation of the child with acute abdominal pain. *Journal of Pediatric Health Care*, 5(5), 251–6.

Fischer, R.G. (1985) Pediatric drug information. *Pediatric Nursing*, 11(3), 215–27.

Foale, H. (1989) Healing the wound. *Paediatric Nursing*, 1(5), 10–11.

Fry, T. (1993) Charting growth, *Child Health*, 1(3), 104–9.

Gartner, J.C., Novak, D. & Schwartz, R. (1992) When abdominal pain strikes a child. *Patient Care*, 26(14), 121–34.

Hamilton, J.R. (1983) Coeliac disease. In *Nelson Textbook of Pediatrics* (eds R.E. Beherman & V.C. Vaughan). W.B. Saunders, Philadelphia.

Hancock, J. (1994) Antegrade Colonic Enemas. *Paediatric Nursing*, 6(1), 22–3.

Herbert, R. (1984) Maintaining the circulating volume. *Nursing*, 2(26), 766–8.

Heubi, J.E. (1992) Evaluating persistent diarrhoea in kids. *Patient Care*, 26(12), 179–98.

Hill, P. (1991) Assessing faecal soiling in children. *Nursing Times*, 87(14), 61–4.

Holden, C. (1991) Home parenteral nutrition. *Paediatric Nursing*, 3(3), 13–15.

Huddleston, K.C. & Ferraro, A.R. (1991) Preparing families of children with gastrostomies. *Pediatric Nursing*, 17(92), 153–8.

Hunsberger, M. & Issenman, R. (1989) Nursing strategies: altered digestive function. In *Family Centered Care of Children* (eds. R.L.R. Foster, M. Hunsberger & J.T.T. Anderson). W.B. Saunders, New York.

Joachum, G. & Hassal, E. (1992) Familial bowel disease in a pediatric population. *Journal of Advanced Nursing*, 17(11), 1310–16.

Johnson, H. (1992) Stoma care for infants, children and young people. *Paediatric Nursing*, 4(4), 8–11.

Jones, T. (1991) Dressed for best. *Paediatric Nursing*, 3(96), 12–15.

Keating, P. (1990) Constipation. *Community Outlook*, 4 November, 4–10.

Kenner, C. & Breuggemeyer, A. (1984) Hirschsprung's disease: current trends and practices. *Neonatal Network*, 3(1), 7–16.

Khatib, H. (1986) Acute gastroenteritis in infants. *Nursing Times*, 23 April, 31–2.

Landman, G.B. (1987) A five year chart review of children biopsied to rule out Hirschsprung's disease. *Clinical Pediatrics*, 26, 288–91.

Lau, C. (1992) Nursing children with intussusception. *Paediatric Nursing*, 4(9), 17–19.

Leape, L.L. (1987) *Patient Care in Paediatric Surgery*. Little Brown Book Company, Boston.

Livesley, J. (1993) Reducing the risks: the management of paediatric intravenous therapy. *Child Health*, 1(2), 68–73.

Livesley, J. (1994) Peripheral IV therapy in children. *Paediatric Nursing*, 6(4), 24–30.

Long, A. (1989) Bottle fed babies. *Paediatric Nursing*, 1(7), 16–17.

MacDonald, C.A. (1989) Biliary atresia. *Journal of Pediatric Nursing*, 6(6), 374–83.

Mackenzie, H. (1991) Caring for a Neonate in Hospital using Roy's Adaptation Model. In *Caring for Children: Towards Partnership with Families* (ed. A. While). Edward Arnold, London.

Martin, L.W. & Torres, A.M. (1985) Hirschsprung's disease. *Surgical Clinics of North America*, 65, 1171–80.

McWade, L.J. (1992) Irritable bowel syndrome: diagnosis and management in school-aged children and adolescents. *Journal of Pediatric Health Care*, 6(2), 82–3.

Metheny, N.M. (1987) *Fluid and Electrolyte Balance: Nursing Considerations*. J.B. Lippincott, Philadelphia.

Milla, P.J. (1988) Gastrointestinal motility disorders in children. *Pediatric Clinics of North America*, 35, 311–30.

Paterson, I. (1990) Baby massage in the neonatal unit. *Journal of Clinical Practice*, 4(23), 19–21.

Peck, S.N. (1992) Paediatric pseudo-obstruction: a case

study. *Society of Gastroenterology Nurses and Associates*, 14(5), 272–3.

Peck, S.N. & Bushby, M. (1992) Alterations in gastrointestinal function. In *Child Health Care, Process and Practice*, 757–808. J.B. Lippincott, Philadelphia.

Pettit, J. (1992) Establishing successful breast feeding in special care. *Paediatric Nursing*, 4(97), 24–5.

Polden, S. & Beadslee, C. (1990) Contacts experienced by neonates in intensive care environments. *Maternal–Child Nursing Journal*, 16(3), 207–26.

Redman, C. (1994) Handling with care: neonatal handling procedures. *Child Health*, 1(6), 177–84.

Russell, J. (1993) Touch and infant massage. *Paediatric Nursing*, 5(3), 8, 10–11.

Rennie, M. (ed) (1992) Infusion equipment. *Intensive Care Britain 1991*, 138–143. Greycoat Pub., London.

Sharrer, V.W. & Ryan Wegner, N.M. (1991) Measurement of stress – coping among school aged children with and without recurrent abdominal pain. *Journal of School Health*, 61(2), 89–91.

Shelton, T., Jeppson, E. & Johnsen, B. (1987) *Family-centred Care for Children with Special Health Care Need*. Association for the Care of Children's Health, Washington DC.

Sidey, A. (1991) The management of gastrostomies. *Paediatric Nursing*, 3(7), 24–6.

Silverman, A. & Roy, C.C. (1983) *Pediatric Clinical Gastro-enterology*. Mosby, St. Louis.

Simmons, M.A. (1984) Using the nursing process in treating inflammatory bowel disease. *Nursing Clinics of North America*, 19, 11–25.

Smith, D.P. (1986) Common day-care diseases: pattern and prevention. *Pediatric Nursing*, 12(3), 175–9.

Smith, J. (1991) Hirschsprung's disease. *Paediatric Nursing*, 3(5), 24–6.

Smith, L.G. (1988) Home treatment of mild, acute diarrhoea and secondary dehydration of infants and small children: an educational programme for parents in a shelter for the homeless. *Journal of Professional Nursing*, 4(1), 60–63.

Sparshott, M. (1991a) Maintaining skin integrity. *Paediatric Nursing*, March, 12–13.

Sparshott, M. (1991b) Reducing infant trauma. *Nursing Times*, 87(50), 30–31.

Stapleford, P. (1989) Formula feeding. *Paediatric Nursing*, 1(4), 14–16.

Stapleford, P. (1990) Parenteral nutrition in children. *Paediatric Nursing*, 2(6), 18–20.

Statler, A.C. (1989) Preventing encopresis. *Pediatric Nursing*, 15(3), 282–84.

Steele, N.F. (1991) The button replacement gastrostomy device. *Journal of Pediatric Nursing*, 6(6), 421–4.

Steward, A. & Fleming, P. (1992) An informed approach may prevent loss: new perspectives on cot death. *Professional Nurse*, 7(5), 329–32.

Sutton, M.M. (1992) Nutritional needs of children with inflammatory bowel disease. *Comprehensive Therapy*, 18(10), 21–25.

Taylor, E. & Watson, A. (1990) Supplementary feeding using a gastrostomy button. *Paediatric Nursing*, 2(10), 16–19.

Tucker, J.A. & Sussman-Karter, K. (1987) Treating acute diarrhoea and dehydration with an oral rehydration solution. *Pediatric Nursing*, 13(3), 169–74.

Turner, A.F. (1991) Encopresis: family support must accompany treatment. In *Child Care – Some Nursing Perspectives* (ed A. Glasper). Wolfe Publishing Ltd, London.

Wallis, M. (1993) Care of the Neonate. In *Manual of Paediatric Intensive Care Nursing* (ed. B. Carter). Chapman and Hall, London.

Walsh, M. & Ford, P. (1989) *Nursing Rituals Research and Rational Actions*. Heinemann Nursing, London.

Watling, R. (1994) Setting off on the right food: good practice in infant nutrition. *Child Health*, 2(1), 16–20.

Webster, P. (1989) Forging a role. *Paediatric Nursing*, 1(6), 8–10.

Whaley, L.F. & Wong, D.L. (1991) *Nursing Care of Infants and Children*, 4th edn. Mosby-Year Book Inc., St. Louis.

White-Taut, R. & Carnier Goldman, M. (1988) Premature baby massage: Is it safe? *Pediatric Nursing*, 14(4), 285–9.

Winch, A.E. & Ouverson, C. (1992) Nursing interventions for thromboembolic complications of chronic ulcerative colitis in children. *American Journal of Maternal Child Nursing*, 17(2), 86–90.

Wright, H. (1990) Nissen's fundoplication. *Paediatric Nursing*, 2(2), 22–3.

Yeo, H. (1993) Expert care at a critical time: surgical repair of gastroschisis in neonates. *Child Health*, 1(2), 74–8.

Younger, J.B. & Hughes, L.S. (1983) No-fault management of encopresis. *Pediatric Nursing*, 9(3), 185–7.

Chapter 23

Nursing Support and Care: Meeting the Needs of the Child and Family with Altered Integumentary Function

Janice Colson

'The eyes are the mirror of the soul: the skin is a canvas on which the psyche reveals itself' (Seville & Martin 1981)

INTRODUCTION

This chapter explores the effects upon the child and family of altered integumentary function.

Burton (1990), making reference to deficits in medical education, stated that 'dermatology does not occupy an important place in the curriculum'. A similar criticism may be levied at the nursing curriculum, although somewhat mistakenly since the skin of a child can tell so much without even an exchange of words.

When reviewing approaches to nursing infants and children with dysfunction of the skin, a number of issues require consideration, in particular the age and developmental level of the child. These factors are important because they will be reflected in the child's ability to understand the nature and cause of the dysfunction. In addition, the child's willingness to co-operate with and possibly participate in treatment will be influenced by their level of cognitive development.

Age is also an important determinant of functions and dysfunctions of the skin. It is for this reason that this chapter will use chronological age to provide a framework from which to explore some of the dysfunctions of the skin which are predominant in infancy and childhood.

The role of the nurse in caring for an infant, child or adolescent with dysfunction of the skin will vary depending on the extent of the problem. The nurse may be engaged as teacher and supporter when the child embarks on a long and arduous course of treatment which necessitates the application of topical preparations or compliance with a dietary regime. Conversely, the nurse's role may be that of providing intensive therapy for the child who has sustained extensive thermal injuries.

Regardless of the problem, an understanding and compassionate approach will be necessary to acquire a full and detailed history about a problem which may have lifelong impact on the child and family. Even in circumstances of a less critical nature, the child and family may be experiencing difficulties in coping with what they perceive as a stressful episode in their lives. Effective communications from the outset will

provide an environment that is conducive to an open and questioning approach for the child, and if they are old enough will enable them to engage in discussion. When the child is too young to participate, parents will need to act as advocates for their child.

Co-operation is an essential component in the majority of instances when dealing with dysfunction of the skin. When parents, or in the case of older children, the child does not co-operate with nursing and medical staff, the treatment is likely to be doomed from the outset. This is mainly because treatment may be over a long period of time, and require changes or adaptations of lifestyle. In addition, current trends mean that children spend the minimal amount of time in hospital whenever possible (Department of Health 1991). They are therefore dependent on parents and carers to comply with treatment regimes and act in their best interests (ASC 1991).

All the features of care previously mentioned will underpin an exploration of some of the many conditions that may cause dysfunction of the skin. In addition to these the nurse should have a sound understanding of both the usual and altered physiology. This will enhance their ability to explain the problems to the parents and child in terms that they can understand. This may in turn encourage them to become involved in restoring function, taking steps to recognize or assist in their adaptation to living to the full, within the confines of the disorder. Knowledge of the structure and function of skin is assumed, but additional information can be obtained from Marieb (1989).

This chapter is divided into three main sections. The first section offers a chronological account of problems relating to the age and stage of development of the child and discusses some of the skin disorders that may occur as a result of everyday living, for example nappy rash during infancy or headlice in the school-age child. It will also include the effects on the skin of the more frequently occurring infectious diseases of childhood such as chickenpox.

The second section is concerned with disorders that may be the result of psychological disturbance and/or the social circumstances in which the child is growing up. Two examples of these are acne and eczema.

The third section addresses trauma of both an accidental and nonaccidental nature; illustrations of these include thermal injury and epidermolysis bullosa and naevi, conditions of genetic origin.

Structure and functions of the skin

The skin is the most extensive organ of the body. The complex structure provides a watertight and air proof barrier between the internal organs and the external environment.

The functions of the skin are:

(1) Protection of internal organs.
(2) Regulation of body temperature.
(3) Elimination of some waste products.
(4) Sensation – particularly early warnings of danger.
(5) Production of vitamin D.
(6) Provision of a store of fat.
(7) Indication of the emotional status.

A CHRONOLOGICAL ACCOUNT OF PROBLEMS AFFECTING THE SKIN

The state of the human skin is constantly changing throughout the life span. The speed and extent of these changes may vary depending on the environment in which the individual lives. The amount of exposure the skin has to environmental conditions, and the care with which the skin is treated, are also important. Old wives' tales should not be dismissed totally.

There is more than an element of truth in the sayings 'as soft as a baby's bottom' or 'as tough as leather' of skin which has been subjected to years of exposure to harsh weather conditions, be they extreme heat or cold. However, regardless of the elements, the skin does undergo specific changes at certain times in life and it is for this reason that some skin abnormalities are more common in infants and children than in adults.

The infant

The skin of the neonate provides an index of growth. Well nourished neonates have clearly defined layers of subcutaneous fat over their bodies, which provide thermoregulation and a barrier against infection. Lack of subcutaneous fat in the neonate may indicate prematurity or malnutrition.

The subcutaneous fat which is evident in the majority of babies born at approximately 40 weeks gestation is deposited mainly in the few weeks prior to term.

All babies in utero have a downy distribution of fine hair over their body. This is known as lanugo, which literally means wool. The word was originally used to describe the fuzz on a peach before being borrowed by human medicine (Morris 1991). Lanugo begins to appear on the fetus at 16 weeks gestation, but gradually disappears from about the 32nd week. It can, therefore, be seen on the pre-term infant in varying degrees depending on the prematurity of the baby. It is mostly found on the shoulders, back, extremities, forehead and temple.

The skin of the pre-term infant is thin with numerous veins and tributaries visible (Harper 1990). Even infants of 34 weeks gestational age have relatively little subcutaneous fat. The skin should be observed closely for breaks as this may be a portal of entry for bacteria.

Due to the thin epidermis the speed of absorption through the skin is dramatically increased. Most compounds placed on the skin of the premature infant can be found in the urine and saliva in a matter of minutes. Topical ointments and other skin preparations, therefore, should not be used without a physician's order. This is particularly relevant when caring for the pre-term infant nursed in a Baby Therm or Ohio crib. The skin will quickly become scaly and dry, increasing the desire to apply moisture creams. This should not be done as it will further destroy the skin due to a 'frying' effect.

The newborn infant will be strongly influenced by the mother's hormones and chemicals. Skin cells are affected by their genetic blueprint, just as other body cells are.

Sebaceous glands are well developed at birth owing to stimulation by the mother's hormones. Newborn 'acne' may result from androgen stimulation of the sebaceous glands in the uterus; some newborn babies may therefore be prone to oily, spotty skin.

As the skin matures the surface becomes acidic, thus providing a medium which discourages the growth of micro-organisms. However, in the early days of life, the pH of the skin is alkaline. Therefore the neonate is more susceptible to infection (Foster *et al.* 1989).

Eccrine glands in the neonate begin to function at two to five days of life and reach mature function at two to three years of age (they are densest on the palms of the hands and soles of the feet). The ability to perspire freely gives the toddler and older child better thermoregulatory function than is possessed by the infant. The evaporation of the sebum also helps to lower the skin pH, thus increasing resistance to skin infections in later childhood. This is particularly important as with increased mobility children come into contact with a wider variety of sources from which they might acquire an infection.

A frequent noninfectious form of skin disorder seen in infancy is napkin dermatitis. This is the most common form of nonallergic irritant contact dermatitis in infancy. The irritation is usually from urine ammonia and inadequate cleansing of the nappy area. The rash tends to be exacerbated by heat, moisture, friction and tight clothing. Although still seen, napkin dermatitis has become less common due to the widespread adoption of the use of disposable nappies as opposed to terry towelling nappies. However, care still needs to be taken even when using disposable nappies.

The incidence of napkin rash is likely to be greatly reduced if some of the modern myths created by the advertising media are dispelled for parents and carers; for example, the use of disposable nappies keeps the baby dry all day. This is an incorrect assumption because the disposable nappy will only keep the baby dry all day if it is changed when urine has been passed or bowels opened. Although disposable nappies reduce wetness by pulling urine to the liner and away from the baby's skin, the urea and ammonia salts that cause the skin to break down are left behind as a residue on the nappy surface. The constant contact of this surface with the infant's skin is therefore the source of the problem.

In order to uphold the manufacturer's claims, the following advice may be helpful. The exact time for changing the infant will vary with individual preferences. However, the activity of changing the infant is usually related to the feeding time. In general, if infants are clean and dry when they are put down to sleep, then the skin covered by the nappy should stay intact and healthy.

Another myth is related to the notion that cream, talcum powder, or baby wipes will suffice instead of soap and water for cleaning the baby. It is argued that the use of baby lotion is messy and talcum powder has no cleansing properties. However, baby wipes may be as effective as soap and water.

General treatment of any nappy rash requires basic nappy and skin care. The area should be kept clean and dry, with prompt, thorough cleansing of the region with mild soap and water or mild baby wipes after each defecation or voiding, to rid the skin of irritant byproducts. The area should be checked every hour in the newborn, and every two hours in older infants.

However, whilst this ideal may be appropriate for the infant who is cared for on a regular basis by his mother, the question arises of how likely this practice is to be maintained for infants and young children being cared for by childminders and in day nurseries. In these situations the ratio of children to carers is often about 4:1, thus making the likelihood of such frequent changes almost impossible. Other circumstances such as situations where there are reduced finances, limited drying facilities for terry towelling nappies and poor understanding of the hygiene needs of the infant, are all contributory factors and should be held in mind when dealing with a family whose child has napkin dermatitis.

Immunoglobulin A antibodies are secreted by the epithelial cells of mucous membranes. Infants and children produce this rather slowly and only at puberty are maximum levels achieved. Diminished ability to produce these antibodies reduces the mucosal resistance to organisms.

One of the most common organisms is candida albicans which is a yeast-like fungus present as a commensal in the gut (Burton 1990). When present in quantity it causes an infection called moniliasis or candiasis. Oral infection is commonly called 'thrush', with spreading milk spot patches and plaques. Sometimes on visual inspection it may appear difficult to distinguish from milk immediately after a feed, but milk can easily be wiped off from the inside of the mouth. Superficial thrush responds rapidly to antimonilial preparations, e.g. Nystatin or Miconazole. Objects mouthed by infants need to be cleaned frequently.

Candida albicans commonly causes secondary infection of eruptions in the area of the genitalia and buttocks. Perianal thrush gives a bright red, confluence rash in the napkin area or around the anus. Typically there are discrete ulcerated satellite lesions lying peripheral to the confluent rash.

Young children should be taught good hand washing at an early age as their hands are often in contact with their mouths, noses and other vulnerable surfaces as they explore their bodies.

Infants in hospital who are not receiving oral fluids are more susceptible to candida, as are all infants and children receiving antibiotics. Broad spectrum antibiotics reduce the normal gut bacteria which in turn allows for excessive proliferation of candida (Burton 1990). These infants and children should therefore be provided with regular and meticulous oral hygiene care which may challenge the ingenuity of parents and nurses. A child with a sore mouth is not usually a co-operative assistant during such procedures.

Infants between the ages of eight and 18 months spend a lot of time on the floor as they learn to crawl and explore every crevice for dust and dirt. This developmental stage means children are particularly vulnerable to bacterial infections of the subcutaneous tissue and dermis. The most common organisms are staphylococci and haemophilus influenzae.

The process of crawling tends to have an irritant effect on hands and knees in the younger child, whilst the accident-prone toddler may provide evidence of a more severe infection with cellulitis, which may have resulted from a minute crack following trauma. In a classic course of cellulitis, a red, tender, warm swelling appears within a day or two of the original skin trauma. The swelling rapidly increases to produce a large, firm area of oedema. The child experiences pain as a result of the intense pressure of the inflammatory exudate on skin tissues. Mild cases of cellulitis may be treated with oral antibiotics. Children with more serious infection are often admitted to hospital for intravenous antibiotic therapy. This is continued until there is noticeable reduction in the redness and oedema.

The pre-school and school child

Children continue to grow and subsequently attend playschool and school where they mix closely with many other children. Bacterial infections such as impetigo, viral infections such as verrucae and chickenpox, infestations such as scabies and lice, and fungal infections such as ringworm and candida, become much more common.

Impetigo as a primary infection is relatively uncommon (Harper 1990) and is most frequently associated with poor hygiene and unsanitary social circumstances. Impetigo is highly contagious. It is most often located around the mouth and nose. Impetigo is superficially caused by staphylococcus aureus or, more rarely, this organism in combination with the haemolytic streptococcus. Fragile blisters or pustules form, which evolve into the characteristic golden yellow crusts. Impetigo

occurs when the organism comes into contact with broken skin, or there may be a precipitating cause, e.g. scabies, head lice or atopic eczema.

The treatment normally involves topical antimicrobial preparations and/or a systemic antibiotic. Impetigo is contagious, therefore children who normally attend nursery or school should remain at home until they have been taking antibiotics for 48 hours and/or the lesions are dry. Contamination among siblings and other family members can be decreased by encouraging thorough hand washing. Towels and face flannels must not be shared.

Treatment aimed to promote healing should include the removal of crusts once or twice daily after soaking in warm salty water. Removing crusts too early, however, will result in recrusting and will prolong healing. Scratching lesions may result in secondary infection. Whilst older children may be prevented from doing this by a variety of methods, mittens may be necessary for the infant.

Health visitors for the pre-school child and the school nurse for older children should be available to provide help and support to families when a child has contracted such an infection.

Certain phage group II staphylococci can cause toxin resulting in staphylococcal scalded skin syndrome (Lyells syndrome). The almost total shedding of superficial epidermis presents considerable nursing problems. This complication almost invariably develops in children under 12 who require hospital admission, fluid replacement, and parenteral antibiotic therapy. Ultimate recovery is usual.

THE CHILD WITH AN INFESTATION

THE CHILD WITH PEDICULOSIS CAPITIS

There are many popular misconceptions concerning headlice, but they are now regarded more of a nuisance than a threat. Infestation with lice became less common in postwar years, but the incidence has recently increased (Buxton 1993). The peak incidence is in pre-school and early school age children. This is thought to be due to the great increase in group activity between the ages of two and four years (Smith 1987), which continues into the early school years and the group activity rises to about 57% of the time when children play out of doors together (Hertz-Lazarowitz *et al.* 1981).

Pediculosis is thought to be more prevalent in Caucasians then in any other ethnic group. This appears to be due to the makeup of the hair shaft (Foster *et al.* 1989). The child can be infected by either direct contact or from objects such as combs, hats and clothing. Human headlice do not jump from head to head unless direct contact has taken place. The louse lives its entire life on the head of the child it infests.

The eggs are called nits and are attached to the hair shaft by a cement-like substance. The nit hatches within a week and the hatched nymph matures into a louse. Within seven to 10 days it punctures the scalp with its hooklike claws, to suck blood. A week after the bite the child develops an allergic response which is evident by intense itching. A mild fever and enlarged occipital glands can appear. Following prolonged exposure, the body's sensitivity is diminished and the child becomes oblivious to the bites (asymptomatic).

The nits can be seen as silvery or greyish-white and are securely attached to the hair shaft near the scalp. They are prominently seen behind the ears and the nape of the neck. The adult louse can be seen as a black speck that moves and jumps on the scalp. During the period of allergic reactivity, the intense scratching can cause secondary infection to occur.

Treatments are both preventative and corrective, and the following advice and information should be given about headlice:

(1) If a louse is injured it lacks the ability to recover. For this reason, twice daily combing of the hair from the roots to the tips and washing with normal shampoo are excellent preventative measures.
(2) Insecticidal shampoos should not be used as a preventative measure as this could lead to the development of resistant lice.
(3) Parents should be advised to inspect their children's hair weekly and look carefully for nits at the hair roots.

Lotions and shampoos can be either prescribed or bought from a local supermarket. Lotions are more effective than shampoos and help delay the emergence of resistant strains of lice. Following shampooing the hair should be allowed to dry naturally (without using a hair dryer). The treatment should be repeated twice with a three day interval between applications. This is to ensure that all louse eggs are dead.

The hair should be combed with a fine toothed comb until all the lice are removed. Dipping the comb in vinegar may help to loosen tightly attached nits. Itching may continue for three to four days after using the insecticide shampoo. Children prone to eczema may have an allergic response to the shampoo. Persistent pruritus may be indicative of more nits which require treatment.

All the child's contacts should be treated simultaneously with the child to prevent immediate re-infestation. Towels and combs should be kept separate, and non-launderable items should be soaked in one of the pediculocidal shampoos for an hour or heated in water. All contactable items that can be laundered should be washed in hot water and dried in sunlight or a clothes drier. Children should be kept away from school until the treatment is complete. The school authorities should be notified of the child's condition.

The treatment of headlice under the Education Act 1944 and the Children Act 1989, is an example of the changing recognition of the rights of children in their treatment.

Under the 1944 Education Act, Section 54 I to VIII, any authorized officer of the education authority may serve a notice on the parents of a pupil requiring the pupil to be treated. If this is not carried out within a specified time, which must not be more than 24 hours, the child may be removed to the cleansing station and treated accordingly (Slack 1978).

The Children Act 1989 suggests that where an inspection includes a physical examination of the child, the examination may be carried out only with the consent of the child where he/she is of sufficient understanding to give or withhold consent.

Nurses should not be complacement where headlice are concerned; they can catch them too! This fact has been realized by many nurses when they have worked in close contact with children who are infected.

THE CHILD WITH SCABIES

The most common infestation encountered is scabies

(Buxton 1993). Scabies is an itchy skin condition caused by the scabies mite which lives under the top layer of the skin, particularly between the fingers, breasts and genitals. It does not occur above the neck. The female mite burrows under the skin to lay her eggs. The developing eggs hatch into larvae within a few days. Intense itching usually occurs two weeks later.

Identification of scabies in children is difficult. Finding the 'burrow', the small ridge (5–10 mm long) caused by the mite, can be difficult as it is often obscured by excoriation from scratching. Without the burrow, diagnosis remains uncertain. It is important, therefore, to find out if there are other members of the household who are also itching. This infestation is only acquired by close contact with infected people.

There are several different preparations that can be used in treatment but care must be taken when using them for children under seven years of age. However, the treatment outlined in Table 23.1 should be adhered to in cases of infestation.

Table 23.1 Treatment procedure for scabies.

(1) Every member of the household should be treated at the same time.
(2) Wash the child well. In the past, a hot bath was advocated; however, this is not now recommended as it is thought to increase absorption of the lotion through the skin.
(3) A thin layer of the prescribed lotion should be applied to the whole body, except for the face and scalp. In children under two years old, however, the head and face should be treated, although great care must be taken to avoid the eyes, mouth and ears.
(4) The treatment should be left on for 24 hours and washed off in a bath or shower.
(5) The nurse should advise the family that although the treatment has been successful it may take several weeks before the itching completely clears.

There is still often a social stigma attached to scabies and the child at times may feel ashamed or guilty. It is important for the nurse to explain to the child the nature of the condition, so giving understanding of why it could have occurred. This in turn may help the child cope with the problem and maintain a positive self image.

This section has provided an overview of the most common skin conditions arising as a result of the child's vulnerable age and/or infestation. The care required has been discussed, and some useful advice to nurses included.

Whilst it has been impossible to include details of all conditions, Tables 23.2, 23.3 and 23.4 summarize other infestations which are experienced during childhood.

THE CHILD WITH DYSFUNCTION OF THE SKIN ARISING FROM INDETERMINATE SOURCES

This section of the chapter will consider disorders that may be the result of psychological disturbance and/or the social circumstances in which the child is growing up. These may arise from a variety of sources, most of which are indeterminate. Attempts at locating the source, however, are an essential aspect of treatment. At the onset these conditions are noninfectious but due to their irritant nature, there is a risk that infection can be introduced.

The conditions which will be considered here are:

(1) Acne.
(2) Eczema.
(3) Psoriasis.

THE CHILD WITH ACNE

A disorder of the skin can be far more of a 'handicap' than is generally realized. Acne is a classic example. A young person with acne may experience considerable suffering; though essentially healthy, young adults may find it particularly difficult to cope with.

At a time when they are most sensitive about their appearance, beginning to discover their own identity and acutely caring what others think, the young adult is especially vulnerable to the social and emotional strains that a condition such as acne can bring. It can affect the way they behave due to self-conscious embarrassment. Acne can restrict the enjoyment of life by influencing relationships within the family, with friends and mem-

Table 23.2 Bacterial infections.

Bacterial infections	Aetiology and incidence	Clinical manifestations	Treatment
Impetigo	(1) Usually a primary condition but can be secondary to eczema, dermatitis, psoriasis or scratching due to scabies. (2) Usually caused by staphylococci or rarely streptococci. (3) Occurs most frequently in children under 10 years of age. (4) Spread by contact easily conveyed person to person.	(1) Incubation period of one to five days. (2) Face, hands, and scalp are commonly involved. (3) The initial small erythematous area enlarges rapidly into a spreading vesicle which bursts and forms a scab.	(1) Relative isolation of the patient is necessary to prevent cross-infection and must be stringent if any babies are in close proximity. (2) Towels, sponges, brushes etc. must not be shared and close contact avoided. (3) Gentle removal of all crusts with saline to ensure penetration of topical antibiotic.
Furunculosis (boils)	(1) An invasion of sebaceous glands and hair follicles usually by pathogenic staphylococcus. (2) Usually occur at site of maceration and recurrent trauma such as chafing and scratching. (3) More common in diabetics and immunological deficient patients.	(1) Usually quite sudden. Skin becomes red around a follicle, tenderness, heat and oedema follow. The centre becomes yellow with pus. (2) Sites commonly affected are back of neck, axillas, buttocks and thighs. (3) Large multiple lesions are called carbuncles.	(1) Local applications are not useful but the painful boil should be protected from trauma by a dressing. (2) Penicillin or a broad spectrum antibiotic may be used. (3) Recurrent boils require treatment for two months after the last lesion has cleared.

bers of the opposite sex. It also affects what toiletries and cosmetics can be used, what foods can be eaten, and the fabrics they are able to wear. In addition, acne may cause such severe psychological stress that achievement at school will be disturbed, thus having an ultimate effect on the young person's career potential. It is therefore important that the severity of the problem is never undermined.

Acne is the classic skin eruption of young adulthood, being a hormonally mediated disease (Harper 1990). It is seen in 40% of this age group. The problem can start at eight years of age and continue into the twenties, but the vast majority who seek medical help are aged between 12 and 18 years (Harper 1990). Acne occurs in the majority of males and 80% of females in varying

degrees. It is a gradual process with an insidious onset, usually affecting the face, chest, back and neck. The pathophysiology of acne is characterized by three mechanisms, as shown in Table 23.5.

Acne is characterized by comedones which occur due to sebum in the glands being held back by horny plugs of keratinized protein. Open comedones are called blackheads. These are found in widely dilated follicles (pores). Although unsightly, they do not progress to inflammatory lesions unless squeezed and manipulated. Closed comedones are termed whiteheads. These are small, nonerythematous papules just under the skin's surface.

As cells and sebum continue to accumulate, they exert pressure which eventually ruptures the follicle

Table 23.3 Viral infections.

Viral infections	Aetiology and incidence	Clinical manifestations	Treatment
Chickenpox	(1) Varicella virus. (2) Highly communicable acquired by direct contact, droplet spread.	(1) Rash appears first on head and mucous membranes then becomes concentrated on body and sparse on extremities. (2) Rash-macules to papules and vesicles to crust within several hours. (3) Itching of lesions may be severe and scratching may cause scarring.	(1) Isolation until all lesions have crusted. (2) Keep child cool, wear loose clothing. (3) Oral antihistamines to decrease pruritus. (4) Calamine lotion applied to skin. (5) Short fingernails to prevent scratching.
Measles	(1) Measles virus RNA containing paramyxo virus. (2) Direct contact with droplet from infected persons.	(1) Fever. (2) Lethargy; 48 hours koplic spots on buccal mucosa.	(1) Bed rest. (2) Darken room if child is photophobic. NB Immunoglobulin is indicated for children at particular risk, for example those who are immuno suppressed.
Rubella	(1) Rubella virus. (2) Droplets or direct contact with infected persons.	(1) Rash. Pinpoint red spots on soft palate (forchheimers spots). Spread to face and downward, covering entire body at end of first day.	(1) Symptomatic.

wall. The follicular contents spill into the dermis causing an inflammatory reaction. Due to the feeling of pressure on the skin as a result of the inflammation, it can be very tempting to squeeze the lesion to alleviate the pressure. This, however, is not effective as there is no channel through which the inflammatory contents can exit and results in further inflammation and predisposition to secondary infection.

Nursing intervention: meeting the young adult's needs

The nurse's role in the treatment of acne is usually one of adviser and supporter. Early treatment is essential and requires careful planning, including the correct medication, counselling and guidance about contributory factors. Common shortcomings in management include too little explanation and counselling, too little concern, a medication regime which is too complex, inappropriate dietary regimes, and dietary manipulation.

Young adults who are aware of the mechanism of acne and have an understanding of the condition and the rationale behind the treatment are most likely to adhere to their treatment regimes. It is important that both the adolescent and family recognize that acne is not a result of uncleanliness and therefore washing the face repeatedly will not cure the problem. There are many creams and lotions available claiming to solve the problem of acne.

Table 23.4   Fungal infections.

Fungal infections	Aetiology and incidence	Clinical manifestations	Treatment
Oral candidiasis (thrush)	(1) Caused by candida albicans. (2) Most frequently seen in newborn babies but may be seen in older infants as a complication of antibiotic therapy. (3) It frequently occurs in children who have a cleft lip and palate. (4) The growth of the organism is favoured in the immunodeficient patient, diabetics, and in contaminated feeding equipment.	(1) The infant develops small plaques on the oral mucous membrane, tongue or gums. The plaques appear like milk curds but cannot be wiped from the mouth.	(1) Good oral hygiene and the oral administration of nystatin in suspension. This should be given following feeds. (2) Teaching parents and junior nurses the importance of cleaning feeding equipment properly.
Candidal nappy dermatitis	(1) It is usually due to prolonged wearing of wet napkins, and less often to the formation of ammonia in the wet napkin as the result of the growth of a saprophytic bacillus.	(1) It is an erythematous and papulovesicular dermatitis which occurs on the buttocks, thighs and lower abdomen and in severe cases may spread to involve chest, face and legs. (2) Generally causes discomfort especially when wetting or changing.	(1) Keep area clean and dry avoiding oil and powders which may retain bacteria. (2) Expose buttocks to fresh air when possible. (3) Topical application of nystatin cream or ointment. (4) Barrier creams to protect the skin, e.g. metonym may also be used.

Table 23.5   Three mechanisms of pathophysiology of acne.

(1) Androgenic hormone and the production of excessive amount of sebum
Rationale: Androgens stimulate the production of sebum by the sebaceous glands and influence keratinization in the pilosebaceous duct (Foster et al. 1989).

(2) Hyperkeratinization
Rationale: Adolescents tend to have narrow follicular orifices which become blocked as a result of hyperkeratinization, thus obstructing the pilosebaceous duct, causing the formation of comedones (Harper 1990).

(3) Bacteria
Rationale: The presence of bacteria, propionbacterium acnes for example, in the pilosebaceous follicle produces mediators which are responsible for the inflammation in acne (Lookingbill & Marks 1986).

Nurses who are involved in the care and support of young people who 'suffer' with acne would do well to familiarize themselves with commercially produced preparations and their claims. In this way they will be able to provide appropriate advice. It is important to consider the ethical issues surrounding the marketing techniques that some companies use to persuade adolescents to purchase their expensive products.

The adolescent should be made aware that using products that dry the skin will further irritate the skin, causing it to produce more oil and so compounding the problem. The face should be washed in lukewarm water using a mild soap. The skin should be cleansed gently using a nonabrasive action. The nurse will need to be supportive of the adolescent commencing treatment. Perseverance is the mainstay in the treatment of acne as it often takes at least a month for physical treatments to start being effective.

The treatment of acne is based on three main aetiological features: increased sebum production, obstruction of the follicle and bacterial infection. Acne is one of the most easily treated diseases of adolescence and with early treatment, scarring can be prevented in most cases. Such treatments require patience, skill and a commitment to good counselling. Table 23.6 shows approaches to treatment.

THE CHILD WHO HAS ECZEMA

It is predicted that five million people or 10% of the population in the UK will develop eczema at some time in their lives (Spowart 1993). This is a common but unpleasant condition. The most frequently occurring symptom is a dry skin but the severity fluctuates according to a variety of circumstances. According to Burton (1992), in the majority of children eczema turns out to be atopic and is often associated with asthma or hay fever.

The children's nurse is most likely to encounter the minority group who are referred to hospital. This means there is the potential for paediatric nurses to have a distorted view of the severity of eczema. In addition, Spowart & Muir (1993) state that whilst health visitors and nurses have heard of eczema, they are apprehensive about treating it due to a lack of understanding. This situation needs to be redressed since these two particular groups of people are in an ideal position to provide extended help and support to the affected child and family.

When considering the different types of eczema, it is important to be familiar with the variety of terminology as it is often interchangeable. According to the National Eczema Society, there are at least eight types of skin disorder which fall under the classification of eczema. Spowart & Muir (1993) contend that a sound understanding of those experienced by children is essential since it will enable nurses to discuss the treatments and long-term implications with children and parents.

Historically differentiations have been made between eczema and dermatitis. Eczema is the term used to refer to inflammation of the skin resulting from events occurring internally. Dermatitis is generally the term applied to inflammation caused by substances affecting the body externally. Currently there is no such clear demarcation, as evidenced by Burton (1992) and Whaley & Wong (1991), and the terms are used interchangeably. Van Bever (1992) summarizes the situation by stating that 'in 66% of patients with atopic dermatitis, there is a family history of atopic diseases but environmental factors seem to have some influence in determining whether the genetic trait manifests itself'.

Eczema, or eczematous inflammation of the skin, refers to a descriptive category of dermatologic diseases and not to a specific aetiology. As mentioned previously, atopic eczema is most common in children up to the age of 11 years. It presents in three forms which can be related to the age of the child and it can be acute, subacute or chronic. Eczema is characterized by erythema, oedema with discrete groups of vesicles, and papules. Combined, these give the appearance of uniform pin head eruptions (Dale 1983).

Infantile eczema is usually seen first in the baby between two and six months of age. Unlike napkin dermatitis, which can be seen in the neonate, atopic eczema usually starts on the cheeks and spreads to distal flexures. This distribution is quite different from that of napkin dermatitis (Shrank 1986).

In the early years of life children have a tendency to thumb sucking, lip licking and dribbling. Additionally, without the appropriate protection they are prone to chapping in extreme weather conditions such as cold and wind. These factors superimposed on the young child who already suffers from atopic eczema will give symptoms of moist or fissured eczema around the

Table 23.6 Common approaches to treatment of acne.

Remedies	Mode of action	Advice
Topical remedies		Effective if lesions are superficial.
Benzoyl peroxide; cream, lotion or gel	Irritant and keratolytic agent. Causes follicular desquamation. Disrupts the compaction within the follicle. Has antibacterial properties. Has minimal effect for established lesions.	Improvement may only be evident after a month or more. Its use should be initiated in a gradual fashion. Initial test application should be made for several hours. Apply a thin film to all acne prone areas, initially every other day and after two to three weeks progress to daily applications. Absorption is increased by moisture so do not apply immediately after washing the face. It is a bleaching agent and can damage clothing.
Vitamin A (Retin A)	Not recommended for dry or fair skin. Creates increased turnover in the pilosebaceous ducts. Decreased stickiness of epidermal cells. Expulsion of existing comedones.	Ensure adherence to treatment. Acne may appear to worsen in the first two weeks. It may take two to three months for the cosmetic improvement to be seen. Cream should be applied gradually. A period of 30 minutes should elapse between washing and application, to avoid moisture. Factor suncreams should be applied liberally when outdoors as this preparation is a photosensitizer.
Other available therapies Ultra violet light	May be effective in reducing acne.	Relapse often occurs after completion of the course.
Comedone extractor	This can be used to remove blackheads.	
Diets		Although these have been popular there is little empirical evidence to suggest they bring about lasting improvement.

mouth. The signs frequently extend beyond the mouth and can become secondarily infected. According to Burton (1992), the activities described above which produce damp soggy skin may have been the source of origin of the condition and where it persists they are almost undoubtedly responsible.

Eczema in childhood may follow on from infantile type, occurring at two to three years of age. Of the children who experience this, approximately 90% will manifest the condition by the time they are five years old (Whaley & Wong 1991). Lesions appear mainly in areas of flexure: the elbows and knees, the neck, wrists, ankles and feet. The child will have small erythematous or flesh coloured papules which may give way to lichenifications.

The skin will be dry and hyperpigmented. In some children, only one site may be involved. The hands may show signs of lesions producing exudate, and changes in the nails are common. Carers should be observant for acute vesiculation, whether generalized or localized, because it may be indicative of a secondary bacterial or viral infection.

In the young adult, the condition begins to manifest at about 12 years of age and may continue for some time throughout adult life. The picture of presentation in this group is very similar to that in later childhood. Lichenification occurs, particularly on the flexures and the hands.

According to Burton (1992), there are a few children who will continue to present with a typical picture of the disease into later adult life. These are people who have pronounced epidermal changes or who have a history of a disturbed psychiatric or home background.

Nursing assessment

A major feature of the nursing assessment will be to obtain a history from the child and family regarding any factors which may be seen to exacerbate the problem; once identified they can usually be eliminated.

Children from all age groups may display one or more of the following physical signs and nurses should be aware of them when undertaking the nursing assessment.

- Intense itching.
- Skin which is not affected is dry and rough.
- Children with darker skins have more papular and/or follicular lesions than white children.
- Lymphadenopathy near to the affected sites.
- Tendency to cold extremities, particularly hands.
- Facial pallor.
- Cutaneous infections.
- Restlessness.
- Irritability.

The onset and pattern of eczema may vary depending on the age of the child. However, the principles of treatment may be applied to all age groups.

Nursing intervention: meeting the child's needs

When considering the aims of care and associated nursing interventions for the child experiencing atopic eczema, it is important to remember that many of the aspects of care are interrelated. Spowart (1993) suggests that the management of eczema should not be confined to the application of skin creams; a holistic approach should be adopted.

The main aim of care will be related to breaking the cycle of pruritis and scratching. When the intense pruritis is relieved, the temptation to scratch will be reduced and hence there will be less risk of introducing secondary infection. This is illustrated in Fig. 23.1.

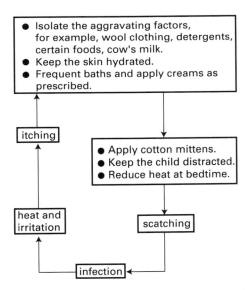

Fig. 23.1   Breaking the cycle of pruritis and scatching.

There are several interventions that will reduce the pruritis, including identification and removal of any causative factors, and increasing the hydration of the skin.

Burton (1990) suggests that the identification and removal of causative factors is one of the most important considerations; for example, sometimes cow's milk allergies result in eczema (David 1994), and thus by eliminating cow's milk from the diet an improvement may be seen. Wool, perfumed soaps and washing powders, if creating pruritis, can be avoided.

The pruritis associated with eczema may be further intensified by the skin being very dry. Therefore parents and children should be involved in care to ensure that the skin remains well hydrated. The most widely accepted practice to maintain skin hydration is that of frequent bathing with the use of suitable emollients such as liquid paraffin preparations (Spowart 1993).

As prescriptions vary it is not intended to discuss in detail the types or frequency of medications, either for topical or enteral use. Individual children will have their own particular prescriptions according to their assessed needs. Where a clinical nurse specialist has been involved, they may have responsibility for determining use of medications.

When carrying out therapeutic baths there are several precautions that should be noted. Parents should be given advice about these. In some areas of the country water is known to be 'hard' and bathing in water without the added emollients can damage the skin. Showers also have a drying effect. The water used should be cool or warm as hot water will increase discomfort.

It is important to supervise children at bathtime, because the use of oils and soap substitutes can be a source of danger since they make the bath very slippery (Spowart & Muir 1993). It should be remembered that the child can drown in very small amounts of water.

In order to counteract some of the drying effects of both water and the atmosphere, the application of preparations that occlude the skin may be beneficial.

Turnbull & Atherton (1994) describe the use of a 'wet wrap technique' for children with atopic eczema. This involves the application of 'two layers of tubular bandage over a suitable cream or ointment', the first layer being moist and the second layer dry. The dressings are left on for about twelve hours. The family and child will receive a demonstration and are given written instruction. Once the child becomes accustomed to the dressings and can begin to see the positive effect of this form of treatment, they usually co-operate and this is undertaken at home.

The prevention of secondary infection is another important aspect of care. Secondary infection will occur directly from the primary lesions as a result of the child scratching and the fissuring of the skin (Harper 1990). Therefore there is a significant relationship between reducing the itch and minimizing secondary infection.

It may be very difficult to prevent a young child from scratching so additional nursing actions can be taken to avoid trauma from scratching, including keeping nails short, clean and devoid of rough edges. This will reduce the risk of introducing dirt into the lesions. Cotton mittens and stockings may also be worn. It must be remembered that these need changing at regular intervals. For the very young child some hours in every day should be spent without them on in order to maintain motor development. Young children can be engaged in supervised play during this time and hence the potential for scratching is minimized.

Parents and carers may need advice about the type and style of clothing chosen for young children. One piece suits with long sleeves and legs in cotton or polycotton are most suitable. Wool should be avoided at all times. Clothes and bedlinen should be washed in nonbiological detergents and care should be taken not to add fabric softener to the water.

In extreme circumstances of exacerbation, elbow splints may be required to prevent the child from scratching. As with the mittens, these need removing to allow the child time to play. Bathtime is ideal as the child will be supervised and can be soothed by the water.

The provision of adequate periods of rest and sleep is an important aspect of care as these children experience frequent disturbance at nights due to the pruritus. Therefore they have a tendency towards being irritable and unco-operative. If the child is overheated the blood flow to the skin increases and makes the itching worse, therefore light cotton sheets and a cool environment may lead to greater comfort at bedtime (Simpson 1992).

Whilst it is acknowledged that the intense regimes of treatment are time consuming and tiring for carer and child, there are several overall strategies which may be adopted to relieve some of the stress. The daily routine should be carefully planned to ensure that treatments are not being given when the child is hungry, tired or the carer is particularly busy. This latter point is frequently transmitted to the child resulting in instant nonco-operation.

The majority of the treatments are carried out in the home environment by the parents. Therefore it is essential that they are made aware from the onset of the importance of such treatments, the methods of implementing them, and the support available when it all seems too much. Support is paramount to a successful outcome. This is discussed at greater length in relation to the case study below.

Emotional stress can become overwhelming during

phases of exacerbation of the eczema. Therefore it is important that all family members have the opportunity to discuss their feelings, which frequently may be negative. By visiting the home the community nurse is able to facilitate discussion and provide reassurance that the feelings are normal. Through discussion, stress can be reduced for both the child and family. This is particularly important since stress aggravates eczema.

The following case study provides an account of the distress experienced by one family when their infant first developed eczema. The involvement of the community paediatric nurse is discussed, and the support emphasized.

Case study

This account illustrates a mother's perception of living with eczema.

'I just couldn't understand why John's skin was so bad. I felt it must be all my fault, that it was something I had done. My other three children had never had any skin problems. I don't know how this happened.

When John's skin was at its worst, he constantly scratched it until it bled. I couldn't seem to stop him. He was always miserable and crying. I tried to cover his skin with clothes and I changed my washing powder but it seemed to make little difference. My husband found it difficult to cope with John. I think in some ways he blamed me. One of the things that hurt the most was that, because his face was so bad, we never liked to take photographs of him.

Every morning I had to change the bed linen as it was always bloody from where John had woken scratching in the night. The doctor gave me some medicine to help John sleep at night, but it seemed to make him sleepy during the day and it didn't stop the night itching. I felt so helpless. I felt the GP thought I was a nuisance and making a fuss over nothing, but it was affecting the whole family.'

John, the youngest of four children, is now 18 months old. His siblings are all well, and there is no family history of atopic disorders. However, at the age of one year, John was referred to the dermatologist at the local district general hospital with severe eczema covering approximately 10% of his total body surface.

At the time of his first visit to the clinic, John's skin was open, bloody and infected. John appeared pale, miserable, and in obvious discomfort. His mother was very anxious and upset by John's appearance. The consultant prescribed aqueous cream and Eumovate ointment (a topical steroid).

John was seen several times during the next few months, but there was little or no improvement in the condition of his skin. A week after his most recent appointment, John was seen as an emergency outpatient due to further deterioration in the condition of his skin. His skin had become infected with a heavy growth of staphylococcus aureus. The areas around his wrists and ankles were ulcerated due to the persistent scratching. His face was bleeding and red. John had a pyrexia of 37.8. He was crying and very miserable.

John's parents were reluctant to have him admitted to the paediatric unit. Therefore the consultant dermatologist requested that the paediatric community nurses visited at home to offer advice, support and assess compliance with the treatment prescribed.

It was established during the PCN's first visit that John had not been receiving the correct dosage of his prescribed antibiotics. His diet was inadequate and his parents had reverted to cow's milk instead of the advised goat's milk. The creams which had been prescribed for topical application were not being applied frequently enough or appropriately. There seemed poor communication between the GP and family and no support had been offered with John's treatment.

John's parents were loving and kind, but totally overwhelmed by John's eczema and its treatment. Communication appropriate to the parents' level of comprehension is an important aspect of the role of the paediatric community nurse. Good communication skills enable the nurse to explain in simple terms the nature of eczema and the importance of giving the correct treatment to help John's skin to improve. This gentle approach aided the family towards compliance with the treatment.

John's mother was then shown step by step how to bathe John effectively by applying aqueous cream to the water and using it as a soap. John was to be bathed twice daily for a minimum of 10 minutes in lukewarm water. His skin was then patted dry and more aqueous cream applied. The Eumovate ointment was then thinly and carefully applied to the areas where it was required.

This information was reinforced in writing and daily visits by the paediatric community nurse were made for the next two weeks. Within this time John's skin dramatically improved and the visits were gradually reduced to once weekly.

John's mother continues her story: 'It was such a relief when the nurse from the hospital came to see us. I felt there was someone who understood how I felt. She explained how to care for John's skin and how to use the creams properly by showing me how to apply netting to his skin. It really helped with the night itching. It has made such a difference to his skin. Even his face is better.

There have been a few times in the last six months when his skin has deteriorated but I feel more confident in how to deal with it and the paediatric community nurse visits more often when this happens so I feel I have some support.'

It may be seen that the source of eczema cannot be completely attributed to either nature or nurture. However, once it becomes established, the way in which the infant or child is nurtured would appear to have significant impact on the success of treatment. It is evident from the case history that the child's debility soon becomes transmitted to the whole family with everyone experiencing stresses ranging from lack of sleep to feelings of dislike for the child because he looks abnormal.

Attitudes to skin complaints such as eczema seem to be rather relaxed and even dismissive of the extent of disability and disruption it might cause the child and family. This is somewhat reflected in John's story in the approach of both the consultant dermatologist and the GP.

The importance of an adequate assessment cannot be overemphasized. When a child is young and totally dependent on the care provided by his parents, the whole family should be involved at all stages.

Through involvement of the whole family, the child is not made to feel isolated and abnormal. In addition, information about the child's condition is received first hand from the doctor, and the other parent, usually the father, is not dependent on the mother for details. Whole family involvement also means that the care, particularly when it is intense as in the case of John, at times of exacerbation can be shared. Older siblings

might not be able to supervise the bath routine or apply creams and lotions, but they can play with and provide distractions for the child, thus helping to reduce the amount of scratching.

A number of other factors may also contribute to increased stress levels within the family. Part of treatment regimes often include a hypoallergenic diet which means that either the whole family change their eating habits or two separate meals have always to be prepared. This can be particularly harrowing for an overstretched mother, especially when the child displays an erratic behaviour at times of extreme exacerbation of the eczema. Furthermore, the implementation of such a diet does not have instant results. Therefore parents need adequate reassurance that the additional trouble will eventually prove worthwhile.

Additional worries that parents and older children may have are about issues such as scarring. They should be assured that scarring will not take place unless the lesions are subject to secondary infection.

Paediatric community nurses can play an important role in support for the child and family and thus prevent the need for hospital admission in most cases.

THE CHILD WITH PSORIASIS

Psoriasis has been documented since the days of Greek mythology almost 2,600 years ago. It is a chronic inflammatory rash with scaling. Although it commonly occurs in adult life, a significant number of people will have experienced onset prior to age fifteen. In this childhood form, males are affected twice as much as females (Hurwitz 1981). Although at present the mode of genetic inheritance is unclear, there is a recognized genetic component. If one parent has psoriasis it is more likely that their children will subsequently develop it. If psoriasis has affected both parents this tendency is significantly higher (Buxton 1993).

The causes of psoriasis are complex but there is evidence that both hormonal and immunological mechanisms are involved at a cellular level. The raised concentrations of metabolites of arichodonic acid in the affected skin are related to clinical changes. Psoriasis affects the stratum corneum in which the usual differentiation and migration of keratinocytes through the layers of epidermal tissue is accelerated. The skin, therefore, fails to shed the cells as quickly as they are produced, so causing accumulation of the stratum corneum cells resulting in scales and inflammation of the dermal layer (Lookingbill & Marks 1986).

The onset can occur following any type of stress, including infection. Lesions may first appear at sites of minor trauma known as the Kobner phenomenon (Burton 1990). When seen in children, the most common is guttate psoriasis. The rash, consisting of many small scaly patches affecting the trunk and limbs and occasionally the scalp, often follows an acute infection, usually by streptococci in the throat. If a child has a tendency to tonsillitis the rash may come back with each episode. In such cases removal of the tonsils may be advised, to minimize and reduce episodes.

Currently there is no definitive cure, only alleviators of the discomfort by adherence to rigorous treatment regimes. Therefore it is important to recognize the effect that diagnosis can have on a child and family. The affected child or siblings may be victims of abuse, bullying or ridicule within the school setting as a result of the ignorance of their peers (Hunter 1992); for example, it is important that the family and child are offered appropriate support and encouragement. They will require information about the condition and its potential progression to enable them to manage the condition effectively at home.

Children will very rarely need to be nursed in hospital. However, if the appropriate support systems, for example paediatric community nurses or health visitors, are not available, a short stay in hospital may be required in order to teach the child and family some of the techniques used in applying creams and dressings.

It is important to promote a positive attitude and assist the family to accept that, although there is no 'cure', with effective treatment they can expect the condition of the skin to improve. They should also be prepared that exacerbation of the disease is often unpredictable and not necessarily linked to aggravating factors. In common with other chronic skin conditions, self blame can have a damaging effect. Therefore the child and family need time to talk through their anxieties and fears. They need to be reassured that the problem has not occurred as a result of any acts or omissions on their part.

Nursing intervention: meeting the child's needs

The mode of treatment prescribed for psoriasis will vary depending on the severity of the disease (Burton 1990). Pastes containing tar in various forms and applied locally are frequently used. Although this form of treatment does actually reduce the rapid cell divisions, so helping to bring about remission, it is messy and can be difficult to apply. Tar preparations are also available in bath form and this may be a more acceptable alternative for young children.

Ultraviolet light is another common form of treatment for guttate psoriasis, the most effective and practical way being exposure to sunlight. However, precautions need to be taken to avoid overexposure as damage to tissue enough to cause exacerbation can occur. In environments where sunlight is not plentiful, ultraviolet light can be prescribed by the dermatologist (Boehncke *et al.* 1992). The dose, however, has to be accurately controlled to give sufficient radiation without burning. Protective goggles, or moist cotton balls, should be worn during treatment to avoid damage to the cornea.

Any treatment should steer a course between overactive or insufficient. Too little treatment and limited improvement will be seen; overzealous treatment and the life of the child and family may revolve around it.

The nurse in the community or hospital has a particular role in evaluating the effectiveness of care; this includes regular, thorough assessment of the child's skin, noting any new lesions, healing of prior lesions and evidence of secondary bacterial infection. This may ascertain whether the treatment prescribed is effective and will act as a monitor, ensuring treatments are applied correctly and with appropriate frequency.

Positive feedback should be given to the child and family when treatments have been adhered to and the condition of the skin has improved. Psychological support to the child and family, as mentioned earlier, should not be underestimated and the nurse can play an important part in promoting a positive body image. The younger child may look upon new outbreaks of the disease as a punishment for previous behaviour and will need a lot of reassurance that new lesions are often not preventable. The child should be encouraged to participate in care as this will enable them to take some 'control' of the disease which has affected their living activities.

Although the majority of children with the dysfunctions of the skin discussed so far are unlikely to require admission to hospital, there may be other challenges associated with the overall management of children with skin problems. There may be shared care between paediatricians and dermatologists and such arrangements sometimes give rise to conflicts of interest when the respective treatment units are not in close proximity. Effective communication may minimize some of these difficulties and the children's nurse has an important liaison role.

Younger children may not be appropriately cared for within the paediatric wards. Older children and adolescents are still on occasions referred to adult specialist skin units. Within the past decade, psoriasis day treatment centres have been developed as another alternative to reduce or avoid hospital admission (Stone & Garibaldinos 1992). These centres provide cost-effective treatment and enable the patients to lead a 'normal' life. In the case of children and young people, this means they can remain in full-time education attending for treatment either before or after school. This is particularly important for adolescents who may already see themselves as being significantly different and apart from their peer group.

It is important to recognize that when the young adult begins to attend an adult specialist skin unit they may realize for the first time that their problem is not necessarily going to resolve with age. At this point the nurse may need to instigate specific support and counselling in order to help them to come to terms with this.

SKIN CONDITIONS THAT ARISE FROM ACCIDENTAL OR NONACCIDENTAL INJURY

Damage to the skin usually occurs as a result of trauma or accidents. When considering accidents it is thermal injuries which most frequently come to mind. However, there is another group of skin conditions which to date are largely unpreventable and occur as a result of what may be termed genetic accidents. An example of these are epidermolysis bullosa and naevi. These will be explored later in the chapter.

THE CHILD WHO HAS SUSTAINED A THERMAL INJURY

This section focuses upon the care of children who have sustained a thermal injury as a result of a scald or burn. It offers classification of the types and frequency of injuries, usually burns and scalds. The first aid measures are outlined and current research into the possible long term effects of thermal injury is discussed.

Whenever a child sustains an accident it is inevitably a traumatic time for both the child and the parents. However, few accidents are likely to provide a lifelong reminder more than a burn or scald.

The types of thermal injury are identified in Table 23.7 but it should be recognized that sunburn could also be included in this category. The nurse has a role to play in providing health education and advice regarding protection of children in the sun (Tait 1992) as prolonged exposure may result in thermal injury, or melanoma in later life.

Table 23.7 Types of thermal injury (data from OPCS 1990)

- Inflammable liquids
- Matches/cigarettes/pipes
- Solid fuel
- Gas and appliances
- Fat/candles
- Electricity and appliances
- Other specified means
- Unspecified means

The method of classification in Table 23.7 was used when assembling data on fatalities resulting from thermal injury.

Until fairly recently there was little national data on thermal injuries and data tended to be extrapolated from local studies. A survey in 1990 (OPCS 1990) reported that 89 children under 15 died as a result of a thermal injury; this represented 15% of the total number burned. The majority of children's nurses will not come into contact with children who have sustained fatal burns injuries unless they take up posts in accident and emergency departments or specialist burn units.

An analysis of burns attributed to an accident in the

home revealed that over 50% of injuries occurred in children under four years old (DTI 1991), with boys cited more frequently than girls. Data on home and leisure accidents and those associated with play were also provided. Overall, the general trend indicates that although the distribution in the cause of burns has not altered significantly over the years, the number of scalds continues to rise. Chisholm (1990) reported that a small scale survey in Nottingham revealed that 'accidents occurring due to hot drinks being spilt are still the largest group'.

Other surveys have been undertaken at a local level to record the number of children seen in the accident and emergency department (Bayram *et al.* 1987; Pearce 1989). Gray (1987) and Gammon & Ogden (1992) found that a large proportion of children sustain their injuries within sight of their parents or carers. This has implications for both the support and counselling required by the parents, and for health education. Overall it would seem that there is still a deficit in health promotion and perhaps by highlighting homogenous groups who may be more prone to accidents preventative measures may be instigated.

Nursing assessment of the child with a minor thermal injury

As already established, any child sustaining a burn or scald will usually be taken to hospital. On admission the child will need to be assessed promptly, efficiently and accurately (Kelly 1994). The nursing assessment will include an appraisal of any first aid measures undertaken, assessment of the degree of injury and a history of the events leading up to the accident. It is important that the nurse has an awareness of the first aid measures that may have been initiated (Table 23.8) as this may influence future care.

Robson & Heggers (1988) stated that it is important to be able to assess the extent of injury and depth of tissue destruction in order to determine what treatment the burn wound requires. The number of cells in the skin that are destroyed or injured is reflected in the functional capacity of the skin. Therefore the vertical depth of the burn is important. Thus burns are usually classified as a degree of injury with a qualifying statement which describes the depth of the injury (Table 23.9).

Sometimes thermal injury is deliberately inflicted and

Table 23.8 First aid measures.

(1) Recognize the development of shock.
(2) Stop the burning process and reduce the pain; this is achieved by removing all materials in contact with the burn area.
Reduce the temperature of the affected area to room temperature by soaking with cold water. Research shows that this is frequent practice (Pearce 1992). However, Walsh (1990) suggests that this is more effective in reducing pain than reducing the temperature.
Cold wet compresses may be applied to small injuries but not extensive ones (Herndon *et al.* 1993). Hypothermia may occur if the compress is left on for more than 15 minutes (Kelly 1994). Give paracetamol (Kelly 1994).
(3) Reduce the potential for introducing infection. Cover the wound with clean linen, preferably material that is nonadherent. Careful handling will avoid breaking blisters.
Provide information and reassurance.

Table 23.9 Classification of burns.

■ *Erytherma, a superficial injury,* will cause the destruction of the epidermis and possibly a small section of the dermis. Providing that the wound remains free of infection, such an injury is likely to heal in 10 to 14 days (Bottomley 1981). There is unlikely to be any lasting disfigurement.
■ *A partial thickness injury* destroys the epidermis and approximately half the dermis. The healing process takes longer, extending from 14 to 21 days. The child should not be disfigured following such an injury. This is extremely painful, as the nerve endings are involved.
■ *A deep injury* destroys the epidermis and most of the dermis. Due to the destruction of the majority of the epithelium, the healing process will take at least 21 days and probably as many as 28. Even with this extended period of time it is unlikely that healing will occur spontaneously. The majority of deep injuries require skin grafts. This type of injury will also leave the victim with some degree of disfigurement.

the sequence of events leading up the injury may alert or allay suspicions. Nonaccidental injury is a feature of 1% to 16% of children presenting to hospital with a burn or a scald. According to Hobbs (1989) two years is the peak age for the child to sustain burns accidentally, whilst in the third year nonaccidental injury is more common.

Although on the surface the nature of the injury may be the same or similar, other factors may arouse suspicion. These include any discrepancy between the nature of the injury and the account provided; frequently the history of the burn is not consistent with the injury (Hobbs 1989) (Table 23.10). Another factor may be inappropriate behaviour, for example misplaced hostility to the nursing staff coupled with a lack of obvious concern or guilt. It is important to recognize that individuals adopt their own unique coping strategies, so behavioural signs alone should not lead one to accusations of abuse.

- Evidence to suggest that parents are unlikely to be able to carry out necessary treatments at home.
- Little confidence that parents and child will attend for follow up appointments.
- The child has sustained significant injury involving face, hands, perineum or feet, or has soft tissue injury, injuries involving the skeletal system or smoke inhalation.
- The child may be at risk from further nonaccidental injury.

Nursing intervention: meeting the needs of the child with a minor thermal injury

Pearce (1992) undertook a small scale study to consider the care children received in the accident and emergency department and identified both similarities and differences in the management of scalds. In the light of this

Table 23.10   Suspicion of nonaccidental injury: nature of the injury.

Burns	Caused by hot, usually metallic objects such as an iron or electric fire. The injury looks like a brand mark or has the shape of the object clearly demarkated.
Friction burns	The result of the child being dragged across the floor.
Cigarette burns	When these are deliberate they form a crater because the injury is deep and full thickness.
Scalds on the bottom of the feet	The child will be unlikely to put both feet into boiling water. The depth of the scald may also be indicative.
Scalds on the buttocks	This may indicate that the child has been forcibly held in very hot water, and arms and legs should be examined for bruising.
Scalds to the face and trunk	There is a difference in the distribution of the scald if water has been thrown at the child in contrast to the child pulling hot water over themselves.
Frequent old injuries	This may indicate repeated abuse, and delay in seeking medical advice.

Those with minor injury, that is fewer than 10%, will be seen on an outpatient basis. However, it is important to assess social circumstances because if any of the following factors are present, admission to hospital may be indicated:

research, it would seem inappropriate to be prescriptive about practice. However, a number of principles indicating good practice have been highlighted:

- The cleansing and deroofing of blisters.
- The application of tulle gras.

- The application of gauze over the tulle gras.
- The application of a Surgi pad for extra protection if the area is blistered.
- Secure the dressing with a bandage and Tubigrip.
- Give an appointment for follow up in 48 hours.
- Give written instructions for aftercare.

The last two points may be particularly important. Follow up appointments will be necessary to make frequent assessments of wound healing and also provide an opportunity to reassess the parents and the child's ability to cope with the injury and care. The nurse should be aware of any signs of stress and should monitor this closely in order to initiate appropriate support. If care is organized so that the same nurse provides continuity of care, parents may be more likely to discuss their anxieties and seek support. This approach could also reduce the incidence of infection and enhance the consistency of the information and advice given to them regarding aftercare. It should be remembered that when individuals are stressed and anxious, their ability to retain information is greatly reduced. This awareness may be particularly important when giving information to these families.

Hutt (1989) undertook a small qualitative study to explore the information given to parents in the accident and emergency department and their subsequent concerns associated with care at home following a burn or scald. It was found that parental anxieties generally centred around wound healing, keeping the dressing in place and pain management. Providing verbal information alone has been found to be unsatisfactory and it is recommended that written information be provided (RCN 1990).

Drawing upon the findings of Hutt's research, Cox (1992) designed an information leaflet to address care related to activities of daily living, including eating and drinking, washing and dressing, playing and sleeping. The leaflet also capitalized on the opportunity to provide first aid and health education advice.

Nursing intervention: meeting the needs of the child with a severe thermal injury

Although the psychosocial components of care are recognized, initially care will be focused on the measures taken to minimize hypovolaemic shock. It is necessary for the nurse to have knowledge of the structure and function of skin in order to identify the child's actual and potential problems. The nurse also needs to understand the principles of shock in order to appreciate the rationale for care during the acute crisis. This knowledge base is assumed and only specific aspects are highlighted.

Immediate care is required for all children under two years of age who have sustained burns covering 10% or more of their total body surface area (TBSA), and children over two who have injuries involving 15% or more of their TBSA. Any child who has even small burns affecting hands, feet, face, perineum and joint surfaces, or those with burns resulting from electrical injuries where deep involvement is suspected, should be admitted to hospital (Herndon *et al.* 1993).

When considering emergency interventions, emphasis is upon the role of the multidisciplinary team, working together to institute care simultaneously.

It is particularly important to:

- Establish airway patency for those children with injury to the face and neck as oedema may occur quite rapidly and create obstruction due to small airways. Smoke inhalation may also cause damage to the airways. Any evidence of respiratory involvement indicates the need for administration of 100% oxygen. Carvajal (1988) emphasizes that children must undergo careful evaluation of respiratory status to assess the need for an artificial airway, for example tracheostomy. All children who are unconscious should be intubated.
- Evaluate cardio-pulmonary status. Children with extensive burns are likely to demonstrate signs of hypovolaemic shock due to sudden loss of plasma and fluid and as a result of the trauma experienced (Strodtbeck & Joyce 1988).

The physiological adaptation to burns

As an effect of heat under destroyed tissue, capillaries dilate leading to increased permeability. There is rapid fluid loss into the extracellular spaces from the plasma (Fig. 23.2). Due to the loss of protein the plasma volume is reduced and this leads to a reduction in circulating volume, and shock. In an attempt to compensate and maintain fluid there is:

- Increased osmosis and withdrawal of fluid from extracellular spaces.

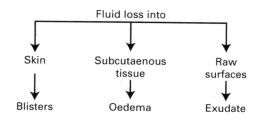

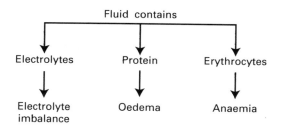

Fig. 23.2 Physiological effect of burns.

- Increased absorption of fluid from the gastro-intestinal tract.
- Concentration of urine by the kidneys.
- Increased thirst.

The main aims of interventions to treat burns may be categorized into three phases, immediate, intermediate and long term.

Immediate:

- Initiate resuscitation measures.
- Replace fluids.
- Prevent respiratory problems.
- Monitor and alleviate shock.
- Relieve pain.

Intermediate:

- Prevent wound infection.
- Promote healing.

Long term:

- Support the child and family in psychosocial adjustment.
- Return the child home as soon as possible.

Immediate phase

The nurse could be said to have a major role in assessing the degree of shock. By observing the child's behaviour and colour and monitoring physiological indices, in particular blood pressure, the nurse is in a prime position to provide information regarding the effectiveness of treatment. The nurse will also be required to assist in the establishment and maintenance of intravenous access.

When recording blood pressure a properly fitting BP cuff is essential. The ideal width of the inflatable bladder of the cuff is 40% of the circumference of the midpoint of the limb to be used. It should be remembered that standard cuff BP techniques are not always reliable for infants and children.

The child's weight is required to calculate fluid replacement. Intravenous fluids will be prescribed for several reasons:

- To compensate for the loss of sodium and water by replacing the sodium deficit.
- To restore the plasma volume.
- To correct electrolyte imbalance, usually acidosis.
- To provide adequate perfusion and maintain renal function.

In an emergency drugs will also be administered intravenously. The nurse has an important role in maintaining accurate records of fluid balance.

If the child is experiencing hypovolaemic shock there will be a delay in gastric emptying, increasing the risk of vomiting and aspiration of stomach contents. An appropriate size of nasogastric tube should be inserted as this will minimize distension and vomiting.

It is recommended that a small amount of antacid is left in the stomach to reduce the potential for the development of stress ulcers (Carvajal 1988). Therefore, once administered, the tube should be spigoted for about an hour. After this time the tube should be left on free drainage, particularly if the child is intubated and ventilated, and regular aspirations should then be made to keep the stomach empty.

There may be difficulty in maintaining body temperature as heat loss can exceed heat production. Rectal temperature should be recorded frequently and measures taken to maintain a warm environment (Bruce 1989).

Reduction in blood pressure and blood flow through

the kidneys may lead to acute renal failure; therefore a catheter should be inserted into the bladder. This will enable initial emptying of the bladder and accurate measurement of further urine production. A complete urinalysis should be made on the first sample produced after the initial catheterization.

Intermediate phase

Once the wounds have been cleaned a more accurate evaluation of the extent of the injury can be made. Carvajal (1988) recommends that a rate of 20 ml/kg fluid of body weight can be administered for up to two hours without any harmful effect. After this time fluid regimes are reviewed.

Although there are a variety of methods for assessing the extent of injury, the most accurate method is that described by Lund & Browder (1944), according to Carvajal (1988). This method takes into consideration appropriate body proportions for age and requires the use of diagrams for mapping the extent of injury. However, it can only be used to evaluate the extent of injury in second and third degree burns. Burns exceeding 60% of TBSA are most appropriately mapped by estimating the nonburned areas. Other methods include the Wallace rule of nines, although it does not take into account age and body proportion (Lowry & Gill 1992).

The issue of pain management is one which involves both the immediate treatment of the child with thermal injury and the continuing care. Historically the concept of the child experiencing pain as a result of injury or illness was strongly denied, particularly by physicians. This meant that children, especially in the younger age group, frequently did not receive adequate analgesia during illness and related treatments (Carter 1994). At best they were prescribed pharmacological preparations in minimal dosage; the rest was left to nursing staff, some of whom may not be experts in the care of children.

This has most often been the case in accident and emergency departments or burns units, where staff are less aware of the needs and reactions of children to pain. Even within the field of children's nursing where nurses are daily confronted with caring for children in pain, the substantive knowledge base about this aspect of care and its effectiveness remains limited (Denyes *et al.* 1991).

Regular analgesia should be given during the initial phase, and assessment and evaluation incorporated into continuing care to measure its effectiveness. Initially analgesia, usually a narcotic, will be administered intravenously as intramuscular injections may have unreliable absorption (Ellis & Rylah 1990) and are most painful. Sometimes Entonox is used (Forshaw & Bottomly 1991).

Significant pain is associated with the post injury treatment of debridement. If the burn is severe, debridement is undertaken using a general anaesthetic. However, many children experience a 'burns bath', which tends to be used more commonly in specialist burns units. This particular treatment is usually carried out at 10 days post injury and is designed to facilitate the removal of the majority of the eschar. It consists of immersing the child in an outsize bath or tank filled with a water and chlorhexadine solution.

Watkins (1993) undertook a study of burns bathing in the USA and suggested that one of the main limitations with the practice was that staff seemed not to appreciate the pain that the children were experiencing, and did not administer sufficient analgesia. This was raised as an important issue and has implications for practice. The children's nurse needs to be familiar with the actions of analgesia so that she/he can ensure that adequate and appropriate doses are prescribed.

In addition to adequate pain management, preparation may also be important to avoid further trauma. Play therapy can be initiated using a doll with cling film applied to the areas corresponding to the injured areas of the child, thus making a false skin. Using the doll's bath the child can be actively involved in placing the doll in the bath, filling the bath with water and helping to remove the skin. Through this medium the play specialist may be able to help the child work through some of their anxieties.

By introducing the child to the bath water gradually, their anxiety may be reduced. It may be effective to fill the bath to an appropriate depth for the size of the child, ensuring that the water temperature is correct. Then, using a hosepipe attachment allowing hot and cold water to mix, still at the correct temperature, continue to trickle water into the bath until the depth required is achieved. In this way the child is more likely to remain relaxed and co-operative.

The child who has sustained burns has specific nutritional needs. This is due to a high metabolic rate due to tissue necrosis, hypothermia and loss of red blood cells, development of infections and the need for multiple skin grafts. Opinions differ as to when enteral feeding should commence. However, perhaps more important than the route of nutrition is the fact that some form of nutrition is instigated. Samba *et al.* (1988) state that major advances in parenteral feeding mean those who have suffered extensively from thermal injury are far more likely to survive than they would have done 15 years ago.

Without the appropriate nutrition a state of malnutrition will rapidly develop, and healing will be delayed. Nutritional requirements include sufficient protein, to avoid protein breakdown, as well as calories to aid the utilization of the proteins and to sustain hypermetabolism.

The majority of children are soon able to eat, and diet should be commenced within 48 hours of the injury. Children who are unable to eat may receive nutrition either via a nasogastric tube or via the parenteral route. The latter route is only used in extreme cases because of the potential for infections, leading to additional complications.

When encouraging oral intake, the nurse will need to consider strategies to provide tempting foods because children are frequently anorexic when confined to bed and feeling generally unwell. In addition, surgical procedures require them to have periods of starvation. Finally, gastro-intestinal complications often mean the ability for oral intake is limited.

In any circumstances an open burn wound, compared with one that is intact, will be more susceptible to infection because the open skin facilitates the access of bacteria (Zuker 1988). The eschar of the wound is a potential source of infection. Therefore the removal of this dead tissue and closure of the wound should be carried out as soon as possible.

Methods of treatment will vary between centres. However, a number of general principles of care may be applied. All wounds require debridement. This may be done as a complete process using skin grafts to cover the wound, or it may be done in stages with regular burns toilets and trimming of eschar as it lifts. Whichever method is used the wound will require dressing.

Two basic techniques are used to dress burns. The open technique is when an antimicrobial ointment is applied and the wound is left exposed. There are a number of disadvantages with this method. The child and family are constantly reminded of the extent of the injury as it is always visible. Movement and close contact with the child are limited because carers fear they will cause the child pain and discomfort. The child will need to be nursed in isolation to reduce the potential for secondary infections, and this is likely to be detrimental to progress and possibly cause developmental regression. These aspects of care will be considered in depth under psychological care. Depending on the age and stage of development of the child, it may be difficult to prevent them from touching the wounds.

The closed technique for dressing burns wounds would appear to be more popular. With this method an ointment is applied as above and then the wound is covered with gauze and a stretch gauze is used to hold the first layer in place. The use of the closed method has also been found to reduce pain experienced from the wounds (Pearce 1992).

Skin grafts are used to achieve closure of full thickness injury. Herndon *et al.* (1993) recommend excision of the wounds and grafting within 24 hours of the burn injury as providing the best possible therapy for the reduction of potential infection. Depending on the extent of injury relevant to TBSA, donor skin may be harvested from the patient. When this is the case additional wound sites will be created and it should be remembered that these can cause as much pain as the burn injury. Alternative sources of skin may be provided from cadaveric allograft or hetero grafts, usually derived from fresh or frozen pigskin.

Francis (1990) argues that parents are already distressed due to the nature of the injury. Their additional anxiety about the treatments which the child has to undergo may further increase the child's own distress. In particular, parents who display acute anxiety and hysteria can affect the child's ability to tolerate pain and treatment.

Dressings frequently cause parents anxiety because inevitably they involve some pain for the child and contribute to reinforcing the parent's guilt feelings (Francis 1990). It is recognized that the presence of parents when a difficult and painful procedure is being carried out on their child can provide additional stresses for nursing staff.

These arguments are sometimes put forward in defence of excluding parents from certain aspects of care. There are, however, very few occasions when a child who is ill or in pain would not want a parent present, although if a child has a nonaccidental injury, the presence of one or both parents may be detrimental and not in the child's best interests. Often these children are withdrawn and do not complain about pain, either from their injury or the treatment. The presence of parents may further restrict the child's expressions of feelings (Hobbs 1989). Conversely the child may be hyperactive, displaying an angry and rebellious approach to both parents and carers. In either circumstance, the child may be reluctant to talk about the nature of their injury.

In most situations it could be argued that, with the appropriate nursing support and preparation, parents can be involved in care. This may have the twofold effect of helping them to manage their anxiety and providing comfort for their child. Furthermore, research suggests that children are more co-operative in the presence of their parents, and parents want to be present (Dearmun 1993).

The concept of family centred care is central to philosophies of care in paediatric settings, and contracts may be developed between parents and carers when they are likely to be in hospital for long periods or when frequent return visits are necessary. George & Hancock (1993) discuss the use of contracts to establish the role of parents' participation in their child's burn treatments. They state that the initial contract is informal and parents have the option to renegotiate at a later date. This situation therefore gives both parents and the care team an opportunity to evaluate the effects of the combined participation in care.

Formal evaluation of the programme to involve parents indicated that it was a positive action. Parents were pleased to be involved with their child's care at this level. They had an enhanced understanding of the healing process and the need for the specific rehabilitation methods. Children had increased feelings of security when parents were present. Finally staff, some of whom expressed negative feelings about the programme initially, changed to feeling positive about it as they witnessed changes in the behaviour of parents.

Factors which should be highlighted from this programme are:

- The commitment to primary nursing, thus establishing a relationship between parents and the child's nurse.
- The need to prepare parents adequately for what will happen during treatments and provide them with the option to change their minds.
- The promises which were made for parents to debrief and be supported after their participation.

- The initial and ongoing education to prepare and support the staff of the multidisciplinary team.

Long term phase

The physical pain which has been discussed above is only the beginning of the burn experience, both for the child and family (Sutherland 1988). The damage caused by the injury is likely to produce long term changes which require determination and resilience in excess of that during the initial period in hospital.

Psychological or emotional support of the child and family should be given parity with any other treatment that the child receives for their injury, because the burned child must be able to return to society as a functional human being (Cooper & Thomas 1988). Regardless of the extent and severity of the injury, the fact that it has happened at all will undoubtedly have caused some degree of trauma to all those involved. Burgdorf (1978) identifies that the family will view the injury as representing a failure in their protective system. Thus every member can be expected to bear a heavy burden of guilt. Although the focus is upon the child who experiences long periods in hospital for the treatment of severe burns, the principles of care may be transferable and can be adapted.

A burn injury is a terrifying and painful experience, particularly for a child whose cognitive developmental level may be such that they are unable to comprehend anything of what has happened. The emergency admission to hospital and the subsequent treatment may also be distressing. Furthermore, the child is removed from all that is familiar – parents, siblings and home – into an unusual and frightening environment. Cooper & Thomas (1988) consider the parents' feelings, stating that they are no longer able to exercise control over what is happening. Undoubtedly the guilt mentioned above is taking hold and parents have an overwhelming sense of helplessness and possibly hopelessness as well.

The injury must be viewed as a crisis for the child and family, the sudden and traumatic nature of which will undoubtedly alter life for the child and their significant others. Those who are caring for children with burns should realize this and should remember it whenever they interact with the child and those closest to them. Adler (1992), highlighting the importance of the multidisciplinary team and the psychosocial meetings to the burned patient's wellbeing, states there is usually a real commitment to those aspects of care within children's nursing settings.

Patients with thermal injury have an extended length of stay in hospital. Whilst the trend in children's nursing has been towards a reduction in the period of hospitalization to approximately three days, the average duration of stay in hospital for the child with thermal injury is 16.7 days (DTI 1991). In addition to this, the child may have to undergo repeated admissions for further corrective surgery. These factors may contribute towards problems of institutionalization as well as the more obvious ones of rehabilitation (Adler (1992).

The incidence of scalds or burns in the very young infant is less. However, when it does happen the sites of injury may have severe detrimental effects on the infant's development; for example, if the injuries are extensive it may be difficult to pick up the child for cuddles. Additionally, if the baby has to spend prolonged periods of time prone, the normal interactions which occur between infants and carers will be restricted.

It has been recognized that when an individual's needs are met by a single organization over an extended period of time, institutionalization is likely to occur. This is because the individual becomes more dependent on the staff and institution, thus relinquishing personal autonomy. If the developing child is striving to gain autonomy, the dependency factor may not be so obvious. However, when the child is admitted to a burns unit at a distance from the family home and parents are unable to remain resident, the child may display signs of greater attachment to the staff than parents. This situation is more likely to occur in the child under five. Where such a situation does arise there can be evidence of rivalry between the child's parents and the unit staff. When staff have a clear understanding of the parental role, they can take measures to help parents readapt to the role of parents to a sick child, thus avoiding the development of this conflict (Rennick 1986).

In addition, staff can negotiate lines of communication with parents, for example by notifying parents of any particular changes in the child's condition be they for better or worse. Parents who are separated from their children for long periods of time also find comfort in reading a diary of the child's daily progress. These actions do not take long to instigate and can considerably reduce the alienation felt by separation.

The support of parents is consistently reported to be a crucial factor in the recovery and rehabilitation of children with thermal injury (Blakeney *et al.* 1993). The child and the multidisciplinary team all look to the parents to provide continuing physical and psychological care. This is particularly relevant once the child is discharged from hospital, when it seems as though parents must become an extension of the care team. Suddenly one or two people are being expected to carry out the care which previously was being undertaken by a team of people.

Blakeney *et al.* (1993) state that the needs of parents when they again become primary care givers after the thermal injury have not been systematically studied. The British literature revealed little on the long-term effects of providing such care. However, some studies do reveal that thermal injuries occur more frequently in families that are already stressed than in the general population (Gray 1987; Levene 1992). Examples are one parent families, families where the mother was pregnant or newly delivered, and families where the child or parent already suffers from ill health (Gray 1987). Levene (1992) states that there are six times as many deaths from thermal injury in households in social class five, compared with social class one. Hazards are more obvious in the environment of social class five households; for example, lack of finance and the power to produce change.

The study by Blakeney *et al.* (1993) identified that the parents of a child requiring extended care following thermal injury tend to experience stress and depression directly related to caring for the child in the two year period immediately after the injury. They identified their children as being demanding, dependent and unhappy, with a tendency to be overactive and restless. This suggests the parents had either minimal or no positive reinforcement from their child. These authors recommend that there are some important family wishes to be addressed, along with the more immediate needs of the child at the time of the injury and in the acute phase. This would seem an essential part of care if the child/parent bond is to endure in the long term.

THE CHILD WITH A SKIN DISORDER AS A RESULT OF A NON-TRAUMATIC ACCIDENT

These problems are either the result of genetic or congenital abnormality. They may be divided into two broad categories: epidermolysis bullosa, the name given to 'a fairly large group of hereditary blistering diseases' (Eady 1989); and naevi, a naevus being defined as 'a circumscribed new growth of the skin of congenital origin' (Harper 1990).

Epidermolysis bullosa is inherited as an autosomal dominant or recessive condition. According to Eady (1989), a mild traumatic incident such as friction may be necessary to induce the blistering. However, in some instances, blisters may develop spontaneously. The incidence of epidermolysis bullosa is very infrequent, tending to vary from country to country. Registers are now being compiled in an attempt to estimate the exact numbers of children experiencing each of the specific types (Carter & Caldwell-Brown 1989). Currently the incidence is thought to be approximately one in a million of the population, who suffer from epidermolysis bullosa simplex. This is the first of the three principal types, the other two being functional and dystrophic.

The nursing care for an infant or child with epidermolysis bullosa presents a challenge to the physical and psychosocial skills of the nursing staff. One of the major factors is that the disease is inherited. Therefore the child and family are living with a chronic illness which may seem to be always in the acute phase.

The main functions of the nurse are related to the teaching and counselling of the child's family and the extended community. Due to the infrequency of the disorder, many people who normally interact with the growing child and family may only have heard of the disease. Therefore it is essential that those experienced in the care of these children liaise closely with the health visitor, local hospital and the child's school.

Epidermolysis bullosa can affect many of the body's other systems, thus increasing the number of health professionals needed to interact with the child and family. Foster (1989) highlights the fact that due to the infrequency of epidermolysis bullosa and the limited number of specialist nurses, there are some aspects of care of which all nurses should be aware. The most important of these is that epidermolysis bullosa is characterized by skin which is susceptible to trauma, therefore normally routine procedures, such as securing dressings or a nasogastric tube, may provide a major challenge in the care of a child sufferer.

One of the main aims of care is to prevent further damage to the already fragile skin. This is achieved through very careful skin treatment and the application of dressings. Foster (1989) writes extensively about the application of dressings, and nurses who are required to provide care for a child with epidermolysis bullosa but who are unfamiliar with the condition, would be well advised to seek help from experienced practitioners or from Dystrophic Epidermolysis Bullosa Research Association (DEBRA), the address of which is provided at the end of this chapter.

Children who are born with, or develop, naevi shortly after birth, will most likely be seen in the community or outpatient department. The majority of these resolve spontaneously given time. When children are admitted to hospital it is for surgical excision but this is usually delayed until the child or young person is of an age to make the decision for themselves.

When a child presents with a naevi, the role of the nurse is one of support and advice. The mongolian spot, which consists of bluish black macules seen over the lumbosacral area and buttocks of most negro and oriental babies (Harper 1990), is perhaps the most frequently encountered form of naevi. The appearance of mongolian spots may be mistaken for bruising, which in turn can result in parents being wrongly accused of nonaccidental injury (Harper 1990). These spots will fade over time and are not of clinical significance.

CONCLUSION

Disorders of the skin have emerged as being more than skin deep. In many instances the child has to learn to live with a lifelong condition which is not only daily evident to them, but often to the world at large. Skin conditions, even if they do not continue to erupt throughout life, leave lifelong reminders in the form of scars. A relatively minor illness, such as chickenpox, can leave scars if the lesions are scratched by the child.

Infancy and early childhood present additional problems of management for the parents and carers because frequently the child is too young to understand the need for co-operation in treatment.

The topical management of skin lesions is only part of the overall care required by the child and family. Psychological and emotional support of the child and other family members if also an important component of care. Children and their families need to know that they are not to blame for the child's problem. Even when the problem has arisen as the result of an accident, parents should be helped to prevent a similar accident in the future, but should not be judged as guilty for what has happened.

All members of the family, in any circumstances, need help in maintaining their self esteem, and motivation to comply with the treatment regimes. This aspect is particularly important when treatments are likely to be required over extensive periods of time, such as following thermal injury (Blakeney *et al.* 1993).

Parents frequently feel the burden of responsibility for the successful outcome of their child's treatment. They rely on the help and support of the health care professionals, even though this may be at a distance. The knowledge that they can telephone the hospital or that they will receive visits from the paediatric community nurse can be a source of great comfort. Additional support can come from specialist support groups. Parents and children who are old enough should be encouraged to make contact with such groups whenever possible. Some of these groups are listed at the end of this chapter.

Children are amazingly resourceful. By being given some degree of control over what is happening to their body, they can often help in the compliance with treatment. This aspect is particularly important when extended regimes of care need to be implemented, as in the case of a child with infected eczema, or one who is recovering from a thermal injury.

The implementation of a nursing model in caring for such a child should prove invaluable. Whilst a number of models immediately come to mind, it might be considered too prescriptive to discuss care within the framework of a particular model. However, the principles encompassed by some of the more popular models have been implicit when discussing modes of care.

Finally, there is evidence to suggest that the subject of nursing care relating to disorders of the skin is an underresearched area in the British Isles, since much of the literature used in support of this chapter is either from medical or American sources. Therefore, without the supporting research, the myths about skin disorders are likely to be precipitated. The majority of children with skin disorders can lead relatively normal lives, but their parents, carers and society at large need to be informed regarding the distress children experience from a problem which, to the nonsufferer, may appear only skin deep.

ACKNOWLEDGEMENT

Kristine Mason, *RGN*, *RSCN*, formerly Paediatric Community Sister, Stoke Mandeville Hospital also contributed to the contents of this chapter.

SUPPORT GROUPS

National Eczema Society (NES), 4 Tavistock Place, London WC1H 9RA. Tel. 0717 388 4097.

Psoriasis Association, 7 Milton Street, Northampton NN2 7JG. Tel. 01604 711129.

Naevus (Birthmark) Support Group, 58 Necton Road, Wheathampstead, Herts. AL4 8AU. Tel. 0582 832853.

Child Accident Prevention Trust, 28 Portland Place, London W1N 4DE. Tel. 0171 636 2545.

Dystrophic Epidermolysis Bullosa Research Association (DEBRA), 1 Kings Road, Crowthorne, Berkshire RG11 7BG. Tel. 01344 771961.

REFERENCES AND FURTHER READING

Adler, R. (1992) Burns are different: the child psychiatrist on the paediatric burns ward. *Journal of Burn Care and Rehabilitation*, 13(1), 28–32.

Adomat, R. (1992) Understanding shock. *British Journal of Nursing*, 1(3), 124–8.

ASC (1991) *Caring for Children in the Health Services: Just for the Day*. Action for Sick Children, London.

Barker, D.J. (1990) *Handbook of Dermatology*. Blackwell Science, Oxford.

Bayram, R., Shattock, S., Blencowe, J., Whiting, M. & Pigott, S. (1987) Burns and scalds in children. *Midwife, Health Visitor and Community Nurse*, 23(11), 494–6.

Blakeney, P., Moore, P., Broemtling, H., Hunt, R., Herndon, D.N. & Robson, M. (1993) Parental stress as a cause and effect of paediatric burn injury. *Journal of Burn Care and Rehabilitation*, 14(1), 73–82.

Boehncke, W.H., Sterry, W. & Kaufman, R. (1994) Treatment of psoriasis by topical photodynamic therapy with polychromatic light. *Lancet*, 343 (8900) 801.

Bottomley, E. (1981) Thermal Injury in Children. *Nursing: The Add On Journal of Clinical Nursing*, 1st Series, 23, 995–8.

Bruce, E. (1989) Thermal injuries in paediatrics. *Paediatric Nursing*, 1(9), 8–9.

Burgdorf, M.M. (1978) Coping behaviours of school age children hospitalized with burns. *Maternal Child Nursing Journal*, 7(1), 11–19.

Burton, J.L. (1990) *Essentials of Dermatology*, 3rd edn. Churchill Livingstone, Edinburgh.

Burton, J.L. (1992) Eczema, lichenification, pairigo and erythroderma. In *Textbook of Dermatology*, 5th edn (eds R.H. Champion, J.L. Burton & F.J.G. Ebling). Blackwell Science, Oxford.

Buxton, P.K. (1993) *ABC Dermatology*. BMJ Publishing Group, London.

Carter, B. (1994) *Child and Infant Pain: principles of nursing care and management*. Chapman and Hall, London.

Carter, D. & Caldwell-Brown, M.D. (1989) The national epidermolysis bullosa registry in *A Comprehensive Review of Classification Management and Laboratory Studies in Epidermolysis Bullosa* (eds G.C. Priestly, M.J. Tidman, J.B. Weiss, R.A.J. Eady). Dystrophic Epidermolysis Bullosa Research Association (DEBRA), Crowthorne, Berks.

Carter, B. & Cooper, D. (1993) Care of the child with polytrauma and thermal injury. In *Manual of Paediatric Intensive Care Nursing* (ed. B. Carter). Chapman & Hall, London.

Carvajal, H.F. (1988) Resuscitation of the Burned Child. In *Burns in Children: Pediatric Burn Management* (eds H.F. Carvajal & D.H. Parks). Year Book Medical Publishers Inc., Chicago.

Chisholm, J. (1990) A rising hazard. *Paediatric Nursing*, 2(9), 26.

Cooper, M.K. & Thomas, C.M. (1988) Psychosocial care of the severely burned child. In *Burns in Children* (eds H.F. Carvajal & D.H. Parks). Year Book Medical Publishers, London.

Coull, A. (1989) Initial treatment of burns. *Nursing*, 3(40), 27–9.

Cox, B. (1992) Research into practice. *Paediatric Nursing*, 4(10), 24–6.

Dale, A. (1983) Nursing in paediatric skin conditions. *Nursing*, 2(10), 267–70.

David, T.J. (1989) Infection and prevention: current controversies in childhood atopic eczema: a review. *Journal of the Royal Society of Medicine*, 82, 820–22.

Dearmun (1993) Towards a partnership in pain management. *Paediatric Nursing*, 5(5), 8–10.

Denyes, M.J., Neuman, B. & Villarruel, A.M. (1991) Nursing actions to prevent and alleviate pain in hospitalized children. In *Issues in Comprehensive Pediatric Nursing*, 14, 31–48.

DoH (1991) *Welfare of Children and Young People in Hospital*. HMSO, London.

Dowding, C. (1986) Nutrition in wound healing. *Nursing*, 3(95), 174–6.

DTI (1991) Department of Trade and Industry Consumer Safety Unit, *Home and Leisure Accident Research: Burns*. HMSO, London.

Eady, R.A.J. (1989)The classification of epidermolysis bullosa. In *A Comprehensive Review of Classification Management and Laboratory Studies* (eds G. Priestly, M.J. Tidman, J.B. Weiss & R.A.J. Eady). Dystrophic Epidermolysis Bullosa Research Association (DEBRA), Crowthorne, Berks.

Ellis, A. & Rylah, T.A. (1990) Transfer of the thermally injured patient. *British Journal of Hospital Medicine*, 44(3), 206–8.

Forshaw, A. (1990) Proven Methods. *Paediatric Nursing*, 2(7), 20–21.

Forshaw, A. & Bottomley, E. (1991) Thermal injuries. In *The Injured Child* (eds D. Mead & J. Sibert). Scutari Press, London.

Foster, P. (1989) Nursing care and management of epidermolysis bullosa. In *Epidermolysis Bullosa: A Comprehensive Review of Classification, Management and Laboratory Studies* (DEBRA) (eds G. Priestly, M.J. Tidman, J.B. Weiss & R.A.J. Eady). Dystrophic Epidermolysis Bullosa Research Association, Crowthorne, Berks.

Foster, R.L.R., Hunsberger, M.M. & Tackett Anderson, J. (1989) *Family Centered Nursing: Care of Children*. W.B. Saunders, Philadelphia.

Francis, A.L. (1990) Support for Parents of Burned Children. *Nursing*, 4(7), 7–10.

Gammon, A.P.J. & Ogden, B. (1992) Child Accident Prevention: role of Hospital and Community. *Auditorium*, 2, 39–43.

George, A. & Hancock, J. (1993) Reducing paediatric burn pain with parent participation. *Journal of Burn Care and Rehabilitation*, 14(1), 104–7.

Gray, G. (1987) Burns: Injured children. *Nursing Times*, 83(21), 49–51.

Harper, J. (1990) *Handbook of Paediatric Dermatology*, 2nd edn. Butterworth Heinemann, London.

Hazinski, M.F. (1990) Shock in the paediatric patient. *Critical Care Nursing Clinics of North America*, 2(92), 309–24.

Herndon, D.N., Rutan, R.L. & Rutan, T.C. (1993) Management of the paediatric patient with burns. *Journal of Burn Care and Rehabilitation*, 14(1), 3–7.

Hertz-Lazarowitz, R., Feitelsen, D., Zahavi, S. & Hartup, W.W. (1981) Social interaction and organisation of Israeli five to seven year olds. *International Journal of Behavioural Development*, 4, 143–55.

Hobbs, C.J. (1989) Burns and scalds. In: *ABC of Child Abuse* (ed R. Meadow). British Medical Journal, London.

Hunter, L. (1992) Applying Orem to skin. *Nursing*, 5(4), 16–18.

Hurwitz, S. (1981) *Clinical Paediatric Dermatology*. W.B. Saunders, Philadelphia.

Hutt, J. (1989) *A Consumer Perspective of Nursing Needs of Pre-school Age Children who have Sustained Thermal Injuries and are Receiving Home Care*. Unpublished dissertation, University of Wales.

Jarrett, P., Sharp, C. & McLelland, J. (1993) Protection of children by their mothers against sunburn. *British Medical Journal*, **306** (6890), 1448.

Kelly, H. (1994) Initial nursing assessment and management of burn injured children. *British Journal of Nursing*, 3(2), 54–9.

Levene, S. (1992) Preventing accidental injuries to children. *Paediatric Nursing*, 4(9), 12–14.

Lookingbill, D.P. & Marks, J.G. (1986) *Principles of Dermatology*. W.B. Saunders, Philadelphia.

Lowry, M. & Gill, A. (1992) Taking the heat out of burns. *Professional Nurse*, 8(1), 26–30.

Lund, C.L. & Browder, N.C. (1944) The Estimation of Areas of Burns. Surgery Gynecology and Obstetrics, 79, 352. Cited in *Burns in Children: Pediatric Burn Management* (eds H.F. Carvajal & D.H. Parks). Year Book Medical Publishers, Chicago.

Marieb, N. (1989) *Human Anatomy and Physiology*, pp. 134–51. Benjamin/Cummings Publishing Company, Redwood City.

McCance, K.L. & Huether, S.E. (1994) *Pathophysiology – The Biological Basis for Disease in Adults and Children*. Mosby, London.

Morris, D. (1991) *Babywatching*. Jonathan Cape, London.

OPCS (1990) *Deaths from Accidents Caused by Fire and Flames in the Home and Communal Establishments: Cause of Accident, Sex and Age Group*. Office of Population Censuses and Surveys, London.

Orton, C. (1981) *Learning to Live with Skin Disorders*. Souvenir Press, London.

Pearce, S. (1989) Researching burns and scalds. *Paediatric Nursing*, 1(8), 13–15.

Pearce, S. (1992) Treatment and care of minor burns and scalds. *Paediatric Nursing*, 4(4), 16–18.

Pegum, J.S. & Baker, H. (1979) *Dermatology*, 3rd edn. Balliere Tindall, London.

Perkins, P. (1993) Prevention through education: a pilot study on skin cancer education in primary schools. *Child Health*, 3, 117–21.

RCN (1990) *Nursing Children in the Accident and Emergency Department*. Royal College of Nursing, London.

Rennick, J. (1986) Re-establishing the parental role in a pediatric intensive care unit. *Journal of Pediatric Nursing*, 1(1), 40–44.

Robson, M.C. & Heggers, J.P. (1988) Pathophysiology of the burn wound. In *Burns in Children, Pediatric Burn Management* (eds H.P. Carjaval & D.H. Parks). Year Book Medical Publishers, Chicago.

Romness Foster, R.L., Hunsberger, M.M. & Tackett Anderson, J.J. (1989) *Family Centered Nursing Care of Children*. W.B. Saunders, Philadelphia.

Samba, W.W., Schindler, R.D. & Carvajal, H.F. (1988) *Nutrition and Metabolism in Burns in Children* (eds H.F. Carvajal & D.H. Parks). Year Book Medical Publishers Inc., Chicago.

Seville, R.H. & Martin, E. (1981) *Dermatological Nursing and Therapy*. Blackwell Science, Oxford.

Shrank, A.B. (1986) Skin problems in infancy. *Maternal and Child Health*, II(4), 122–6.

Simpson, C. (1992) Eczema in Children. *Paediatric Nursing*, 4(5), 16–18.

Slack, P.A. (1978) *School Nursing*. Balliere Tindall, London.

Smith, P.K. (1987) A longitudinal study of social participation in pre-school children: solitary and parallel play re-examined. *Developmental Psychology*, 14, 517–23.

Smith, P.K. & Cowie, H. (1991) *Understanding Children's Development*, 2nd edn. Blackwell Publishers, Oxford.

Spowart, K. (1993) Management of eczema in children. *Paediatric Nursing*, 5(8), 9–12.

Spowart, K. & Muir, M. (1993) *A Guide to Eczema. Management for community nurses and health visitors*. The National Eczema Society, London.

Stobert, L. (1994) Nurse aid management of burns. *British Journal of Nursing*, 3(9), 469–72.

Stone, L. & Garibaldinos, T. (1992) Apply daily. *Nursing*, 5(4), 8–10.

Strasburger, V.C. & Brown, R.T. (1991) *Adolescent Medicine: A Practical Guide*. Little, Brown and Company, Boston/Toronto/London.

Strodtbeck, F. & Joyce, B. (1988) Shock in newborns and children. *Critical Care Nursing Quarterly*, 11(1), 75–83.

Sutherland, S. (1988) Burned adolescents' descriptions of their coping strategies. *Heart and Lung*, 17(2), 150–56.

Tait, A. (1992) Children in the sun. *Paediatric Nursing*, 4(5), 21–3.

Torrance, C. (1986) The physiology of wound healing. *Nursing*, 3(5), 162–8.

Turnbull, R. & Atherton, D. (1994) Use of wet wrap dressings in atopic eczema. *Paediatric Nursing*, 6(2), 22–6.

Urquhart, S. (1989) Nursing a serious scald. *Paediatric Nursing*, 1(8), 16–17.

Van Bever, H.P. (1992) Recent advances in the pathogenesis of atopic dermatitis. *European Journal of Paediatrics*, 151, 870–73.

Wallace, E. (1993) Nursing a teenager with burns. *British Journal of Nursing*, 2(5), 278–81.

Walsh, M. (1990) *Accident and Emergency Nursing*, 2nd edn. Heinemann, Oxford.

Watkins, P.N. (1993) This one's for Billy. *Journal of Burn Care and Rehabilitation*, 14(1), 58–64.

Whaley, L.F. & Wong, D.L. (1991) *Nursing Care of Infants and Children*, 4th edn. Mosby Year Book, London.

Wilding, P.A. (1986) *Burns Nursing* (5), 184–7.

Zuker, R.M. (1988) Initial management of the burn wound in psychosocial care of the severely burned child. In *Burns in Children* (eds H.F. Carvajal & D.H. Parks). Year Book Medical Publishers, London.

Chapter 24

Nursing Support and Care: Meeting the Needs of the Child and Family with Altered Mobility

Annette K. Dearmun and Anne Taylor

INTRODUCTION

This chapter will consider the experiences of the child and family resulting from alterations in usual mobility, and will examine the particular contribution of the children's nurse in meeting the needs of such families.

Many of the general principles of children's care – the impact of illness on the family, play and preparation, growth and development and pain management – have been discussed elsewhere in this book and apply equally to the child with an alteration in mobility. A philosophy underpinning the care of children will be assumed and only specific principles will be applied.

Although an alteration in mobility may result from congenital or acquired 'conditions', the fundamental problems for the child and family are broadly similar. All the activities of daily living may be affected, and tasks for parents include long term care for a child with a plaster of Paris cast or traction, entertaining a child with restricted mobility, and assisting a child to maintain, maximize or regain movement and independence.

Differences might lie in the child's and family's approach to dealing with these problems. To a great extent this will be an individual response determined by previous experience or social circumstances, but it may also be influenced by the aetiology of the 'condition'; for example, whether it is an isolated deficit or whether the mobility dysfunction is part of a more complex condition, or whether the dysfunction is temporary, more long term or permanent. Furthermore, a child who has a recognized mobility problem at birth may have differing needs and a different experience from a child who sustains a fractured femur as a result of an accident.

It may also be seen that an alteration in mobility, in many cases, will affect a child for a considerable period of time. It may lead to the child developing new skills, for example eating and dressing with one hand for six weeks following a fractured radius and ulna. It may necessitate parents taking on new or additional responsibilities; for example, if the child has osteomyelitis, learning to give intravenous antibiotics so that time spent in hospital can be minimized.

The first section will explore the needs of the infant with congenital dysfunction evident from birth. It will examine the care required for the child with a talipes and congenital dysplasia of the hips. The nurse's role in providing care for the child with a plaster of Paris cast, Gallows/Pugh's traction and a hip spica will be highlighted. These principles of care may be applied to caring for the child with an application of a plaster cast following trauma.

The second section will address some of the needs of the child admitted with osteomyelitis. The role of the nurse in teaching the parents technical skills will be mentioned.

The third section will focus on the care required for the child with a fractured femur, to discuss the care required following an accidental injury, traction, application of an external fixator and prolonged immobility. This will focus on the nurse's role of direct care giver, and the principles may be applied to the care of the child following any orthopaedic trauma.

The fourth section considers surgical intervention for scoliosis and will include reference to the role of the nurse as advocate.

The final section will give an overview of other general considerations for a child with a mobility problem.

A certain level of prior knowledge will be assumed; for example, an understanding of the normal embryology of the musculoskeletal system, the structure and function of the skeleton, development of bones, classification of fractures, wound and bone healing and the features of physiological shock. Therefore preliminary reading would be useful.

NURSING CARE OF THE CHILD WITH A CONGENITAL LOWER LIMB DEFORMITY

The child born with a limb deformity may also have a syndrome or other rare anomaly. As the critical stage of limb development occurs simultaneously with the development of other body systems, a teratogen will affect the development of other sensitive tissues. Thus the child may have deficiencies associated with other congenital abnormalities, in particular the genito-urinary and cardiovascular systems. Some children may also have a degree of learning disability and alterations in other daily activities.

Talipes, or 'club foot', the most common lower limb deformity, is associated with neural tube malformations, for example meningomyelocoele, and therefore the initial correction may be one of a series of medical interventions.

These parents may be in need of particular support because they may have considerations that go beyond just caring for their infant with a lower limb plaster.

Nursing assessment

The infant with talipes will be seen to have an obvious deformity of their foot at birth. This endorses the importance of the nursing assessment in order to determine the child's and family's particular needs, and to co-ordinate often quite complex care. The nurse may also need to draw upon the knowledge and expertise of other members of the multiprofessional team, including dieticians and physiotherapists to obtain optimal developmental progress.

The problems may have been detected by either the parents, midwife or other health care professionals during health screening. This obvious visible defect of the foot may force the parents to face reality, and sometimes the health care professionals present at the delivery lack the necessary knowledge of current approaches to be able to provide the immediate reassurance required by the family; this may increase the parents' anxieties.

The family will usually see a specialist on a regular basis. This may involve frequent outpatient visits, travelling long distances and other inconveniences associated with being 'followed up' over a long period of time. The nurse may co-ordinate the efforts of other members of the team to meet the parents' need for a combination of psychological, social and financial support. This may enable the family to adapt more effectively to the situation, grieve the loss of the normal child they expected, define a new role for themselves and maintain contact with their family and friends.

Nursing intervention: meeting the child's needs

One of the main aims of care for the child with talipes of both feet is maintaining optimal position of the limb or joint by use of plaster of Paris or splints. Stretching and serial plastering is often commenced early and continues for the first three months. The aim of this is to maintain the correct anatomical position of the foot. It should be remembered that it may be potentially distressing for

the family to see this 'deformity', and parents may have anxieties about their child's ultimate ability to walk.

If the conservative approach is unsuccessful, surgical intervention and/or oesteomoties to release soft tissue or oesteotomies may be required. This introduces other dimensions of care in addition to the general post operative considerations.

The infant may experience pain which may be exacerbated by swelling and a plaster that is applied too tightly. Pain may also be indicative of developing circulatory impairment. As a goal of care is to ensure that the infant is pain free and therefore as comfortable as possible, nursing measures are related to reducing swelling and providing appropriate levels of analgesia.

Sometimes nonsteroidal anti-inflammatory drugs are prescribed in addition to analgesics immediately post operatively, although only three doses are given to babies. Paracetamol or a caudal block may also be effective in minimizing pain.

Swelling, and thus pain, may be reduced for about 4–6 hours by elevation of the leg, for example on a gamgee roll or a small pillow, acknowledging the need to ensure safety. Particular attention should be given to the circulation and digits should be checked for colour and warmth, although the estimation of sensation may be difficult in the pre verbal child. Occasionally the plaster will need to be split to allow for swelling, it is then bandaged in place. This is usually carried out by the technician in conjunction with medical advice.

Following an oesteotomy the surgical incision is obscured by the plaster. Thus initial haemorrhage or delayed wound healing may not be readily detected. In relation to post operative bleeding parents need to be reassured that plaster of Paris tends to soak up blood and so even a small amount can look alarming. Drawing around the mark left by the blood will enable assessment of blood loss with greater accuracy.

Unusual discharge or odour may herald a complication in wound healing. Information regarding this could be incorporated into the aftercare advice, as the parents may be the first to notice alterations of this nature.

Although this discussion has been related to talipes, the principles of care of plaster may be applied to other situations; for example, when the child sustains a fracture and has a plaster cast applied. However, it should be noted that following trauma, increasing pain and inability to extend and flex the fingers may be indicative of a build up of pressure and complications, commonly 'compartment syndrome'. This should be reported immediately to avoid permanent damage.

Many children's wards offer general principles and aftercare advice about caring for a child with a plaster cast (Table 24.1).

abduction of one leg, asymmetrical gluteal folds, unequal knee lengths, toe walking or an abnormal gait and they will bring it to the attention of the health visitor. They may experience frustration if their concerns do not appear to be taken seriously. It is recognized that

Table 24.1 Aftercare advice for parents whose child has had a plaster of paris cast applied to a limb (Oxford Radcliffe Hospital, Oxford).

Do's	Don'ts
Encourage your child to exercise fingers/toes, shoulder and elbow joints as often as possible as instructed by the physiotherapist/nurse. Elevate the plastered limb on a cushion or pillow, when sitting down or asleep and wear the sling at all other times. Use the crutches as instructed by the physiotherapist.	Do not stand or press on the plaster for 48 hours, as it takes this long to dry properly. Do not write on the plaster until it is dry. Do not use felt tip pens as they make the plaster soggy, or ball point pens as they crack the plaster. Do not get the plaster wet as it will crumble and not set properly. Do not put anything down inside your plaster.

If any of the following occur, you need to seek medical advice immediately by returning to the accident and emergency department:

(1) Sudden severe pain.	(5) Numbness or pins and needles.
(2) Swelling of areas you can see.	(6) The plaster cracks.
(3) Blueness or discolouration of fingers and toes.	(7) The plaster goes soft.
(4) Inability to move fingers and toes.	(8) The plaster becomes uncomfortable.

NURSING CARE OF THE CHILD WITH CONGENITAL DYSPLASIA OF THE HIPS

Nursing assessment

Assessment for congenital dysplasia of the hips is also part of routine surveillance of the newborn baby. According to Department of Health statistics, 15–20 per thousand live births have hip instability (LeMaistre 1991). Many babies with this dysplasia are detected through this early screening, the application of Barlow and Ortolani tests, and classical signs of limb shortening and limited abduction. Ultrasound may also be used to screen a population considered 'at risk' (LeMaistre 1991).

Sometimes the parents are the first to notice limited

parents may express their disappointment in terms of anger and this is a difficult emotion to cope with, as often it is directed towards the health care professionals. The nurse may need to draw on their knowledge of counselling skills to deal sensitively with the parents in this situation.

Awareness programmes (Lee 1991) for health care professionals may reduce the number of children presenting over the age of six months, may minimize the number of children requiring hospitalization and lead to more effective utilization of resources (Lee 1991).

Nursing intervention: meeting the child's needs

An exploration of the care of a child with congenital dysplasia of the hips serves to highlight further nursing considerations related to caring for a child in a plaster hip spica. When detected early, again the initial approach will be conservative and a Von Rosen splint, plaster of Paris or harness will be applied for about six to eight weeks to maintain an optimal position of hip abduction and flexion. Because of the position of the splint parents may request particular advice on skin care. Nappy changing will be more frequent in an attempt to ensure that the skin is kept dry beneath the splint. If a harness has been applied it should be kept on for 24 hours per day; however, the chest strap may be released when washing the child. Parents will be advised to use limited soap and water because if used excessively it may wet the harness and lead to irritation of the skin (LeMaistre 1991).

If the hips are dislocated or the problem is detected late, splinting alone may be insufficient to correct the problem and lengthy and more complex treatment is necessary. This involves planned admission to hospital and a period of up to three weeks on traction, followed by surgery and three to four months in a hip spica.

Two main types of skin traction are used: Gallows and Pughs (Figs. 24.1 and 24.2). The medical staff use criteria to determine the most suitable, generally related to age and previous level of mobility.

Gallows traction is reserved for infants/children with dislocated hips who are not yet walking, and it can also be used in children below one year who have sustained a fractured femur. Pughs traction is used for toddlers and

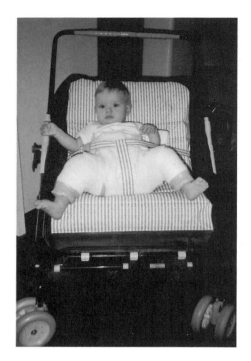

Fig. 24.2 Infant in a hip spica.

children who have already started to walk. The common features in both these approaches is that the child has to become accustomed to an unusual position when the traction is applied. This may adversely affect all activities of living, for example sleeping, eating and drinking, passing urine and stools and hygiene.

Approximately 50% of all children have some form of sleep problems (White 1990). This can be particularly prevalent amongst children with learning and physical disabilities and may include a reduction in rapid eye movement (REM) and nonrapid eye movement (NREM) sleep. It may be further exacerbated if the child is unable to sleep and wake when they wish, and if usual bedtime routines are disrupted, for example the child is unable to have their usual bath prior to bedtime.

White (1990) concludes that hospitalized children can lose 20–25% of their expected sleep time as a result of delay in sleep onset, and this aspect is also discussed by Bullard (1980). This lack of sleep may be compounded by the child's limited mobility; they use less energy and become less tired. Organizing care to maintain as many aspects of the child's usual routine as possible, and providing adequate stimulation during

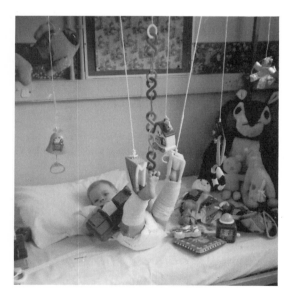

Fig. 24.1 Infant in Gallows traction.

waking hours, may minimize this problem. In some situations if the child is unable to settle they may be given sedation at night but it has been suggested that resolving sleep problems with medication is not desirable and is often unsuccessful (Pfeil 1993).

Eating and drinking and ensuring an adequate and balanced diet may become a particular challenge. Between the ages of one and five years early food habits are consolidated and independence in food and eating is gained (Wagner 1989). The unusual positioning of the child in traction may disrupt this process. As gastric capacity is small snacks may be required between meals; these can include finger foods such as raw vegetables, biscuits or fruit. This will enable the child to maintain their independence in eating.

At least 250 ml of whole milk should be consumed daily (Holmes 1991), although high intake of milk is a poor iron source and may result in iron deficiency. Fluid intake should be increased to minimize constipation and a teacher beaker will help to maintain the child's independence in drinking.

Passing urine and stools may also be problematic, especially for the toddler who is establishing continence. If the child is on Pugh's traction they can be taken off to use the potty; but knowing this, if they are anxious they may be less inclined to ask. If the parents are not present the nurse should be vigilant in order to anticipate the child's need to pass urine and stools. It may be considered expedient to put the child back into nappies, but usual routines should be acknowledged to minimize disruption to developmental progress.

Maintaining hygiene, especially skin care, is of particular importance when the baby is on Gallows traction. When they are in an optimal position they will be lying on their back with legs suspended in the air and it should be possible to slide a hand under their bottom. The position can be adjusted by adding additional weights or adjusting the cord. Maintaining this traction leads to pressure on the back, particularly the shoulders, see Fig. 24.1. Particular attention should be paid to checking the pressure points for redness. It should also be recognized that prolonged exposure to excrement may lead to skin breakdown and additional padding may be necessary in the nappy to prevent seepage of urine. The skin traction, adhesive or nonadhesive, will be bandaged into position. The bandages should be removed regularly to check the skin condition.

A hip spica (Fig. 24.2) is applied following surgery to

the hips and is commonly used for congenital dysplasia or Perthes disease, to maintain an optimal position of the head of the femur in the acetabulum. A review of current British literature revealed very little empirical research regarding the care of the child in a hip spica cast. However, a research study conducted in America by Shesser & Kling (1986) offered some pertinent findings.

The study evaluated the care for a child in a hip spica cast using parental input. There were 21 children below the age of five years placed in a cast for a minimum of four weeks. Five were continent and 16 were still in nappies. All parents were shown a short slide tape and received verbal advice and 'hands on' demonstrations from a clinical nurse specialist. The points highlighted by the slide tape addressed all the activities of living and included advice on the following:

- *Elimination* – Applying waterproof tape around the perineal opening to act as a barrier against the absorption of urine and stool. Elevating the child's head and chest by propping them on pillows or a bean bag to allow gravity to pull the urine and stools away from the cast. There is little consensus regarding the application of nappies; for example, Shesser & Kling (1986) suggest using smaller nappies and tucking them between the baby's skin and the cast with the plastic backing next to the cast's inside surface, to minimize soiling, securing the nappy with an elastic belt that encircles the waist and comes between the legs.

  In contrast STEPS (Congenital Dislocated Hips Association) advise putting nappies over the plaster, using non-absorbent cotton wool which must be disposed of with each nappy change, and changing the nappies more frequently. If the child is continent a 'wick' can be constructed with toilet paper to redirect the urinary stream into the toilet.
- *Eating and drinking* – Selecting a diet with increased fluids, fruit and vegetables and roughage to prevent constipation.
- *Mobility* – Handling the child in the cast, with particular guidance on turning them from front to back to inspect the condition of the skin and observe the plaster for cracks, dents or increasing tightness.
- *Dressing and hygiene* – Using baking soda or baby powder on the cast to diminish odours.
- *Safety and comfort* – Preventing small objects from getting down into the cast.

There was also advice about when to seek further assistance; for example, in situations where there is an unexplained fever, odour and unexplained discharge coming from beneath the cast, and swelling and poor circulation.

During subsequent follow up at outpatients the odour, soiling and general overall condition of the plaster was noted. The size of the perineal opening seemed to be a significant factor in the handling of the nappies and maintenance of a clean cast. As a result of this study guidelines were developed for the application of a cast with specific reference to the size and cutting of the perineal opening in the cast, and there was a reduction in the number of cast and skin problems.

This study may provide evidence of the effectiveness of the educational and teaching role of the nurse, particularly with regard to the particular considerations related to elimination and mobility at home.

Specific considerations in discharge planning are raised by the Community Care Act 1992 which stresses the need to plan from admission to discharge. This is supported by the second charter from the Action for Sick Children (formerly NAWCH) which states that: 'Parents have responsibility for their children and shall receive positive and appropriate support to care for their sick child both at home and in hospital'.

Apart from the aftercare advice already discussed, other aspects may include discussion of any practical difficulties in caring for their child at home. These may be related to door widths, stairs and height of the child's bed.

It may be obvious that as the child will be nonweight-bearing on the affected leg, so steps will need to be taken to maintain a level of mobility at home. The child will be heavy to carry, and to avoid injury parents should be taught safe lifting and handling skills. Depending on the amount of living space available, some children will be able to use a board on wheels or reclining wheelchair to increase their mobility. However, special considerations should be given to all living conditions at home and liaison with health visitors and social services may be required, to make adaptations.

Creative approaches to safe transportation of the child may need to be explored in the light of the child restraint laws. When the child is sent home an adapted car seat may be needed because they will probably not fit their present seat. Unfortunately these are scarce but are known to be available in Sweden.

The emphasis has been upon identifying knowledge that the nurse may acquire in order to offer appropriate advice to parents regarding aftercare at home. With the exception of perhaps long periods in traction, the length of stay in hospital will be minimal and therefore much of the care will fall to the parents at home. Even for the child in traction there are examples of successful attempts to nurse these children at home with the appropriate community services.

Occasionally a child has to remain in hospital for the two to three months they are in plaster, because of difficulties with the physical living space at home. In this case needs for play and education should be considered and this will be discussed later.

Although distressing for the family these problems are generally not of a life threatening nature and very often corrective treatment is conservative. If surgery is required the infant or child is admitted to hospital on an elective basis.

NURSING CARE OF THE CHILD ADMITTED WITH OSTEOMYELITIS

The child with infection in their bone or joint, osteomyelitis or septic arthritis, will usually be admitted to hospital via the GP or outpatient clinic as an emergency.

Nursing assessment

They will be generally unwell, may be refusing to eat and drink, may be irritable, may limp or be reluctant to move the affected limb or joint, and there will be a rise in temperature, indicative of infection.

Nursing intervention: meeting the child's needs

One of the main aims of care will be to maintain the temperature within acceptable limits to minimize the effects associated with a raised temperature. In addition to recording the temperature at regular intervals, the pulse and respiratory rate should also be monitored as the temperature will have an influence on heart rate and breathing. An antipyretic such as paracetamol may be given to reduce temperature, and if it continues to rise consistently other measures may be employed, for example fan therapy and tepid sponging.

This has created interesting debate, with some hospitals devising policies which only allow these methods to be used with written instructions, or others which ban them altogether on safety reasons. The contra indications associated with these therapies should be fully recognized and regular monitoring of temperature should always be maintained throughout. A dramatic fall in temperature may lead to hypothermia and shock.

Offering adequate fluids, usually half a cup (100 ml) per hour will reduce the temperature. The medical staff will take a blood test to confirm the proposed diagnosis and will site an intravenous infusion to ensure the child receives adequate fluids and to administer antibiotic therapy. Wound infection increases the demand for energy, reduces iron and zinc absorption and increases the excretion of vitamins B_2 and C. This knowledge is useful when giving the parents advice about their child's dietary needs.

Usually due to the infection, the child requires long term intravenous antibiotic therapy, sometimes eight weeks or more; in this case a Hickman line may be inserted. This has several advantages: it is less likely to become dislodged or fall out, reducing the need for repeated venepunctures, and it is less obtrusive than a peripheral cannula.

Pain will limit movement and thus analgesia and careful positioning of the affected limb with strategically placed pillows will minimize discomfort. Sometimes a plaster of Paris back slab, or occasionally traction, will be applied to ensure that the child is unable to move the affected joint.

Sometimes surgical incision is required to debride the infected bone and this will result in an open wound. It seems that there is little research in wound care in children and much practice is based on ritual rather than empirical evidence. There appears to be no one single product which may be considered ideal for all wounds (Jones 1991). Principles are that the wound should be cleaned using an aseptic technique and attention should be given to any drains that may have been inserted to draw out exudate and infection.

Preparation for home care once again involves the nurse in a teaching role. The parents will be given instructions regarding care of the Hickman line. A protocol is usually developed to ensure that the information and advice is consistent (Sidey 1989).

There may be ethical issues when home care is discussed as an option. This was debated by Charles-Edwards & Casey (1992). They suggested that home care can often be predicted when parents agree to a treatment option which will shorten their child's stay in hospital; for example, surgery and application of a plaster cast. In such cases they are seen to be consenting to the subsequent care as well as the surgery, and should thus be fully informed of the implications of their decisions and the subsequent care.

In situations where home care is unforeseen – for example, in the case of a child being discharged with a Hickman line and having to have intravenous antibiotics for up to eight weeks three or four times per day – they argue that parents should be allowed time to adjust to the new situation and should feel they can opt out if they want to.

It is also recommended that parents sign to confirm that they have been instructed in a particular technique and that they accept responsibility for performing the procedure on the child at home. However, Dimond (1990) is more cautious of this as a way of releasing the health professional from their obligations. It is suggested that a signed consent form does not exempt the nurse or health authority from liability for negligence if the child suffers any harm as a result.

NURSING CARE OF THE CHILD FOLLOWING MINOR TRAUMA

Following an accident resulting in a soft tissue injury or fracture, the child's attendance to hospital will be unforeseen, unplanned and may constitute an emergency. There will be minimal time for preparation.

A fracture usually occurs as a result of an accidental or nonaccidental injury. Jackson & Wilkinson (1976, cited in Almond 1993) describe accidental injury in children as 'the most important epidemic in the western world today'. Statistics collected by the Child Accident Prevention Trust (Levene 1992) suggest that accidental injury causes 700 deaths in children per year in England and Wales. Interestingly, it appears that accidents are more prevalent in the north of England and in socially disadvantaged children.

It is recognized that accidents may be prevented and there are three principles related to this:

(1) Primary intervention to prevent the accident happening, for example the provision of safe road play schemes.

(2) Secondary intervention to ameliorate injuries in an accident, for example fitting a seat belt in the car.

(3) Tertiary intervention, which involves optimal treatment of injuries to ensure a complete recovery or minimal residual disability.

Towner & Barry (1993) discuss the Health of the Nation and provide further discussion of effective strategies to reduce the number of accidents.

Although nurses have a role in all these aspects, often the focus is the nurse's contribution to tertiary aspects.

Nursing assessment

On arrival in the accident and emergency department the child will be assessed and immediate treatment provided. The comprehensive assessment should include a report of the events surrounding the accident and the perceived coping ability of the family. It is also important to review the child's immunization records in order to ascertain whether a tetanus toxoid vaccination is required. Brown & Evans (1989) monitored the immunization status of children attending accident and emergency departments and found that a considerable number of children had incomplete immunizations.

Nursing intervention: meeting the child's needs

If the injury is relatively minor, in medical terms, the treatment will include cleaning and suturing the wound or putting on a plaster, sling or bandage. The nurse should be available to support the child and family by preparing the child and providing appropriate information regarding treatment and aftercare.

It is recommended that details of all children under 16 years of age who attend the accident and emergency service, should be recorded and reported to a liaison health visitor (DoH 1992). The nurse should also record the child's attendance on the parent-held record, if available.

NURSING CARE OF THE CHILD FOLLOWING MAJOR TRAUMA

An exploration of the needs for a child with a fractured femur provides an opportunity to discuss the physiological processes associated with trauma, and the use of this knowledge to consider the role and responsibility of the nurse in assessment and implementation of care during the initial stages when the child may experience the effects of physiological instability.

Nursing assessment

Children who have experienced this major injury will usually be transported by ambulance to the accident and emergency department. The injury may be isolated or multiple and may lead to alteration of other bodily functions; for example, a deterioration in consciousness level may indicate a head injury, or abdominal pain, pallor and bleeding may suggest a ruptured spleen or kidney. By undertaking a systematic assessment, including details regarding the circumstances of the accident, the nurse will be able to identify any immediate potentially life threatening problems. It is important to ascertain the child's tetanus toxoid status and to administer this if necessary.

Even if other injuries are not present the child will usually be distressed and anxious due to pain, and will be sweating and pale due to vasoconstriction, indicative of physiological shock, which is likely to be exacerbated by severe pain.

Nursing intervention: meeting the child's needs

Immediate care in the accident and emergency department will be aimed at supporting the child and family, reducing the child's pain by administering analgesia and immobilizing the leg, and minimizing the effects of physiological shock. If the fracture is mid shaft or lower third a Thomas splint will often be used to support the child's leg. Following X-rays and measurement of the unaffected leg, appropriate traction will be applied.

A fractured femur will result in bleeding; sometimes up to 400 ml of blood is lost and so there is a reduction in blood volume and circulating haemoglobin and oxygen. This will lead to a reduction in oxygen to the tissues, and breathlessness. In an attempt to compensate there will be a redirection of blood from the skin and hence a reduction in oxygen to the skin and wound; ultimately this may delay healing.

Pain may cause the child to hyper or hypo ventilate, precipitating electrolyte imbalance. This alters the usual physiology and has an influence on heart rate and blood pressure, creating tachycardia and hypotension.

The nurse's main role is in assessing and monitoring these vital signs in order to evaluate the effectiveness of care being prescribed. The nurse will also need to support the child and family during cannulation, which may be made more difficult as a result of the vasoconstriction mentioned previously, of the child's anxiety and of the lack of opportunity to apply EMLA cream and wait for it to become effective due to the urgency of needing to obtain venous access. Parents may have difficulty in maintaining their parenting role due to their own helplessness and anxiety.

Following the initial care the child will be transferred to the ward where he/she will continue to be regularly assessed and care will be implemented to minimize pain and prevent complications associated with, initially, shock, and later on the effects of prolonged immobilization.

Initially physiological shock may increase the risk of hypothermia; the child may also lose heat during examinations and X-rays. After a few days a rise in temperature may indicate infection, particularly osteomyelitis which may occur following a compound fracture.

If there is an open fracture, intravenous prophylactic antibiotics are usually prescribed and these should be given at regular intervals to maintain therapeutic levels. If the wound is visible the nurse should observe and report signs of redness, warmth or swelling around the wound site. These signs, together with reports of increasing pain and a rise in temperature, may indicate an inflammatory response. Prolonged inflammation may lead to coagulation of blood, necrosis of the tissue, infection and delayed healing. Optimal healing may also be reduced by disruption of the vascular supply to the damaged tissues and reduction in wound temperature.

A reduction in blood volume will affect blood pressure which in turn influences the blood flow through the kidneys. A reduction in blood flow through the kidneys leads to oliguria. The nurse who is aware of this will understand the need to maintain accurate fluid balance records. Sugar may be detected in the urine due to stress.

The child may be reluctant to move due to pain and hence may be unwilling or unable to use a bedpan. A degree of urinary retention is not uncommon. This may be particularly distressing for the child and family and the nurse will need to support them during the initial difficult stages. The nurse should endeavour to obtain accurate pain assessment and offer adequate analgesia. Once pain-free, the child will be more co-operative in many other aspects of their care, including hygiene.

Physiological stress has several effects on the nutritional status of the child with a fractured femur. These are mainly linked to effects of shock. The liver converts glycogen to glucose to provide additional energy. The reduction in blood flow to the mesenteric artery leads to delay in gastric emptying and therefore the child may not digest their last meal. Stimulation of the vagus nerve causes vomiting. This knowledge has implications if surgical intervention is required to stabilize the fracture. The anaesthetic may be hazardous and it is particularly important to ascertain the last time the child had anything to eat.

Finally, an increase in metabolic rate leads to a breakdown of protein and lyposis. Protein deficiency inhibits the basic phases of wound healing, and it impairs humeral and cell mediated antibody responses and decreases phagocytosis. Particular attention should be paid to the child's dietary needs to promote optimal healing.

Appetite usually provides the best guide to food requirements (Holmes 1991) but the child in traction may have less control over food consumption, and a varied diet should be available. Mills *et al.* (1993) conducted a survey of 14 children aged nine to eleven years on an orthopaedic ward, to look at a child's dietary intake whilst in hospital. The findings indicated that most children had 'quite a good awareness of what constitutes a healthy diet, but this did not influence their actual dietary intake'. They appeared to eat more 'junk food' in hospital, which concurred with the actual food discovered in the child's locker. The nurse can educate the parents about their child's dietary needs whilst in hospital.

Vitamins A and C are required for normal epithelialzation and as the latter is not stored, food containing vitamin C should be encouraged daily. Vitamin E and additional calcium are also required.

The child will usually remain in traction for four to six weeks. Regular X-rays will monitor the degree of bone healing and when callous is formed and the bone is stable, the traction will be removed and the child will be helped to mobilize on crutches. For the child on traction it is usually a period of unnatural enforced rest. Some of the considerations related to sleep, hygiene, elimination and diet were discussed in relation to the child in Gallow's traction, so specific points will be raised here.

The type of traction will be decided by the orthopaedic surgeon but the nurse should have sufficient knowledge of the principles of traction to ensure that traction is effective at all times in enabling the fracture to heal in the correct position (Andrew & Pudner 1985). This includes ensuring that the alignment is correct, and checking weights to ensure that they are free of restriction. Short cords should not be joined by knots as they will not run freely through pulleys and if incorrectly secured may slip and come undone. There should be a degree of flexion at the knee to prevent stiffness, and padding of the Thomas splint to maximize comfort. A pain in the thigh or a muscle spasm may indicate that the traction is inadequate. Sometimes antispasmodic drugs are given, in addition to analgesia, to reduce muscle spasm.

As already mentioned, immobility may lead to a deterioration in the child's skin, and the Thomas splint may cause friction around the groin and should be inspected regularly. Skin covered by traction should be assessed for signs of dryness or allergic reaction. The neurovascular status of the child's limb should be assessed regularly as increased pressure on nerves and blood vessels may lead to temporary or permanent damage. A monkey pole may be used to enable the child to lift their bottom off the bed; they should be encouraged to use this to relieve pressure.

Due to inactivity the child may experience generalized muscle wastage and contracture of the Achilles' tendon. This 'foot drop' may be prevented by generating play activities which will encourage the child to exercise all freely moveable joints and undertake ankle and foot exercises.

Inability to use the bedpan and immobility may lead to constipation. This may be minimized by ensuring that the child has drinks available all day, and offering a diet high in roughage. However, it should be recognized that

a high fibre diet may also disrupt the absorption of minerals, namely iron and calcium, and the latter is required for bone healing. Sometimes a mild aperient will be prescribed.

Exercise of the unaffected limbs will commence as soon as possible, but once the child's fracture is stable the nurse will liaise with the physiotherapist and rehabilitation will begin. When the child first takes to crutches this can be both an exciting and challenging time for the family. The nurse can assist the child by negotiating goals with the child regarding the distance they will walk, and providing incentives and appropriate encouragement.

Although this section has identified some of the issues related to caring for the child who has sustained a fractured femur, the overall principles related to assessment and management can be equally applied to any child confined to bed for long periods in hospital or at home.

NURSING CARE OF THE CHILD WITH AN EXTERNAL FIXATOR

Although the focus in this section is upon the care of a child with an external fixator, the principles of care can be applied to care of the pin sites for a child on skeletal traction. External fixators may be applied for the treatment of a fractured leg, for straightening of deformity and for adjusting leg length discrepancies. There are different types of fixator, such as Orthofix, Illizarov, but a major consideration in both is pin site care and body image.

These pins, inserted through the skin into the bone, are a potential site for infection and possible osteomyelitis (Nichol 1993). Following adequate analgesia the initial dressing should be removed 24 hours after surgery. Sometimes the dressing is soaked off. If the fixator gets wet it should be dried adequately afterwards. A shower with warm water will assist in soaking the dressing off. Pin sites should then be cleaned aseptically and covered with a light nonadhesive keyhole dressing around the pin, which is taped in place.

There appears to be little agreement regarding the best solutions to use and the best way to dress pin sites (Draper 1985). Sproles (1985, cited in Wallis 1991) provides no physiological evidence but suggests that crusts should be allowed to form around the skeletal pin sites. A contrasting view is offered by Celeste *et al.* (1984), who contend that once primary healing has occurred at the pin site any crusts around the pin site should be removed because fluid accumulated beneath the crust can become trapped and result in secondary bacterial infection.

Nichol (1993) reviewed the literature and found no consistent research about the best solutions to use for pin sites cleaning. Some writers argued that antiseptics hinder healing (Ryan 1993), and a solution of normal saline is often used successfully. Draper (1985) suggests the use of hydrogen peroxide to debride and remove necrotic tissue which may create a focus for infection, but this can cause skin irritation and Wallis (1991) suggests that a crust should be allowed to form. Although it is often assumed that any wound care should be carried out using aseptic techniques, Ryan (1985, cited by Nichol 1993) found that an emphasis on hand washing and using a clean technique was easier for encouraging compliance and did not compromise the wound safety. Cold solutions on the pin site may reduce the temperature and delay healing (Wallis 1991).

A fixator may be worn for up to nine months depending on how much lengthening or straightening is required. Therefore the child and family need to be educated to undertake the pin site care at home. Mount (1993) applied Orem's 1985 model to the care of the child undergoing leg lengthening, and devised a 'patient directed learning plan' with particular attention to pin site care. The plan involves teaching basic principles such as standards of hygiene and asepsis in treatment. Videos and photographs of previous children undergoing similar procedures are shown. Advice is given regarding the optimal time of day to clean the pins, for example after a shower or before bed.

Within 72 hours any changes such as inflammation, discharge and severe pain local to the pin site should be reported as this may be indicative of pin reaction or adverse tissue response. After this time infection is more likely and a swab for culture and sensitivity should be taken; antibiotics are then usually prescribed. Once the discharge from the pin site has ceased the area could be left without a dressing.

NURSING CARE OF THE CHILD WITH IDIOPATHIC SCOLIOSIS

Idiopathic scoliosis is a problem commonly found in young adults following the adolescent growth spurt (Tanner 1978).

Nursing assessment

The scoliosis (curvature of the spine) may be detected by the school nurse during health screening. Once discovered the parents may experience a degree of guilt as, although the cause is generally unknown, there is thought to be a familial tendency. They may need support and reassurance during the long treatment regime.

Nursing intervention: meeting the child's needs

There are many treatment options available, from wearing braces or a plaster jacket and performing a series of regular exercises, to surgical intervention to achieve partial correction. Each treatment pathway will have an emotional, physical and social impact upon the young adult and their family.

The young adult may be required to wear a brace in an attempt to control the curve externally and prevent progression. A key consideration is their co-operation and this may be influenced by their stage of psychological and social development, in such areas as developing their identity and self esteem and their acceptance by peers. If they are allowed to 'contract' the number of hours they wear the brace and are able to continue physical sports, this may enhance their compliance.

Sometimes surgical intervention is necessary to prevent further deterioration. All decisions regarding treatment options should be made taking individual preferences into account and based upon accurate knowledge of the surgical procedures and risks involved. The nurse has a role in supporting both the young adult and their family in their decision making and could introduce them to others who have had similar surgery.

There are two main aims of surgery: to prevent further progression and to gain partial correction of the spinal curve. The specific aspects of care prior to surgery and afterwards will be highlighted, together with an exploration of the experience for the child and family.

Before surgery a number of investigations will need to be undertaken. These include:

- ISIS (Intraged Shape Imaging System) scan and spinal X-ray to define the extent of the curvature.
- Chest X-ray and lung function tests to assess respiratory function.
- Collection of urine for Labstix (Lloyd 1993) and mid stream urine to identify any abnormalities and infections.

The nurse has a particular role in preparing the young adult for these tests and discovering their concerns and alleviating them. Body image and preservation of dignity are considerations for all people but are perhaps more pertinent for the young adult in hospital. The X-rays and scan will require removal of their clothes and they may be very conscious of their deformity, especially if it is pronounced. Providing a mid stream urine specimen, if they are not given privacy, may prove embarrassing.

The nurse can offer support and explanation and can above all act as an advocate ensuring that other members of the health care team recognize the particular concerns of this age group. Burr (1993) and Shelley (1993a) discuss the health care provision for adolescents and outline their special needs.

Preparation for surgery may also include opportunities to practise log rolling – a special technique for changing position without flexing the spine – using a bed pan or urinal, eating and drinking whilst lying flat, and getting up from a supine position whilst maintaining a straight spine. Post operatively the nurse may assume a more direct care giving role.

Enforced restricted mobility due to spinal surgery and associated pain may lead to difficulty in maintaining a comfortable position in which to sleep. This may be exacerbated by noise and unfamiliar surroundings. The young adult may be offered their own room to reduce noise from younger children. Comfort may be increased by encouraging them to log roll from side to side and by placing pillows vertically either side of the body and under the back. Moving their arms and legs may minimize joint stiffness.

Anterior procedures are in close proximity to the abdominal region, so to avoid paralytic ileus food and drink are usually restricted until bowel sounds are present. Sometimes there is a decreased appetite following surgery, and it may be further affected by pain. Other factors may influence the child's willingness to drink; for example, previous experience of using a bedpan, and lack of privacy.

As soon as they are able, the child should be encouraged to eat and drink and should be given free choice of beverages and food with provisions brought in from home if desired. When at home the young adult often has erratic eating problems, but they often require additional nutritional requirement to maintain a steady pattern of growth and development. At this age, when provided with explanations they are usually able to understand and appreciate the reasons for certain actions and this may increase their compliance with care.

The key emotion will be one of self consciousness and embarrassment. Initially a urinary catheter may have been inserted and this may feel uncomfortable. Once it is removed, if they remain flat they may be unable to use a bedpan. After several days there is a potential of constipation due to reduction of roughage and fibre in their diet. This will be exacerbated by wanting to wait until they are more mobile and so able to use the toilet.

It is essential to maintain privacy and dignity. Once allowed out of bed they may use a commode, and a raised toilet seat may be useful to avoid having to flex the spine too much. Burr (1993) undertook a small study into the perceptions of adolescents and discovered that all those who were on the children's ward commented on the 'poor facilities for personal hygiene, and lack of privacy'. 'There were no facilities provided for the disposal of sanitary towels and no locks on the toilet doors'.

There is a potential for incorrect balance of fluid and electrolyte requirements due to vomiting and lack of adequate dietary intake. An intravenous infusion is usually maintained until drinking and eating resumes. Anti-emetics may be given to alleviate vomiting associated with the anaesthetic; this may be particularly important as vomiting may create further discomfort and cause back strain.

There is a potential of difficulty with breathing due to lying flat, and due to pain which may lead to shallow breathing in an attempt to minimize movement of the intercostal muscles and the diaphragm. Blood may be lost during surgery, reducing the circulating blood volume and leading to hypovolaemic shock.

Deep breathing should be encouraged to loosen secretions and reduce the risk of pulmonary infection or pneumonia. Presence of a raised temperature may indicate a urinary, chest or wound infection.

Pain, especially in shoulders, ribs and spinal muscles, may be due to surgery. This pain can be alleviated by using patient controlled analgesia (PCA) containing morphine, although it should be remembered that opiates reduce gastric motility and lead to constipation (Carter 1994). Nonsteroidal anti-inflammatory drugs are also successful if used on a regular basis. Analgesic drugs can be reduced according to the child's own report of their pain, bearing in mind that the pain can worsen when the child begins to stand and walk.

Once the child is mobilized after surgery, there may be stress associated with being unable to carry out usual physical activities and the problems of having to wear a plaster cast jacket for three to six months following surgery.

Educating the child and their family about the reasons for the immobility and for wearing a plaster cast, providing advice about how to disguise it under baggy clothes, and if possible introducing them to another child who might have a similar experience, are all strategies that may help to minimize the psychological impact of this.

Schilder (1935, cited by MacGinley 1993), defines body image as 'the picture of our own body which we form in our own mind, that is to say the way in which the body appears to ourselves'. It is recognized that surgery can alter a person's body image, and Price (1986, cited by MacGinley 1993) suggests that patients should be involved in their own care and should receive information about altered body image. As a result they will be more likely to come to terms with their altered body image and will be able to adapt to it.

The primary role of attending school is interrupted for at least two weeks due to hospitalization. There are reports that some schools do not allow the child to re-attend until the jacket has been removed. There may also be changes in role of family members, especially if the family live far away; for example, in who looks after any younger members of the family.

The young adult is usually more dependent on peer relationships and is accustomed to being independent from the family. The hospital stay has the potential for altering this because they will become more dependent on others for their physical and personal care. Burr

(1993) identified that adolescents place great importance on 'having someone of their own age to talk to', and thus visitors are very important.

Through a consideration of the needs of the child with scoliosis the principles of care needs of the young adult which may be applied to other situations have also been identified.

OTHER CONSIDERATIONS

There are several common factors associated with the care required by the child with a mobility dysfunction. They are largely related to the elective nature of most surgery and the prolonged immobility. They include the opportunity for preparation for events, discipline of the child, and particular needs for play and education.

As many orthopaedic procedures are elective there is an ability to plan the admission. This has several advantages, not least the opportunity afforded for pre admission preparation for the child and family. Eiser (1990) argues that very young children are often poorly informed and unprepared for hospital, and parents may experience more anxiety than their child. It is recognized that anxiety may be transmitted to the child. Many children's wards adopt pre admission programmes using videos, books and visits to departments within the hospital (Glasper & Stradling 1989), although setting up these schemes has resource implications and evaluation into their effectiveness should be carried out.

Specific preparation for children having orthopaedic surgery may include providing children with opportunities to play with and mould plaster of Paris, applying it to dolls and hoisting teddies into traction. The benefits of using play to prepare children for events is well documented (Diverty 1992). Whiting (1993) discusses the role of therapeutic play both before and after surgery. Whilst this is a role of the children's nurse, a play specialist will organize suitable activities to promote development and assist the child in coping with experiences in hospital. They can also give parents information about appropriate play materials. The child in traction will have energy which is suppressed and this may be displaced by encouraging 'messy play' with water, modelling materials, cooking and painting.

The parenting role in relation to discipline may be affected when the child is immobile or in hospital for long periods of time. This was discussed by Brykczyńska (1989). These challenges may be heightened when the child is confined to bed because if there is lack of privacy the parents can be observed by all those present on the ward.

The common form of punishment – time out – involves the parent imposing a certain amount of temporary social distancing and may not seem appropriate. If parents distance themselves they may feel guilt, leaving their child at a time when they perceive they need them.

Some of the child's challenging behaviour may be averted by ensuring that they are offered opportunities to be involved in decisions about their care and appropriate stimulation and play. This reduces the chance that the child will become frustrated and bored. It was suggested that 'all disciplinary measures should be age appropriate, consistent and fairly applied', and the nurse can support the parent to enable them to correct undesirable behaviour.

When the hospital stay is extended or the child is sent home encased in plaster, using a wheelchair or crutches and unable for whatever reason to attend school or socialise with peers, then a major problem for the child becomes one of boredom.

Wiles (1987) suggests that education of the hospitalized child is adequate. NAWCH (1984) discovered that 50% of wards did not employ a teacher despite the Warnock Report (DES 1978) recommendations that education should be arranged as soon as possible after admission.

There appear to be no specific policies regarding the education of children in hospital. Wilson (1993) recognized that hospital schools are under the influence and control of the local education authorities (LEAs) but several Education Acts – 1944, 1981 – have suggested that LEAs have a power but not a statutory duty to provide education in hospital. It is recommended that links should be made between home and hospital teaching in order to share resources (Wilson 1993). The nurse can liaise with the hospital teacher on discharge to arrange home tuition.

CONCLUSION

Whatever the situation, it may be appropriate to consider a nursing philosophy in which the overall aims of

nursing are seen to be synonymous with enabling the child and family to become self sufficient.

Pearson & Vaughan (1986) discuss various nursing frameworks which seem to express this concept in different ways; for example, Roper *et al.* (1980) refer to maximizing independence. Orem (1985) and Casey (1993) identify the goal of nursing as supporting the self care activities of the child and family. Roy (1980) defines the nursing activity in terms of supporting adaptation of the child and family to maintain optimal functioning. Taking all these into account there has been an emphasis in this chapter on the supporting and teaching function of the children's nurse in relation to the child with an alteration in usual mobility.

ACKNOWLEDGEMENT

Christina Laurie, *RGN*, *RSCN*, Senior Staff Nurse, Paediatric Surgical Ward, Oxford Radcliffe Hospital also contributed to the contents of this chapter.

REFERENCES AND FURTHER READING

Acharya, S. (1992) Assessing the need for pre-admission visits. *Paediatric Nursing*, 4(9), 20–22.

Adomat, R. (1992) Understanding shock. *British Journal of Nursing*, 1(3), 124–8.

Alderson, P. (1991) Children's consent to surgery. *Paediatric Nursing*, 3(10), 10–13.

Alderson, P. (1993) *Children's Consent to Surgery.* Open University Press, Buckingham.

Almond, P. (1993) Putting safety first. *Child Health*, 1(3), 97–100.

Andrew, R.J. & Pudner, R. (1985) Fractures. *Nursing*, 2(44), 1293–7.

Bell, E. (1989) Treatment of a fractured femur. *Paediatric Nursing*, 1(8), 6–8.

Benz, J. (1986) The adolescent in a spica cast. *Orthopaedic Nursing*, 5(3), 22–3.

Brosnan, H. (1991) Nursing management of the adolescent with idiopathic scoliosis. *Nursing Clinics of North America*, 26(1), 17–25.

Brown, G. & Evans, S. (1989) Immunisation uptake study. *Paediatric Nursing*, 1(4), 18–19.

Brunt, M. (1982) *Physiology in Nursing*, pp. 103–8. Harper and Row, London.

Brykczyńska, G. (1989) The art of discipline. *Paediatric Nursing*, 1(9), 6.

Bullard, W. (1980) A good night's sleep. *Nursing*, 3(20), 866–9.

Burr, S. (1993) Adolescents and the ward environment. *Paediatric Nursing*, 5(1), 10–13.

Campbell, J. (1993) Making sense of shock. *Nursing Times*, 89(5), 34–6.

Carter, B. (1994) *Child and Infant Pain: principles of nursing care and management*. Chapman and Hall, London.

Casey, A. (1993) Development and use of the partnership model of nursing care. In *Advances in Child Health Nursing* (eds E.A. Glasper & A. Tucker). Scutari Press, London.

Celeste, C., Folicik, M., Dumas, K. (1984) Identifying a standard for pin site care using the quality assurance approach. *Orthopaedic Nursing*, 3(4), 17–24.

Charles-Edwards, I. & Casey, A. (1992) Parental involvement and voluntary consent. *Paediatric Nursing*, 4(1), 16–20.

Cuddy, C.M. (1986) Caring for the child in a spica cast: parents perspective. *Orthopaedic Nursing*, 5(3), 17–21.

David, J. (1986) Wound Healing. *Paediatric Wound Care*. Martin Dunitz, London.

Davis, P. (1989) The principles of traction. *Nursing*, 3(34), 5–8.

DES (1978) *Special Educational Needs*. Report of the committee of enquiry into the education of handicapped children and young people (Warnock Report). HMSO, London.

DoH (1992) *The Health of the Nation – a strategy for health in England*. HMSO, London.

Dimond, B. (1990) Treatment of the Adolescent. *Paediatric Nursing*, 2(4), 21–22.

Doverty, N. (1992) Therapeutic use of play in hospital. *British Journal of Nursing*, 1(2), 77–81.

Draper, M. (1985) Make the dressing fit the wound. *Nursing Times*, 81(41), 32–35.

Eiser, C. (1990) *Chronic Childhood Disease*. Cambridge University Press, Cambridge.

Finchan Gee, C. (1990) Nutrition and wound healing. *Nursing*, 4(18), 26–8.

Flanagan, M. (1992) Outside influences. *Nursing Times*, 88(36), 72–8.

Foale, H. (1989) Healing the wound. *Paediatric Nursing*, 1(5), 10–11.

Glasper, A. & Stradling, P. (1989) Preparing children for admission. *Paediatric Nursing*, 1(5), 18–21.

Griffiths, R. (1988) *Community Care Agenda for Action*. HMSO, London.

Herbet, R. (1984) Maintaining the circulating volume. *Nursing*, 2(26), 76–8.

Heywood Jones, I. (1990) Making sense of traction. *Nursing Times*, 86(23), 39–41.

Hinchcliff, S. & Montague, S. (1988) *Physiology for Nursing Practice*. Bailliere Tindall, London.

Holmes, S. (1991) Nutrition in childhood and adolescence. *Paediatric Nursing*, 3(3), 10–12.

Jones, T. (1991) Dressed for best. *Paediatric Nursing*, 3(6), 12–15.

Lee, A. (1991) Screening for Congenital Dislocated Hip. *Paediatric Nursing*, 3(4), 12–13.

LeMaistre, G. (1991) Ultrasound and dislocation of the hip. *Paediatric Nursing*, 3(4), 13–21.

Levene, S. (1992) Preventing accidental injuries to children. *Paediatric Nursing*, 4(9), 12–14.

Lloyd, C. (1993) Making sense of reagent strip urine testing. *Nursing Times*, 89(48), 32–6.

MacGinley, K.J. (1993) Nursing care of the patient with altered body image. *British Journal of Nursing*, 2(22), 1098–1102.

Marieb, E.N. (1992) *Human Anatomy and Physiology*, 2nd ed. The Benjamin/Cummings Pub. Co. Inc, London.

Mason, G. (1993) Partners in care. *Child Health*, 1(1), 38–42.

Mason, K.J. (1991) Congenital orthopedic anomalies and their impact on the family. *Nursing Clinics of North America*, 26(1), 1–16.

Mead, D. (1989) The injured child. *Nursing Times*, 85(36), 28–32.

Mills, L., Magill, L. & Allen, S. (1993) Children's Dietary Needs in Hospital. *Paediatric Nursing*, 5(8), 17–19.

Mount, M. (1993) Self care to home care, the way forward. *Paediatric Nursing*, 5(5), 20–23.

Müller, D.J., Harris, P.J., Wattley, L. & Taylor, J.D. (1992) *Nursing Children. Psychology, Research and Practice*, 2nd edn. Chapman & Hall, London.

NAWCH (1984) *Charter for Children in Hospital*. National Association for the Welfare of Children in Hospital (now Action for Sick Children), London.

Nichol, D. (1993) Preventing infection. *Nursing Times*, 89(13), 78–80.

Orem, D.E. (1985) *Nursing: Concepts of Practice*, 3rd edn. McGraw Hill, New York.

Pearson, A. & Vaughan, B. (1986) *Nursing Models for Practice*. Heinemann Nursing, London.

Pfeil, M. (1993) Sleep disturbance at home and in hospital. *Paediatric Nursing*, 5(7), 14–17.

Roper, N., Logan, W. & Tierney, A. (1980) *The Elements of Nursing*. Churchill Livingstone, Edinburgh.

Roy, C. (1980) The Roy adaptation model. In *Conceptual Models for Nursing Practice*, 2nd edn (eds L.J.P. Rich & C. Roy). Appleton-Century Crofts, New York.

Ryan, D. (1993) Preventing infection. *Nursing Times*, 89(13), 78–80.

Secretaries of State for Health and Social Security (1989) *Caring for people: Community care in the next decade and beyond.* HMSO, London.

Shelley, H. (1993a) Adolescent needs in hospital. *Paediatric Nursing*, 5(9), 16–18.

Shelley, P. (1993b) Giving children a voice – the profile of Action for Sick Children. *Child Health*, 2(1), 21–4.

Shesser, L.K. & Kling, T.F. (1986) *Orthopaedic Nursing*, 5(3), 11–15.

Sidey, A. (1989) Intravenous home care. *Paediatric Nursing*, 1(3), 14–16.

Tanner, J.M. (1978) *Fetus into Man: Physical Growth from Conception to Maturity.* Open Books, Exeter.

Torrance, C. (1986) The physiology of wound healing. *Nursing.*, 3(5), 162–8.

Towner, E. & Barry, A. (1993) Accidental injury in childhood. *Paediatric Nursing*, 5(10), 10–12.

Wagner, V. (1989) A healthy start. *Paediatric Nursing*, 1(3), 16–18.

Wallis, S. (1991) An agenda to promote self-care nursing care of skeletal pin sites. *Professional Nurse*, 6(12), 715–20.

Watling, R. (1994) Setting off on the Right Foot. *Child Health*, 2(1), 16–20.

Webb, J.T. (1985) Orthopaedic conditions affecting children. *Nursing*, 2(44), 1306–10.

White, M. (1990) Sleep onset latency and distress in hospitalised children. *Nursing Research*, 39(3), 134–9.

Whiting, M. (1993) Play and surgical patients. *Paediatric Nursing*, 5(6), 11–13.

Wiles, P. (1987) The school teacher on the hospital ward. *Journal of Advanced Nursing*, 12, 631–40.

Wilson, K. (1993) Education of the hospitalised child. *Paediatric Nursing*, 5(4), 24–6.

Chapter 25

Nursing Support and Care: Meeting the Needs of the Child and Family with Altered Neuromuscular Function

Carolyn Evans and Tony Andrews

'I have plaster on my feet and I'm getting my new leg splints soon. I'm allowed to use my electric wheelchair to go round the ward and the physio department. In the ward school it fits under the desk with the computer. The play therapist has special scissors which I can use and we're making paper decorations for the ward. The pain control nurse promised I would not have any pain. She gave me tablets and they really worked. Mum and Dad took it in turns to stay with me and I ate some of the food they cooked in the parents' kitchen. But the hospital food is OK ... sometimes!' (Andrew, aged 10, post minor surgery – he has Duchenne muscular dystrophy)

INTRODUCTION

There are over 60 different neuromuscular conditions. They vary widely in terms of severity, age of onset, type of muscle affected, pattern of genetic inheritance and their effect on life expectancy. The common features include their tendency to involve weakness and wasting of muscle, their rarity, and the fact that, at the time of writing, there is no known cure although significant advances in medical research are being made.

There will be a focus on two of these disorders: Duchenne muscular dystrophy and Werdnig Hoffman's disease, also known as spinal muscular atrophy type 1. They are among the most common and the most severe of the neuromuscular conditions. Others that nurses may encounter might be very different and nurses will need to familiarize themselves with the individual characteristics at the time of coming into contact with an affected child. There will nearly always be problems caused by weakness of muscles controlling movement, but with some of the conditions other bodily functions might also be affected.

As the conditions are so rare, most nurses, as with any other professionals, will only see a very small number in their whole career. It is therefore unreasonable to expect them to be familiar at the outset with all the needs of these children, and yet an understanding of the more unusual needs can make all the difference to the successful outcome of nursing care. This chapter will provide some helpful guidance. Of course, as with any other condition, the parents and often the children

themselves will be the most valuable source of detailed and reliable information about care needs.

THE NURSING ENVIRONMENT

The most suitable environment for any child to be nursed in is usually their home as this is the setting most accommodating to their physical, intellectual, emotional and social wellbeing. However, there are times when admission to hospital may be unavoidable and a child-centred environment can make their stay in hospital a more pleasant experience.

A newborn baby with a suspected neuromuscular disorder (e.g. spinal muscular atrophy) may well be admitted to the special care baby unit (SCBU) or transferred from the maternity hospital to a paediatric department. A side ward or single cubicle with facilities for the parent(s) to stay is ideal, giving privacy as well as maintaining bonding. Very often a child with a (suspected) neuromuscular disorder will first have contact with the hospital via the children's outpatients department. Future attendance may well depend on the family's experience at this first visit.

Parking for people with disabilities should be available close to the entrance of the outpatients department. These parking bays should be larger than the standard size parking bay to enable wheelchairs to be manoeuvred from the vehicle. Level or ramped access into the outpatients department is vital, with door widths accommodating wheelchairs. Doors should be easy to open and preferably automatic. All rooms within the outpatient department, or the children's ward itself, should be wheelchair accessible and have good circulation space. Examination couches should be height adjustable and weighing scales should be of the type a child can sit on. A hoist should be available to lift the child from wheelchair on to scales and/or couches.

Toilet facilities should have space for a wheelchair beside and in front of the lavatory in order to facilitate transfers. A Closomat wash/dry lavatory pan will allow good hygiene as well as enabling dignity to be maintained. Washbasins should be inset into a worktop, preferably height adjustable, 600 mm from wall to front of worktop, allowing the child in a wheelchair to get right up to the basin without the foot plates hitting the pipes or wall at the rear. The basin itself should be flush with the worktop, with easy to operate level taps so that the child can slide his or her arms across the surface into the basin.

Toys and games suitable for children with weak muscles should be available in the waiting area. A play worker empathetic to the needs of a child with a muscle weakness is vital (Muscular Dystrophy Group).

If a child has to be admitted to hospital, parent(s) should be actively encouraged to stay, preferably in a single room with the child. A partnership between parents and staff should be actively encouraged to enable the most appropriate care for the child (Casey 1988).

Apart from wheelchair accessibility and circulation space, specialized equipment can make the difference between an independent child integrating with the ward and an unhappy child confined to bed. A four-section height adjustable electric bed allows the child to sit up or lie down independently and allows wheelchair transfers and care to be given more easily. A turning bed may be useful to reduce the need for manual changing of position through the night, enabling the carer to get more rest as well as giving the child a less interrupted night of sleep.

The locker should be accessible to the child whenever possible; it should certainly be within view. A height adjustable bed table will enable a child to do school lessons or to play, providing it is positioned correctly. A few millimetres can make the difference between these children participating in activities or being left out. The nurse-call button should be within the child's reach, pinned on to clothing if appropriate or attached to the tray or bedtable. The cord should be straight as a coiled one tends to spring away easily.

Lifting can be made easy by the use of a ceiling or portable hoist. Bath aids such as the Mermaid Ranger allow a child access to a bath (which should preferably be en suite to the bedroom), easing aches and joints as well as enabling personal hygiene. Showers are often disliked by children with neuromuscular conditions as they cannot move under the water jet and therefore get cold very quickly.

Some of these children will bring their own equipment into hospital, such as powered wheelchairs, toilet seats, standing frames, etc. This should be taken into consideration when planning their stay, as it will increase their independence and their self-esteem. Powered wheelchairs need to be charged up in a safe, well-ventilated area, preferably away from the sleeping area. Space for standing frames, and/or suitable work surfaces and correctly positioned trays and tables, allow the child to participate in lessons and play as well as stretching joints and maintaining good posture. Children with neuromuscular conditions tire easily and have short spans of concentration, which should be taken into consideration when planning activities.

If intensive care is required special consideration must be given to the child's muscle weakness and reduced lung capacity. Frequent change of position and physiotherapy will be required.

It is important to remember that children with neuromuscular conditions are usually nursed at home by their family, who know and understand their needs and their limitations of movement. For these children even a few millimetres out of reach means an unbridgeable chasm. If hospital staff work with the family they can provide care more effectively and enable a child's stay in hospital to be a more enjoyable experience.

NURSING CARE OF THE BABY WITH ACUTE SPINAL MUSCULAR ATROPHY

Werdnig Hoffman's disease, or spinal muscular atrophy (SMA) type 1, is one of a group of genetically determined neuromuscular disorders in which there is a degeneration of the anterior horn cells of the spinal cored, and the bulbar motor neurons, with early onset either *in utero* or within the first two to three months of life. Spinal muscular atrophy is inherited through an autosomal recessive mechanism; the gene has been identified on the longer arm of chromosome 5. Pre-natal testing and diagnosis is available to parents at certain regional genetic centres.

Babies affected by SMA have marked generalized weakness and many assume a characteristic frog posture when laid on their backs, with abduction and external rotation of their legs. Their legs are frequently totally immobile. They may have a little more movement in their arms with the ability to move their hands and fingers, but they are generally unable to raise their arms against gravity. The trunk is severely affected and there is marked head lag. The baby's respiratory muscles are weak; the abdomen may be distended and the baby may demonstrate a spinal scoliosis. These children are never able to raise their heads or roll over, and are often likened to a rag doll.

Difficulties relating to sucking, swallowing and breathing may present at an early age, along with a poor weight gain and a general failure to thrive. Yet, for all this, these babies are intellectually normal and are bright and alert. Sadly, however, they do not usually survive beyond the age of two years. This poor prognosis distinguishes them from the three other types of spinal muscular atrophy: intermediate type 11 SMA; mild/type 111 SMA; and SMA of adult onset. Babies affected by other neuromuscular conditions, such as congenital muscular dystrophy, the congenital myopathies and the mitochondrial myopathies, may demonstrate some symptoms similar to those described in acute spinal muscular atrophy.

Nursing assessment

The nurse's role in assessing the baby with SMA in many ways starts with assessing the way the family, the parents in particular, respond to and cope initially with the diagnosis and then with the rest of the baby's life. The way in which parents respond to the news of the potential and inevitable death of their baby varies widely, and is greatly affected by the degree of skill and sensitivity shown by the doctor and the nurse. The nurse needs to appreciate that the parents and family begin to grieve for the loss of a healthy baby from the time of diagnosis and some families grieve before the diagnosis is officially made.

In assessing the parents' understanding of the diagnosis, the nurse must be aware of the emotional turmoil which is being experienced by the parents and family. Feelings will inevitably vary from a sense of outrage through to anger, guilt, and an overwhelming sense of sadness. It is important that the nurse should constantly be aware of the family's fragile emotional state. The nurse must ensure that they are fully appraised about the nature of the diagnosis and should be available to give honest and accurate information, practical help and emotional support. The cost to these families is enormous in physical, psychological, social and spiritual terms; they have a great deal less time for themselves, their partner, their other children, their work and leisure activities. One parent may feel the need to give up work

and assume the full time responsibility for promoting the child's survival. They may tend to overprotect and indulge their baby or exclude their partner and family.

As the baby deteriorates and its care needs increase, the parents may feel physically exhausted and the nurse needs to be sensitive to the possibility of referral to such services as the community paediatric nurse, a children's hospice or social services home care support. Help with household tasks, the provision of quality care for the other children, and the services of a 'night sitter' can be very supportive to families, should they choose to care for their baby at home.

The comprehensive nature of nursing assessment of babies with SMA should not be underestimated and must consider a range of physical (Fig. 25.1) and psychological needs. Babies with a severe neuromuscular condition will be unable to move themselves without help. The nurse will need to assess ways in which the baby's comfort may be maximized by considering a variety of supportive postures – from being laid supine on a sheepskin mattress to sitting in a supportive seat with a tray to facilitate play. This will enable the child to enjoy a variety of light colourful toys which, along with music, mobiles, and story tapes, can give interest, pleasure and comfort to a baby who is unlikely to be able to move independently and who may often become fractious because of frustration and boredom rather than physical pain. As the baby's needs increase, as its condition progresses, it may be too weak to sustain a sitting position and will need a soft mattress or a sheepskin rug on which to rest.

The nurse needs to appreciate that activities of daily living for babies with SMA are radically altered because of their severe muscle weakness. The baby's respirations will be compromised in certain positions and the nurse needs to discuss positioning and lifting techniques with the parents, to ensure that appropriate care is taken. Inappropriate handling of the baby may well bring on a choking attack and make breathing more difficult. Careful assessment is also required of the baby's feeding pattern, in that sucking and swallowing reflexes are affected and feeding via breast or bottle can be a tiring and lengthy procedure. The baby's weight needs to be carefully monitored, and many of these babies eventually require their nutrition to be provided via a nasogastric tube.

In assessing the care needs of the baby the nurse needs always to appreciate that the parents are intimately

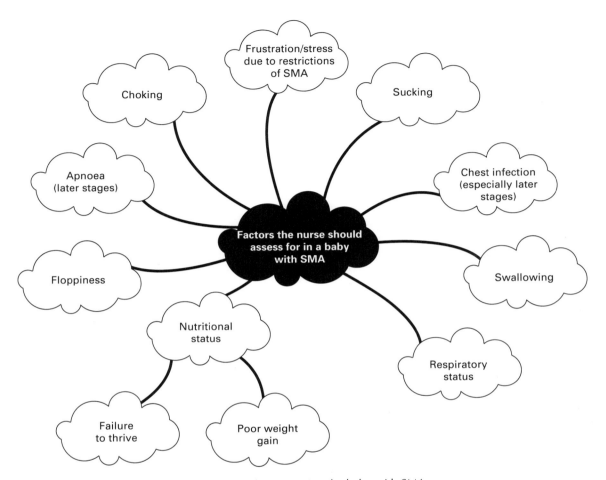

Fig. 25.1   Factors the nurse should consider when assessing the baby with SMA.

aware of their baby's needs. The nurse must share and learn both from the parents and with the parents at every opportunity.

Due to the fact that the baby will have undergone invasive and potentially traumatic investigations, such as muscle biopsy, nerve conduction studies, haematological investigations and X-rays, the impact that these have had on both the baby and the parents needs to be assessed as they are likely to have been distressing to both parents and child.

Nursing intervention: meeting the baby's needs

The parents may ask the nurse many difficult questions relating to their baby's condition and the inevitable outcome. The nurse needs to fully inform herself/himself of the baby's medical condition and seek advice and guidance from colleagues as appropriate. Throughout their sick child's life parents may question their attitudes towards parenthood and talk about their lack of experience in caring for a sick child and their fears for the future. The 24 hour responsibility of caring for their child may seem overwhelming. They may find it difficult to share their feelings with each other and with other family members. They need assurance that they are not alone and that there is expert care available to give support and direction. The nurse's capacity to provide a supportive framework in which the parents can work out the ways in which they wish their baby to be cared for will, hopefully, give them strength to act in the best interests of their baby and family.

The urge to take control, sometimes encouraged by the family's traditional expectation of the nurse's role, needs to be resisted in the awareness that it is always more difficult to give families choices and allow them sometimes to make mistakes. This demands a level of commitment and involvement on the part of the nurse and may be frowned upon by some good intentioned people. The needs of siblings can, however, be easily overlooked. The main focus of the literature has been on the sick child and the parents to the detriment of other family members. Attempts by the nurse to strengthen the parents' awareness of the needs of the siblings, and attempts to develop a friendly and informed dialogue with siblings, if this is possible, is likely to help them to confront any fantasies they may have, and so be supportive.

The nurse must ensure that all necessary equipment is available to support the parents in the care of their baby at home or in hospital. A (portable) suction machine, a supportive seat with a tray, suitable pram/pushchair, bathing aids, and the provision of as stimulating an environment as possible, will require the nurse to refer to and liaise with local community health and social services. The nurse needs to become proficient in all aspects of the baby's nursing care. Efforts to accurately inform community staff of the baby's care needs and attempts to act as the family's advocate by steering away all but the most necessary and trusted of professional callers, will be greatly appreciated by the family.

The nurse's awareness of DSS benefits relating to the total care needs of the baby and those benefits also available to carers may be of vital assistance to the family, particularly as one parent may have given up paid work to care for the sick baby. Knowledge and information needs to be continually assessed and revised, in the light of the progressive nature of acute spinal muscular atrophy.

In implementing specific care, the nurse's approach should be concrete and supportive. Hopefully, a good caring relationship will quickly be established enabling the nurse to perform effectively in a role with which the family feel comfortable. As previously highlighted, the baby severely affected by a neuromuscular condition will be slow to feed and may be distressed by frequent choking episodes. The sheer effort of sucking, associated with a poor weight gain, may be such that feeding via a nasogastric tube is recommended. The nurse will be required to pass the tube, to give milk feeds, to maintain

oral hygiene and teach and support the parents, so that they feel confident to feed the child themselves. All reflexes and muscle tone associated with swallowing, feeding and the clearing of secretions will be impaired, such that frequent pharyngeal suction is required, particularly as the baby reaches the terminal stages. The technique of pharyngeal aspiration needs to be thoroughly understood by the nurse, so that by demonstration and education the family are able to use suction effectively themselves.

Consultation with the family regarding the most appropriate way to handle their baby is vital. These babies are extremely floppy and need careful handling so as not to compromise their respiratory status. They cannot sit up unaided or move their legs, and will require a variety of supported seating positions to ensure their comfort and give variety and interest to their day. The weakness of the baby may be such that they need to be nursed in the supine position. A soft mattress, padding or a sheepskin to promote comfort would need to be provided. Attention to safety is also vital, in that all chairs should have a strap provided, yet it is important to ensure that the style of the strap/harness does not inhibit the function of the child's respiratory muscles.

As the baby deteriorates, admissions to hospital may increase for the treatment of chest infections and support in the event of choking and apnoea attacks. Intensive suction to the oropharynx and nasopharynx may be required as the muscles to the upper body fail. The family need to be assured that they can return to hospital or have access to additional community support whenever problems arise.

Families need to be prepared for the possibility of sudden death. Parents are afraid that their baby will choke, suffocate and fight for breath at the time of death. Changes in the baby's colour, the development of stridor, signs of pulmonary oedema and changes in the respiratory pattern, should be explained, and assurance given that analgesia will be available should the baby be distressed or in pain. Implementing terminal care sensitive to the baby's life-limiting condition and the rate of progression, may involve the nurse negotiating with medical staff as to when aggressive medical treatment is no longer appropriate. Attempts at resuscitation and ventilation for respiratory failure should not be attempted, as it is virtually impossible to wean these babies off a ventilator. The nurse needs to be sensitive to the ethical issues surrounding these discussions and should encourage an honest yet gentle dialogue between the parents and the doctor.

On the death of the baby the nurse needs to stay nearby as the parents say their goodbyes. Touch, attentiveness, explanations and listening, and a respect for the child as a person, will prove more effective than words alone, as the nurse continues to implement supportive care at bereavement. An awareness of the child's family's particular religious and cultural beliefs is particularly vital at this time. Insensitivity to the wishes and feelings of the parents, as to how they would like their baby's body to be cared for, can be profoundly damaging:

'I still see in nightmare fashion the nurse trundling off outside to the morgue with Jennifer in the tattiest pram you have ever seen... She had the most beautiful baby equipment when she was alive and it broke my heart to see her in such a scruffy thing.'

Because of the rapidly progressive nature of acute SMA, the nursing care of the baby should be regularly reviewed in consultation with the parents. The baby's physical wellbeing and comfort should always be of paramount importance. In attempting to evaluate the care given, a consideration of the whole environment in which the baby and family is cared for may prove helpful: the staffing levels on the ward, the degree of privacy offered to the baby and family, the equipment used, the inter-agency support and collaboration. Such aspects of care may enable the nurse to appreciate the value of family centred care.

Research shows that early counselling and support is crucial to parental attachment and adjustment of loss. Yet care for the family does not end on the death of the baby. Both hospital and community staff should consider the value of inviting the family back to the hospital to discuss the care provided to them and their baby. The parents may wish to revisit the ward where the baby died or had been nursed. They may wish to thank particular staff or they may need to cry, to be angry, or to remonstrate with staff regarding a particular incident or aspect of care. An opportunity to fulfil these needs can be immensely therapeutic to families, and a learning experience for staff, if handled sensitively and with care. Staff may wish to consider the value of a bereavement support group.

Caring for dying babies/children and their families brings nurses face to face with their personal feelings and experiences of death and bereavement. Their need for professional support and supervision in such situations is crucial and in evaluating the care given, the nurse needs to assess the quality of the support given to the care team. This support needs to include an awareness of the nurse's personal involvement and sense of vulnerability.

NURSING CARE OF THE CHILD WITH DUCHENNE MUSCULAR DYSTROPHY

Duchenne muscular dystrophy is a progressive degenerative wasting disease which mainly affects boys. Both skeletal and cardiac muscle are involved without any associated structural abnormality in the peripheral nervous system. Life expectancy is late teens/early twenties. It is genetically determined as an X linked recessive disorder. The abnormal gene is located on the short arm of the X chromosome known as band p 21. The effect is a complete absence of the protein dystrophin in the muscle cell.

Most of the clinical features of Duchenne muscular dystrophy are from involvement of skeletal muscle but the disease may affect other systems including the cardiovascular genito-urinary tract and gastro-intestinal tract. There is evidence that a degree of intellectual or speech impairment may be present. The nurse must realize that the severity and rate of deterioration varies considerably between individual children. Some boys retain their subcutaneous fat and muscle bulk whereas others become thin and atrophic.

There is considerable variation in their age of death. Some boys die as early as eight years while others survive into their mid-twenties. The age at death does not seem to correlate with the age of onset but does correlate with the age at which boys need to use a wheelchair permanently. Most boys die of respiratory failure at a mean age of between 16 and 17 years, while others die suddenly from arrhythmias secondary to a cardiomyopathy.

While recognizing that the severity and rate of deterioration varies considerably in individual cases, generally it can be said that there is a characteristic pattern occurring in three stages.

First stage
During this first stage the child maintains a high

degree of independence. This period can extend from the age of 18 months until approximately seven to eight years of age. Initially the child appears to lead a near normal life. There may be some obvious signs of muscle weakness. The lower limbs are affected more than the distal muscles. The child tends to walk on his toes and develops a lumbar lordosis. This gait is to compensate for the muscle weakness. In all cases boys are unable to run properly and have difficulty in climbing stairs. In this first stage at approximately four to five years old the child will demonstrate the classic Gowers manoeuvre when they will 'climb up' their thighs using their hands in order to extend their hips and push up the trunk. They are unable to rise from a sitting position on the floor if they have their arms folded. Weakness of the upper limbs, although not obvious, may be observed by an attempt to lift the child by grasping them under the arms; there is a tendency for them to slide through. This will affect the way nursing staff handle children with Duchenne dystrophy.

Second stage

This period can extend from approximately seven to 12 years of age when independent walking becomes impossible. There is progressive muscle weakness with more pronounced lumbar lordosis and the 'waddling gait' increases. Walking is very precarious and unstable. During this stage more obvious orthopaedic deformities can occur, with further shortening of the Achilles' tendon, asymmetry, and weakness of muscles at the hip joint with possible pelvic obliquity. Scoliosis may develop and respiratory function will begin to deteriorate.

Third stage

Most boys with Duchenne dystrophy will have to use a wheelchair permanently by the age of 13. Muscle weakness becomes more profound and the involvement of the upper limbs is more obvious, with shoulder, elbow

and wrist movement becoming more restricted. Respiratory function deteriorates after walking stops, and many boys develop a progressive scoliosis. In the end stages there is loss of head control. Swallowing becomes difficult and breathing is severely restricted due to a decrease in lung capacity and weakness of all thoracic muscles including the intercostals and the diaphragm. Movement is severely restricted. Some boys only retain slight movement of their fingers.

Nursing assessment

Apart from problems relating directly or indirectly to dystrophy, most affected boys have very few other health problems. Their admission to hospital, other than for emergency treatment, is usually for planned specific orthopaedic procedures such as release of contractures or surgical instrumentation of the spine. In the later stages they may need to be admitted for treatment of respiratory problems.

Since the condition is so variable in its relentless progression, which can last over 15–20 years, it is important that nursing staff liaise with all members of the multidisciplinary team who may be involved in the care of the child and his family. This enables the nurse to establish which physical stage each child has reached, and will avoid increasing the child's and parents' stress by a lack of awareness in using negative and inappropriate comments. Due to the nature of this condition the child and family may be involved in a multidisciplinary team (MDT) of carers (Fig. 25.3).

The most important source of vital knowledge for the nursing staff is the child and his parent/carer. They live and cope with the disability 24 hours a day. What might be judged as overprotective or even interfering for an otherwise healthy child, can in the case of a child with dystrophy prove to be the correct way of managing.

0		7	10		20
Walking phase (yrs)			Wheelchair phase (yrs)		
'normal' life	decrease walking		scoliosis 80% respiratory decrease 100%		terminal stage

Fig. 25.2 The main phases and features of Duchenne muscular dystrophy.

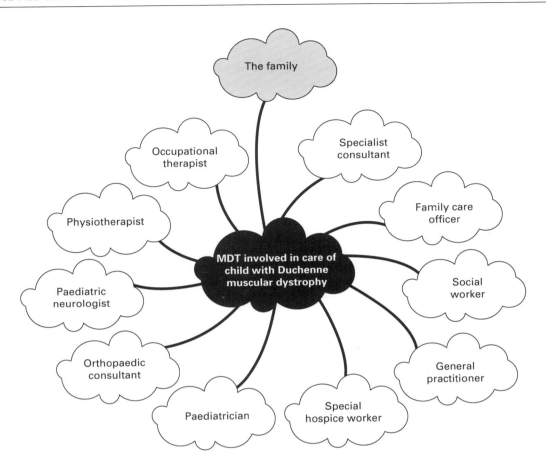

Fig. 25.3 Members of multidisciplinary team (MDT) involved in holistic care of child with Duchenne muscular dystrophy.

Although both medical and nursing staff may be the professionals, parent and child are usually the experts.

Parents are subject to enormous stress. They will from the day of diagnosis have been going through a form of bereavement which may have to last for over 15 years. Grief in all its different forms will be part of their lives. Boys with Duchenne muscular dystrophy, and their parents, have to deal with a multiplicity of emotions as the condition deteriorates: frustration, rebelliousness, resentment, bewilderment, envy, anger, depression, hopelessness and fear.

Nursing staff must be sensitive to this when they are assessing the needs of the child and his parents. It is important to respect the individual ways different families live and cope with this relentless progressive wasting disease for which, at this point, there is no cure. It is vital not to impose their own beliefs and attitudes on how it should be done. This becomes even more important in the later stages when our own fears may overshadow how we can help.

Nursing intervention: meeting the child's needs

Meeting the needs of a child and their family with Duchenne muscular dystrophy requires a multidisciplinary approach as the medical, physical and psychological problems are constantly changing. Nurses should appreciate that parents usually live with this condition in a restricted time limit of their own coping abilities, which may be from day to day. Any intervention care plans should be sensitively handled. Goals should be established (Table 25.1) as soon as the diagnosis is made and a holistic approach is ideal. Psychosocial, educational, vocational and independent living needs are as important as the treatments of the medical and musculoskeletal conditions.

Table 25.1 Main goals for the long term care of the child and their family.

- To establish an effective overall management plan based on careful evaluation.
- To maintain activities of daily living and ambulation as long as possible.
- To anticipate complications and prevent crisis.
- To facilitate supportive counselling to the child and his family.
- To assist the child to lead a life as 'normal and positive' as possible regardless of current medical prognosis.

In stage one the specific nursing goals should include advice on genetic counselling and family planning, advice to help understand procedures that can delay loss of function, and information concerning prevention of complications. In stage two the nurse includes advice on maintaining activities of daily living, prevention of spinal deformity and support and advice on wheelchair mobility. There will be specific goals relating to the treatment of musculoskeletal problems such as weakness, contractures, deformity and functional ability, and these need to be discussed with the multidisciplinary team. Goal setting in stage three involves symptomatic management of medical complications, and enhancing and facilitating nursing care.

The main goal for nurses caring for the terminal stage of dystrophy should be to provide an environment which is safe and private, with people to help and support who will show respect for the child's and their family's own individual needs, preferences and desires.

Nurses may be involved in the care of a boy with Duchenne dystrophy at any stage of his life and at different stages of the condition. As stated, the child and family may be part of a multidisciplinary care team which will involve different professionals being involved

at particular times of need. A holistic approach to all aspects of care is ideal and a partnership of care is essential. The Roper, Logan and Tierney model allows the nurse and family to highlight problems related particularly to Duchenne muscular dystrophy. These are relevant to principles of nursing care in specific procedures such as general medical and chest management, tendon releases, spinal fusion, and care of the child at the terminal stage. The child and their parent will have developed the most suitable way to lift and nurses should be guided by them. Nurses need to be aware of the degree of muscle weakness and this may not always be obvious if the child uses a wheelchair. Special consideration of supporting their head and limbs should be made when lifting the child. The correct use of suitable hoists with special slings can be helpful but it is not appropriate to introduce this method in a hospital environment if the child is not comfortable with this way of being lifted. Boys with muscular dystrophy feel very vulnerable as they lose muscle control. Prevention of pressure sores is important and the use of special cushions and mattresses should be considered.

Communication

Some boys with Duchenne dystrophy have a degree of learning difficulties and associated impairment of verbal intelligence. It is helpful if nurses are aware of this. The nurse should not underestimate the child's level of awareness of their condition or their intelligence. Boys can appear to be quiet and withdrawn but this may be part of their particular way of dealing with their condition. The nurse should not presume to instigate discussion about the child's problems but should be prepared to listen and answer any questions honestly. It may be appropriate to involve the help of others, such as the family care officer or psychologist if there are particular concerns. As boys become weaker it may be physically impossible for them to talk loudly or for long periods. Nurses should ensure that there is an effective call button for them to use, which is suitable for their restricted mobility.

Breathing

Duchenne muscular dystrophy is associated with respiratory muscle weakness and cardiomyopathy. Respiratory problems include impaired muscle strength, reduction in lung volumes and development of a scoliosis. Obesity will also restrict breathing. The nurse should liaise with the physiotherapist to help promote an effective chest management programme of breathing exercises and to help with particular treatments such as effective coughing and postural drainage. The aim of treatment is to help clear the lungs of secretions effectively in the shortest possible time without causing fatigue, and so improve lung function. When surgery is required particular attention should be paid to respiratory function, pre and post operatively.

In later stages the ability to take a deep breath is very limited. It is worth considering the use of intermittent positive pressure breathing to help improve the ventilation of the base of the lungs. This will facilitate the removal of secretions in those who cannot do so unaided. Recurrent chest infections need to be treated early with antibiotics which can be administered intravenously at home. Many boys in the end stages of the disease die of respiratory infections. Many families prefer their child to be allowed to die at home as this can alleviate any distress a hospital admission may cause. Ventilatory support using noninvasive methods may be helpful, to alleviate respiratory distress.

Eating and drinking

A healthy diet to control weight is important. Obesity can cause respiratory problems and can also mean premature cessation of walking. Encouraging a good diet in the early stages can improve the mobility of the child in the later stages. It can allow parents to have a positive nurturing pattern rather than a compensatory way of dealing with the diagnosis and condition. Boys may need help to cut up food, and strategic positioning with height adjustable tables will allow independence.

In the later stages nutritional supplements can be beneficial. Smaller meals given more often can be easier to tolerate. Swallowing becomes difficult. Some boys have been helped with advice and exercise from a speech therapist. Reduction in fluid intake can cause problems with respiratory, cardiac and gastro-intestinal functions. Fluids should be encouraged. Some boys will try and reduce their fluid intake as they become less mobile, and an awareness of this with introduction of appropriate aids and accessibility to toilet areas can eliminate this problem. Advice from the dietician is useful. Constipation can be a problem through lack of mobility and early measures with a good diet and plenty of fluids can help. Gentle laxatives may be needed under supervision.

Personal cleansing and dressing

Eventually boys will be dependent on carers for all activities, therefore it is important to encourage independence as long as possible. Initially this may be achieved by correct positioning of the child and with clothes and toilet articles in easy reach. Safety is the key aspect as balance becomes more precarious. As upper limbs become weaker more help is needed to wash their faces and comb their hair. Introducing small aids such as longer handles and lightweight brushes will enable them to continue with their own toileting. An electric/battery operated toothbrush is recommended. Height adjustable surfaces are essential. Contractures can cause problems with tight fitting clothes, and if the child is using orthosis, larger sizes will be better.

Eliminating

Incontinence is not a usual feature of Duchenne muscular dystrophy, though some boys will present with some problems. If this occurs the nurse should consider discussing this with relevant health professionals. As boys lose their mobility in their upper limbs they will need help to put their penis into a urinal. In the later stages the use of a convene can be helpful. Catheterization, as a temporary measure, is usual following spinal surgery. Suitable adaptions to the child's environment may be necessary to allow maximum independence, to retain dignity and to give carers help. The problems of accessible toilets can cause restrictions in the social life of these boys. Greater accessibility should be promoted at all times.

Controlling body temperature

Usual methods of control of pyrexia are suitable for boys with Duchenne dystrophy. It has been noted that some boys demonstrate a high temperature following surgery. Four hourly observations of temperatures are therefore recommended.

Mobility

In the early stages careful and regular assessment of the child's mobility should be undertaken. This enables any intervention needed to enhance independent ambulation to be performed at the optimal time. This may involve the use of orthosis, e.g. leg bracing or variable centre of gravity swivel walkers. Surgical procedures may be necessary to release contractures. In order to facilitate these options, early mobilization is essential and physiotherapy involvement is an important part of any treatment. Particular care should be taken, when positioning boys in bed, not to restrict any movement and to give support to joints and limbs. Stretching exercises must continue and parental involvement with any treatment is important.

As mobility decreases decisions will have to be made as to the benefits of therapeutic walking. The introduction of a wheelchair is a major crisis for the child and family; it must be handled sensitively. The value of the correct wheelchair at the right time can be immense. A wheelchair should enhance function and aid independence. There are several different chairs available which are suitable for boys with dystrophy. A full assessment, involving the child, his family and his therapist, is important. It should take into consideration all the different environments the chair will be used in. To enable mobility some boys have bizarre positioning and individual movement of particular limbs. This may appear at odds with their overall functional ability.

As the condition deteriorates mobility will decrease. There will be further involvement of the upper limbs and eventually loss of head control. It is important to be aware of this lack of movement in order to facilitate comfort when positioning. Boys who are in bed will need turning regularly. They will also need their limbs moved regularly as sometimes even a few inches can help to overcome a cramped stiff feeling.

Working and playing

Children with Duchenne dystrophy have the same expectations from life and should have the opportunity to have the same experiences. This includes going to school. Mainstream schools can provide him with equal opportunity and the benefit of developing relationships with children in his local community. Advice from specialists will be needed for schools to help with integration. Suitable play and educational toys are available for children with weak muscles. A computer is an essential piece of equipment to a boy with dystrophy. It is something he can learn at an early age and will help to develop his communication skills. He can use it for play and schoolwork and it can be adapted for use when mobility decreases.

Expressing sexuality

Boys with Duchenne dystrophy will have the same needs as any other boys. Nurses should be sensitive when handling boys to prevent any embarrassment or anxiety over intimate procedures. Parents should be encouraged to give their child privacy. Boys with dystrophy will have erections and may need their hands to be put in a position where they are able to masturbate. Relationships should be encouraged to develop. Practical problems can be helped with suitable aids and adaptions, and referral to disability advice groups such as SPOD (an association to aid the sexual and personal relationships of people with a disability) may be appropriate.

Sleeping

A major problem of caring for a child with Duchenne dystrophy is the necessity of turning. Many children will need turning frequently at night, and this is exhausting for both the child and family. Suitable beds with comfortable supportive mattresses can help. Adjustable beds can enable a child to be more independent. Sleep disturbances are recognized in boys with dystrophy and there is ongoing research into this problem. In the terminal stage the child will sleep for long periods as he becomes weaker.

Dying

Some boys may die suddenly from cardiac involvement, but usually death is the end of a slow deterioration over many months – the inevitable conclusion to this wasting disease. Many families choose to care for their child at home, but others may choose for the child to die in a hospice. Nurses should be supportive and sensitive. They must respect the child's and family's own individual needs, preferences and desires. Any intervention must be discussed with the child, when possible, the family and the nursing team. It is not usually appropriate for any emergency resuscitation for children with Duchenne muscular dystrophy. Pain relief and relief of respiratory distress may require administration of morphine and oxygen. This should be with the full agreement and understanding of the parents.

Support for the family after the death may need to continue for a long time. This can involve the family care officer or hospice staff.

Evaluation of care

Evaluation of care for boys with Duchenne dystrophy will be continuous and ongoing through the different stages of the condition. The emphasis is on the multidisciplinary team approach with direct involvement of the child and his family. Regular clinic assessments and liaison with all other professional agencies involved are important. Nurses should continually refer to the goals established, while recognizing the need to be flexible and adaptable. This will help to ensure a good overall effective management that will be supportive to the child and his family through the various stages of this condition and the long road they have to travel.

CONCLUSION

In caring for children with neuromuscular problems, a number of key points need to be considered as they can help to provide a quality service for the child and their family. It is sometimes the little points of care that can be forgotten or overlooked and which are particularly important for the child and their family. The nurse should always listen to the advice of carer and child on general management and should seek advice from specialist staff whenever possible.

The child's actual level of motor weakness may not be obvious when they are sitting up in bed or in their wheelchair, but should be taken into consideration when positioning the child's toys, food and call button. The child may also have difficulty in adjusting their own clothing and their bedclothes, so it is important to ensure that they are comfortable. Careful and appropriate lifting techniques and the use of appropriate resources should be employed and particular care should be taken when lifting the limbs and in supporting the child's head. The child should always have access to their own wheelchair and the nurse should ensure that it is charged overnight and ready for the child to use. Prolonged bed rest and inactivity should be avoided and the support of the physiotherapist and occupational therapist should be sought at an early stage of the child's admission. The nurse should also remember that the muscular dystrophy group is a prime resource and will provide information and encourage them to contact colleagues with relevant expertise for further advice and help.

At the time of writing, parents, nurses and other professionals are providing care for children with neuromuscular conditions in the knowledge that there is currently no cure. They try to strike a balance between encouraging a positive attitude, finding a basis for hope and ensuring that families have accurate information.

As cures for the various neuromuscular conditions are developed, hopefully in the not too distant future, there are likely to be interim periods when access to a cure or to its preceding clinical trials will not be universally available throughout the UK. The eventual discovery of cures, therefore, has complex implications for the care and counselling of children and their families that are both exciting and challenging. This is an area requiring further study and research. Nurses will play as vital a part in the development of effective ways of caring for children when cures become available, as they have now at the current stage of medical research.

ACKNOWLEDGEMENTS

The following people also contributed to the contents of this chapter:

Jennifer Baker, *RGN, CMB Part I, HV Cert, FPA Cert, FWT Cert*, Family Care Officer, Muscular Dystrophy Group, Manchester.

Carol Cole, *RGN, BNurs, HV Cert, DN Cert*, Family Care Officer, Muscular Dystrophy Group, Manchester.

Rhona Currie, *RGN, RSCN, HV Cert, BA*, Family Care Officer, Muscular Dystrophy Group, London.

Oonagh Morrison, *RGN, ONC, CMB, HV Cert*, Family Care Officer, Muscular Dystrophy Group, Northern Ireland.

REFERENCES AND FURTHER READING

Casey, A. (1988) A partnership with child and family. *Senior Nurse*, 8(4), 8–9.

Casey, A. (1993) Development and use of the partnership model of nursing care. In *Advances in Child Health Nursing* (eds E.A. Glasper & A. Tucker), pp. 183–93. Scutari Press, London.

Dubowitz, V. (1980) Clinics in Developmental Medicine No. 76 – *The Floppy Infant*, Spastics International Medical Publications. William Heinemann Medical Books, London and J.B. Lippincott, Philadelphia.

Dubowitz, V. (1989) *A Colour Atlas of Muscular Disorders in Childhood*. Wolfe Medical Publications, London.

Evans, M. (1991) Caring by parents. in *Child Care: Some Nursing Perspectives* (ed. A. Glasper), pp. 244–9. Wolfe Publishing Ltd, London.

Galasko, C.S.B. (1987) *Neuromuscular Problems in Orthopaedics.* Blackwell Science, Oxford.

Longo, D.C. & Bond, L. (1984) Families of the handicapped child: research and practice. *Family Relations*, 33, 57–65.

Myers, B.A. (1983) The informing interview. *American Journal of Disease in Childhood*, 137, 572–7.

Powell, T.H. (1987) *Brothers and Sisters: How Children Cope When a Sibling Has a Muscle Disease.* Siblings Information Network, Connecticut's University Affiliated Programme. Storr, Connecticut.

Muscular Dystrophy Group. *Suitable Toys for Children with Muscle Weakness.* Muscular Dystrophy Group. Hammersmith Hospital, London.

Wilson-Barnett, J. & Raiman, J. (1988) *Nursing Issues and Research in Terminal Care.* Wiley Series on Developments in Nursing Research, Vol. 6. John Wiley, Chichester.

Appendices

Appendix 1
Normal Values

The data in this section are drawn from a large number of sources in the paediatric literature. In many cases the tables presented are a composite of what has been published elsewhere, and no references are therefore given.

VITAL SIGNS

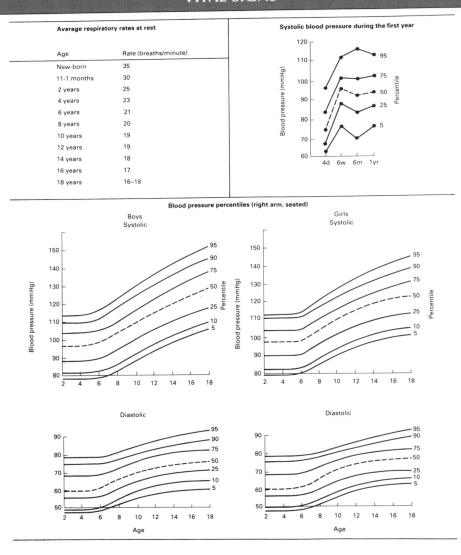

Average respiratory rates at rest

Age	Rate (breaths/minute)
New-born	35
11-1 months	30
2 years	25
4 years	23
6 years	21
8 years	20
10 years	19
12 years	19
14 years	18
16 years	17
18 years	16–18

Systolic blood pressure during the first year

Blood pressure percentiles (right arm, seated)

Boys
Systolic

Girls
Systolic

Diastolic

Diastolic

Heart rate.	
Age	Heart rate (BPM)
Newborn	120–150
Neonate	110–140
Infant	100–120
Toddler	90–110
Preschool	85–105
School	65–100
Adolescent	60–95

Normal range of body temperature for one year and older.

Method	Acceptable Range
Oral	36.4°–37.4°C
Rectal	36.2°–37.6°C
Axilla	35.9°–36.5°C

CONVERSION CHART

	Pounds (lb)							
Ounces	1	2	3	4	5	6	7	8
0	454	907	1361	1814	2268	2722	3175	3629
1	482	936	1389	1843	2296	2750	3204	3657
2	510	964	1418	1871	2325	2778	3232	3686
3	539	992	1446	1899	2353	2807	3260	3714
4	567	1021	1474	1928	2381	2835	3289	3742
5	595	1049	1503	1956	2410	2863	3317	3771
6	624	1077	1531	1985	2438	2892	3345	3799
7	652	1106	1559	2013	2466	2920	3374	3827
8	680	1134	1588	2041	2495	2948	3402	3856
9	709	1162	1616	2070	2523	2977	3430	3884
10	737	1191	1644	2098	2552	3005	3459	3912
11	765	1219	1673	2126	2580	3033	3487	3941
12	794	1247	1701	2155	2608	3062	3515	3969
13	822	1276	1729	2183	2637	3090	3544	3997
14	851	1304	1758	2211	2665	3119	3572	4026
15	879	1332	1786	2240	2693	3147	3600	4054

Conversion of pounds and ounces to grams. To convert pounds and ounces to grams, read the pounds value on the horizontal axis and the ounces value on the vertical axis. The point at which the two values intercept in the bulk of the table is the equivalent value in grams, e.g. 4 lb 6 oz is equivalent to 1985 grams.

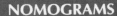

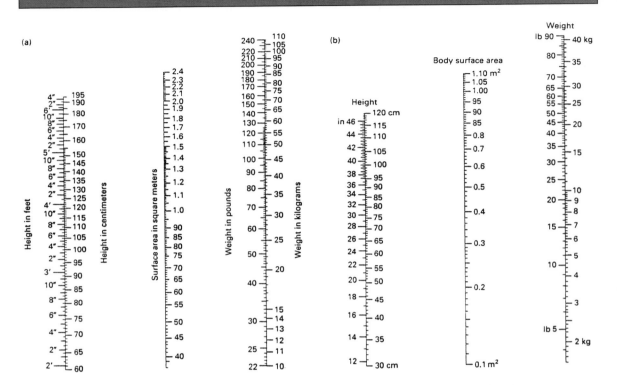

Nomograms for determination of body surface area from height and weight (a) adults (b) children (*After Lentner, 1982*).

Action for Sick Children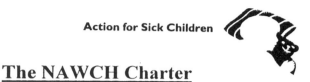

The NAWCH Charter

1

Children shall be admitted to hospital only if the care they require cannot be equally well provided at home or on a day basis.

2

Children in hospital shall have the right to have their parents with them at all times provided this is in the best interest of the child. Accommodation should therefore be offered to all parents, and they should be helped and encouraged to stay. In order to share in the care of their child, parents should be fully informed about the ward routine and their active participation encouraged.

3

Children and their parents shall have the right to information appropriate to their age and understanding.

4

Children and their parents shall have the right to informed participation in all decisions involving their health care. Every child shall be protected form unnecessary medical treatment, and steps taken to mitigate physical and emotional distress.

5

Children shall be treated with tact and understanding and at all times their privacy shall be respected.

6

Children shall enjoy the care of appropriately trained staff, fully aware of the physical and emotional needs of each age group.

7

Children shall be able to wear their own clothes and have their own possessions.

8

Children shall be cared for with other children of the same age group.

9

Children shall be in an environment furnished and equipped to meet their requirements and which conforms to recognised standards of safety and supervision.

10

Children shall have full opportunity for play, recreation and education suited to their age and condition.

One voice for sick children

Appendix 3

The United Nations Convention on the Rights of the Child

Gerison Lansdown

BACKGROUND TO THE CONVENTION

The concept of children's rights is a comparatively new one and draws on both the recognition that every individual by virtue of being human is entitled to enjoy the full range of human rights, and the recognition that children should be treated as people in their own right and not merely as the property of adults who have responsibility for them.

The first real international recognition of children's rights was contained in the Declaration of Geneva put forward in 1924 by the then Save The Child Fund International Union. This first attempt to codify children's rights was endorsed by the League of Nations. However, these principles were exclusively concerned with the needs of children for welfare and protection. The Declaration was couched in terms of what must be done for children and described children as objects of concern but with no actual rights to any services. It contained no language detailing civil or political rights and was protective of children rather than empowering them. It was only with the Declaration on the Rights of the Child adopted by the General Assembly of the United Nations (UN) in 1959 that the first international commitment to civil and political rights appeared and then only in relation to the right to a name and nationality from birth.

A Declaration is a statement of principles to be accepted by Government but carrying no specific obligations. The UN convention on the Rights of the Child, then, which was adopted by the General Assembly in 1989 represented a turning point in the international movement on behalf of children's rights. It was a turning point in two respects. *First*, it provides a comprehensive framework which addresses rights relating not only to children's need for care, protection and adequate provision but also for participation. *Second*, a convention is binding requiring an active decision by States to ratify it and until the Convention on the Rights of the Child was adopted, there was no binding international instrument which brought together States' obligations towards children.

The history behind the convention is that on the eve of the International Year of the Child, Poland put forward a proposal for a Convention on the Rights of the Child. A Working Group was set up by the UN Commission on Human Rights with representatives of the 43 member States of the Commission, including the United Kingdom (UK), and the Group produced a draft text over the next 10 years. The draft was adopted by the General Assembly on 20 November 1989, just 30 years after the adoption of the Declaration on the Rights of the Child.

The Convention was officially opened for signature on 26 January 1990 and an unprecedented 61 countries signed on that day. The signing of a document indicates a State's willingness to give serious consideration to ratification of the document and as soon as 20 States have ratified, the Convention enters into force an international law for those States. In this case, it was 20 September 1990 that the Convention came into force. It was ratified by 174 countries in June 1995, a level of commitment unprecedented in the history of the UN. No other international treaty has achieved a comparable support and UNICEF are now optimistic that universal ratification can be achieved. The Convention, once ratified, is binding under international law and governments are obliged to comply with its provisions.

CONTENT OF THE CONVENTION

The Convention is a wide ranging treaty addressing the rights of children, and consequent obligations on governments, in every sphere of their lives. Its articles can be categorized as follows:

General measures of implementation:
> **article 4**, the duty to take all possible measures to ensure implementation of the Convention,
> **article 42**, the duty to make the principles of the Convention widely known to children and adults,
> **article 44.6**, the duty to make countries' reports on progress towards implementation widely available.

Definition of the child:
> **article 1**, the Convention applies to everyone under the age of 18 years.

General principles:
> **article 2**, non-discrimination,
> **article 3**, best interests of the child,
> **article 6**, the right to life, survival and development,
> **article 12**, respect for the views of the child.

Civil rights and freedoms:
> **article 7**, name and nationality,
> **article 8**, preservation of identity,
> **article 13**, freedom of expression,
> **article 17**, access to appropriate information,
> **article 14**, freedom of thought, conscience and religion,

> **article 15**, freedom of association and of peaceful assembly,
> **article 16**, protection of privacy,
> **article 19**, protection from violence, abuse and neglect,
> **article 37(a)**, the right not to be subjected to torture or other cruel inhuman or degrading treatment.

Family environment and alternative care:
> **article 5**, parental guidance,
> **article 18**, parental responsibilities,
> **article 9**, separation from parents,
> **article 10**, family reunification,
> **article 27(4)**, recovery of maintenance,
> **article 20**, children deprived of a family environment,
> **article 21**, adoption,
> **article 11**, illicit transfer and non-return,
> **article 25**, periodic review of placement.

Basic health and welfare:
> **article 18**, child care services and facilities,
> **article 23**, disabled children,
> **article 24**, health and welfare,
> **article 26**, social security,
> **article 27**, standard of living.

Education, leisure and cultural activities:
> **article 28**, education,
> **article 29**, aims of education,
> **article 31**, leisure, recreation and cultural activities.

Special measures of protection:

(a) Children in situations of emergency
> **article 22**, refugee children,
> **article 38**, children in armed conflicts,
> **article 39**, physical and psychological recovery and social reintegration.

(b) Children in conflict with the law
> **article 40**, the administration of justice,
> **article 37(b), (c), (d)**, children deprived of liberty including imprisonment, detention or placement in custodial settings,
> **article 37(a)**, sentencing of juveniles, in particular, the prohibition of capital punishment and life imprisonment.

(c) Children in situations of exploitation
    article 32, economic exploitation,
    article 33, drug abuse,
    article 34, sexual exploitation and abuse,
    article 35, sale, trafficking and abduction.

(d) Children belonging to a minority or indigenous group
    article 30, right to respect for culture, language and religion.

IMPLEMENTATION OF THE CONVENTION IN THE UK

The UK government ratified the Convention in December 1991. Having ratified it is required to report after two years and subsequently every five years to the UN Committee on the Rights of the Child on its progress towards implementation of the rights contained in the Convention. This Committee is a body established under the terms of the Convention to act as an international monitor on the rights it contains. The Committee examined the UK Government in January 1995 and produced a number of recommendations on how law, policy and practice might be developed to further enhance the rights of children in this country. These are reported in the Eighth Session Committee on the Rights of the Child, concluding observations of the Committee on the Rights of the Child: United Kingdom of Great Britain and Northern Ireland.

RECOMMENDED READING

UK Agenda for Children (1994) Children's Rights Development Unit, London.

Implementing the UN Convention on the Rights of the Child within the health service: a practitioner's guide (1995) BACCH, RCN and CRDU.

Building Small Democracies: Civil rights of children in families (1995) Children's Rights Office, London.

Making the Convention work for children (1995) Children's Rights Office, London.

All above are available from the Children's Rights Office, 235 Shaftesbury Avenue, London WC2H 8EL.

Appendix 4

Hospital Play Specialists: Professional Role and Training

Pamela A. Barnes

'Play in hospital has a special significance. It promotes a continuation of normal development for children and helps them to cope with the particular stresses and problems arising from hospital admissions. It gives children an opportunity to express in an appropriate and familiar way some of the apprehension arising from the stress of illness in a completely unfamiliar situation. Play is one of the few elements of normal life in an abnormal situation'

Quality Management for Children,
Play in Hospital publication,
Play in Hospital Liaison Committee 1990.

The value of play in the development of children is fully recognized by the experts and the need for play in hospital is considered an integral part of the treatment they receive.

Hospital Play Specialists are now an established group of professionals operating within the National Health Service. As members of the multidisciplinary paediatric team they offer a complementary service to medical and nursing care, in the recovery of the sick child.

Pioneers in the field of hospital play therapy were the late Susan Harvey, David Morris and Hugh Jolly. With their encouragement the National Association of Hospital Play Staff (NAHPS) was set up in 1975. The aims

of the Association were to have their work recognized as valuable within the health care setting; to become a professional group, and have a recognized training with a national qualification.

National Association of Hospital Play Staff initiated the Hospital Play Staff Education Trust, known as the Hospital Play Staff Examination Board (HPSEB) to establish the education and training structure for hospital play specialists. The Hospital Play Staff Education Trust was established in 1985. The course offered is designed as a post qualifying course for experienced persons to develop professional competence in the field of therapeutic play for children and young people, individually and in groups, in the hospital setting. The Board issue certificates and registration to successful students. The qualification is recognized as the required professional training for hospital play specialists. The Board is recognized by the Department of Education as an awarding body. Some of the present courses now offered in the UK are jointly validated with HPSEB and Business and Technology Education Council (BTEC) qualifications. Registration however can only be acquired through the HPSEB, this being the only recognized qualification.

The hospital play specialist must work co-operatively with all members of the health care team. There must be consultations concerning treatment plans, family concerns, reactions to medical procedures and the complications of diagnoses. With this information the hospital play specialist is able to design a suitable programme of play to meet the needs of the child and young person in hospital.

The hospital play specialist is able to extend the channels for normative play and inventiveness and helps to elevate the play into a way of learning, not only in normal play experiences, but also in medical play and preparation for treatments through play. Through observations in the playroom or by the bedside the hospital play specialist can make a valuable contribution to the diagnostic process.

· Training in child development and observation is required along with competence in family dynamics, interpersonal and communicative skills, as well as a good understanding of a child's reactions to illness and hospitalisation.

The role of the hospital play specialist also reaches out into the community, liaising here with the community paediatric team. The benefits of enabling children through play to master their own situations is extremely therapeutic and a valuable part of all treatment plans.

REFERENCES AND FURTHER READING

Barnes, P. A. (1992) *Provision of Play for Children in Hospital.*

Barnes, P. A. (1995) 30 years of Hospital Play. *Article OMEP International Journal.*

PHLC (199) *Quality Management in Children's Play in Hospital.*

Save the Children Fund (1989) *Hospital: A Deprived Environment for Children.*

Sylva K. (1993) Play in Hospital: When and Why It's Effective: Current Paediatrics.

ADDRESS FOR INFORMATION

HPSEB, Thomas Coram Foundation for Children, 40 Brunswick Square, London WC1N 1AZ.

NAHPS, Thomas Coram Foundation for Children, 40 Brunswick Square, London WC1N 1AZ.

Index